'It is a pleasure to introduce a book which I have found both good reading and a stimulus to think more about the non-organic mental misery which is so common and often so remediable, in old age. I see this volume as a timely exercise in stocktaking. Depression, not dementia is still the commonest mental disorder of old age.' From the foreword by Tom Arie.

Psychiatry in old age is no longer a field solely concerned with the 'Everest of Dementia'. Until now, however, the literature has sadly neglected the broad field of mental illness in the elderly which, lacking a demonstrable organic basis, has tended to be called 'functional'. Professor Chiu and Dr Ames provide us with the first comprehensive text to deal with all the nondementing psychiatric disorders in a practical guide with exhaustive reference for practitioners from all clinical disciplines related to geriatric psychiatry.

'It is the functional illness in the elderly that we should be able to help now. This text clearly outlines our 'core knowledge' about the clinical problems, discusses appropriate treatments and also describes gaps in the knowledge where future research is needed'. From the concluding overview by Brian Davies.

This multidisciplinary work is of international significance. It links psychiatry and somatic medicine and confronts issues of comorbidity. Mood disorders are the commonest psychiatric illnesses encountered in the elderly and as such they receive the greatest coverage, but the text also focuses on the controversial area of late life paranoid disorder and schizophrenia, the neglected field of neurosis in old age and the emerging problem of substance abuse in the older patient. Several chapters feature case histories to bring the subject into lively focus. All chapters are neatly cross-referenced and rich in practical advice for the multidisiplinary team.

FUNCTIONAL PSYCHIATRIC DISORDERS OF THE ELDERLY

FUNCTIONAL PSYCHIATRIC DISORDERS OF THE ELDERLY

Edited by

EDMOND CHIU

Academic Unit in Psychiatry of Old Age, University of Melbourne, Victoria, Australia

DAVID AMES

Academic Unit in Psychiatry of Old Age, University of Melbourne, Victoria, Australia

CAMBRIDGE
UNIVERSITY PRESS

CAMBRIDGE UNIVERSITY PRESS
Cambridge, New York, Melbourne, Madrid, Cape Town, Singapore, São Paulo

Cambridge University Press
The Edinburgh Building, Cambridge CB2 2RU, UK

Published in the United States of America by Cambridge University Press, New York

www.cambridge.org
Information on this title: www.cambridge.org/9780521431606

First published 1994
This digitally printed first paperback version 2006

A catalogue record for this publication is available from the British Library

Library of Congress Cataloguing in Publication data
Functional psychiatric disorders of the elderly / edited by Edmond
Chiu and David Ames.
p. cm.
Includes an index.
ISBN 0-521-43160-3 (hardback)
1. Geriatric psychiatry. 2. Aged – Mental health. I. Chiu,
Edmond. II. Ames, David.
[DNLM: 1. Mental Disorders – in old age. WT 150 F979 1994]
RC451.4.A5F86 1994
618.97′689 – dc20
DNLM/DLC
for Library of Congress 93-33740 CIP

ISBN-13 978-0-521-43160-6 hardback
ISBN-10 0-521-43160-3 hardback

ISBN-13 978-0-521-02676-5 paperback
ISBN-10 0-521-02676-8 paperback

This book is gratefully dedicated to those psychiatrists in every continent, who have pioneered the work of geriatric psychiatry, paving the way for our generation.

Contents

List of contributors

Kristine J. Alexander BAppSci (OT)
Formerly Senior Occupational Therapist, Geriatric Psychiatry Services, Eastern Suburbs Geriatric Centre, Melbourne, Australia

George S. Alexopoulos MD
Professor of Psychiatry, Cornell University Medical College, White Plains, New York, USA

Osvaldo P. Almeida MD
Institute of Psychiatry, Section of Old Age Psychiatry, London, UK

David Ames BA, MD, MRCPsych, FRANZCP
Senior Lecturer in Psychiatry of Old Age, University of Melbourne, Australia

Kaarin Anstey BA (Hons)
Research Officer, Academic Department of Psychogeriatrics, Prince Henry Hospital, Sydney, Australia

Tom Arie MA, BM, FRCP FRCPsych, FFPHM, FRCP
Professor of Health Care of the Elderly, University of Nottingham, UK

Nancy Bailey LCSW
NorthWestern Memorial Hospital, Chicago, USA

Rotimi Bajulaiye MD, MPH
Assistant Professor of Psychiatry, Cornell University Medical College, White Plains, New York, USA

Sube Banerjee MBBS, MRCPsych
Research Fellow in Psychiatry, United Medical and Dental School, Guy's Hospital Campus, London SE1, UK

Barbara Beats MBBS, MRCP, MRCPsych
Senior Registrar, Maidstone Hospital, Kent, UK

Susan Benbow MB, ChB, MSc, MRCPsych
Consultant Psychiatrist for the Elderly, Central Manchester Health Authority, Manchester Royal Infirmary, Manchester, UK

Karen Berte PhD
NorthWestern Memorial Hospital, Chicago, USA

Martin Blanchard BSc, MRCPsych
Senior Registrar, Maudsley Hospital, London, UK

Diane Brauer LCSW
NorthWestern Memorial Hospital, Chicago, USA

Ruth Bright AM, BMusc, RMT
Music Therapist, Wahroonga, New South Wales, Australia

Henry Brodaty MBBS, MD, FRACP, FRANZCP
Professor of Psychogeriatrics, University of New South Wales, Australia

Graham Burrows AO, MD, ChB, BSc, DPM, FRANZCP, FRCPsych
Professor/Director, University of Melbourne Department of Psychiatry, Austin Hospital, Melbourne, Australia

Peter Burvill MD, FRANZCP, FRCPsych, FRCPE, MFCM
Professor of Psychiatry, Department of Psychiatry and Behavioral Sciences, Queen Elizabeth II Medical Centre, Perth, Australia

Edmond Chiu AM, MBBS, DPM, FRANZCP
Associate Professor, Academic Unit in Psychiatry of Old Age, University of Melbourne, Australia

Brian Davies MD, FRCP, FRACP, FRANZCP, FRCPsych, DPM, DCH
Emeritus Professor of Psychiatry, University of Melbourne, Australia

Robin Eastwood MD, FRCP(C), FRCPsych
Professor of Psychiatry, Professor of Preventive Medicine & Biostatistics, University of Toronto, Director, Neuroepidemiology Research Unit, Clarke Institute, Toronto, Canada

Sanford I. Finkel MD
Director, Gero-Psychiatry Services, NorthWestern Memorial Hospital, Chicago; Associate Professor NorthWestern University Medical School; Associate Director Buehler Center on Aging of NorthWestern University

Medical School and Past President, International Psychogeriatric Association, USA

Marshal F. Folstein MD
Professor and Chairman, Department of Psychiatry, Tufts University School of Medicine, Boston, USA

Hans Förstl MD, MADAC
Head of the EEG-Laboratory, Director Alzheimer's Disease Research Program, Central Institute of Mental Health, Mannheim, Germany

James Gandy DO
NorthWestern University Medical School, Chicago, USA

Thirunavukarasu Ganesvaran MBBS, DPM, FRCPsych
Consultant Psychiatrist, North Eastern Metropolitan Psychiatric Services, Melbourne, Australia

Chris Gilleard PhD
Head of Psychology Services, Springfield Hospital and Senior Lecturer in Psychology of Old Age, St. George's Hospital Medical School, London, UK

Heinz Häfner MD, PhD, Drs. hc
Professor of Psychiatry at the University of Heidelberg, Head of the Central Institute of Mental Health in Mannheim, Germany

Martin Hambrecht MD, PhD
Clinical Psychiatrist and Senior Scientist, Central Institute of Mental Health in Mannheim, Germany

Robert Howard MA, MBBS, MRCPsych
Lecturer, Section of Old Age Psychiatry, Institute of Psychiatry, London, UK

Fiona Judd MBBS, DPM, MD, FRANZCP
Associate Professor, University of Melbourne, Department of Psychiatry, Austin Hospital, Melbourne, Australia

John Kellett MA (Cantab), MB, BChir, DPM, FRCP, FRCPsych
Division of Geriatric Medicine, St George's Hospital, London, UK

Barbara Knothe MBBS, DPM, FRANZCP
Consultant Psychiatrist, Melbourne, Australia

Brian Leonard PhD, DSc, MRIA
Professor of Department of Pharmacology, University College, Galway, Ireland

Raymond Levy PhD, FRCP, FRCPsych
Professor of Old Age Psychiatry, Institute of Psychiatry, London, UK

James Lindesay MA, DM, MRCPsych
Professor of Psychiatry for the Elderly, University of Leicester, UK

Anthony Mann MD, MPhil, FRCP, FRCPsych
Professsor of Epidemiological Psychiatry, Institute of Psychiatry and Royal Free Hospital School of Medicine, London, UK

Peter McArdle MB, BS, DPM, FRANZCP
Former Director of Geriatric Psychiatry, Eastern Suburbs Geriatric Centre, Melbourne, Australia

Joan M. McMeeken DipPhysio, BSc(Hons), MSc, MAPA
Professor and Head, School of Physiotherapy, University of Melbourne, Australia

Paul Metler PsyD
Clinical Psychologist, NorthWestern Memorial Hospital, Chicago, USA

Elizabeth Ozanne BA, Dip Soc Studs, MSW, MA, PhD
Senior Lecturer, School of Social Work, University of Melbourne, Australia

Godfrey Pearlson MBBS
Director of Division of Psychiatric Neuro-imaging and Professor, Departments of Psychiatry and Mental Hygiene, Johns Hopkins University School of Medicine, Baltimore, USA

Michael Philpot BSc, MBBS, MRCPsych
Consultant and Senior Lecturer in Psychogeriatrics, Guy's and St Thomas' NHS Trust, London, UK

Brice Pitt MD, FRCPsych
Professor, Academic Unit in Psychiatry of Old Age, St Charles Hospital, London, UK

Peter Rabins MD
Associate Professor of Psychiatry, Johns Hopkins University School of Medicine, Baltimore, USA

Joel Sadavoy MD, DipPsych, FRCP(C)
Associate Professor of Psychiatry, University of Toronto, Head, Division of Geriatric Psychiatry, University of Toronto, Canada

Norman Sartorius MD, MA, DPM, PhD, FRCPsych.
Director, Division of Mental Health, World Health Organization, Geneva, Switzerland. President-Elect, World Psychiatric Association.

Ajit Shah MB, ChB, MRCPsych
Consultant Psychiatrist, North Eastern Metropolitan Psychiatric Services, Melbourne, Australia

Kenneth I. Shulman MD, SM, FRCPsych, FRCP(C)
Head, Department of Psychiatry, Sunnybrook Health Science Center, University of Toronto, Canada

John Snowdon FRANZCP, FRCPsych, FRACP, MPhil
Area Director of Psychogeriatric Services,Central Sydney Health Service, Australia

Stephen Ticehurst MBBS, FRANZCP
Director, Psychogeriatric Services, Hunter Area Health Service, Clinical Lecturer in Psychiatry, University of Newcastle, UK

John Tiller MD, MB, ChB, BSc, DPM, FRACP, FRANZCP
Associate Professor, Department of Psychiatry, University of Melbourne, Australia

Jan Tinney RPN, RN
Nurse Unit Manager, Geriatric Psychiatry Service, Royal Park Hospital, Melbourne, Australia

T. Bedirhan Üstün MD
Scientist, Division of Mental Health, World Health Organization, Geneva, Switzerland

Wendy Wasson PhD
NorthWestern Memorial Hospital, Chicago, USA

Karen D. B. Webster BAppSc,(Physiotherapy), Grad Dip Movement & Dance, Grad Dip Health Education, MAPA
Senior Physiotherapist, Heatherton Hospital, Heatherton, Victoria, Australia

Sid Williams MBBS, FRANZCP
Lidcombe Hospital, Sydney, Australia

Preface

The Geriatric Psychiatry Section of the World Psychiatric Association held its 1990 Symposium in Melbourne, Australia, with the theme of 'Functional Psychiatric Disorders in the Elderly'. Having regard to the constant exposure of dementia in recent conferences all over the world, it was noted that the functional psychiatric disorders had received far less attention. As any practising clinician in geriatric psychiatry can readily attest to the number of patients whose functional psychiatric disorder requires attention, such a situation of neglect requires some redress.

Cambridge University Press, through the perspicacity and energy of Dr Richard Barling noted this conference theme and requested E. C. to make a proposal for the publication of a multi-authored volume on this subject. D. A. agreed to be a co-editor to accomplish the task. Some individual chapter authors were recruited on the basis of papers presented at the Melbourne Symposium, while others who had been unable to attend that meeting were invited to contribute because of their acknowledged expertise in particular areas which the editors considered pertinent to the theme of this text.

The editors are very grateful to the chapter authors, who took to the task given to them with goodwill and enthusiasm.

In the process of planning this book the term 'functional' exercised our minds as, in the context of geriatric psychiatry, such terms give rise to considerable debate. As early as 1971, Tom Arie noted 'There is nothing to be gained and a lot to be lost by thinking separately of organic and functional disorders; even were such a distinction always clinically realistic, which it is not'. We sought suggestions for alternative titles from all chapter authors but there was clear consensus that at present there is no term that can easily replace the word 'functional'. Other terms suggested were more cumbersome, inelegant and lacked clarity. Therefore, until a better term emerges (as it inevitably will) we have chosen to keep this word in temporary usage.

We hope that this volume will provide the first book to deal exclusively with all the non-dementing psychiatric disorders for practitioners from all clinical disciplines related to geriatric psychiatry. We have aimed the book to help clinicians in their day-to-day practice. Thus there is an extensive section devoted to multidisciplinary management strategies, which in other volumes have not been given such prominence. We have also attempted to highlight the interface between psychiatry, somatic medicine and the issues of co-morbidity which confront clinicians. The relative lack of information in the area of neurosis in the elderly is highlighted by the chapter authors, while the chapters on psychotherapeutic treatment strategies address an area which has suffered marked neglect to date. Most authors have indicated potential directions for future research, and as academic geriatric psychiatrists, we will feel privileged if this book prompts further research on the functional psychiatric disorders of old age.

It would delight us if this book rapidly became outdated as geriatric psychiatry advances towards a more sophisticated and dynamic understanding of these disabling disorders.

Edmond Chiu
David Ames
Melbourne

Reference

Arie, T. (1971). Morale and the planning of psychogeriatric services. *British Medical Journal*, 3, 166–70.

Introduction: A personal note

TOM ARIE

This book originates in Australia, but it is of international significance. Deriving from a World Psychiatric Association meeting hosted in Melbourne, this is no mere text of conference proceedings; Edmond Chiu and David Ames have used the theme of that conference as the basis for a carefully planned series of commissioned contributions to a well-structured book.

The early years of psychogeriatrics were dominated, rightly and inevitably, by the 'Everest of dementia'. It is evidence of the maturity and confidence of this branch of psychiatry (now an official subspecialty in the United Kingdom) that it here steps back from its concern with the insistent burden of the organic psychosyndromes, and focuses on the hugely important functional disorders of old age. Dementia in its most obvious manifestations obtrudes itself in a way which is hard (though too often still not impossible) to ignore; the sometimes more personal misery of functional mental disorders is too easy to overlook, or to confront inadequately amid the pressure of the needs of sufferers from the organic disorders and those who look after them.

Yet there were times when it was to functional illness that most of the attention of those working in the field of old age mental disorder was being given; prognosis here is generally better, the course often (not always) shorter, and the gratifications of successful treatment more direct. Today, the nettle of the dementias has generally been firmly grasped, but most 'psychogeriatricians' now see themselves as psychiatrists to the elderly, dealing with organic and functional disorders alike, and recognizing that both types of disorder (and sorting the components of one from the other) are part of the responsibility of good old age psychiatry services.

A much earlier World Psychiatric Association symposium, which took place well before old age psychiatry had become defined as a discrete branch of psychiatry, focused on the mental disorders of old age, and in a book (which is now a collector's item) arising out of that meeting, attention was given alike to the functional and organic disorders (WPA 1965). A quarter of a century later, psychogeriatric services have developed with vigour in most developed countries

– even as they are beginning to do in the third world (as I write a request arrived for help with planning psychogeriatrics in Indonesia).

Research too has moved apace, and is by no means confined to clinical psychiatry. It is clear that the relevant basic sciences have a crucial contribution, as do the many other applied specialties and professions which have contributed richly to the growth of knowledge. Progress has of late been greater in understanding the organic disorders of old age, and in the functional disorders the basic science disciplines have so far contributed rather less, and are consequently less prominent in this book than they would have been in a text on the dementias; yet it is surely reasonable to expect that the basic sciences will soon be contributing as richly to this field as they have already done towards unravelling the organic syndromes.

Several chapters in this book are concerned with the relationship between functional and organic factors in the brain disorders in old age. Much of what we took for granted about the relationship, for example, of depression and organic brain disorders has had to be rethought, and few firm conclusions are yet available. It is clear that research in this area will be much aided by greater access to powerful new techniques, ranging from molecular biology to brain imaging. Thus, new light has begun to be shed on the role of organic brain changes in paranoid states in old people: long reported, this has only of late been the subject of study by the newer imaging techniques.

At the other pole from basic science research is practical provision of services. This book is strong on this topic, both in its emphasis on, and in the range of contributions from, the different members of the mixed team. Like most research, services are rarely effective if they are not rooted in teamwork: this text is in some measure a handbook of good teamwork.

Perhaps these introductory words should mention a topic which impinges on several of the book's themes. I refer to the 'graduates' – the chronic psychotics who have 'graduated' into old age with their disease, often over decades spent in large institutions, or hovering around their edges. The natural history of schizophrenia as the sufferer ages, and the implications and options for local services – and the sometimes vexed question whether this large group of elderly people should all be wholly looked after by local psychogeriatric services – all these are important questions. This topic has recently been well tackled by Campbell (1991), and there is not much at present that can now be added; but the issue persists.

I see this volume as a timely exercise in stocktaking. Depression, not dementia, is still the commonest mental disorder of old age – and despite the inroads of dementia at very high ages, the prevalence of depression remains as high among the 'old old' as the 'young old'. This book is important as a reminder of these matters, and as evidence of the enormous growth in interest and knowledge in the quarter of a century since that 1965 WPA symposium in London. It is satisfying that the book should have originated from the initiative of colleagues in Australia, where psychogeriatrics flourishes and where developments move hand in hand with those in the rest of the world, as the list of contributors demonstrates. But the invitation to introduce the book is particularly gratifying to one who has been able to follow, and even share a little, in the development of our discipline in Australia and New Zealand from its beginnings. Five years ago I had the good fortune to be present at the inauguration of the Specialist Section on Old Age Psychiatry in the Royal Australian and New Zealand College of Psychiatrists, and I am grateful for the frequent and generous hospitality of colleagues in those countries. It is a pleasure to introduce a book which I have found both good reading, and a stimulus to think more about the non-organic mental misery which is so common, and often so remediable, in old age.

References

Campbell, P. G. (1991). Graduates. In *Psychiatry in the Elderly*, ed. by R. Jacoby & C. Oppenheimer, Oxford: Oxford University Press.

World Psychiatric Association (1965). *Psychiatric Disorders in the Aged*. Manchester: Geigy.

Tom Arie
Professor of Health Care of the Elderly
University of Nottingham
Past Chairman, Geriatric Psychiatry Section, World Psychiatric Association

Acknowledgement

Dr Richard Barling of Cambridge University Press has been, since the conception of this volume, most supportive and encouraging. Mrs Roz Seath has tirelessly liaised with chapter authors, organized material received and typed the manuscript and gave unstinting support, especially to E. C. Mrs Yvonne Liddicoat provided excellent secretarial support to D. A.

Part 1

Classification

1

Functional psychiatric disorders in ICD-10

NORMAN SARTORIUS T. B. ÜSTÜN

Introduction

This chapter reviews the so-called 'functional' psychiatric disorders in the mental and behavioral disorders section of International Classification of Disorders 10th Revision (ICD-10). It describes the clinical characteristics of these disorders in the elderly and discusses their classification in the ICD-10, using the following outline:

1. General structure of ICD-10
2. Overview of functional disorders in ICD-10 (Organic versus functional: The concept of functional disorders in ICD-10.)
3. Special features of functional disorders in the elderly: selected examples are given for each section of ICD-10 Chapter V.

Section F0:	Mild cognitive disorder
Section F1:	Psychoactive substance use disorders
Section F2:	Late paraphrenia
Section F3:	Depressive disorders
Section F4:	Anxiety disorders
	Adjustment disorders
	Neurasthenia
Section F5:	Physiological disorders
Section F6:	Disorders of adult personality and behavior

General structure of ICD-10

The production of an international classification of diseases is a constitutional task for the World Health Organization (WHO). The organization took on this task in 1948 and since then has prepared five revisions of the International Classification of Diseases. The tenth version (ICD-10) was adopted in 1990 by the World Health Assembly which is the supreme decision making body of the WHO formed by representatives of the 183 Member States of the Organization. The classification began to enter into use in the member states on 1 January 1993.

ICD-10 has 22 chapters, each dealing with different groups of conditions which have to be classified and reported to public health authorities. The chapters provide a classificatory structure for groups of diseases or syndromes, causes of death, reasons for contact with health services and other health-related information.

Chapter V of ICD-10 dealing with 'Mental and Behavioral Disorders' is the only chapter in ICD-10 which has brief definitions for each of the categories of the classification. These definitions were first introduced in the ICD-8 (Sartorius et al. 1993; Sartorius 1991*a*). Their development was a component of a special program dealing with the standardization of psychiatric diagnosis and classification launched in the early 1960s. It was felt that such a program was necessary because of the vast differences which existed between psychiatric schools, the vagueness of categories and allied difficulties, which were making communication in the field of mental health extremely difficult. The program was successful: it raised awareness of public health and alerted psychiatric communities to difficulties in making reliable diagnoses and recording them; it developed methods for the exploration of these differences and it prepared an internationally acceptable classification of mental disorders and a glossary describing its categories (Kramer et al. 1979; Shepherd, Brooke & Cooper, 1968).

Mental disorders in the elderly were given a special emphasis in this program. One of the seven scientific meetings held to discuss proposals for ICD-8 focused on mental disorders of old age such as involutional melancholia 296.0 and involutional paraphrenia 297.1 (Stengel, 1958; Averbuch, E. S. et al., 1970; WHO, 1977). The meeting recommended inclusion of new categories (e.g. the depressive syndrome linked to organic brain damage in the elderly) and urged the WHO to develop a multidiagnostic or multiaxial classification for work in psychogeriatrics. It also drew attention to the need to better define methods for the assessment of severity of cognitive deficit and related disability. Some of the recommendations of the program were implemented in making the ICD-8: others led to research (e.g. to the current WHO coordinated comparative studies of dementia and the development of a battery of neuropsychological tests); some remain valid and may be taken up by WHO in the future.

In the development of ICD-10, WHO introduced several innovative features. These included an alphanumeric designation of codes (which resulted in a significant expansion of the number of categories available to each group of diseases). The alphanumeric coding scheme also allows discrimination between the content of different chapters (e.g. letter 'A' designates 'certain infectious and parasitic diseases' whereas letter 'F' signifies 'mental disorders'. The digits after the letter specify the individual categories. However, not all of the digits are being used. In this way, it will be possible not only to adapt to advances in the scientific

Table 1.1. *ICD-10 Chapter V diagnostic categories*

F0	Organic, including symptomatic mental disorders
F1	Mental and behavioral disorders due to psychoactive and other substance use
F2	Schizophrenia, schizotypal and delusional disorders
F3	Mood (affective) disorders
F4	Neurotic, stress related and somatoform disorders
F5	Behavioral syndromes and mental disorders associated with physiological dysfunction
F6	Disorders of adult personality and behavior
F7	Mental retardation
F8	Disorders with onset specific to childhood
F9	Behavioral and emotional disorders with onset usually occurring in childhood and adolescence

knowledge but also to maintain a continuity between the successive versions of the classification without disruptions in the coding scheme. The categories in ICD-10 are meant to apply to all age groups with the exception of categories reserved for disorders which only appear at a certain age. Thus depression in children will be coded in the same category as all depressive disorders, while disorders specific to childhood and adolescent problems are given separate categories.

The mental and behavioral disorders in ICD-10 have been classified into ten major groups by broad clinical similarity (Cooper, 1988). Table 1.1 shows the major groupings.

Experience from different countries made it obvious that the various groups of users of a classification have different needs (Sartorius 1991*a*). Therefore the mental disorder classification in the ICD-10 has been prepared in several versions for use by clinicians, researchers and primary health care workers. A multiaxial presentation as well as special 'fascicles' for special groups of users have also been prepared. Each of these versions is based on the 'core ICD-10' classification and is compatible with other members (see Table 1.2).

Table 1.2. *ICD-10 Chapter V family of documents*

Member	Primary Audience
ICD-10 Clinical descriptions and diagnostic guidelines	Clinicians
ICD-10 Diagnostic criteria for research	Researchers
ICD-10 Psychiatric adaptation	Medical record librarians and statisticians
ICD-10 Primary care adaptation	PHC practitioners
ICD-10 Neurological adaptation	Neurologists
ICD-10 Multiaxial presentation	Researchers and epidemiologists
ICD-10 Lexicon of terms	All users

ICD-10 Terminology: What is organic and what is functional?

In current psychiatric use, a differentiation is usually made between 'organic' and 'functional' disorders. An 'organic' disorder is characterized by certain symptoms and by structural or otherwise identifiable changes in the central nervous system. The word 'functional' is used to describe conditions in which a different set of symptoms is present and current methods of investigation have been unable to prove structural damage or identifiable (e.g. humoral) change that could account for the condition. 'Functional' usually includes the psychogenic disorders (e.g. dissociative disorders),as well as mood disorders, schizophrenia and related disorders. Recent years have brought evidence of structural change and neuro-physiological derangement in several of the 'functional' disorders and it is probable that both the terms 'functional' and 'organic' will soon be a thing of the past. WHO has maintained the term 'organic' disorders in the ICD-10 because of its wide current use; it does not use the term 'functional' as a descriptor for a category or a group of categories.

There are a few categories which are referred to as 'nonorganic' e.g. 'F51 nonorganic sleep disorders' or F52 'sexual dysfunction not caused by organic disorder or disease'. When used, the words 'nonorganic' in these categories, have been employed because they allow the placement of such categories in the chapter of mental and behavioral disorders, the 'organic' counterpart term being placed in other chapters of the ICD-10 (organic sleep disorders for example are classified in neurological disorders).

Special features of functional disorders in the elderly

Although there are no mental disorders within the ICD-10 Chapter V that are seen only in old age, mental disorders in the elderly have certain unique features. In this section these features are briefly reviewed within the context of the ICD-10 classification focusing on selected examples. (As with all other diagnostic categories in ICD-10, these diagnoses apply to any age group and are not intended for application in the elderly only.)

F0: Mild cognitive disorder (MCD)

Epidemiological findings (Basset & Folstein, 1991) and clinical reports in the area of cognitive disorders have resulted in the inclusion of a new category as 'F06.7 Mild cognitive disorder'(MCD) in ICD-10 (Division of Mental Health, 1992). This category covers the spectrum of disorders which are not as severe as dementia and delirium but do display a decline in cognitive performance. MCD are frequently

Table 1.3. *General criteria defining organic disorders in ICD-10 diagnostic criteria for research*

G1.	Objective evidence (from physical and neurological examination and laboratory tests) and/or history of cerebral disease, damage or dysfunction, or of systemic physical disease known to cause cerebral dysfunction, including hormonal disturbances (other than alcohol or other psychoactive substance-related) and nonpsychoactive drug effects.
G2.	A presumed relationship between the development (or marked exacerbation) of the underlying disease, damage or dysfunction, and the mental disorder, the symptoms of which may have immediate onset or may be delayed.
G3.	Recovery or significant improvement of the mental disorder following removal or improvement of the underlying presumed cause.
G4.	Absence of sufficient or suggestive evidence for an alternative causation of the mental disorder, e.g. a highly loaded family history for a clinically similar or related disorder.
	If criteria G1, G2, and G4 are met, a provisional diagnosis is justified; if, in addition, there is evidence of G3, the diagnosis can be regarded as certain.

encountered in the course of other diseases such as cerebral or systemic infections. A variety of diseases can cause an impairment in functioning, mainly in the areas of attention, information processing, language, learning and recall, abstracting and other cognitive domains.

Boundaries of the concept of MCD pose a problem of definition (Henderson, 1992). The concept is so far recognized by exclusion of cases who are normal and those cases with cognitive impairment who already meet diagnostic criteria for dementia, delirium and other categories. Definition of a middle spectrum is never easy. Patients given this diagnosis suffer from a variety of conditions heterogeneous in etiopathogenesis, associated symptoms and outcome.

There are also other issues which arise with the introduction of this new category. How should subjective complaints of cognitive dysfunction be assessed? How much change in cognitive function can be expected in normal ageing? Moreover, verification of complaints by objective tests, and relationship of the cognitive disorder with other medical conditions also pose a question: what will be acceptable as the required 'evidence' of association?

As we have discussed in the second section of this chapter, the discrimination between organic versus functional is somewhat arbitrary and vague. The distinction mainly depends on our capacity to find the organic basis of the signs. If one is confronted with complaints of cognitive difficulty that fulfil the criteria as outlined in Table 1.3 (e.g. in medical or surgical wards, in patients after a viral infection) the diagnosis may be easy to make. On the other hand, in some elderly patients who complain about increasing forgetfulness, it may be difficult to establish the 'organic' etiological link. There is no 'functional counterpart' of MCD category as a formal diagnosis in ICD-10. Subjective complaints of cognitive dysfunction shoud therefore lead diagnosticians to explore also: F39 Unspecified mood disorder, F48.9 Neurotic disorder, unspecified; or F59 Unspecified behavioral syndromes associated with physiological disturbances and physical factors.

F1: Psychoactive substance use disorders

Patterns of drug use change with age. While some drug use (e.g. heroin, cocaine and hallucinogens) is mainly seen in younger age groups, the elderly more often abuse alcohol and other legally permissible substances (e.g. medical drugs). The elderly often use several such substances at the same time, in a stereotyped way. Old people may be more prone to intoxication and other harmful consequences of substance use because of changes in the metabolism of substances in old age. 'Tolerance' to psychoactive substances may be diminished and low amounts of the substance may lead to significant behavioral or toxic effects.

When 'functional' disorders are seen in conjunction with substance use disorders and are due to such use they are coded in Section F1, such as a psychotic disorder (F1x.5), Personality or Behavior disorder (F1x.71), Residual affective disorder (F1x.72), other persisting cognitive impairment (F1x.74).

F2: Late paraphrenia

Paraphrenia was included in ICD-9 as a formal diagnostic category (297.2), and discontinued in ICD-10. Kraepelin (1896) had defined paraphrenia as a category which falls between paranoia and dementia praecox. As later used by Roth (1955), the term referred to a delusional disorder that does not show the personality disintegration associated with early-onset schizophrenia. Affectivity should be well preserved and there should be no 'schizophrenic' symptoms such as inappropriate affect, loosening of associations, incoherence, and overtly disorganized behavior. Today, there is a growing tendency to see this category as being composed of several disorders. Cases previously diagnosed as paraphrenia are now placed within the boundaries of either 'paranoid schizophrenia' (Quintal et al., 1991; Hymas, Naguib, & Levy, 1989), 'delusional disorder' or 'organic delusional disorder' (Flint, Rifat & Eastwood, 1991; Holden, 1987; Miller et al., 1986; Gold, 1984). In view of this, paraphrenia was dropped from ICD-10 as a main entry; however, since some clinicians still use this category, it has been retained as an inclusion term for schizophrenia and delusional disorders. ICD-10 does not specify an upper age limit for the initial occurrence of schizophrenia or related disorders. Therefore it is possible to classify some of these cases as late onset schizophrenia or a delusional disorder. There is no provision of a separate code for 'age of onset' in the ICD-10.

Table 1.4. *F32 General criteria depressive episodes*

G1 The depressive episode should last for at least two weeks.
G2 Absence of hypomanic or manic symptoms sufficient to meet the criteria for hypomanic or manic episode (F30.–) at any time in the subject's life.
G3 Most commonly used exclusion criteria: the episode is not attributable to psychoactive substance use (F1) or any organic mental disorder, in the sense of F0.

F32.0 Mild depressive episode
A The general criteria for depressive episode (F32) must be met.
B At least two of the following three symptoms:
1. Depressed mood to a degree that is definitely abnormal for the subject, present for most of the day and almost every day, largely uninfluenced by circumstances, and sustained for at least two weeks.
2. Loss of interest or pleasure in activities which are normally pleasurable.
3. Decreased energy or increased fatiguability.

C An additional symptom or symptoms from the following to give a total of at least four:
4. Loss of confidence, and self-esteem.
5. Unreasonable feelings of self-reproach or excessive and inappropriate guilt.
6. Recurrent thoughts of death or suicide, or any suicidal behavior.
7. Complaints or evidence of diminished ability to think or concentrate, such as indecisiveness or vacillation.
8. Change in psychomotor activity, with agitation or retardation (either subjective or objective).
9. Sleep disturbance of any type.
10. Change in appetite (decrease or increase) with corresponding weight change.

However, researchers are free to add a code for the categories in question (e.g. as the fifth or sixth digit) to facilitate retrieval of data for further investigation. The ICD-10 dedicated WHO instruments; Schedules for Clinical Assessment in Neuropsychiatry (SCAN) (WHO, 1992) and Composite International Diagnostic Interview Core Version (CIDI) (Division of Mental Health, 1990) for clinical and research use have provisions for the coding of age of onset for this purpose.

F23: Acute and transient psychotic disorders

These may be seen in the elderly under stress. These are cases in which symptoms develop suddenly (within hours to two weeks) and total duration is less than three months (schizophrenia-like symptoms lasting less than one month). A careful evaluation is necessary for differential diagnosis from F0 organic disorders (e.g. delirium) or F1 substance use (e.g. withdrawal state).

Table 1.5. *Somatic syndrome*

To qualify for the somatic syndrome, *four* of the following symptoms should be present:
(1) marked loss of interest or pleasure in activities which are normally pleasurable;
(2) lack of emotional reactions to events or activities that normally produce an emotional response;
(3) waking in the morning two hours or more before the usual time;
(4) depression worse in the morning;
(5) objective evidence of marked psychomotor retardation or agitation (remarked on or reported by other persons);
(6) marked loss of appetite;
(7) weight loss (5% or more of body weight in the last month);
(8) marked loss of libido.

F3: Depressive disorders

ICD-10 employs a generic description for depressive disorders for all age groups (Table 1.4). Although depression may be more frequent in the elderly and has some special features (e.g., increased suicide rates, increased importance of dysphoric symptoms and probable linkage to psychosocial factors occurring in old age such as retirement and object loss), the groups reviewing the evidence did not feel that depression in the elderly should be given a special category.

Involutional melancholia

Kraepelin (1896) described this as a disorder with severe agitated depression, delusions of nihilism, guilt, grandiosity and hypochondriasis beginning after menopause in women and during late adulthood in men. It 'survived' as an independent category in ICD-9. The findings of some research that the elderly report more somatic symptoms, may be an artefact due to coexisting physical illness. In controlled studies, melancholia in hospitalized populations was found to be symptomatically similar to depression in the middle-aged (Blazer, Bachar & Hughes, 1987). Consequently, ICD-10 retained the term among inclusion terms but removed the category, unconvinced that 'involutional depression' is a separate disease entity. The notion of 'melancholia' (which implies a sort of 'biological basis' in depression), has been recognized by providing a category for *somatic syndrome* in ICD-10 (Table 1.5). Terms such as biological, vital, melancholic or endogenomorphic are used for this syndrome in other classifications.

The diagnosis of depression in the elderly may be problematic. Many systemic diseases and some drugs may cause depression in late life. Depressive disorders following stroke (Robinson et al., 1984) and other diseases such as Parkinson's Disease are common (Ring & Trimble 1991; Fleminger, 1991). When diagnosed, these conditions should be coded as organic depression (F06.3) with an additional code to specify the associated disease. In addition, comorbidity with physical disease may make the depressive disorder more severe and more difficult to treat.

Another important point in the diagnosis of depression in the elderly is the differential diagnosis between pseudodementia and coexisting dementia and depression. In pseudodementia, patients may have depression (F32) or another mental or physical illness presenting with apathy and apparent cognitive decline which may be confused with dementia; however, the cognitive impairment resolves when the affective disorder or other illness is successfully treated. In coexisting dementia and depression, patients have two diagnoses – both dementia (F00 to 03) and depression (F32) – and when the depression is treated, there is usually improvement in mood but not in cognitive impairment.

F4: Neurotic, stress-related and somatoform Disorders

These disorders in the elderly are similar to those occurring in earlier life. The old are considered to be more prone to adjustment disorders (F43.2) due to psychosocial factors. Life events (such as object loss, physical illness and changes in the social status,) may interfere with social functioning and the performance of the individual. The diagnosis of adjustment disorder in the ICD-10 system depends on findings from an evaluation of the relationship between:

(i) form, content and severity of symptoms;
(ii) previous history and personality; and
(iii) presence of stressful event, situation, or life crisis.

The criteria require that the presence of stress factors should be clearly established and that there should be strong, presumptive, evidence that the disorder would not have arisen without them. If the stressor is relatively minor, or if a temporal connection (less than three months) cannot be demonstrated, the disorder has to classified elsewhere, according to its presenting features. ICD-10 also allows the user to code the stressor by means of one of the Z codes (Chapter XXI).

Neurasthenia

A category for the classification of Neurasthenia (F48.0) is included in ICD-10. While research carried out in various settings has demonstrated that a significant proportion of cases diagnosed as neurasthenia have symptoms which would make it possible to classify them under depression or anxiety, there are also cases in which the clinical picture does not fit any other disease definition (Sartorius, 1991*b*). In the elderly the decline of the motor capacity or slowing of motor functions should be carefully evaluated before making a diagnosis in this category.

Section F5: Nonorganic insomnia

Complaints about difficulty in falling asleep, maintaining sleep, or nonrefreshing nature of sleep are common in old age. They can be classified as nonorganic insomnia in ICD-10 if the sleep disturbance occurs at least three times per week for at least one month, and results in marked personal distress or interference with personal functioning in daily living. The criteria draw attention to the fact that insomnia is a common symptom of other mental disorders; to the fact that total sleep time decreases with age; and to the finding that the most frequent cause of insomnia is pain, which is common in old age. The ICD-10 diagnosis of 'nonorganic insomnia' is therefore unlikely to be made frequently in the elderly.

Abuse of nondependence producing substances (F55)

This is a new category in the ICD-10. For services dealing with problems of the elderly this may be an important category since the old are prone to use a wide variety of medicinals, proprietary drugs and folk remedies for their physical illnesses. Although the medication may have been medically prescribed or recommended in the first instance, older people often continue taking unnecessary medication, sometimes in excessive dosage. Abuse is facilitated since many substances likely to be used by the elderly are easily available without medical prescription. Three particularly important groups are:

(i) psychotropic drugs which do not produce dependence, such as antidepressants,
(ii) laxatives, and
(iii) analgesics that can be purchased without medical prescriptions, such as aspirin and paracetamol.

F6: Disorders of adult personality and behavior

There is evidence that some personality traits diminish with age and can therefore cease to appear as a cause for personal or social distress. For example, dissocial or emotionally unstable and borderline personality types are known to 'calm down' with age. Failure of adaptive mechanisms, due to dementia and other physical or mental disorders, may, on the other hand, make some personality traits more prominent and disturbing. Since the definition of personality disorder is based on longstanding traits, these factors may influence the categorical definition because the number of criteria fulfilling the threshold for the specified category may change.

Other personality changes such as enduring personality change after psychiatric illness (manifested by: two years or more excessive dependence, persistent complaints of being ill, dysphoric mood, significant impairment in social and occupational functioning compared with the premorbid situation) is classified as F62.1 and enduring personality changes after bereavement or chronic pain personality syndrome are classified in F62.8.

Elaboration of physical symptoms for psychological reasons (F68.0)

This may also be seen in the elderly more frequently because of their physical health status and their psychological state (e.g. for attention-seeking).

Conclusion

Although mental disorders in the elderly may have unique features, there are no separate diagnostic categories specific for this group in ICD-10 Chapter V. Diagnostic concepts such as late (involutional) paraphrenia or involutional melancholia are no longer cited as titles for the categories in the ICD-10 classification although a provision is made for coding them when they are used.

The review of diagnostic criteria for ICD-10 categories, however, supports the need for special knowledge and skills to diagnose and classify mental disorders in the elderly.

ICD is a uniaxial classification but its format can be revised to assume the shape of a multiaxial classification (Sartorius, 1991*a*). This may be particularly useful for the old. Furthermore, the concept of the ICD-10 as a 'Family of Documents' allows the development of specific application modules to meet the needs of geriatric psychiatry services and research and to develop a specific adaptation of ICD-10 for the coding of information important for the elderly patients, including that applying to physical disorders, environmental factors, and psychosocial stressors.

References

Averbuch E. S., Melnik E. M., Serebrjakova Z. N., Schachmatov N. F. & Sternberg, E. A. (1970). *Diagnosis and Classification of Mental Disorders in Old Age (In Russian)*. Leningrad: Ministry of Public Health.

Basset S. S. & Folstein, M. (1991). Cognitive impairment and functional disability in the absence of psychiatric diagnosis. *Psychological Medicine*, **21**, 77–84.

Blazer, D., Bachar, J. R. & Hughes, D. C. (1987). Major depression with melancholia: a comparison of middle-aged and elderly adults. *Journal of the American Geriatrics Society*, **35**, 927–32.

Cooper, J. E. (1988). The structure and presentation of contemporary psychiatric classifications with special reference to ICD-9 and 10. *British Journal of Psychiatry*, **152**, (Suppl. 1), 21–8.

Division of Mental Health (1990). *Composite International Diagnostic Interview Core Version 1.0 November 1990*. Geneva: World Health Organization.

Division of Mental Health (1992). *The ICD 10 Classification of Mental and Behavioral Disorders – Clinical Descriptions and Diagnostic Guidelines.* Geneva: World Health Organization.

Division of Mental Health (1992). *Schedules for Clinical Assessment in Neuropsychiatry.* Geneva: World Health Organization.

Fleminger, S. (1991). Left-sided Parkinson's disease is associated with greater anxiety and depression. *British Journal of Psychiatry,* **21**, 629–38.

Flint, A. J., Rifat, S. L. & Eastwood, M. R. (1991). Late-onset paranoia: Distinct from paraphrenia? *International Journal of Geriatric Psychiatry,* **6**, 103–9.

Gold, D. D. J. (1984). Late age of onset schizophrenia: present but unaccounted for. *Comprehensive Psychiatry,* **25**, 225–37.

Henderson, A. S. (1992). Mild cognitive disorder in ICD-10. Paper Presented in *WPA Symposium* May 25 1992, Palermo, Italy.

Holden, N. L. (1987). Late paraphrenia or the paraphrenias? A descriptive study with a 10-year follow-up. *British Journal of Psychiatry,* **150**, 635–9.

Hymas, N., Naguib, M. & Levy, R. (1989). Late paraphrenia – a follow-up study. *International Journal of Geriatric Psychiatry,* **4**, 23–9.

Kraepelin E. (1896). *Psychiatrie. Ein Lehrbuch fur Studierende und Aertze.* V Auflage. Leipzig: Hirch.

Kramer, M., Sartorius, N., Jablensky, A. & Gulbinat, W. (1979). The ICD-9 Classification of Mental Disorders: a review of its development and contents. *Acta Psychiatrica Scandinavica,* **59**, 241–62.

Miller, B. L., Benson, D. F., Cummings, J. L. & Neshkes, R. (1986). Late-life paraphrenia: an organic delusional syndrome. *Journal of Clinical Psychiatry,* **47**, 204–7.

Quintal, M., Day Cody, D. & Levy, R. (1991). Late paraphrenia and ICD 10. *International Journal of Geriatric Psychiatry,* **6**, 111–16.

Ring, H. A. & Trimble, M. R. (1991). Affective disturbance in Parkinson's disease. *International Journal of Geriatric Psychiatry,* **6**, 385–93.

Robinson, R. G., Kubos, K. I., Starr, L. B., Rao, K. & Price, T. R. (1984). Mood disorders in stroke patients: importance of location of lesion. *Brain,* **107**, 81–93.

Roth, M. (1955). The natural history of mental disorder in old age. *Journal of Mental Science,* **101**, 281–301.

Sartorius, N., Jablensky, A., Cooper, J. E. & Burke, J. D. (1988). Psychiatric Classification in an International Perspective. *British Journal of Psychiatry,* **152**, Suppl. 1, 3–52.

Sartorius N. (1991*a*). The Classification of mental disorders in the tenth revision of the international classification of diseases. *European Psychiatry,* **6**, 315–22.

Sartorius, N. (1991*b*). Phenomenology and classification of Neurasthenia. In *Mental Disorders in Primary Care.* ed. M. Gastpar and P. Kielholz. New York, Toronto, Bern, Gottingen: Lewingston.

Sartorius, N., Kaelber, C. T., Cooper, J. E., Roper, M. T., Rae, D. R., Gulbinat, W., Üstün, T. B., & Regier, D. A. (1993). Progress toward achieving a common language in psychiatry. Results from the field trial of the clinical guidelines accompanying the World Health Organization classification of mental and behavioral disorders in ICD-10. *Archives of General Psychiatry,* **50**, 115–24.

Shepherd M., Brooke E. M., & Cooper J. E. (1968). An experimental approach to psychiatric diagnosis. An international study. *Acta Psychiatrica Scandinvavica*, Suppl., **201**, 7–89.

Stengel E. (1958). Classification of mental disorders. *Bulletin of the WHO*, **21**, 601–63.

Venkoba Rao, A. & Madhavan, T. (1981). 'Late paraphrenia' (a report from the geropsychiatric clinic, Madurai, India). *Indian Journal of Psychiatry*, **23**, 291–7.

World Health Organization (1967). *International Classification of Diseases, 8th Revision*. Geneva: WHO Publication.

World Health Organization (1977). *International Classification of Diseases, 9th Revision*. Geneva: WHO Publication.

World Health Organization (1992). *International Statistical Classification of Diseases and Related Health Problems, 10th Revision*. Geneva: WHO Publication.

2

The classification of functional psychiatric disorders in the elderly in DSM-III-R and DSM-IV

PETER RABINS MARSHAL FOLSTEIN

Introduction

Classification systems have varied over the centuries. Their differences reflect the changing purposes of classification and the varying ethos of the time periods in which they are developed. The DSM-III-R (American Psychiatric Association, 1987) and DSM-IV (American Psychiatric Association, 1991), structured upon the approach developed by Emil Kraepelin (1915) at the end of the nineteenth century, were devised to provide reliable, operationalized criteria for the diagnosis of psychiatric disorder. The issue of age differences is rarely explicitly addressed in either set of criteria but the texts of both books do make reference to age-related issues. This chapter will review the classification of the functional psychiatric conditions common in later life in these two sets of criteria.

As will be evident in the discussion that follows, many of the strengths and weaknesses of DSM-III-R and DSM-IV reflect the basic assumptions Kraepelin made a century ago. Three of these are highlighted in this chapter.

1. Kraepelin adopted the syndromic approach of Thomas Sydenham (McHugh & Slavney, 1973). He and the DSM-III-R cluster psychiatric signs and symptoms into recognizable syndromes that are assumed to be diseases. However, because no underlying bodily abnormality has been found in most cases of functional psychiatric disorder, these categories should remain tentative until valid markers are identified.
2. Kraepelin employed a hierarchical approach to mental illness. He believed that intact cognitive status is necessary for a functional disorder to be diagnosed and that both cognitive status and 'functional' status need to be intact before disorders in the personality disorder/neurotic realm can be considered. This hierarchical approach has the strength of separating brain diseases with known pathology from disorders without neuropathology. One weakness of this viewpoint is its assumption that disorders cannot simultaneously occur at several levels. In fact, Kraepelin (1915) himself recognized that disorders could coexist at different levels and noted that affective disorder occurred together with both Huntington's disease and stroke more often than

chance would predict. The DSM-III-R, however, adopts the hierarchical approach without compromise and does not allow a diagnosis of schizophrenia or affective disorder if an identifiable brain disorder or lesion is present.

3. Kraepelin emphasized that the course of an illness, i.e. its progression or lack thereof, is an important determinant of and validation for distinct syndromes. As Berrios (1985) notes, Kraepelin was not the first person to use prognosis in this way but his emphasis on its importance as a feature distinguishing dementia praecox (schizophrenia) from manic-depressive insanity has profoundly influenced modern diagnostic practice.

Kraepelin did recognize the need to seek sources of validation other than course. For example, he went to Java to determine whether symptomatology might vary by culture. This openness to the variability of symptoms within a syndrome and his willingness to revise his views in succeeding editions of his textbook bespeak our need to continue refining criteria based on validated, objective data.

Classification can be criticized on many grounds including efficiency, usability and humanness. One general critique is that classification obscures individual differences and diminishes the power of measurement to identify relevant dimensions because it considers only categories of people already known. That is, it assumes complete knowledge in a field where most mechanisms and causes remain unknown. Category-based classification also disregards the graded nature of some aspects of mental life. It demands single cut points (i.e. present or absent) even for dimensional traits and behaviors. These criticisms have particular relevance to the elderly because they have been less studied as a group and because as longitudinal studies are beginning to demonstrate that, variability among individuals is a hallmark of the aging process (Baltes, 1991).

Population-based epidemiologic studies provide an important data source for validating or refuting existing schema such as the DSM-III-R and for revising them when appropriate. They are a means of determining whether standard classes apply to the elderly and whether age differences in symptomatology need to be taken into account in classificatory schema. They provide data from large representative populations of elderly with methods that do not presume a particular classification. The epidemiological catchment area (ECA) study provided such data.

The prevalence of functional psychiatric disorders in the elderly

The ECA study was a five site community-based epidemiologic study of psychiatric disorder in the US. Data were derived from the administration of the Diagnostic Instrument Schedule (DIS) in the households (Eaton et al., 1984). In Baltimore a subsample underwent an additional reexamination or clinical reappraisal by psychiatrists who adapted Present State Examination (PSE) questions into algorithms for making DSM-III-R diagnoses (Romanoski et al., 1992).

Lower prevalence rates for both DIS lay interviewer-derived and PSE clinician-derived diagnoses were obtained for major depression, the anxiety disorders, schizophrenia, substance abuse disorders and personality disorders in the elderly (Anthony & Aboraya, 1992). The prevalence of cognitive disorder increased after age 65.

Methodologic questions have been raised about these findings (Jarvik, 1986). Since the examination was carried out by lay interviewers it has been suggested that they misattributed somatic complaints that derived from psychiatric disorder to physical illness. Other potential sources of age bias include using the same criteria across the age span without their being validated in all age groups; differential rates of participation in the study based on age; cohort differences that might affect symptom reports; and a masking of functional disorders by the development of cognitive impairment. Few of these critiques can be directly refuted at present. None-the-less, there are a number of potential interactions between age and the syndromic classification of functional psychiatric disorder. Two general questions are addressed in the sections that follow. First, are there aspects of ageing which broadly affect the application of classification schema to the elderly? Second, are there age-related differences in symptomatology within specific psychiatric syndromes?

General obstacles to the application of classified schema to the elderly

Medical comorbidity

The elderly are much more likely than other age groups to suffer from one or more 'medical' diseases in addition to an identifiable psychiatric disorder (Kramer, 1983). For example, the likelihood of having cancer in addition to depression increases over the lifespan because the prevalence of cancer rises with age. This concurrence of the two disorders makes it difficult to assign a symptom that commonly occurs in both, for example, weight loss, to only one of the two categories. Thus the use of this symptom in the classification of depression (in essence the specificity of the symptom) may be compromised in the elderly because the prevalence of cancer causing weight loss rises with age. On the other hand, excluding 'physical' complaints from the criteria of depression will lower their sensitivity. While one study which compared patients with stroke with and without major depression found that DSM-III-R major depression 'breeds true' even when it occurs in a medical disorder with which it shares symptoms (Lipsey et al., 1986), comparisons with other diseases are necessary before this concern can be eliminated.

Presumed comorbidity may mask the identification of causal links between the two disorders. For example, major depression and stroke are often seen in the same individual (Post, 1965). Only by studying groups of patients meeting criteria for both disorders and comparing them to appropriate control groups can one determine whether this is a causal, coincidental or imagined association. Classification systems must be structured to allow such studies and not prematurely exclude possible relationships.

DSM-III-R made just such an error by not allowing diagnoses of schizophrenia and mood disorder to be made when an 'organic' condition is present. This is a heritage of the hierarchal approach bequeathed by Kraepelin. DSM-IV attempts to resolve the issue in two ways. It provides a code for 'secondary' disorder to denote that a psychiatric syndrome is caused by an identifiable etiology and it allows diagnoses of both the 'functional' and the 'organic' disorder to be made when a causal relationship has not been established or does not exist.

Social dysfunction criteria

Several DSM-III-R and DSM-IV categories include in their criteria clinician judgments about the social competency of subjects. The diagnosis of schizophrenia, for instance, requires impairment of social relations, occupational function or self-care. Several problems arise in making such judgments in the elderly. One major difficulty is that accurate measures of social function in the elderly have not been developed. Also, social criteria are more difficult to apply to older persons. For example, the elderly are more likely than the young to live in conditions of relative isolation and restricted social activity that impose changes in interaction patterns. Comorbid medical conditions also impair social functioning and it may not be possible to ascribe a change in social activity solely to the medical or psychiatric condition in a reliable fashion. Finally, it is generally not possible to use changes in occupational status as a guideline since most old people are retired.

Another consideration in applying social dysfunction criteria is the potential for abuse when they are applied to a group that is often stigmatized and disadvantaged economically. Particular care must be taken to avoid diagnosing members of such a group as having a mental disorder because they are not functioning well socially.

Cohort effect

The term cohort effect refers to the persisting effects of an exposure to an identifiable condition during a specific time period. For example, living through the great depression of the 1930s shaped the economic views of many of those who lived at that time and these views have been carried through their lifespan. If the economic views of this group differ from the values of individuals who were born later and not exposed to the depression the difference can be ascribed to this 'exposure' and the group referred to as a 'cohort'. One aspect of late life mental experience and psychiatric disorder that might be influenced by cohort issues is the lower likelihood of the elderly to admit to psychological symptoms (Butler, 1975). However, since this has not been definitely linked to a cohort phenomenon, it remains possible that it is age-related rather than exposure related.

A cohort issue that does affect the presentation of 'functional' and 'organic' psychiatric disorders in the current group of elderly is their lower exposure to education. This may explain why individuals reared at the turn of the century, especially in deprived circumstances, have higher rates of limited cognitive capacities that appear unrelated to any diagnosable psychiatric illness including identifiable brain diseases such as Alzheimer's disease (Bergmann et al., 1971; Basset & Folstein, 1991). Low levels of education in the current elderly cohort have also been linked to the likelihood of having depression-induced cognitive impairment (Post, 1975; Pearlson et al. 1989*a*; Rabins & Pearlson, in press) and of being diagnosed as having Alzheimer's disease (Zhang et al., 1990).

Another potential cohort issue affecting the elderly is the rate at which they report somatic complaints. Older individuals have more physical complaints than the young, but it remains unclear whether this is explained by a higher prevalence of explainable physical illness (Costa & McCrae, 1985), as a culturally sanctioned complaining style that was more prevalent when the current cohort was young, or as an age-related, culturally sanctioned behavior. The DSM-III-R and DSM-IV criterion for somatoform disorder that requires lifelong complaints can help the clinician distinguish between somatoform disorder and late-life onset conditions like major depressive disorder in which somatic complaints develop anew. However, if no other informant is available the criterion is not always easy to apply.

Cohort effects might explain the lower prevalence rates of major depressive disorders in the elderly. While the ECA found lower rates of major depression after age 65 (Regier et al., 1988), recent reanalyses of symptom data from the ECA study demonstrate that minor depression and atypical depression are more common in the elderly (Blazer et al., 1988; Romanoski et al., 1992, Heithoff, 1992). These studies show that the prevalence of depressive disorder does not decline in late life when the rates of minor and major depression are added together. This could well reflect cohort patterns of symptom reporting but it could also be a developmental issue (i.e. an issue intrinsically related to an ageing process) or reflect the fact that comorbid diseases which occur more commonly in late life (such as frailty, atherosclerotic cerebral vascular disease, and hip fracture) changed the patterns of symptom reporting in the elderly.

Cognitive impairment

The higher prevalence of cognitive disorder in late life presents several obstacles to the application of a single set of diagnostic criteria to all age groups. Dementia is predominantly an illness of the elderly (Gruenberg, 1978) and delirium is much more likely to occur in late life (Erkinjuntti et al., 1986; Levkoff et al., 1992). As noted above, the DSM-III-R does not allow a functional illness to be diagnosed when a cognitive disorder is present. In addition to the issues raised above, this hierarchical approach is problematic for the elderly for several reasons. The old have higher rates of coexisting affective and cognitive impairment than the young (McHugh & Folstein, 1979). This cooccurrence has been variously called the dementia syndrome of depression (Folstein & McHugh, 1978), pseudodementia (Wells, 1979), cognitive-affective disorder (Ancill, 1989), and depression-induced cognitive impairment (Rabins & Pearlson, in press). Several follow-up studies suggest that a specific neuropathologic process such as stroke or Alzheimer's disease is present and probably causative of the cognitive disorder in at least half of these individuals while the affective disorder appears to be the primary etiology of the cognitive impairment in the other half (Reding et al., 1984; Rabins, Merchant & Nestadt, 1984; Reynolds et al., 1986;) see Chapter 18(*b*). At initial presentation, however it is often not clear which etiology is primary. DSM-III-R attempted to solve this issue by establishing the category 'organic affective disorder' but provided no specific criteria for this separate category. The DSM-IV category of secondary major depressive disorders (for patients in whom an identifiable brain disease is likely causal of the major depressive disorder) and its sanctioning of making two diagnoses (major depressive disorder and dementia) is an appropriate solution in the opinion of this chapter's authors.

Approximately 20% of patients with Alzheimer's disease suffer from depression (Rovner et al., 1989). The DSM-III-R has a code for primary degenerative dementia of the Alzheimer type with depression but no specific criteria are provided. DSM-IV also provides a code for dementia of the Alzheimer's type (DAT) with depressed mood but requires that separate codes for DAT and major depressive disorder be used when criteria for the latter are reached. The reliability of diagnostic criteria for major depressive disorder in patients with DAT however is yet to be established. Therefore, the appropriateness of this coding schema needs to be assessed empirically. Reliable classification of depression coexisting with a primary dementing illness is important because the depression is a treatable source of morbidity in both patient and caregiver. Reliable classification is also important because it could foster research into the study of the underlying neural basis of depressive symptoms and advance our understanding of the pathophysiology of idiopathic forms of mood disorder (Zweig et al., 1988).

Aging issues in specific DSM-III-R disorders

Affective disorders

As noted above, the ECA finding that rates of major depression are lower in individuals 65 and over has been challenged by many practitioners. They suggest that the DSM-III-R criteria and the methodology used to elicit specific symptoms led to a spuriously low ascertainment rate in the elderly. Might there be anything structural in the DSM-III-R approach that could affect rates of disorder differentially across the age span? As noted in the discussion of the cohort effect, three studies suggest that requiring four symptoms in addition to dysphoric mood for the diagnosis of major depression might be too high a 'threshold' for major depression in the elderly. Blazer et al. (1988) applied a factor analytic approach to the ECA data and demonstrated higher rates of a cluster of 'atypical' depressive symptoms among the elderly than other age groups. Heithoff (1992) used a latent class analytic approach to demonstrate that lowering the number of symptoms needed to meet criterion B of DSM-III-R equalizes rates of depression across the adult years. Romanoski et al. (1992), using data from the Clinical Reappraisal Study of the ECA (the part of the study which relied on clinician interviews and diagnoses rather than lay interviewer and instrument-generated diagnoses) also found higher rates of 'minor' depression in the elderly and noted that when 'major' and 'minor' depression are added together there is no decrease in prevalence across the age span. Thus, a general critique of DSM-III-R is that it provides no means of recognizing these 'sub threshold' cases. DSM-IV will address this problem by adding a category of 'minor depression' and setting a lower threshold for it. This however, still implies a difference between 'minor' and 'major' depression that has not been empirically demonstrated.

Schizophrenia, schizophreniform disorder, delusional disorder and psychosis not otherwise specified

The US/UK study demonstrated a wide disparity in the criteria used to diagnose schizophrenia in America and Britain pychiatrists (Kendell et al., 1971). Bridge and Wyatt (1980) pointed out that there were also major differences between American and European views on later life onset schizophreniform conditions. The introduction of DSM-III in 1981 brought American practice closer to the restrictive British and German approach but did not allow a diagnosis of schizophrenia to be made if the symptoms began after age 45. This exclusion criterion was withdrawn in DSM-III-R and a category of schizophrenia with late onset was added.

One tradition in diagnosing schizophrenia-like disorders that begin in later life dates back to the work, Roth and Morrisey (1952). They resurrected the term 'paraphrenia' that was first used by Kraepelin (1915) to describe individuals of any age with schizophrenia-like symptoms who lacked personality deterioration. Kay and Roth (1961) used the label 'late-paraphrenia' to refer to a late-onset disorder in which hallucinations and delusions are vivid, affective and cognitive symptoms are lacking and in which intact personality and lack of thought disorder are usual. A similar view was offered by Felix Post (1966). He suggested there might be three forms of late-life schizophreniform disorder ranging from a disorder in which paranoia was the predominant symptom to a condition with prominent delusions, hallucinations and first rank symptoms. As Chapters 18 parts I and II of this volume illustrate, many unresolved questions about the classification of these disorders remain.

The DSM-III-R contains four categories that share similarities with the conditions referred to as late-onset paraphrenia or late-onset schizophrenia. *Schizophreniform disorder* is the most appropriate diagnostic category when hallucinations and delusions predominate, mood and cognitive symptoms are lacking, the symptoms have been present for less than six months and there is no deterioration in interpersonal relationships or self-care. The category of *delusional disorder* is used when delusions are prominent and there are no mood or cognitive impairments. Hallucinations can be present if they are 'minor' but 'minor' is not operationalized. For a diagnosis of *schizophrenia with late onset* to be made, the DSM-III-R requires persistence of delusions and hallucinations for longer than six months, no primary mood symptoms, no identifiable somatic etiology and impairment in social or occupational function. The category entitled *psychosis not otherwise specified* is used by some authors (e.g. Lesser et al., 1992) to diagnose patients with various hallucinatory and delusional symptoms who do not meet the criteria of the other syndromes discussed in this paragraph.

Neither DSM-III-R nor DSM-IV contain the category paraphrenia. Since thought disorder is not a required criterion for the diagnosis of a schizophrenic, its uncommon occurrence in the late-onset condition (Kay & Roth, 1961; Pearlson et al., 1989*b*) does not rule out the use of this category. In spite of evidence that there is little personality deterioration or social dilapidation in late-onset schizophrenia (Pearlson et al., 1989*b*), premorbid personality traits do differ from those of the affectively ill (Kay et al., 1976). Stable cognitive disorder has been demonstrated in late-onset schizophreniform disorder (Naguib & Levy, 1987; Cullum, Heaton & Nemiroff, 1988). Its equivalence to the cognitive impairment seen in younger individuals with schizophrenia has not been demonstrated. Until long-term follow-up studies determine whether personality deterioration develops at rates similar to the early onset condition (Harding et al., 1987) it seems more prudent to remain open-minded about the classification of the conditions that have been labelled late-onset paraphrenia.

Neuroses and personality disorders

Personality disorders have been understudied in the elderly. The DSM-III-R codes personality disorders on a separate axis (Axis II) and does not address possible age changes or age effects on diagnoses. Several potential age confounds are plausible. Descriptions of premorbid personality from other observers are not always available to determine if a behavioral pattern is lifelong and this can complicate making a personality disorder diagnosis. Furthermore, environmental circumstances (e.g. group or nursing homes), new physical illness or retirement may be so different from the person's usual circumstances that they induce new persisting behavior patterns.

A large body of data support the persistence of personality traits over the lifespan (Costa & McCrae, 1988). Thus, it is surprising that personality disorder is diagnosed less frequently among the elderly in both community ascertained (Nestadt et al., 1990) and clinically derived (Rabins et al., 1983) samples. The reasons for this declining prevalence are unknown and a fertile ground for study.

DSM-III-R takes a categorical approach to personality disorder diagnoses. Although the DSM-III-R does not require impairment in social and work functioning as a criterion for diagnosis, the discussion section notes that such impairment is almost invariably present. Occupational impairment is generally not applicable to the elderly since most are retired and medical comorbidity may induce social or interpersonal disability.

There is also no recognition in either DSM-III-R or DSM IV that the enduring patterns of behavior on which the concept of personality disorder is based may manifest differently in late life. For example, unexplained somatic complaints may first become prominent in a dependent or narcissistic person late in life. Nor do the DSM-III-R or DSM-IV recognize that disordered behavior may be determined in part by personality traits which have been present life long but become manifest only in specific circumstances that are more common in late life such as hospitalization or institutionalization (the predisposition-provocation paradigm). The DSM-III-R category of adjustment disorder not otherwise specified is most applicable in such circumstances but it does not allow the symptoms or behaviors to be present for longer than six months.

Conclusions

The operationalized criteria of DSM-III-R and DSM-IV enable researchers to develop reliable diagnoses and to compare samples accumulated at different sites and different times periods. They allow clinicians to communicate with each other by providing a standardized set of definitions. These are important strengths of syndromic classification. Whether these are the most reliable and valid sets of criteria however, are questions for empirical study. It remains unclear whether the single sets of criteria in DSM-III-R and DSM-IV can be applied reliably across the lifespan. This issue deserves study since the potential confounds outlined in this chapter could diminish the validity of these classification schema when applied to the elderly. DSM-IV appears to be an improvement upon DSM-III-R by allowing disorders at both the 'organic' and 'functional' levels to be diagnosed simultaneously and by its addition of a code indicating that a disorder is secondary when an etiology is identified. Questions about the criteria for major depressive disorder and schizophreniform disorder in late life however remain.

References

American Psychiatric Association (1987). *DSM-III-R: Diagnostic and Statistical Manual of Mental Disorders.* 3rd edition, revised. Washington, DC American Psychiatric Association.

American Psychiatric Association (1991). *DSM-IV: Diagnostic and Statistical Manual of Mental Disorders – draft.* 4th edition. Washington, DC American Psychiatric Association.

Ancill, R. J. (1989). Cognitive-affective disorders: the copresentation of depression and dementia in the elderly. *Psychiatric Journal of the University of Ottawa*, **14**, 370–1.

Anthony, J. C. & Aboraya, A. (1992). The epidemiology of selected mental disorders in later life. In *Handbook of Mental Health and Aging*, ed. J. E. Birren, R. B. Sloane & G. D. Cohen. San Diego: Academic Press, Inc.

Baltes, P. B. (1991). The many faces of human ageing: toward a psychological culture of old age. *Psychological Medicine*, **21**, 837–54.

Bassett, S. S. & Folstein, M. F. (1991). Cognitive impairment and functional disability in the absence of psychiatric diagnosis. *Psychological Medicine*, **21**, 77–84.

Bergmann, K., Kay, D., W. K., Foster, E. M., McKechnie, A. A. & Roth, M. (1971). A follow-up study of randomly selected community residents to assess the effects of chronic brain syndrome and cerebrovascular disease. In *Psychiatry: Proceedings of the Fifth World Congress of Psychiatry*, ed. R. de la Fuente & M. N. Weisman, pp. 856–865, Amsterdam: Excerpta Medica.

Berrios, G. E. (1985). 'Depressive pseudodementia': or 'Melancholic dementia': a 19th century view. *Journal of Neurololgy, Neurosurgery and Psychiatry*, **48**, 393–400.

Blazer, D., Swartz, M., Woodbury, M., Manton, K. G., Hughes, D. & George, L. K. (1988). Depressive symptoms and depressive diagnoses in a community population: use of a new procedure for analysis of psychiatric classification. *Archives of General Psychiatry*, **45**, 1078–84.

Bridge, T. P. & Wyatt, R. J. (1980). Paraphrenia: paranoid states of late life. II. American research. *Journal of the American Geriatrics Society*, **28**, 201–5.

Butler, R. N. (1975). Psychiatry and the elderly: an overview. *American Journal of Psychiatry*, **132**, 893–900.

Costa, P. T. & McCrae, R. R. (1985). Hypochondriasis, neuroticism, and aging. *American Psychologist*, **40**, 19–28.

Costa, P. R., Jr. & McRae, R. R. (1988). Personality in adulthood: a six-year longitudinal study of self-reports and spouse ratings on the NEO personality inventory. *Journal of Personality and Social Psychology*, **5**, 853–863.

Cullum, C. M., Heaton, R. K. & Nemiroff, B. (1988). Neuropsychology of late-life psychoses. In *Psychiatric Clinics of North America*, eds. DV Jeste and S. Zisook. Philadelphia: W. B. Saunders Company.

Eaton, W. W., Holzer, C. E., VanKorff, M., Anthony, J. C., Helzer, J. E., George, L., Burnam, M. A., Boyd, J. H., Kessler, L. G. & Locke, B. Z. (1984). The design of the epidemiologic catchment area surverys. *Archives of General Psychiatry*, **41**, 942–8.

Erkinjuntti, T., Wikstrom, J., Palo, J. & Autio, L. (1986). Dementia among medical inpatients: evaluation of 2000 consecutive admissions. *Archives of Internal Medicine*, **146**, 1923–6.

Folstein, M. F. & McHugh, P. R. (1978). Dementia syndrome of depression. In *Dementia*, Vol. 7, ed. R. Katzman, R. D. Terry, & K. L. Bick. New York: Raven Press.

Gruenberg, E. M. (1978). Epidemiology of senile dementia. In *Advances in Neurology*, ed. B. S. Schoenberg. New York: Raven Press.

Harding, C. M., Brooks, G. W., Ashikaga, T., Strauss, J. S. & Breier, A. (1987). The Vermont longitudinal study of persons with severe mental illness. II. Long-term outcome of subjects who retrospectively met DSM-III criteria for schizophrenia. *American Journal of Psychiatry*, **144**, 727–35.

Heithoff, K. A. (1992) Depression in late-life: *Analysis of data from the NIMH epidemiologic catchment area (ECA) program*. Dissertation. Baltimore: School of Hygiene and Public Health, Johns Hopkins University.

Jarvik, L. (1986). Cited in O'Connor. Elderly need more MH services under Medicare. *Psychiatric Times*, November 21.

Kay, D. W. K. & Roth, M. (1961). Environmental and hereditary factors in the schizophrenias of old age ('late paraphrenia') and their bearing on the general problem of causation in schizophrenia. *Journal of Mental Science*, **107**, 649–85.

Kay, D. W. K., Cooper, A. F., Garside, R. F., & Roth, M. (1976). The differentiation of paranoid from affective psychoses by patients' premorbid characteristics. *British Journal of Psychiatry*, **129**, 207–15.

Kendell, R. E., Cooper, J. E., Gourlay, A. J., Copeland, J. R. M., Sharpe, L., & Gurland, B. J. (1971). Diagnostic criteria of American and British psychiatrists. *Archives of General Psychiatry* **25**, 123–30.

Kraepelin, E. (1915). *Clinical Psychiatry*. (Ed. and trans A.R. Diefendorf). New York: Macmillan.

Kramer, M. (1983). The continuing challenge: the rising prevalence of mental disorders, associated chronic diseases and disabling conditions. *American Journal of Social Psychiatry*, **3**, 13–24.

Lesser, I. M., Jeste, V. J., Boone, B. B., Harris, M. J., Miller, B. L., Heaton, R. K. & Hill-Gutierrez, E. (1992). Late-onset psychotic disorder, not otherwise specified: Clinical and neuroimaging findings. *Biological Psychiatry*, **31**, 419–23.

Levkoff, S. E., Evans, D. A., Liptzin, B., Wetle, T. T., Reilly, C. H., Pilgrim, D. M., Schor, J. & Rowe, J. (1992). Delirium: the occurrence and persistence of symptoms among elderly hospitalized patients. *Archives of Internal Medicine*, **152**, 334–40.

Lipsey, J. P., Spencer W. C., Rabins, P. V. & Robinson, R. G. (1986). Phenomenological comparison of poststroke and functional depression. *American Journal of Psychiatry*, **4**, 527–9.

McHugh, P. R. & Folstein, M. F. (1979). Psychopathology of dementia: implications for neuropathology. *Research Publication of the Association for Research in Nervous and Mental Diseases*, **57**, 17–30.

McHugh, P.' R. & Folstein, M. F. (1973). Address to the American Academy of Neurology, *Recent Advances in Dementia*, April (unpublished).

McHugh, P. R. & Slavney, P. R. (1973). *The Perspectives of Psychiatry*. Baltimore: Johns Hopkins University Press.

Naguib, M. & Levy, R. (1987). Late paraphrenia: neuropsychological impairment and structural brain abnormalities on computed tomography. *International Journal of Geriatric Psychiatry*, **2**, 83–90.

Nestadt, G., Romanoski, A. J., Chahal, R., Merchant, A., Folstein, M., Gruenberg, E. M. & McHugh, P. R. (1990). An epidemiological study of histrionic personality disorder. *Psychological Medicine*, **20**, 413–22.

Pearlson, G., Rabins, P. V., Kim, W. S., Speedie, L. J., Moberg, P. J., Burns, A. & Bascom, M. J. (1989*a*). Structural brain CT changes and cognitive deficits in elderly depressives with and without reversible dementia ('pseudodementia'). *Psychological Medicine*, **19**, 573–84.

Pearlson, G. D., Kreger, L., Rabins, P. V., Chase, G. A., Cohen, B., Wirth, J. B., Schlaepfer, T. B. & Tune, L. E. (1989b). A chart review study of late-onset and early-onset schizophrenia. *American Journal of Psychiatry*, **146**, 1568–74.

Post, F. (1965). *The Clinical Psychiatry of Late Life*. Oxford: Pergamon Press.

Post, F. (1966). *Persistent Persecutory States of the Elderly*. Oxford: Pergamon Press.

Post, F. (1975). Diagnosis of depression in geriatric patients and treatment modalities appropriate for the population. In *Depression: Behavioral, Biochemical, Diagnostic and Treatment Concepts*, ed. D. M. Gallant & G. M. Simpson, New York: Spectrum Publications.

Rabins, P. V., Lucas, M. J., Teitelbaum, M., Mark, S. R. & Folstein, M. (1983). Utilization of psychiatric consultation for elderly patients. *Journal of the American Geriatrics Society*, **31**, 581–5.

Rabins, P. V., Merchant, A. & Nestadt, G. (1984). Criteria for diagnosing reversible dementia caused by depression: validation by 2-year follow-up. *British Journal of Psychiatry*, **144**, 488–92.

Rabins, P. V., & Pearlson, G. D. (In press). Depression-induced cognitive impairment. In *Dementia*, ed. A. Burns & R. Levy, London: Chapman & Hall.

Reding, M. J., Haycox, J., Wigforss, K., Brush, D. & Blass, J. P. (1984). Follow-up of patients referred to a dementia service. *Journal of the American Geriatrics Society*, **32**, 265–8.

Regier, D. A., Boyd, H. J., Burke et al. (1988). One month prevalence of mental disorders in the United States. *Archives of General Psychiatry*, **45**, 977–86.

Reynolds, C. F., Kupfer, D. J., Hoch, J. J., Stack, J. A., Houck, P. R. & Sewitch, D. E. (1986). Two year follow-up of elderly patients with mixed depression and dementia. *Journal of the American Geriatrics Society*, **34**, 793–9.

Romanoski, A. J., Folstein, M. F., Nestadt, G., Chahal, R., Merchant, A., Brown, C. H., Gruenberg, E. M. & McHugh, P. R. (1992). The epidemiology of psychiatrist-ascertained depression and DSM-III depressive disorders. *Psychological Medicine*, **22**, 629–56.

Roth, M. & Morrisey, J. (1952). Problems in the diagnosis and classification of mental disorders in old age. *Journal of Mental Science*, **98**, 66–80.

Rovner, B., Broadhead, J., Spencer, M., Carson, K. & Folstein, M. (1989). Depression in Alzheimer's disease. *American Journal of Psychiatry*, **146**, 350–3.

Wells, C. E. (1979). Pseudodementia. *American Journal of Psychiatry*, **136**, 895–900.

Zhang, M., Katzman, R., Salmon, D., Jin, H., Cai, G., Wang, Z., Qu, G., Grant, I., Yu, E. & Levy, P. (1990). The prevalence of dementia and Alzheimer's disease in Shanghai, China: impact of age, gender and education. *Annals of Neurology*, **27**, 428–37.

Zweig, R. M., Ross, C. A., Hedreen, J. C., Steele, C., Cardillo, J. E., Whitehouse, P. J., Folstein, M. F. & Price, D. L. (1988). The neuropathology of aminergic nuclei in Alzheimer's disease. *Annals of Neurology*, **24**, 233–42.

Part 2

General epidemiology

3

Epidemiology in the study of functional psychiatric disorders of the elderly

ROBIN EASTWOOD

Introduction

This chapter deals with the contribution that epidemiology has made to our understanding of the functional psychiatric disorders in the elderly. To start with two terms should be defined. First, what is epidemiology? Descriptions range from the succinct 'study of disease as a mass phenomenon' by Greenwood (1934) to seven uses (Morris 1957) to five point definitions (Shepherd 1987). Practically speaking, nowadays, epidemiologists think in terms of four areas: rates of illness, correlates of caseness, risk factors and evaluating treatment and management. These can be addressed with relatively modest budgets and time frames. Other enterprises like longitudinal studies and field trials of new classifications, although fascinating, must be considered expensive and exceptional. Secondly, what does 'functional' mean? The Concise Oxford Dictionary (1982) defines functional in the case of mental illness as '*having no discernable organic cause*'. While modern textbooks do not attend to this definition, the Mayer-Gross, Slater and Roth textbook gave it two pages in 1969. There, 'functional' is used '*to denote psychiatric disturbances unassociated with cerebral pathology or identifiable somatic disease*'. There was thought to be relatively small overlap between 'organic' and 'functional'. In the section on mental diseases of the aged, in the language of the day, the authors include manic-depressive disorder, chronic schizophrenia, late onset paraphrenia, neuroses and allied disorders and character disorders, including paranoid states.

The utility of epidemiology will be looked at through the perspectives of history, textbooks and recent publications. Being brief, the reviews cannot be comprehensive and fully representative.

A brief historical perspective

Psychiatric epidemiology is a recent discipline. The first professor, Ernest Gruenberg was appointed in 1958 and only died in 1991. Nevertheless mental health statistics were seen as useful as long ago as the early nineteenth century. This led Ray (1849) to say that:

'statistics has (sic) become a favorite instrument for developing truth';

but then followed with a lengthy caveat showing that mental hospital data, for example, did not even approximate to the truth:

'That they form very suitable data for an opinion ... but a candid consideration of the subject must convince us, that such an opinion is no more likely to be exact, than a shrewd conjecture founded upon one's general impressions of his own experience.'

Budding epidemiologists however were not deterred and health statistics reports abounded in the 19th century. These caused May (1913) of New York State, in commenting on statistical studies of the insane, to complain that comprehensive classification of illness had only started in 1909. Prior to that,

'"statistical results" are usually characterised by striking irregularity of methods of classification in the various localities'.

By 1927 Elkind felt confident enough to ask whether mental illness was on the increase. He thought not, since hospital figures were defective, and the extent of mental illness in the community was unknown. Later (1936), examining 1917–34 data, albeit with the same caveat, he found no increase in the psychoses, except possibly for that associated with arteriosclerosis. Pollock (1945), reviewing the development of mental health statistics in the United States during the previous century, cited Pliny Earle (1848) who collected asylum data from 1821 to 1844. Earle had found rates to be highest between 20 to 40 years of age and then to rapidly diminish with age. Pollock saw these 'as unwarranted conclusions' and thought the rate of mental disease increased with advancing age. Shades of future discussions of incidence versus prevalence and whether mental illness rises or falls with increasing age! Despite these epidemiological efforts, Munroe writing on the 'Aging of Population' in the *New England Journal of Medicine* (1953) stated that

there is no area (among the health problems of aging people) where information is less factual or more tinged with emotional bias than geriatric neuropsychiatry. My statistics suggested that the majority of old people have mental disorders, but what is a normal standard? Possibly few people pass their 55th year without feeling that they are losing mental competence or that others are beginning to think so; the retirement crisis intensifies this fear 10 years later ... Most disorders of mental health in old people stem from struggles with their environment. For want of a better term, I have called them reactive depressions – that is, states of inferior mental and physical performance arising from inhibitions due to disease or to losses ... treatment of such depressions taxes the ingenuity and patients or the clinician able to see them, but much can be accomplished ... only one must not be content with halfway measures, for then the next reaction leads to nursing home and custodial care, and solutions must be arrived at with full respect for the patient and with his willing co-operation.

Shortly after, this opinion gave way to fact and the methodologists took over. Forty years ago an epidemiological study of major importance took place (Roth, 1955). Roth examined the natural history of mental disorder in old age and made the critically significant finding that affective psychosis, senile psychosis, paraphrenia, acute confusion and arteriosclerotic psychosis have different presentations, durations and risks. Thus

if the findings reported here are correct it will be evident that the category of illness is an essential prerequisite towards accurate prognosis of mental illness in old age.

Furthermore, in the study there was a preponderance of affective psychosis giving lie to the then popular notion that old age psychiatry was synonymous with the dementias. This study, carried out at the dawn of modern pharmacological treatment, was almost an experiment in nature (apart from electroconvulsive therapy) and used the best statistic, namely predictive validity. **The speciality of geriatric psychiatry has been based upon these findings.** Other statistics, like reliability and consensual validity, have been used to effect in the last four decades but never with the same force. To complete the adumbration of events in the field, particularly the increasing sophistication, come the studies emphasizing reliability of diagnosis. The US/UK Cross National Study of Diagnosis of the Mental Disorders of Psychiatric Patients (Copeland et al., 1975) is a case in point. By using a standardized clinical interview, it was possible to show that the putative differences between the two countries in admission rates for dementia and depression did not occur when the patients were examined in a reliable and standardized fashion. Such interviews, particularly the Geriatric Mental Status schedule (Copeland, Dewey and Griffiths-Jones 1986) developed in detail following the above study, have now become commonplace.

This brief history of geriatric psychiatric epidemiology tells us that mental health statistics have been analyzed for the past 150 years; but serious methodology only started at the beginning of the century and impressive professional involvement and research findings at mid-century. The next step is to see what body of knowledge has been incorporated in the textbooks.

A teaching perspective

By happy coincidence major textbooks on psychiatric disorders in the elderly appear roughly every decade, which makes it easy to chronicle changes in knowledge and attitude over the last quarter century.

The first book worthy of mention is *Clinical Psychiatry* written by Mayer-Gross, Slater and Roth. The third edition was published in 1969. It has chapters on ageing, the mental disorders of the aged, the affective disorders, symptomatic psychoses, schizophrenia, alcoholism and drug addiction, the epilepsies, mental disorder in trauma, infection and tumor and, finally, social psychiatry. There, epidemiology is specifically discussed.

The association between sociology and clinical variables defined by epidemiological research ... rarely permits an unequivocal interpretation (but) the epidemiological approach has brought greater methodological rigour into the field of psychiatry as a whole. The insistence on careful design of enquiries and on precise definition of terms, the development of objective and reliable indices for the phenomena under investigation which have been characteristic of the best of epidemiological work have contributed to self criticism and discipline in clinical and scientific work.

Martin Roth and colleagues have made some outstanding contributions to the epidemiology of geriatric psychiatry and it is intriguing to go back to 1969. Due note is made of the 12% of the population aged 65 and over and prospective increases. Concern is expressed about the social, economic and medical problems that will arise and the services that will be required. First admission rates to hospital for mental illness are used to predict a rapid rise in future years. The authors see this as being due to socioeconomic factors, the destigmatization of admission to psychiatric hospitals, physical treatments and the increasing treatment of functional depressive and paranoid illnesses of the elderly. While the population over 65 in England and Wales increased by 1% between 1951 and 1960, admissions increased by over 40%. The authors argue that the growth in admissions was not due to a greater incidence of senile psychosis in the elderly. They clearly state that hospital data are not representative and cite seven community prevalence studies, done between 1948 and 1964, which give a range between 1.1 and 4.2% for major functional disorders and 8.7 to 17.6% for moderate to severe neuroses and character disorders. Importantly, they describe the Newcastle-upon-Tyne study (Kay, Beamish & Roth, 1962, 1964*a*, *b*) which surveyed community and institutional samples starting in 1960. Severe or moderate functional psychiatric disorders, including character disorders, were found in 15%, and chronic schizophrenia in 1% of those living at home. Affective disorders and neuroses made up 10% and mild disorders a further 16%. Five per cent had late onset affective disorders. Most cases were not being treated.

The authors dealt with the vexed issue of diagnoses and pointed out that geriatric psychiatry had started in a rudimentary way at the beginning of the century with the differentiation of senile dementia, arteriosclerotic dementia, presenile psychoses and other psychoses like neurosyphilis. However, affective and paranoid disorders were not properly distinguished from senile psychosis. Roth & Morrisey (1952, 1955) looked at the categories of affective disorder, late paraphrenia, delirium, senile psychosis (dementia) and arteriosclerotic psychosis and found distinct mortality and discharge patterns. Significantly, neurotic depression was at least as important as endogenous depression. They go on to say that follow-up studies revealed a guarded prognosis for affective disorder; that neurotic illnesses had previously been neglected; and that the schizophrenia-like illness, called late onset paraphrenia, was mainly confined to women and made up 8 to 9% of all female first admissions over 65. In summary, the epidemiology known in 1969 stated that most late-life functional psychiatric disorder existed in the community and was untreated. Much of it was neurotic disorder coexisting with physical disease. The functional and organic psychoses could be distinguished by presentation but, more critically, on outcome and mortality.

The second book is the *Handbook of Mental Health and Aging* edited by Birren and Sloane (1980). There is a specific chapter on epidemiology and mentions in the chapters for specific disorders. Chapter 2, entitled 'Epidemiology of Mental Disorders amongst the Aged in the Community', is by Kay and Bergmann. The aims of epidemiology were said to be utilitarian, clinical or scientific. Previous surveys had at least one of the following aims: planning and evaluation of services, social characteristics, early stages of illness, age distribution of illness, genetics, disease expectation and comparative rates. Prevalence and incidence rates have been determined from case registers, general practice settings and field surveys. The prevalence for total psychiatric morbidity derived from case registers, shows an accumulation of cases with age. In contrast, incidence starts early in life for schizophrenia and the neuroses and declines with age; affective psychoses peak in middle age and decline thereafter, whereas dementia starts late and increases enormously in old age. Specifically, prevalence rates of schizophrenia, paranoid psychoses and affective psychoses vary from 1.2 to 3.7% and must include both hospital and community cases. Incidence studies show that schizophrenia can start after 45 and importantly there may be underreporting with functional and organic psychoses being confused. The prevalence of neuroses and personality disorders ranges from 4.8 to 27% which must indicate methodological problems. Needless to say these illnesses are poorly understood. A striking feature is that much of the neurosis of old age is depressive. Bergmann (1971) suggests that, in depression, men may be responding to physical illness and women to personality. Loneliness seems to be important.

In summary, the book makes some valuable conclusions when it says that the studies in the 1950s and 1960s were able to highlight the high prevalence of especially hidden psychiatric morbidity, but were unable to do comparative, etiological and incidence studies. As it appeared then (1980) better work had been done with dementia than with functional disorders and too little was known about the neuroses. Future research would have to focus on services for the demented, incidence studies and normal brain aging.

The third book is *Psychiatric Disorders in America* edited by Regier and Robins (1991). While not specifically dealing with functional disorders of the elderly it describes the epidemiological catchment area (ECA) studies carried out in the United States in the late 1970s and early 1980s. This was the first time that DSM-

III criteria had been used in major field surveys. In 1980 five areas were surveyed and 20000 people were examined. The result was a large prevalence study and ranking of all the major DSM-III diagnoses by demographic variables. A disadvantage was that other epidemiological studies had used ICD diagnoses, whereas the ECA studies not only used DSM-III but also the somewhat idiosyncratic concept of 'lifetime prevalence', which some see as having dubious utility.

The ECA teams found a lifetime prevalence for all psychiatric disorders of 32% and an annual prevalence of 20%. Most disorders started in the first half of life and only dementia contributed to any extent later. Depression, obsessive compulsive disorder, panic and phobic disorders had the longest risk periods, but most illnesses had started by 50 years of age. The average duration for all disorders was around 10 years. It is obvious to clinicians that the functional disorders can occur at any time of life but the ECA studies act as a watershed in reminding us that these illnesses strike at the young and have long durations. Since it is known that they are associated with premature death (Murphy et al., 1987), both natural and unnatural, then geriatric psychiatrists deal with the survivors. Nevertheless it is a moot point whether mental illness increases or decreases in old age. Snowdon (1990) argues against the findings of the ECA studies for not including institutional cases and taking symptoms like phobias at face value when depression may also be present. Since most epidemiology studies are in agreement on the decline with age, this suggests that case finding is not at fault. Nevertheless, the finding offends the popular belief that the old live in misery. There are two other myths worth noting. One says that common sense dictates that with age *and* increasing infirmity, people must be more vulnerable to depression. This does not appear to be true (Eastwood & Corbin, 1986). The other suggests that the old must be poor. Again, this is no longer true (Preston, 1984).

The fourth book is *Psychiatry in the Elderly* edited by Jacoby and Oppenheimer (1991). Epidemiology is addressed by specific disorders. Baldwin, in the depressive illness section, indicates that international studies have similar findings with 10 to 15% of subjects having depressive symptoms and 3% depressive illness. Symptoms are commoner amongst females but this difference is less so for illness. He cites the findings of the Duke University group (Blazer & Williams, 1980) who, in accordance with Bergmann (1971), see such illness as being divided into depressive illness and dysphoria secondary to physical illness and personality. Jacoby addresses mania and indicates that it may start at any time of life but there seems to be no simple relationship between incidence and hospital admission. Overall, mania has a modest prevalence and makes up 5% of all geriatric admissions to psychiatric facilities.

Lindesay attends to anxiety disorders and makes the point that only since ICD-9 and DSM-III has anxiety had its own nosology. It is now divided into generalized anxiety, phobic and panic disorders. The period prevalence varies by study and is

1.4 to 7.1% for generalized anxiety, up to 10% for phobic disorders and apparently rare for panic disorders. Both incidence and prevalence of anxiety disorders are low in the elderly but insufficiently studied. Anxiety can be co-morbid between its own categories, with depression and with some physical illnesses.

Paranoid states in the elderly are dealt with by Naguib and Levy. These illnesses have been going through nosological changes in the ICD and DSM series and in ICD-10 and DSM-IV run the risk of being muddled with early onset schizophrenia. This will make the epidemiology of these disorders much harder to research. As it is, getting accurate data is difficult since these patients are often suspicious and reclusive. The best estimates suggest an annual incidence figure of 17 to 26 per 100000 for late paraphrenia. Meanwhile, 10% of geriatric psychiatry first admissions are for late onset paranoid disorders.

The last book is *Geriatric Psychiatry* edited by Busse and Blazer for the American Psychiatric Press (1989). Blazer specifically looks at the epidemiology of psychiatric disorders in later life. He quotes Roberts (1977) who suggested that:

> epidemiology is not only the basic science of preventive and community medicine but also may serve as the basic science of clinical practice.

In this chapter Blazer looks at the uses of epidemiology according to Morris. These are identification of cases (symptoms versus syndromes in the elderly); the distribution of psychiatric disorders in the populations; the historical trends of mental illness amongst the elderly (cohort effects); the etiology of psychiatric disorders in late life and the use of health services by the elderly.

In the same volume there are chapters devoted to affective disorders in late life; late life schizophrenia and paranoid disorders; and anxiety in the elderly. Blazer discusses his own Duke University study (1987) and states that, in his community sample, while 27% reported depressive symptoms, only 2% had a dysthymic disorder, 0.8% a major depressive episode and 1.2% a mixed depression and anxiety syndrome. Since there have been differences, however between this and other studies (for example in the Mid-town Manhattan study, both in 1954 and 1974, the elderly had higher rates of mental impairment) he argues for a cohort effect wherein a birth cohort retains its diathesis towards depression throughout life. Coming to schizophrenia and paranoid disorders he quotes a San Francisco elderly community study indicating that 2.5% exhibited suspicousness and 2% paranoid delusions. In Blazer's own study 4% of the elderly had generalised persecutory ideation. The epidemiologic catchment area (ECA) prevalence studies, perhaps because of the idiosyncrasies of DSM-III, found few elderly schizophrenics. Finally, the piece on anxiety in the elderly cites the ECA finding showing that anxiety and phobic disorders for adults are the commonest psychiatric conditions in the United States. Nevertheless, the elderly showed less anxiety and panic disorders and no somatization disorder.

Busse and Blazer make it clear that there is a great deal of ECA data available. In effect, psychiatric epidemiology is now commensurate with the ECA studies in the US and this may happen worldwide. This trend is clearly going to cause a great deal of controversial discussion.

Recent publications

Going back a decade on a Med-line search most likely picks up the pertinent English language literature. This section deals with the drift of recent work and any apparent gain in knowledge. It is not always easy to disentangle population-based studies and clinical studies (extra care has to be taken in North America since drug trials are now called clinical epidemiology).

There have been some longitudinal or quasilongitudinal studies. Christie & Wood (1990) had the idea of repeating Roth's seminal work (he first published in 1952) and comparing hospital cohorts. Christie emphasized that others had tried this in other settings. He was impressed that most patients in the recent cohorts could be placed in Roth's original five categories. As a proportion of admissions the functional psychoses had dropped: for paraphrenia this was thought to be due to better and more tolerant community care and for affective disorder to improved antidepressant treatment. (A caveat for affective disorder is that mortality remains high implying definite room for improved treatment.) So bed requirements for functional cases have obviously dropped, stabilizing at six beds per 100 at two-year stay. Dementia bed requirements have shot up. In a community cohort study in Iceland, Helgason & Magnusson (1989) showed that the expectancy rate of developing a mental disorder increased from 34% at 61 to 67% at 81 years. While most cases were of dementia, there were more functional cases observed than expected. Elsewhere, Yassa et al. (1988) made the piquant finding in elderly Canadians that marital discord could precipitate mania for the first time!

Staying with community work, Kay et al. (1985) from Hobart, Australia, saw the need for refinement of case criteria. Nevertheless, others went ahead. In London, Lindesay, Briggs and Murphy (1989) found 13.5% to be depressed and the same number anxious or phobic; Livingston et al. (1990) obtained 15.9% for depression in the same city. Copeland et al. (1987) found depressive illness to be more or less equally common in the elderly in London and New York; Cohen, Tesesi & Holmes (1988) showed that the elderly homeless in the Bowery, New York were one-quarter psychotic and one-third depressed. Finally O'Connor, Pollitt and Roth (1990) in Cambridgeshire demonstrated that 5% of the demented were also depressed, compared with 9% of the nondemented. Snowdon and Donnelly in Australia (1986) and Kivelä, Lehtomäki and Kivekäs (1986) in Finland found depression in up to one third of the elderly in institutions. Ames et al. (1988) found that dementia and depression accumulated in Part III homes in London with little recovery for depression on follow-up. Interestingly, Jorm (1987) has shown that historically the sexes only differ for depression in middle age. Nevertheless, Kivelä, Pahkala, Laippala (1988) found elderly women in care to be prime subjects for depression. Proceeding from there, Kivelä et al. (1988) and Lindesay et al. (1989) concurred in showing that affective illnesses were related to dependency rather than class. While there is a great deal of geriatric depression in institutions, and major geriatric depression may be increasing (Eagles & Whalley 1985), this is not reflected, apparently, in the community. In a thoughtful review, Blazer (1989) argues for a cohort effect with younger generations being more susceptible to depression. The suggestion that the elderly suffer from less affective disorder is heeded since it is supported by the influential ECA studies. The arguments relate to whether the elderly differ in depressive syndromes and symptoms, and whether their affective illnesses are masked by somatic complaints and frank physical illnesses. An Australian group (Brodaty et al., 1991) recently reviewed in depth the relationship between age and depression. From a study of referrals of all ages to a mood disorder unit they deduced that the elderly with unipolar major depression were more likely to be psychotic and agitated, and less prone to personality problems and inherited depression, than younger patients. Early and late onset depressed geriatric patients, however, had similar phenomenology. This was a useful qualitative rather than quantitative study. Another contentious area is outcome which is discussed in Chapter 8 (Cole, 1990; Burvill et al., 1989).

Psychiatrists, probably in lieu of biological validators, are great classifiers and nosologists. Nowhere is the 'new lamps for old' effect, and its converse, seen more than in paranoid states in the elderly. While there is little epidemiological research here (there is some clinical investigation) there are numerous articles on what to call and how to treat the beast (Stoudemire and Riether 1987; Munro, 1988; Flint, Rifat & Eastwood, 1991; Munro, 1991 and Hassett et al., 1992). Without writing yet a further article, it is possible to succinctly restate what has happened this century. Kraepelin distinguished paranoia and paraphrenia from dementia praecox. Some of his paraphrenics, however, were said later to become schizophrenics. Mid-century, Roth described the condition called late paraphrenia and this concept has persisted, particularly in Britain. Paraphrenia may occur throughout adult life and is associated with preservation of personality. There is divided opinion as to whether paraphrenia is a type of schizophrenia and whether schizophrenia itself can actually start later in life. With elderly paranoid states care has to be taken to separate them from affective disorder and dementia. The Americans with their DSM series are more influential than the international ICD series and have given insufficient attention to these paranoid illnesses. They did forego the idea that schizophrenia stops at 45 in DSM-III-R but paranoid illnesses, regardless of age, are lumped together. While paranoia has been reified as delusional disorder, paraphrenia is not accepted and awaits timidly in the wings.

Munro has recommended a spectrum disorder, which is very sensible, since so many medical variables are continuous. Nevertheless, unlike diabetes, for example, the medical and heuristic value of the spectrum of paranoid ideation has to be tested.

There are few recent population-based or even clinical studies. Christenson and Blazer (1984) demonstrated that 4% of a community sample had persistent persecutory delusions with most not being treated. Clinically, Grahame (1984) and Holden (1987) have attempted to debunk the concept of paraphrenia. Holden sees it as being of many parts and Grahame as being part of schizophrenia. Elsewhere Flint et al. (1991) see paranoia and paraphrenia as distinct as based on CT scan evidence of strokes and less treatment response in the former. However, Jeste et al. (1987) and Naguib and Levy (1987) have other 'organic' findings. Etiological factors like gender, isolation, deafness and premorbid personality have been suspected. Deafness has been evaluated at some length (Eastwood et al., 1985; Corbin & Eastwood, 1986).

Paranoid disorders in the elderly are discussed in detail in Chapter 18.

Conclusions

Has epidemiology helped in the study of the functional psychiatric disorders? In 1985 we asked the same question (Eastwood & Corbin 1985) and answered by applying the MacMahon criteria (1960). These referred to first, descriptive epidemiology dealing with the distribution of disease; secondly, the formulation of hypotheses to explain the distribution; thirdly, analysis to test the hypotheses by observation; and fourthly, experiments to test these hypotheses if supported by observation. In the summary we concluded that, among psychiatric syndromes, little is known about associations and etiological factors. The functional disorders are now fairly well described and merit attention for their natural histories, onset and outcomes, and the bearing they have on other morbidities and causes of death.

Specifically for *major affective disorders* in the elderly in 1985 the observed rate was known but not the treated and outcome figures. Early and late onset cases were not properly distinguished. Much of this has been redressed and hypotheses are being stated if not yet tested. For *neuroses* and *personality disorders* the subject was stuck at the descriptive level. At least for the neuroses the classification has probably improved. As a matter of conjecture, rather than experiment, personality and illness may be involved in the development of neurosis. *Schizophrenia* and *paranoid disorders* of late life are important when the sub-illness paraphrenia is considered. It can be investigated along the MacMahon lines more than most geriatric psychiatric illnesses. Sensory deficits, personality and isolation are all involved and can be tested.

The functional disorders are well described and their correlates, natural histories, morbidity and mortality risks are better understood, nowadays, by the profession if not the public. Curiously, the paranoid disorders are not being well handled in the present classifications of disease. Far more is known about the prevalence than the incidence and risk factors of the functional disorders. In this respect the epidemiology of mental disorders in old age is well behind that for cancer and vascular disease. The burden of care research is, however not as backward.

While biological markers are not imminent, great hope must lie in the refreshing number of young investigators committed to the field. Epidemiology and pathology are the twin pillars of geriatric psychiatry and have successfully defined clinical syndromes. Neuroepidemiology by defining risk factors and neuropharmacology by defining drug effects, will take us to the next stage.

References

Ames, D., Ashby, D., Mann, A. H. & Graham, N. (1988). Psychiatric illness in elderly residents of Part III homes in one London borough: prognosis and review. *Age and Ageing*, **17**, 249–56.

Bergmann, K., (1971). The neuroses of old age. *In Recent Developments in Psychogeriatrics*. ed. D. W. K. Kay & A. Walk, pp. 39–50, Ashford: Headley Bros.

Birren, J. E. & Sloane, R. B. (eds.). (1980). *The Handbook of Mental Health and Aging* (1980) Inglewood Cliffs, New Jersey: Prentice-Hall Inc.

Blazer, D. & Williams, C. D. (1980). Epidemiology of dysphoria and depression in an elderly population. *American Journal of Psychiatry* **137**, 439–444.

Blazer, D. (1989). The epidemiology of depression in late life. *Journal of Geriatric Psychiatry*, **22**, 35–52.

Blazer, D., Hughes, D. C., George, LK (1987). The epidemiology of depression in an elderly community population. *Gerontologist*, **27**, 281–7

Brodaty, H., Peters, K., Boyce, P., Hickie, I., Parker, G., Mitchell, P. & Wilhelm, K. (1991). Age and depression. *Journal of Affective Disorders* **23**, 137–49

Burvill, P., Hall, W., Stampfer, A. & Emmerson, J. (1989). A comparison of early-onset and late-onset depressive illness in the elderly. *British Journal of Psychiatry*, **155**, 673–9.

Busse, E. W. & Blazer, D. G. (1989) (eds.). *Geriatric Psychiatry*. Washington DC: American Psychiatric Press.

Christenson R. & Blazer D. (1984). Epidemiology of persecutory ideation in an elderly population in the community. *American Journal of Psychiatry*, 141:1088–1091.

Christie, A. B. & Wood, E. R.(1990). Further changes in the pattern of mental illness in the elderly. *British Journal of Psychiatry*, **157**, 228–31.

Cohen C. I., Teresi J. A., & Holmes D. (1988). The mental health of old homeless men. *Journal of the American Geriatric Society*, **36**, 492–501.

Cole, M. (1990). The prognosis of depression in the elderly. *Canadian Medical Association Journal*, **143**, 633–9.

The Concise Oxford Dictionary (1982). Oxford: Oxford University Press.

Copeland, J. R. M., Kelleher, M. J., Kellett, J. M., et al. (1975) Cross-national study of diagnosis of the mental disorders: a comparison of the diagnoses of elderly psychiatric patients admitted to mental hospitals serving Queens County, New York, and the former Borough of Camberwell, London. *British Journal of Psychiatry*, **126**, 11–20.

Copeland, J. R. M., Dewey, M. E. & Griffiths-Jones, H. M. (1986) A computerized psychiatric diagnostic system and case nomenclature for elderly subjects: GMS and AGECAT. *Psychological Medicine*. **16**, 89–99.

Copeland, J. R., Gurland, B. J., Dewey, M. E., Kelleher, M. J., & Smith, A. M. (1987) Is there more dementia, depression and neurosis in New York? A comparative study of the elderly in New York and London using the computer diagnosis AGECAT. *British Journal of Psychiatry*, **151**, 466–73.

Corbin, S. L. & Eastwood M. R. (1986). Sensory deficits and mental disorders of old age: casual or coincidental associations? *Psychological Medicine*, **16**, 251–256.

Eagles, J. M. & Whalley, L. J. (1985). Ageing and affective disorders: The age at first onset of affective disorders in Scotland, 1969–1978. *British Journal of Psychiatry*, **147**, 180–187.

Eastwood, M. R., Corbin, S. L., Reed, M., Nobbs, H. & Kedward, H. B., (1985). Acquired hearing loss and psychiatric illness: an estimate of prevalence and co-morbidity in a geriatric settings. *British Journal of Psychiatry*, **147**, 552–6.

Eastwood, M. R. & Corbin, S. L. (1985). Epidemiology of mental health disorders in old age. In *Recent Advances In Psychogeriatrics*, ed. Arie T., Churchill Livingstone, UK.

Eastwood, M. R. & Corbin, S. L. (1986). The relationship between physical illness and depression in old age. In *Affective Disorders in the Elderly*, ed. Murphy E., Edinburgh: Churchill Livingstone.

Elkind, H. B. (1927). The epidemiology of mental disease: A preliminary discussion. Is mental disease on the increase? *American Journal of Psychiatry*, **VI**, 623–40.

Elkind, H. B. & Taylor M. (1936) The alleged increase in the incidence of the major psychoses. *American Journal of Psychiatry*, **92**, 817–25.

Flint, A. J., Rifat, S. L., Eastwood, M. R. (1991). Late-onset paranoia: distinct from paraphrenia? *International Journal of Geriatric Psychiatry*, **6**, 103–109.

Grahame, P. S. (1984). Schizophrenia in old age (late paraphrenia) *British Journal of Psychiatry*, **145**, 493–5.

Greenwood, M. (1934). Preventive Aspects of Medicine, *Lancet*, **1**, 201–5.

Harris M. J. & Jeste D. V. (1988) Late onset schizophrenia: an overview. *Schizophrenia Bulletin*, **14**, 39–55.

Hassett, A. M., Keks, N. A., Jackson, H. J., & Copolov D. L. (1992). The diagnostic validity of paraphrenia. *Australian & New Zealand Journal of Psychiatry*, **26**, 18–29.

Helgason, T. & Magnusson, H. (1989). The first 80 years of life: a psychiatric epidemidogical study *Acta Psychiatrica Scandinavica*, **79**, (suppl. 348) 85–94.

Holden, N. L. (1987). Late paraphrenia or the paraphrenias? A descriptive study with a 10-year follow-up. *British Journal of Psychiatry*, **150**, 635–9.

Jacoby, R. & Oppenheimer, C. (eds.) (1991). *Psychiatry in the Elderly*. Oxford: Oxford University Press.

Jeste, D. V., Harris, M. J., Cullum, C. M., Zweifach, M., Thal, L. J. & Grant, I.(1987). Late onset schizophrenia: neuropsychology and MRI (new research abstract number NR76), Presented at the 140th Annual Meeting of the American Psychiatric Association.

Jorm, A. F. (1987). Sex and age differences in depression: a quantitative synthesis of published research. *Australian & New Zealand Journal of Psychiatry*, **21**, 46–53.

Kay, D. W. K. (1962) Outcome and cause of death in mental disorders of old age: a long-term follow-up of functional and organic psychoses. *Acta Psychiatrica Scandinavica*, **38**, 249–549.

Kay, D. W. K., Beamish, P. & Roth, M. (1964*a*). Old age mental disorders in Newcastle-upon-Tyne, part I, a study of prevalence. *British Journal of Psychiatry*, **110**, 146–58.

Kay, D. W. K., Beamish, P. & Roth, M. (1964*b*). Old age mental disorders in Newcastle-upon-Tyne, Part II: a study of possible social and medical causes. *British Journal of Psychiatry*, **110**, 668–82.

Kay, D. W. K., Henderson, A. S., Scott, R., Wilson, J., Rickwood, D., & Grayson, D. A. (1985). Dementia and depression among the elderly living in the Hobart community: the effect of the diagnostic criteria on the prevalence rates. *Psychological Medicine*, **15**, 771–88.

Kivelä, S.-L., Lehtomäki & Kivekäs, J. (1986). Prevalence of depressive symptoms and depression in elderly Finnish home nursing patients and home help clients. *International Journal of Social Psychiatry*, **32**, 3–13.

Kivelä, S.-L., Pahkala, K. & Laippala P. (1988). Prevalence of depression in an elderly population in Finland. *Acta Psychiatrica Scandinavica*, **78**, 401–13.

Lindesay, J., Briggs, K. & Murphy, E. (1989). The Guy's/Age Concern Survey: prevalence rates of cognitive impairment, depression and anxiety in an urban elderly community. *British Journal of Psychiatry*. **155**, 317–29.

Livingston, G., Hawkins, A., Graham, N., Blizard, B. & Mann, A. (1990). The Gospel Oak Study: prevalence rates of dementia, depression and activity limitation among elderly residents in Inner London, *Psychological Medicine*, **20**, 137–46.

MacMahon, B., Pugh, T. F. & Ipsen, J. (1960). *Epidemiologic Methods*. Toronto: Little, Brown & Company.

May, J. (1913). Statistical studies of the insane. *American Journal of Insanity* **70**, 427–39.

Mayer-Gross, W., Slater, E. & Roth, M. (1969). *Clinical Psychiatry*. 3rd. edn. London: Bailliere, Tindall & Cassell.

Monroe, R. T. (1953). The effect of aging of population on general health problems. *New England Journal of Medicine*, **249**, 277–85.

Morris, J. N. (1957). *Uses of Epidemiology*, Edinburgh and London: E.& S. Livingstone Ltd.

Munro, A. (1988). Delusional (paranoid) disorders. *Canadian Journal of Psychiatry*, **33**, 399–404.

Munro, A. (1991). A plea for paraphrenia. *Canadian Journal of Psychiatry*, **36**, 667–72.

Murphy, J. M., Monson, R. R., Olivier, D. C., Sobol, A. M. & Leighton, A. H. (1987). Affective disorders and mortality: a general population study. *Archives of General Psychiatry*, **44**, 473–80.

Naguib, M. & Levy, R. (1987). Late paraphrenia: neuropsychological impairment and structural brain abnormalities on computed tomography. *International Journal of Geriatric Psychiatry*, **2**, 83–90.
O'Connor, D. W., Pollitt, P. A. & Roth, M. (1990). Co-existing depression and dementia in a community survey of the elderly. *International Psychogeriatrics* **2**, 45–53.
Pliny Earle (1948). *History, Description and Statistics of the Bloomingdale Asylum for the Insane*, New York: Egbert, Hovey & King.
Pollock, H. M. (1945) Development of statistics of mental disease in the United States during the past century. *American Journal of Psychiatry*, **102**, 1–17.
Preston, S. H. (1984). Children and the Elderly in the US *Scientific American*, **251**, 44–9.
Psychiatric Disorders in America. The Epidemiologic Catchment Area Study (1991) eds. Robins L. N. and Regier D. A. New York: The Free Press.
Psychiatry in the Elderly (1991). ed., R. Jacoby & C. Oppenheimer, Oxford: Oxford University Press.
Ray, I. (1849). The statistics of insane hospitals. *American Journal of Insanity*. **6**, 23–52.
Robins L. N. & Reiger D. A. (eds.) (1991). *Psychiatric Disorders in America. The Epidemiologic Catchment Area Study*, New York: The Free Press.
Roberts, C. J. (1922). *Epidemiology for Clinicians*. London: Pitman Medical Publishing
Roth, M. & Morrissey, J. D. (1952). Problems in the diagnosis and classification of mental disorder in old age: with a study of case material. *Journal of Mental Science*, **98**, 66–80.
Roth, M. (1955). The natural history of mental disorder in old age. *Journal of Mental Science*, **101**, 281–301.
Shepherd, M. (1987). Epidemiology of Psychogeriatric Disorders. In *Psychogeriatrics: An International Handbook*, ed. M. Bergener. New York: Springer Publishing Company.
Shepherd, M. (1990). *Conceptual issues in psychological medicine: Collected papers of Michael Shepherd*, London :Tavistock/Routledge.
Snowdon, J. & Donnelly, N. (1986). A study of depression in nursing homes. *Journal of Psychiatric Research*, **20**, 327–33.
Snowdon, J. (1990). The prevalence of depression in old age. *International Journal of Geriatric Psychiatry*, **5**, 141–4.
Stoudemire, A. & Riether, A. M. (1987). Evaluation and treatment of paranoid symptoms in the elderly: a review. *General Hospital Psychiatry*, **9**, 267–74.
Yassa, R., Nair, V., Nastase, C., Camille, Y. & Belzile, L. (1988). Prevalence of bipolar disorder in a psychogeriatric population. *Journal of Affective Disorders*, **14**, 197–201.

Part 3

Neuroses

4

Panic disorder in the elderly

FIONA K. JUDD GRAHAM D. BURROWS

Introduction

Anxiety disorders have been named and classified in various ways; often the diagnostic label chosen has reflected the patient's most prominent symptom. Examples include Da Costa's syndrome, neurasthenia, effort syndrome, soldier's heart, cardiac neurosis, and autonomic epilepsy (Judd & Burrows, 1985). Early descriptions of anxiety disorders did not differentiate 'chronic nervousness' from recurrent 'anxiety attacks' (Sheehan, 1982). Contemporary diagnostic systems (DSM-III-R, ICD-9) view anxiety disorders in dissimilar ways. In the ICD9 (World Health Organization, 1978) panic and generalized anxiety are grouped together as anxiety states. The DSM-III-R (American Psychiatric Association, 1987) contains separate categories of panic and generalized anxiety disorder.

Clinical features

Panic disorders are characterized by spontaneous attacks of anxiety which occur suddenly, without warning, for no apparent reason and not in response to a particular environmental stimulus. Commonly described symptoms include dyspnoea, palpitations, chest pain or discomfort, shortness of breath or smothering sensations, dizziness, vertigo or unsteady feelings, depersonalization and derealization, paresthesia, sweating, faintness, trembling or shaking. Prominent cognitive symptoms include fear of dying, fear of going crazy, and fear of losing control. A variety of additional symptoms may occur, at times influenced by coexisting medical illnesses. These include muscle aches and pains, urinary frequency and diarrhea, fear of urination and defecation, blurred vision, buzzing in the ears, nausea and vomiting. The DSM-III-R criteria for panic disorder are shown in Table 4.1.

Spontaneous attacks usually occur against a background of generalized anxiety.

Table 4.1. *Diagnostic criteria for panic disorder DSM-III-R*

A. At some time during the disturbance, one or more panic attacks (discrete periods of intense fear or discomfort) have occurred that were:
   1. unexpected, i.e. did not occur immediately before or on exposure to a situation that almost always caused anxiety, and
   2. not triggered by situations in which the person was the focus of others' attention.

B. Either four attacks, as defined in criterion A, have occurred within a four-week period, or one or more attacks have been followed by a period of at least a month of persistent fear of having another attack.

C. At least four of the following symptoms developed during at least one of the attacks:
   1. shortness of breath (dyspnea) or smothering sensations
   2. dizziness, unsteady feelings, or faintness
   3. palpitations or accelerated heart rate (tachycardia)
   4. trembling or shaking
   5. sweating
   6. choking
   7. nausea or abdominal distress
   8. depersonalization or derealization
   9. numbness or tingling sensations (paresthesias)
   10. flushes (hot flushes) or chills
   11. chest pain or discomfort
   12. fear of dying
   13. fear of going crazy or of doing something uncontrolled

   Note: Attacks involving four or more symptoms are panic attacks; attacks involving fewer than four symptoms are limited symptom attacks.

D. During at least some of the attacks, at least four of the C symptoms developed suddenly and increased in intensity within ten minutes of the beginning of the first C symptom noticed in the attack.

E. It cannot be established that an organic factor initiated and maintained the disturbance, e.g. amphetamine or caffeine intoxication, hyperthyroidism.

This state of apprehensive tension and restlessness may persist chronically for days or weeks when no panic attacks have occurred. Patients usually identify this anxiety as secondary to the anticipation of another panic attack. Attacks usually last from a few seconds to five minutes, but occasionally last an hour or more. They occur with variable frequency, most commonly two to four times per week, but may occur weeks or months apart, or be repeated in intense bursts for hours or days at a time (Sheehan, 1983).

Fears of physical, psychological or social disaster occurring during a panic attack are characteristically reported (Hibbert, 1984). Fear of dying, going crazy, or doing something embarrassing such as losing control of bladder or bowel, shouting out or taking off clothes are common. Fear of being trapped and unable to escape or obtain help is characteristic.

Following the onset of panic a number of secondary problems may occur. The most frequent of these is the development of phobic avoidance. Klein (1981), and Sheehan (1983), suggested that this occurs by a process of classical conditioning, in which patients develop fear and avoidance of situations in which attacks occur most often. In a group of approximately 500 patients with panic, 79.6% described agoraphobia, 15.4% limited phobic avoidance, and only 5% no phobic avoidance (Ballenger et al., 1988). Secondary depression is also common, occurring in approximately 50% of patients with panic (Woodruff, Guze & Clayton 1972; Delay et al., 1981, Ballenger et al., 1988). Patients with secondary depression have a more severe and chronic course. The third major complication of panic is addiction to alcohol, sedatives and tranquillizers. These are used to alleviate anticipatory anxiety, but often have little effect on panic. It is estimated that 5–10% of patients with panic develop secondary alcohol and drug abuse (Quitkin et al., 1972). Additional problems are those common to many chronic disorders, such as marital and family dysfunction, occupational impairment and social withdrawal.

Epidemiology

Studies of anxiety states conducted prior to the use of specified diagnostic criteria have shown a current prevalence rate of 2–4.7/100 (Marks & Lader, 1973). Disorders were more prevalent in women, particularly those aged between 16 and 40 years old. Four studies using research diagnostic criteria (RDC) (Spitzer, Endicott & Robins, 1975) or DSM-III (American Psychiatric Association, 1980) criteria have now been reported (Angst & Dobler-Mikola 1985; Myers et al., 1984; Robins et al., 1984; Uhlenhuth et al., 1983; Weissman, Myers & Harding, 1978), allowing the study of specific disorders (Table 4.2). With the exception of the Zurich study (Angst & Dobler-Mikola, 1985), the prevalence rates for panic are similar. Applying diagnostic hierarchies to the Zurich study data, reduces the prevalence of panic to 0.2/100. The ECA data show similar rates across five sites (0.6–1.0/100). The rates were higher in women. There was no strong relationship with age, although rates were higher for those aged 22–45 years, and generally lower in those 65 years and older. Examination of data from three sites showed an increase in onset of panic attacks in the group aged 15–19 years, and the onset of panic after age 40 to be rare (Von Korff, Eaton & Reyl, 1985). This is consistent with data drawn from clinical samples where mean age of onset occurs in the mid-twenties (Sheehan, Sheehan & Minichello, 1981; Thyer et al., 1985), and onset after age 40 is rare.

The epidemiology of panic in the elderly has been little studied. Lindesay, Briggs & Murphy (1989) assessed prevalence rates of cognitive impairment, depression and anxiety in a sample of 890 people aged 65 years and over living in the community. Nobody met DSM-III criteria for panic disorder, and only one subject

Table 4.2. *Prevalence of panic disorder*

Study	Sample	Diagnostic criteria	Prevalence period	Rate/100
1975 New Haven survey (Weissmann et al., 1978)	Community survey $N = 511$	RDC	1 month	0.4
1979 National survey of psychotherapeutic drug use (Uhlenhuth et al., 1983)	$N = 3161$	DSM III*	1 year	1.2
1982 Epidemiologic catchment area survey (Myers et al., 1984; Robins et al., 1984)	Community Survey $N \simeq 15000$	DSM III	6 months (lifetime)	0.6 (New Haven) (1.4) 0.9 (St. Louis) (1.5) 1.0 (Baltimore) (1.4)
Zurich study (Angst & Dobler Mikola, 1985)	Community Sample $N = 500$	DSM III	1 year	3.1

* Panic with agoraphobia.

had experienced a panic attack in the month prior to interview. The prevalence rate of agoraphobia was 7.8%, and of social phobia was 1.3%. No documentation of medication use is given, and patients were asked only if they had experienced panic attacks in the previous month. It is possible that these methodological features resulted in an underestimate of the prevalence of panic. This suggestion is supported by the ECA data which showed a six-month prevalence rate for panic of 0% for men aged over 65 years, but rates for women over 65 of 0.1% (St Louis), 0.2% (Baltimore), and 0.4% (New Haven) (Myers et al., 1984).

Although it appears that onset of panic in the elderly is uncommon, it is nevertheless well documented. Kenardy, Oei & Evans (1990) studied age of onset in a sample of 261 patients attending an anxiety disorder clinic. Mean age of onset was 30 years, with a range from 10 to 69. Four patients first developed symptoms after the age of 60 years. Luchins & Rose (1989), reported three cases of panic with onset after the age of 65 years, drawn from their practice in a geriatric psychiatric service. All three patients were women. In two cases panic first began at age 75, the third at 87. Hassan and Pollard (1990) reported that retrospective chart review of all patients over 60 years with DSM-III panic seen within a three-year period yielded ten patients who reported initial onset of panic after age 60. Patients were aged 62–81 (average 66) years, the majority were women (8/10).

The setting in which the patient is evaluated may significantly influence the findings regarding prevalence of panic. Patients with panic are commonly found in general medical clinics. Katon et al., (1986), found 6.5% of 195 randomly assessed primary care patients met DSM-III criteria for panic alone, and a further 6.5% met criteria for panic and depression. Von Korff et al., (1987) found 1.4% of predominantly middle and old-aged internal medicine patients assessed in a primary care epidemiologic study suffered from panic disorder. Beitman, Kushner and Grossberg (1991), in a study of 187 cardiology patients with chest pain and no evidence of coronary disease, found 91 patients (49%) suffered from DSM-III-R panic disorder. Twenty-seven patients aged 65 years and older were identified. Of these, nine (33.3%) met DSM-III-R criteria for panic. Mean age of onset of panic in this group was 62.4 ± 22.8 years. The age range for seven of the nine patients was 62–83, of the remaining two, one began experiencing panic when aged 12, the other at 40.

Paucity of data precludes detailed comparison of early and late onset panic. In their study of patients with chest pain, Beitman, et al. (1991) compared panic patients over 65 with those less than 65. The older group were more likely to be widowed, of lower socioeconomic status, and female. The two groups did not differ on self-report psychological symptomatology. Sheikh, King & Taylor (1991) examined differences in phenomenology of early (< 55 y) and late (> 55 y) onset panic attacks in a sample of volunteers assessed by self-report mailed questionnaire. Seventy-five subjects aged 55 or older were identified. Of these, 57 reported that the panic began before age 55, 18 that panic first began after age 55. Respondents with late onset panic attacks had significantly fewer symptoms and less avoidance behavior than those with early onset attacks.

Assessment of the elderly with panic

Clinically, panic in the elderly will be seen in two situations. Panic is a chronic episodic disorder, thus the elderly patient presenting with panic may have a history of many years duration of similar symptoms. Another diagnosis such as neurasthenia, irritable heart, or hyperventilation syndrome may previously have been made. Secondly, and less commonly, an elderly patient may complain of the recent onset of panic attacks. Here, the diagnosis of panic disorder is less likely than it would be in a younger person, and alternative diagnoses should be considered.

Panic attacks may occur as a feature of other psychiatric illnesses, most commonly depression. Patients with depression with secondary panic attacks have a later age of onset of panic attacks than patients with panic disorder only, or panic disorder with secondary depression (Van Valkenberg et al., 1984).

The symptoms of panic disorder may affect almost every system of the body, and may mimic many medical illnesses. High rates of physical illness in patients referred for psychiatric treatment are well documented (Koranyi, 1979; Hall et al., 1980). The physical illness may cause the psychiatric illness, may be an

Table 4.3. *Medical conditions which may present with panic-like episodes*

Cardiovascular
- cardiac arrythmias especially PAT
- mitral valve prolapse
- angina

Endocrine
- hyperthyroidism or hypothyroidism
- hypoglycemia
- phaeochromocytoma
- carcinoid syndrome
- Cushing's syndrome
- Hypoparathyroidism

Respiratory
- asthma
- hyperventilation syndrome
- chronic obstructive airways disease

Neurological
- temporal lobe epilepsy
- vestibular disorders: Menière's disease
acute labyrinthitis

Substance related
- intoxication: caffeine, cocaine, amphetamine, hallucinogens
- anticholinergic agents, sympathomimetics, steroids, digitalis, appetite suppressants
- withdrawal: alcohol, barbiturates, benzodiazepines, narcotics

exacerbating factor, or may simply coexist with it. Medical conditions which may present with panic-like episodes are shown in Table 4.3.

Complaints referable to the cardiovascular system are frequent concomitants of panic attacks. Arrythmias, anginal chest pain and mitral valve prolapse syndrome (MVPS) may all be confused with panic attacks. Patients with panic have a higher incidence of MVPS than the general population (Pariser et al., 1979; Kantor, Zitrin & Zeldis, 1980; Ventkatesch et al., 1980). Patients are prone to extrasystoles, syncope, tachycardia, palpitations, cardiac awareness, dyspnoea, fatigue and atypical chest pain. Patients with chest pain and normal coronary arteriograms present a challenging problem. Panic disorder is commonly diagnosed in patients presenting with chest pain and no evidence of coronary artery disease (Beitman et al., 1991), and atypical chest pain (Mateos et al., 1989). At the same time, cardiologic studies have shown some such patients have a dynamic abnormality of coronary blood flow reserve in arteries too small to be seen during angiography (microvascular angina) (Cannon et al., 1983). Roy-Byrne et al. (1989) compared clinical characteristics in patients with microvascular angina (MVA) and with panic disorder. They found similar sex distribution between the two groups. MVA patients were older, panic patients had been ill significantly longer, and had a much earlier onset of their chest pain. Panic disorder diagnostic criteria were met by 40% of MVA patients. As has been suggested for the association between panic and mitral valve prolapse, MVA may also consist of two subgroups, those with small vessel abnormalities due to primary cardiac disturbance, and those with centrally mediated abnormalities resulting from the autonomic dysregulation associated with panic (Wielgosz, 1988).

Panic attacks may be characterized by prominent neurological symptoms; giddiness, dizziness, vertigo, depersonalization and derealization. Determining that panic-like symptoms are not related to neurological dysfunction may be difficult. Partial seizures may mimic panic (Stern & Murray, 1984) and may not be detectable by standard EEG. Edlund, Swann & Clothier (1987) described a series of patients presenting with atypical panic attacks presenting with hostility, irritability, severe derealization and social withdrawal, and EEG abnormalities involving the temporal lobes. Coyle & Sterman (1986) found 19 of 350 patients referred for evaluation of focal neurological symptoms had panic attacks as the underlying cause. Hyperventilation was thought to account for the symptoms in half the group studied.

Dizziness and unsteadiness are prominent symptoms in the panic attacks of many patients. Vertigo was recognized as a prominent symptom in the earliest descriptions of anxiety. Thus an association between vestibular function and panic has been sought. Phobic anxiety states have been described in patients with documented vestibular lesions (Pratt & McKenzie, 1958), and abnormal responses to vestibular and audiological tests demonstrated in patients with panic disorder (Jacob et al., 1985)

Hyperventilation is a common symptom of panic, and may itself be the cause of several other symptoms. Chest pains occur in 40–50% of cases, most commonly due to spasm and strain in the muscles and joints of the precordium (Ker, Dalton & Gliebe, 1937). Air hunger, the need to take a deep satisfying breath together with a feeling of difficulty in inflating the lungs, is due to the characteristic overinflation of the chest. Dizziness, unsteadiness and blurred vision result from cerebral vasoconstriction and hypoxia. These symptoms are frequently seen in patients with organic respiratory problems (e.g. chronic obstructive airways disease, asthma) and anxiety.

Abnormalities of endocrine function may present with symptoms of anxiety. Hyperthyroidism may present with nervousness, palpitations, sweating, heat intolerance and diarrhoea, and clinical signs may be few, particularly early in the course of the disorder. Although uncommon, pheochromocytoma is an important organic cause of anxiety. Hypoglycemia produces acute anxiety with prominent symptoms of sweating, tremor, hunger and fatigue.

In most cases a careful history (including family history, collaborative history from others), physical examination and laboratory screening (e.g. blood count, blood chemistry, thyroid function tests, electrocardiogram) will lead to the diagnosis of an organic condition. The presentation of an organic illness however, may be modified in the elderly, particularly where there are other coexisting medical conditions, or where the patient is taking a variety of medications. Where there is diagnostic uncertainty, more sophisticated medical investigations (e.g. 24 hour Holter monitor, cerebral CT scan, EEG) or referral for a specialist physician opinion are indicated.

Treatment

Management of the elderly patient with panic begins with a thorough and comprehensive assessment. Where the elderly patient is presenting with panic of recent onset, in the absence of a past history of similar problems, attention must first be directed to ensuring that the panic attacks are not secondary to some other psychiatric or medical illness. More commonly, the patient will have a past history of similar symptoms, and factors causing an exacerbation of the disorder should be sought. Coexisting medical illness, prescribed medications, or the development of secondary depression are commonly identified. Life events viewed as uncontrollable, undesirable and causing extreme lowering of self esteem have been shown to precede the onset of panic (Roy-Byrne, Geraci & Uhde, 1986). The elderly are particularly at risk for these types of events.

Once the diagnosis of panic disorder has been established, treatment should focus on control of the panic attacks, followed by treatment of the secondary complications. These include phobic avoidance, depression, alcohol and drug abuse, family and marital dysfunction, and social isolation.

Control of panic attacks

Psychological techniques

A variety of strategies are available for the treatment of the panic attacks. Attention to modifying specific stressors which are exacerbating anxiety, together with instruction in general stress reduction strategies are important first steps. Patients should be taught general relaxation techniques, which can be used to lower anticipatory anxiety. Hyperventilation control techniques include breathing retraining to improve chronic hyperventilation, and rebreathing to deal with acute attacks.

Cognitive strategies are based on the cognitive models of anxiety and panic (Clark, 1986; Beck, 1976). Beck's (1976) model proposes that individuals with anxiety systematically overestimate the danger inherent in a given situation. This results in changes in autonomic arousal, and selective scanning of the environment for possible sources of danger. The cognitive model of panic (Clark, 1986) suggests that individuals experience panic attacks because they have a persistent tendency to interpret a range of bodily sensations in a catastrophic fashion (e.g. palpitations as a sign of impending heart attack). Patients become hypervigilant and repeatedly scan their body making them aware of sensations most people do not notice. These sensations are then assumed to be evidence of serious disease. Treatment aims to teach patients how to identify, evaluate, control, and modify their negative danger-related thoughts (Clark, 1989). Typically the thoughts involve the assumption that the somatic symptoms of panic signify serious physical disease. These strategies have been well researched in groups of young patients, but their efficacy has not been evaluated in elderly patients, where cognitive impairment and coexisting medical illnesses may cause difficulties in their use. However the efficacy of cognitive therapy has been demonstrated for depression in the elderly (Gallagher & Thompson, 1983), suggesting that evaluation in anxiety is warranted.

Pharmacological treatments

Where symptoms are persistent and severe, and psychological strategies are not sufficient to control the panic, medication may be appropriate. Efficacy of a variety of medications for the control of panic has been demonstrated (Judd, Norman & Burrows, 1990). The most commonly used agents are the antidepressants and the benzodiazepines (Norman et al., 1988).

Several factors should be considered when prescribing psychotropics in the elderly. Ageing is associated with altered pharmacokinetic disposition of psychotropic drugs (see Chapter 25). All four main aspects of pharmacokinetics, absorption, distribution, metabolism and clearance, are altered. The function of hepatic microsomal enzymes which cause Phase I oxidative drug metabolism may be significantly impaired in old age, leading to reduced total drug clearance and higher steady-state plasma concentrations with multiple dosage (Greenblatt, Sellers & Shader, 1982). Altered CNS pharmacodynamic response to drugs may make the elderly more sensitive to the effects of drugs than younger patients. Concomitant physical illness and the treatment of such illness may alter the patient's response to psychotropic medications. Compliance may be poor, with both the omission of prescribed doses and ingestion of extra tablets.

Tricyclic antidepressants and monoamine oxidase inhibitors

Since Klein & Fink (1962) first suggested imipramine was effective in the treatment of panic anxiety, and West & Dally (1959) noted the efficacy of monoamine oxidase inhibitors (MAOIs) in the treatment of neuroses characterized by panic attacks and phobic symptoms, the efficacy of both groups of drugs has been extensively studied. Findings of these studies have been reviewed elsewhere (Judd, Norman & Burrows, 1990). Care should be taken in applying the results of these studies to the elderly, as patients included in studies have generally been aged below 65 years.

In younger populations, doses of tricyclics have usually been in the 150–300 mg range, and of MAOIs the 45–90 mg (phenelzine) range. Elderly patients who are generally more sensitive to side-effects than younger adults, should be started on a low dose of antidepressant. Doses should be increased cautiously, while ensuring that sufficient dose is prescribed to achieve a therapeutic effect. In particular, anticholinergic side-effects (e.g. constipation, dry mouth, urinary retention), postural hypotension and confusion may be troublesome.

Benzodiazepines

Generally longer acting benzodiazepines (elimination half-life > 50 hours) have been favored in the treatment of panic (e.g. diazepam, chlordiazepoxide, clorazepate, clobazam). Their metabolism is primarily by phase I oxidation, and so it is prolonged in later life. Cumulation may be marked and slow, and impairment of cognitive and psychomotor function develops insidiously. Intermediate acting drugs (e.g. oxazepam, clonazepam, lorazepam) with half-lives of 12–18 hours and no active metabolites are metabolized by phase II conjugation, which is generally unimpaired in the elderly, and so are considered more suitable for this age group. The most studied of the benzodiazepines in the treatment of panic is the triazolobenzodiazepine alprazolam (Chouinard et al., 1982; Ballenger et al., 1988). Although metabolized by oxidation, it has minimally active metabolites and a relatively short half-life (11–15 hours) (Barbee & McLaulin, 1990). These features suggest it may be suitable for the treatment of panic in the elderly. Altered pharmacodynamic responses may render the elderly more sensitive to the sedative and psychomotor effects, and thus the use of lower doses than those recommended in younger populations (e.g. mean daily dose 5.7 mg/day in the Cross National Collaborative Panic Study, Ballenger et al., 1988) should be considered. The possible development of benzodiazepine tolerance, dependence and withdrawal must be recognized when using these drugs.

Other agents

A variety of other medications have been used for the treatment of panic. The most frequently used of these is propranolol. The efficacy of beta blockers in panic continues to be debated, with some positive (Noyes et al., 1984; Munjack et al., 1985) studies suggesting they have a role. Clonidine, an α-adrenoreceptor agonist is also suggested to be of value in the treatment of panic (Liebowitz et al., 1981). Both drugs may produce significant hypotension, and should be used cautiously in the elderly. Early studies suggest the selective serotonin reuptake blockers fluvoxamine (Den Boer & Westenberg, 1988) and fluoxetine (Schneier et al., 1990) are also effective in the control of panic. The side-effect profile of these drugs may render them more suitable for use in the elderly than the tricyclics and MAOIs.

Many patients will require a combination of pharmacological and psychological treatments. When medication is used, the minimum dose to achieve therapeutic effect should be prescribed. Patients should be reviewed regularly, and particular care taken to monitor the development of side effects. Where possible, doses of medication should be reduced as the patient improves, and increased reliance is placed on the use of nonpharmacological treatment measures. Cessation of medication should be cautious and gradual, particularly for the benzodiazepines, in order to avoid withdrawal effects.

Together with the treatment of the panic, secondary problems should be addressed. Phobic avoidance may require the use of in vivo exposure techniques; depression, alcohol and drug abuse may necessitate the use of a variety of therapies, as will marital and family dysfunction.

Conclusions

The elderly patient with panic may have a long history of panic disorder, or may present with the recent onset of panic attacks. Careful assessment is required to ensure panic attacks are not secondary to, or exacerbated by another psychiatric disorder or medical illness. If a diagnosis of panic disorder is confirmed, treatment should focus on control of the panic attacks, together with management of the secondary complications. For the treatment of panic a combination of psychological and pharmacological strategies will usually be required. Altered pharmacokinetic disposition of psychotropics in the elderly renders them more sensitive to the effects and side-effects of drugs, so they should be used with caution and close monitoring.

References

American Psychiatric Association (1980). *Diagnostic and Statistical Manual of Mental Disorders*, 3rd edition, Washington DC: American Psychiatric Association.

American Psychiatric Association (1987). *Diagnostic and Statistical Manual of Mental Disorders*, 3rd edition (revised) (DSM-III-R), Washington DC: American Psychiatric Association.

Angst, J. & Dobler-Mikola, A. (1985). The Zurich Study: anxiety and phobia in young adults. *Archives of Psychiatry and Neurological Sciences*, **235**, 171–8.

Ballenger, J. C., Burrows, G. D., DuPont, R. L., Lesser, I. M., Noyes, R. Pecknold, J. C., Rifkin, A. & Swinson, R. P. (1988). Alprazolam in panic disorder and agoraphobia: results from a multicentre trial. *Archives of General Psychiatry*, **45**, 413–22.

Barbee, J. G. & McLaulin, J. B. (1990). Anxiety disorders: diagnosis and pharmacotherapy in the elderly. *Psychiatric Annals*, **20**, 439–45.

Beck, A. T. (1976). *Cognitive Therapy and the Emotional Disorders*. New York: International Universities Press.

Beitman, B. D., Kushner, M. & Grossberg, G. T. (1991). Late onset panic disorder: evidence from a study of patients with chest pain and normal cardiac evaluations. *International Journal of Psychiatry in Medicine*, **21**, 29–35.

Cannon, R. O., Watson, R. M., Rosing, D. R. & Epstein, S. E. (1983). Angina caused by reduced vasodilator reserve of the small coronary arteries. *Journal of the American College of Cardiology*, **1**, 1359–64.

Chouinard, G., Annable, L., Fontaine, R. & Solyom, L. (1982). Alprazolam in the treatment of generalized anxiety and panic disorders: a double-blind placebo controlled study. *Psychopharmacology*, **77**, 229–33.

Clark, D. M. (1986). A cognitive approach to panic. *Behavior Research and Therapy*, **24**, 461–70.

Clark, D. M. (1989). Anxiety states: panic and generalized anxiety. In *Cognitive Behavior Therapies for Psychiatric Problems: A Practical Guide*, ed. K. Hawton, P. M. Salkovskis, J. Kirk & D. M. Clark, pp. 52–66. New York: Oxford University Press.

Coyle, P. K. & Sterman, A. B. (1986). Focal neurologic symptoms in panic attacks. *American Journal of Psychiatry*, **143**, 648–9.

Den Boer, J. A. & Westenberg, G. M. (1988). Effect of a serotonin and noradrenaline uptake inhibitor in panic disorder: a double-blind comparative study with fluvoxamine and maprotiline. *International Clinical Psychopharmacology*, **3**, 59–74.

Delay, R. S., Ishiki, D. M., Avery, D. H., Wilson, L. G. & Dunner, D. L. (1981). Secondary depression in anxiety disorders. *Comprehensive Psychiatry*, **22**, 612–18.

Edlund, M. J., Swann, A. C. & Clothier, J. (1987). Patients with panic attacks and abnormal EEG results. *American Journal of Psychiatry*, **144**, 508–9.

Gallagher, D. E. & Thompson, L. W. (1983). Effectiveness of psychotherapy for both endogenous and nonendogenous depression in older adult outpatients. *Journal of Gerontology*, **38**, 707–12.

Greenblatt, D. J., Sellers, E. M. & Shader, R. I.(1982).Drug disposition in old age. *New England Journal of Medicine*, **306**, 1081–8.

Hall, R. C. W., Gardner, E. R., Stickney, S. K., LeCann, A. F. & Popkin, M. K. (1980). Physical illness manifesting as psychiatric disease: analysis of a state hospital in-patient population. *Archives of General Psychiatry*, **37**, 989–95.

Hassan, R. & Pollard, C. A. (1990). Late-life onset of panic disorder. *American Journal of Psychiatry*, **147**, 1103–4.

Hibbert, G. A. (1984). Ideational components of anxiety: their origin and content. *British Journal of Psychiatry*, **144**, 618–24.

Jacob, R. G., Moller, M. B., Turner, S. M. & Wall, C. (1985). Otoneurological examination in panic disorder and agoraphobia with panic attacks: a pilot study. *American Journal of Psychiatry*, **142**, 715–20.

Judd, F. K. & Burrows, G. D. (1985). Classification of anxiety and panic disorders. *Australian Family Physician*, **14**, 865–70.

Judd, F. K., Norman, T. R. & Burrows, G. D. (1990). Pharmacotherapy of panic disorder. *International Review of Psychiatry*, **2**, 399–409.

Kantor, J. S., Zitrin, C. M. & Zeldis, S. M. (1980). Mitral valve prolapse syndrome in agoraphobic patients. *American Journal of Psychiatry*, **137**, 467–9.

Katon, W., Vitaliano, P. P. & Russo, J., Cormier, L., Anderson, K. & Jones, M. (1986). Panic disorder: epidemiology in primary care. *Journal of Family Practice*, **23**, 233–9.

Kenardy, J., Oei, T. P. S. & Evans, L. (1990). Neuroticism and age of onset for agoraphobia with panic attacks. *Journal of Behavior Therapy and Experimental Psychiatry*, **21**, 193–7.

Ker, W. J., Dalton, J. W. & Gliebe, P. A. (1937). Some physical phenomena associated with anxiety states and their relation to hyperventilation. *Annals of Internal Medicine*, **2**, 962–7.

Klein, D. F. & Fink, M. (1962). Psychiatric reaction patterns to imipramine. *American Journal of Psychiatry*, **119**, 432–8.

Klein, D. F. (1981). Anxiety reconceptualized. In *Anxiety: New Research and Changing Concepts*. ed. D. F. Klein & J. Rabkin, pp. 235–65, New York: Raven Press.

Koranyi, E. K. (1979). Morbidity and rate of undiagnosed physical illness in a psychiatric clinic population. *Archives of General Psychiatry*, **36**, 414–49.

Liebowitz, M. R., Fyer, A. J., McGrath, P. & Klein, D. (1981). Clonidine treatment of panic disorder. *Psychopharmacology Bulletin*, **17**, 122–3.

Lindesay, J., Briggs, K. & Murphy, E. (1989). The Guy's/Age Concern Survey Prevalence rates of cognitive impairment, depression and anxiety in an urban elderly community. *British Journal of Psychiatry*, **155**, 317–29.

Luchins, D. J. & Rose, R. P. (1989). Late-life onset of panic disorder with agoraphobia in three patients. *American Journal of Psychiatry*, **146**, 920–1.

Marks, I. & Lader, M. (1973). Anxiety states (anxiety neurosis): a review. *Journal of Nervous and Mental Disease*, **156**, 3–18.

Mateos, J. L. A., Perez, C. B., Carrasco, J. S. & Olivares,D. (1989). Atypical chest pain and panic disorder. *Psychotherapy and Psychosomatics*, **52**, 92–5.

Munjack, D. J., Rebal, R., Shaner, R., Staples, F., Braun, R. & Leonard, M. (1985). Imipramine versus propranolol for the treatment of panic attacks: A pilot study. *Comprehensive Psychiatry*, **26**, 80–9.

Myers, J. K., Weissman, M. M., Tischler, G. L. et al. (1984). The prevalence of psychiatric disorders in three communities: 1980–1982. *Archives of General Psychiatry*, **41**, 959–70.

Norman, T. R., Judd, F. K., Marriott, P. F. & Burrows, G. D. (1988). Physical treatment of anxiety: the benzodiazepines. In *Handbook of Anxiety, Vol 1, Biological, Clinical & Cultural Perspectives*. ed. M. Roth, R. Noyes, G. D. Burrows, pp. 355–384. Amsterdam: Elsevier Science Publishers.

Noyes, R., Anderson, D. J., Clancy, J., Crowe, R. R., Slyman. D. J., Choneim, M. M. & Hinricks, J. V. (1984). Diazepam and propranolol in panic disorder and agoraphobia. *Archives of General Psychiatry*, **41**, 287–92.

Pariser, S. F., Jones, B. A., Pinta, E. R., Young, E. A. & Fontana, M. E. (1979). Panic attacks: diagnostic evaluations in 17 patients. *American Journal of Psychiatry*, **136**, 105–6.

Pratt, R. T. C. & Mckenzie,W. (1958). Anxiety states following vestibular disorders. *Lancet*, **ii**, 347–9.

Quitkin, F. M., Rifkin, A., Kaplan, J., Klein, D. F. & Oaks, G. (1972). Phobic anxiety syndrome complicated by drug dependence and addiction. *Archives of General Psychiatry*, **27**, 159–62.

Robins, L. N., Helzer, J. E., Weissman, M. M., Orvaschel, H., Gruenberg, E., Burke, J. D. & Regier, D. A. (1984). Lifetime prevalence of specific psychiatric disorders in three sites. *Archives of General Psychiatry*, **41**, 949–58.

Roy-Byrne, P. R., Geraci, B. S. N. & Uhde, T. W. (1986). Life events and the onset of panic disorder. *American Journal of Psychiatry*, **143**, 1424–7.

Roy-Byrne, P. R., Schmidt, P., Cannon, R. O., Diem, H. & Rubinow, D. R. (1989). Microvascular angina and panic disorder. *International Journal of Psychiatry in Medicine*, **19**, 315–25.

Schneier, F. R., Liebowitz, M. R., Davies, S. O., Fairbanks, J., Hollander, E., Campeas, R. & Klein, D. F. (1990). Fluoxetine in panic disorder. *Journal of Clinical Psychopharmacology*, **10**, 119–21.

Sheehan, D. V. (1982). Panic attacks and phobias. *New England Journal of Medicine*, **307**, 156–8.

Sheehan, D. V. (1983). *The Anxiety Disease*. New York: Charles Scribner's Sons.

Sheehan, D. V., Sheehan, K. H. & Minichello, W. E. (1981). Age of onset of phobic disorders: a re-evaluation. *Comprehensive Psychiatry*, **22**, 544–53.

Sheikh, J. I., King, R. J. & Taylor, C. B. (1991). Comparative phenomenology of early-onset versus late-onset panic attacks: a pilot survey. *American Journal of Psychiatry*, **148**, 1231–3.

Spitzer, R. L., Endicott, J. & Robins, E. (1975). *Research Diagnostic Criteria*. New York: New York State Department of Mental Hygiene.

Stern, T. A. & Murray, G. B. (1984). Complex partial seizures presenting as a psychiatric illness. *Journal of Nervous and Mental Diseases*, **172**, 625–7.

Thyer, B. A., Parish, R. T., Curtis, G. C., Nesse, R. M. & Cameron, O. G. (1985). Ages of onset of DSM-III anxiety disorders. *Comprehensive Psychiatry*, **26**, 113–22.

Uhlenhuth, E. D., Balter, M. B., Mellinger, G. D., Cisin, I. H. & Clinthorne, J. (1983). Symptom checklist syndromes in the general population. *Archives of General Psychiatry*, **40**, 1167–73.

Van Valkenberg, C., Akiskal, H. S., Puzantian, V. & Rosenthal, A. (1984). Anxious depressions. Clinical, family history and naturalistic outcome – comparisons with panic and major depressive disorders. *Journal of Affective Disorders*, **6**, 67–82.

Ventkatesch, A., Pauls, D. L., Crowe, R., Noyes, R., Valkenberg, C. V., Martins, J. B. & Kerber, R. E. (1980). Mitral valve prolapse in anxiety neurosis (panic disorder). *American Heart Journal*, **100**, 302–5.

Von Korff, M., Eaton, W. & Reyl, P. (1985). The epidemiology of panic attacks and disorder: results from 3 community surveys. *American Journal of Epidemiology*, **122**, 970–81.

Von Korff, M. V., Shapiro, S., Burke, J. D. et al. (1987). Anxiety and depression in a primary care clinic. Comparison of diagnostic interview schedule, general health questionnaire and practitioner assessments. *Archives of General Psychiatry*, **44**, 152–6.

Weissman, M. M., Myers, J. K. & Harding, P. S. (1978). Psychiatric disorders in a US urban community. *American Journal of Psychiatry*, **135**, 459–62.

West, E. D. & Dally, P. J. (1959). Effects of iproniazid in depressive syndromes. *British Medical Journal*, **i**, 1491–4.

Wielgosz, A. T. (1988). Connecting the locus ceruleus and the coronaries. *American Journal of Cardiology*, **62**, 308–9.

Woodruff, R. A., Guze, S. B. & Clayton, P. J. (1972). Anxiety neurosis among psychiatric outpatients. *Comprehensive Psychiatry*, **13**, 165–170.

World Health Organization (1978). *Manual of The International Statistical Classification of Diseases, Injuries and Causes of Death*. Rev. 9, Vol.1. Geneva: WHO

5
Obsessive–compulsive disorder in the elderly

JOHN TILLER

Introduction

Obsessive–compulsive disorder (OCD) has been a hidden disease. It was thought to be uncommon, largely untreatable when it occurred, and was thought to be treated mostly in specialty units. It was believed possible to be helped when depression was associated with OCD in that treatment of depression was often associated with remission of the OCD. In recent years, epidemiological studies have suggested a general population prevalence of about 2% for OCD. Previous data had relied on numbers of patients attending specialist facilities, while ignoring morbidity in the general community. Furthermore, new and more effective psychological and physical treatments have resulted in renewed interest in diagnosing and treating this disabling disorder.

Almost nothing has been written about OCD in the elderly. This is despite the fact that it would be expected that approximately 2% of the elderly would be affected by OCD and that it is both disabling and potentially treatable. The failure to diagnose OCD in the elderly may reflect the general way in which this is a hidden disorder. Many patients are embarrassed and reluctant to talk about the problem, or reveal it, even to people close to them. Elderly sufferers may lead relatively restricted lives without their OCD being challenged and made manifest by the need to cope with a job and raise a family. As the disabilities would have waxed and waned over the course of their lives, there may also have been an assumption on the patient's part, as well as that of their attending doctors, that any symptoms are simply 'the way that person is', or assumed to be a personality trait, rather than reflecting a disorder which is eminently treatable.

This chapter highlights the importance of considering a diagnosis of OCD in the elderly, establishing the diagnosis, and instituting effective treatment.

Obsessive and compulsive symptoms

Obsessive symptoms are common in many psychiatric disorders. They may be manifest in depression, where they tend to remit following treatment; in dementia, especially early dementia when they reflect a response on the patient's part to try and retain some order and control in their lives; in schizophrenia; and as an element of organic disorders such as delirious states which impair mental functioning. Obsessive–compulsive symptoms may also be apparent in obsessive–compulsive personality disorder (anakastic personality disorder) which is a lifelong characteristic way of perceiving and responding and is distinct from obsessive–compulsive disorder.

Diagnosis

It is important to consider the possibility of a diagnosis of OCD and to specifically inquire of a patient when the diagnosis is suspected. Many patients will not volunteer symptoms. Symptoms and signs may need to be elicited by detailed questioning and careful observation.

Diagnostic criteria for OCD from the *Diagnostic and Statistical Manual of the American Psychiatric Association*, third edition, revised (*DSM-III-R*) are as follows.

The patient has either obsessions or compulsions:

Obsessions

1. Recurrent and persistent ideas, thoughts, impulses, or images that are experienced, at least initially, as intrusive and senseless, e.g. a parent having repeated impulses to kill a loved child, a religious person having recurrent blasphemous thoughts.
2. The person attempts to ignore or suppress such thoughts or impulses or to neutralize them with some other thought or action.
3. The person recognizes that the obsessions are the product of his or her own mind, not imposed from without (as in thought insertion)
4. If another Axis 1 disorder is present, the content of the obsession is unrelated to it, e.g. the ideas, thoughts, impulses, or images are not about food in the presence of an eating disorder, about drugs in the presence of a psychoactive substance use disorder, or guilty thoughts in the presence of a major depression.

Compulsions

1. Repetitive, purposeful and intentional behaviors that are performed in response to an obsession, or according to certain rules or in a stereotyped fashion.
2. The behavior is designed to neutralize or to prevent discomfort or some dreaded event or situation; however, either the activity is not connected in a realistic way with what it is designed to neutralize or prevent, or it is clearly excessive.

3. The person recognizes that his or her behavior is excessive or unreasonable (this may not be true for young children; it may no longer be true for people whose obsessions have evolved into overvalued ideas).

   The obsessions or compulsions cause marked distress, are time consuming (take more than an hour a day), or significantly interfere with the person's normal routine, occupational functioning, or usual social activities or relationships with others.

Differential diagnosis

The important differential diagnostic considerations in someone presenting with symptoms of OCD are of depression, schizophrenia, dementia, or another organic disorder.

Other conditions that may give rise to symptoms like those in OCD include hypochondriasis, phobias, panic disorder, generalized anxiety disorder, delusional disorder, impulse control disorder, trichotillomania, and obsessive–compulsive personality.

Epidemiology

OCD is frequently quoted as having a prevalence of 0.05% or thereabouts. That figure has been derived from surveys of hospitalizations and psychiatric facilities, reflects the more severely affected, and does not indicate the prevalence of the disorder in the community at large. Myers et al., (1984) in the Epidemiologic Catchment Area Survey (ECA survey), suggested, in persons aged 18 years and over, a 1–2% six-month prevalence, and a 2–3% lifetime prevalence for OCD (Robins et al., 1984). There are approximately equal numbers of male and female OCD sufferers. This is unusual as most psychiatric disorders have a predominance of women affected.

Transient obsessions or compulsions are very common. During childhood, there are phases when children will not walk on cracks or will develop certain rituals which are evanescent and soon go. In adulthood, there can be appropriate checking that a door is locked, a car is properly prepared and mechanically sound, or documents are at hand when about to travel. Others might have a particular piece of music which they have on their mind and tends to persist. This is sometimes referred to as 'having a tune on the brain'. A common characteristic of such an experience is that the theme or piece of music is perceived initially as pleasurable, then has a dysphoric quality as the person tries to get rid of it yet it persists. Eventually it goes spontaneously. These features do not constitute OCD because the transient thought or the behavioral activities are not characteristic for that individual.

These occasional obsessional and compulsive symptoms should be seen as the person being careful in daily activities, or reflecting a transient developmental phase. Furthermore, these characteristics are generally advantageous rather than disabling.

Etiology

The etiology of obsessive–compulsive disorder is unknown. There is probably a genetic component though the genetics are, as yet, not well defined. If a family member has OCD, the risk of a relative suffering the disorder is increased. Because of the recent data from the ECA survey (Myers et al., 1984) suggesting the community prevalence of OCD is about 2% rather than 0.05%, old calculations using actual versus expected prevalence in families must now be in doubt.

Brown (1942) reported obsessional neurosis in 8% of parents and 7% of siblings, higher than community rates, compared with 0% from controls with other anxiety disorders. These data support some family component but there is argument whether this and other studies reflect a genetic element, or learnt behaviors. Beliefs of a low frequency for OCD have precluded effective twin studies to date. The population prevalence of 2% suggests twin studies are now feasible.

Learning etiologies have been proposed (Rachman & Hodgson, 1980; Foa, Steketee & Ozarow 1985) including that OCD symptoms represent that the patient has learnt specific (OCD) patterns of behavior within the family, in the social setting with particular reference to religious upbringing, and/or following certain life experiences.

Some OCD sufferers have structural changes in their brains. This may be seen when OCD follows a congenital deficit, develops after trauma to the brain such as a head injury (Jenike & Brandon, 1988) or a more generalized assault such as after encephalitis (Ravenholdt & Foege, 1982).

Positron emission tomography and other neuro-imaging studies of OCD are in their early stages. Studies reported to date have methodological difficulties including the probability of type 2 error in the small samples which have been reported. Mediating OCD symptoms appears to involve dysfunction in the prefrontal cortex and caudate nucleus (Baxter et al., 1990).

Biochemical hypotheses of OCD suggest a relative deficiency of serotonergic activity in the brain (Zohar & Insel, 1987). This theory predominantly arises from the response to certain medications which increase synaptic serotonin (5-hydroxytryptamine, 5-HT). However, this view is probably oversimplistic. It does not explain why one patient will respond to one 5-HT uptake inhibitor and not to another. There is probably a complex set of neuromodulatory actions which occur.

In the clinical arena, Rapoport (1989) reported that 20% of OCD children had chorea-like movements, implying deficits in the extrapyramidal system.

Some 50% of people with Gilles de la Tourette's Syndrome are reported to have

OCD symptoms (Frankel et al., 1986). These patients were also reported to have basal ganglia deficits on PET scanning. This may imply the possibility of a dopamine component to the syndrome in addition to a serotonin component. Baxter et al. (1987), in a PET scanning study with fluorodeoxyglucose, reported functional deficits in the left orbital gyrus and caudate nucleus. The caudate to hemisphere activity normalized after clomipramine treatment.

Further evidence of caudate involvement in OCD comes from Luxenberg et al. (1988) who reported from computerized tomography scanning that the caudate volumes of OCD sufferers were reduced.

Hypothalamic pituitary adrenal (HPA) axis dysfunctions are not reported to occur in OCD (Coryell et al., 1989). This would appear to separate OCD from mood disorders and anxiety disorders which do have HPA axis dysfunction (Tiller et al., 1987, Maguire et al., 1987, Schweitzer et al., 1987).

Serotonin hypothesis

In 1984, Insel et al., noted that 5-hydroxyindole acetic acid (5-HIAA) was elevated in the cerebrospinal fluid of OCD patients. Following treatment with zimelidine (a specific 5-HT uptake inhibitor) the elevation of 5-HIAA was reduced. Flament et al. (1987) also noted that platelet 5-HT was reduced after successful treatment. The 5-HT antagonist metachlorphenylpiperazine (mCPP), was reported as worsening OCD (Zohar & Insel, 1987). As lactate, yohimbine and caffeine all worsen anxiety without of themselves worsening OCD, Zohar and Insel argued that this was not just an anxiety effect. Metergoline, another 5HT antagonist also, in some instances, worsens OCD (Benkelfat et al., 1989). Metergoline did not worsen untreated OCD but only worsened OCD after there had been some improvement following clomipramine therapy.

Clinical course of OCD

After an onset ranging from the teenage years to the forties, the disorder tends to wax and wane (Rasmussen & Eisen, 1990).

Approximately two-thirds of patients improve to a degree over a 12-month period though the outcome is variable (Goodwin, Guze & Robins, 1969).

The majority of sufferers have the typical clinical course of exacerbations and remissions (American Psychiatric Association, 1987). Such patients are rarely free of the disorder. A smaller proportion estimated at about 5% have periods of OCD interspersed with periods in which they are relatively asymptomatic. About 13% have a persisting disability affecting their personal life, and their interpersonal, social and occupational functioning (Rasmussen & Tsuang, 1986).

There are no current specific data on the clinical course of OCD in the elderly, with the assumption based on clinical experience rather than scientific data, that OCD continues in later years as in young adulthood.

Evaluating the severity of OCD

While it is usually sufficient to estimate severity in a general sense with a clinical global impression, it is also useful to be more specific in the assessment of the patient's disability. The progress of specific obsessions and compulsions and their response to elements of behavior therapy and pharmacotherapy can be monitored. Behavior therapy in particular, is directed at specific symptoms rather than at the patient's overall state.

In monitoring progress, it is useful to rate the severity of each obsession, and each compulsion separately because treatments can then be tailored in response to the patient's detailed progress. Reduction in obsessional thoughts (regarding contamination for example) with medication, may not necessarily be associated with a reduction in compulsive washing. If monitoring shows this dissociated response, it may indicate the need for additional behavior therapy such as response prevention targeted against the washing behaviors.

In addition to the specific rating of individual obsessions and compulsions, there are evaluations for the patient's OCD as a whole. A widely used scale is the Yale Brown Obsessive–compulsive Scale (Y-BOCS), an adaptation of which is listed in the Appendix.

Comorbidity

There is a wide range of comorbid DSM III-R axis 1 (clinical syndromes) and axis 2 (development disorders and personality disorders) disorders found with OCD which can lead to misdiagnosis as detailed by Rasmussen and Eisen (1992) (see Table 5.1).

Treatment

Psychoanalytical therapies

Psychoanalytical therapies relate more to characteristics of obsessive–compulsive personality disorder than obsessive–compulsive disorder. Characteristic defence mechanisms associated with OCD include defective repression, displacement, reaction formation, isolation, undoing, and rigidity. The latter is not strictly speaking a defense mechanism but is commonly associated. While these concepts may assist the understanding of the behaviors of people with OCD, including the elderly, they have not proved especially useful in formal treatment studies.

Table 5.1. *Coexisting Axis 1 Diagnoses in Primary OCD (N = 100)*†

Diagnosis	Current (%)	Lifetime (%)	
	Semistructured (N = 100)	Semistructured (N = 100)	From SADS (N = 60)
Major depressive disorder	31	67	78
Simple phobia	7	22	28
Separation anxiety disorder	—	2	17
Social phobia	11	18	26
Eating disorder	8	17	8
Alcohol abuse (dependence)	8	14	16
Panic disorder	6	12	15
Tourette's syndrome	5	7	6

* Abbreviations: OCD = obsessive-compulsive disorder
SADS = Schedule for Affective Disorders and Schizophrenia
† From Rasmussen and Eisen (1988), with permission.

Supportive psychotherapy

Supportive psychotherapeutic measures are common to almost all treatments for OCD including pharmacotherapy. The effects of such measures have not been adequately tested to date. With any treatment, the patient will be given some form of explanation, hope for a favorable outcome, emotional support, a sympathetic hearing, and other general therapeutic measures.

Cognitive therapy

Cognitive behavior therapy (CBT) aims to reduce anxiety and symptoms by teaching patients how to identify, evaluate, control, and modify their negative thoughts which are usually danger-related thoughts and associated behaviors. This may include learning how to deal with anticipatory, or residual, anxiety, to make more realistic cognitive appraisals of rısks and the individual's ability to cope. This approach results from the idea that obsessions and rituals in compulsions result from unrealistic cognitive appraisals of risks (Greist, 1992).

The effectiveness of cognitive therapies alone have yet to be well demonstrated in OCD, with the limited number of studies suggesting no effect, marginal effect or having methodological problems. Patients with OCD generally have well preserved-insight, recognize that their thoughts are 'crazy' and have done their utmost to try and control those. Given this situation, it seems unlikely that shifting cognitions alone will suffice for treatment.

Behavioral therapies, especially those including prolonged exposure and response prevention have been shown to be effective in treating OCD. One of the earliest reports of this approach was from Meyer (1966). Though about a quarter of patients refuse, or do not complete behavior therapy (Marks, 1981), some 75% of those who pursue this treatment approach improve. Thus approximately 50% of patients presenting for behavioral therapy are helped and 50% are not. Improvement is shown with a reduction in compulsions and a lessening of the obsessions. Imaginal exposure is useful to maintain the gains achieved with exposure in vivo even though it is a fairly weak treatment in its own right. Foa et al., (1985) have shown that the combination of exposure and response prevention yielded a 70% reduction in obsessions and compulsions in 51% of patients who complied with those treatment techniques. An additional 39% of patients had reductions of obsessions and rituals ranging from 30% to 69%.

An important element of behavior therapy is that of persisting improvement following treatment. The work of Pato et al., (1988), Pato, Hill & Murphy (1990) shows that 76% of patients in at least one study remained moderately improved or better at follow ups ranging from months to years. This contrasts with the rapid relapse seen after ceasing the 5-HT uptake inhibitors.

Poor response to behavior therapy is said to be most likely to occur in patients who are depressed, those using CNS depressing drugs (such as benzodiazepines) because of the impairment of state-dependent learning and those who are noncompliant through the use of mental rituals which are invoked to decrease the discomfort associated with exposure tasks.

Pharmacotherapy

The most effective treatments are inhibitors of the uptake of serotonin into the presynaptic nerve terminal (Zohar & Insel, 1987; Turner et al., 1985; Goodman et al., 1989*a*). The most extensively studied of these medicines is clomipramine, though others include fluoxetine, fluvoxemine, sertraline, paroxetine, and citalopram. Zimelidine had been subject to some studies but was withdrawn worldwide in 1983. Clinically, there is the impression that clomipramine is the most effective of these agents.

Clomipramine has been shown to be significantly superior to placebo (Goodman et al., 1989*bc*). In these studies, the Y-BOCS scores decreased 35% to 42% from baseline in the clomipramine groups but only 2% to 5% for the placebo groups.

It should be noted that pharmacotherapy does not eliminate all symptoms of OCD. For many patients, the effect of pharmacotherapy is to reduce a level of severity from that which is unable to be managed by the patient to a level which the patient can control using additional behavioral techniques.

Although clomipramine is effective, the elderly are especially intolerant of the side-effects of such tricyclic antidepressants (see Chapter 25). Potential cardiotoxicity may limit use in those with cardiovascular disease when arrhythmias or conduction impairment are prominent. Postural hypotension may be dose limiting. The hypotensive effects can be especially troublesome to the old, who have a propensity to faint and fall. This is a particular issue at night, only a few hours after dosing, when the patient may wake, get out of bed to urinate, and fall. Such a situation might be avoided by divided dosing over the day to reduce peak drug levels. Although sedative effects can limit the tolerated dose, there is a fairly rapid development of tolerance to some of the sedative effect, and with gradual dose escalation the patient may eventually tolerate doses which would previously have caused intolerable sedation. Sedation may also impair attention, concentration and memory and worsen confusion. The anticholinergic (antimuscarinic) effects also cause confusion in some elderly patients. Furthermore, anticholinergic effects may add to prostatic problems in elderly men and can result in acute urinary retention, as well as potentially precipitating acute angle glaucoma in those who are predisposed with a narrow anterior chamber. All tricyclic antidepressants can lower the convulsive threshold leading to the emergence of, or exacerbation of fitting.

Overdose safety should be considered, recognizing that clomipramine can be fatal in overdose, and the elderly represent 25% of all suicides with overdose being especially common as the mode of suicide for elderly women (see Chapter 14).

These problems with side-effects and toxicity are compounded because the doses of clomipramine needed for the treatment of OCD are frequently higher than those needed for the treatment of depression. To offset some of the need for higher doses, drug metabolism in the old is reduced compared with younger adults so that lower doses (100 to 200 mg) may nevertheless be clinically effective in the elderly. If clomipramine is to be used, it is useful to start with a low dose (say) 25 mg at night and slowly increase by 25 mg each 2 to 7 days depending on how the patient tolerates the medicine.

Fluoxetine is better tolerated than clomipramine. It has fewer anticholinergic side-effects and sedation tends not to occur, though symptoms of nausea and dizziness may be dose limiting factors. Agitation is a reason some people have to cease the medication and in the elderly, who may not in some instances have a good appetite, the tendency for fluoxetine sometimes to decrease appetite might preclude its use. As with the other new 5-HT uptake inhibitors, fluoxetine is relatively safe in overdosage compared with the tricyclics.

Fluoxetine may need to be gradually increased to a dose range of 20 to 80 mg per day. Because of its long half life (about 4 days) and the long half-life of its active metabolite norfluoxetine (about 7 days), it takes almost 4 weeks before a plateau is reached in plasma drug levels. The strong protein binding of fluoxetine may displace other concomitant medications so that the doses of other drugs may need to be adjusted.

Fluvoxemine 100 to 300 mg per day, has also been shown superior to placebo (Greist, 1991) in the treatment of obsessive–compulsive disorder.

Which uptake inhibitor in OCD?

There do not appear to be marked differences in efficacy amongst the serotonin uptake inhibitors. An example of such comparisons is that between clomipramine and fluoxetine reported by Pigott et al. (1990).

The cost of pharmaceuticals can be an important consideration for the elderly, many of whom are on limited and fixed incomes. The newer agents may only be approved for depressive illness and not for OCD. In countries with pharmaceutical benefits schemes, the cost of such medicines for OCD in the absence of depression may thus be prohibitive for some old people.

The choice of drug to treat OCD must be made on the basis of efficacy, tolerability (which relates to side-effects especially those noted of particular relevance to the elderly), safety in overdosage (considering the risk of depressive comorbidity and the risk of overdosage), and the availability and cost when assessed in the context of the individual's clinical status, medical condition and other treatments.

The duration of treatment needs to be for a minimum of 10 to 12 weeks. Clinically adequate response may take several weeks, often longer than the response to antidepressants for depression. The normal duration of treatment will be six to twelve months if there is a satisfactory response to medication. After such a period of reasonable clinical remission, one can attempt a gradual reduction of the medication dosage.

The relapse rate following discontinuation of 5-HT uptake inhibitors is high, nearly 90% being reported within two months by Pato et al. (1988). There are no data on relapse rates following discontinuation in the elderly. It is not known whether a gradual reduction in medication over a long period of time produces a lower relapse rate or not. At least one report (Pato et al., 1990) suggests that patients can be maintained successfully at lower doses than those required to produce initial treatment response.

There is a limited role for pharmacological combination treatment for OCD. If the patient is anxious, there may be a role for the addition of buspirone and in some instances benzodiazepines can be helpful in relieving episodic acute anxiety, but benzodiazepines may inhibit the response to behavior therapy. If the patient has recurrent depressions, lithium may be a useful adjunctive mood stabilizer. When the patient has delusional qualities, or in the presence of tics a neuroleptic particularly haloperidol might be helpful. In the presence of depressive illness, other antidepressants might be useful, and occasionally electroconvulsive therapy (ECT).

Combination therapy

In clinical practice, a combination of pharmacotherapy, particularly using the serotonin uptake inhibitors, and behavior therapy can prove most useful in helping patients (Perse, 1988). The medications can assist some patients in commencing behavior therapies when without pharmacotherapy they were too disabled to engage in such treatments. On the other hand, behavior therapy may facilitate a response at a lower dose of medicines than might otherwise have been necessary.

Psychosurgery

There remains a limited role for psychosurgery in those patients who have failed to respond to intensive behavioral and pharmacotherapies including a period of intensive inpatient treatment. About 20% of patients do not respond to behavior therapy, pharmacotherapy, or the combination (Perse, 1988). While these 20% may seem candidates for psychosurgery, the ideal neurosurgical treatment has not been defined (Chiocca & Martuza, 1990). Cingulotomy and subcaudate tractotomy have been used (Bartlett, Bridges & Kelly, 1981; Ballantine & Giriuonas, 1981) and improvements reported range from 50–100%. The numbers of patients studied are relatively few (192 in a total of ten studies from 1952), and there remains great scope for further detailed evaluation. The permanent nature of neurosurgical interventions, reluctance on the part of some patients and clinicians, and the effect of legislative constraints, will leave this as a minor area of treatment, though still a significant therapy for the few very disabled sufferers unresponsive to other treatments.

Obsessive–compulsive personality disorder

Historically it has been common for people to confuse obsessive–compulsive personality disorder (anakastic personality disorder) with obsessive–compulsive disorder. The characteristics of the personality disorder are that the person is perfectionistic, has a preoccupation with detail, wishes others to submit to their ways, tends to be devoted to work and work activities rather than friends and friendships, has a characteristic quality of being indecisive, over-conscientious and rather moralistic, taking to themselves the quality that their moral attitude is the correct one. It is claimed that people with this personality disorder tend to have a rather restricted expression of emotions, tend to lack generosity and to be rather retentive. Unlike OCD, this personality characteristic is said to be more common in men than women (American Psychiatric Association, 1987).

This disorder is different from OCD and is not coincidental with it. Lewis (1936) noted that 33% of people with obsessive–compulsive personality disorder did not have OCD while Pollitt (1957) noted that the outcome for these people was a tendency to depressive illness rather than to develop OCD. Rasmussen & Tsuang (1986) found that 50% of a sample of patients with OCD did not have obsessive–compulsive personality.

Summary

The central role for the clinician regarding OCD in the elderly is to recognize the disorder, to exclude other possible causes of obsessive and compulsive symptoms, and to institute effective treatment. Treatment should recognize the patient's age and the potential for adverse medication effects. It is helpful to monitor the patient's progress and recognize that a combination of pharmacotherapy and behavior therapy may be the most successful. Scales such as the Y-BOCS (see Appendix) can be helpful in tailoring treatment and monitoring the patient's overall status.

References

American Psychiatric Association (1987). *Diagnostic and Statistical Manual of Mental Disorders, Third Edition Revised.* Washington DC: American Psychiatric Association.

Ballantine, H. T. & Giriuonas, I. E. (1981). Treatment of intractable psychiatric illness and chronic pain by stereotactic cingulotomy. In *Operative Neurosurgical Techniques: Indications, Methods and Results*. Vol. 2, ed. H. H. Schmidek & W. H. Sweet, pp. 1069–1075. New York: Harcourt Brace Jovanovich.

Bartlett, J., Bridges, P. & Kelly, D. (1981). Comtemporary indications for psychosurgery. *British Journal of Psychiatry*, **138**, 507–54.

Baxter, L. R., Phelps, E., Mazziotta, J. C., Guze, B. H., Schwartz, J. M. & Selin, C. E. (1987). Local cerebral glucose metabolic rates in obsessive–compulsive disorder: a comparison with rates in unipolar depression and in normal controls. *Archives of General Psychiatry*, **44**, 211–18.

Baxter, L. R., Schwartz, J. M., Guze, B. H., Borgaman, K., Szuba, M. P. (1990). Neuroimaging in obsessive-compulsive disorder. *Journal of Clinical Brain Imaging*, **1**, 10–17.

Benkelfat, C., Murphy, D. L., Zohar, J., Hill, J. L., Grover, G. & Insel, T. R. (1989). Clomipramine in obsessive–compulsive disorder: further evidence for a serotonergic mechanism of action. *Archives of General Psychiatry*, **44**, 23–8.

Brown, F. W. (1942). Heredity in the Psychoneuroses. *Proceedings from the Royal Society of Medicine*, **35**, 785–97.

Chiocca, E. A. & Martuza, R. L. (1990). Neurosurgical therapy of obsessive–compulsive disorder. In *Obsessive–Compulsive Disorder: Theory and Management*. Ed. M. A. Jenicke, L. Baer & W. E. Minichiello. Chicago: Year Book Medical Publishers.

Coryell, W. H., Black, D. W., Kelly, M. W. & Noyes, R. (1989). HPA axis disturbance in obsessive–compulsive disorder. *Psychiatry Research*, **30**, 243–51.

Flament, M. F., Rapoport, J. L., Murphy, D. L., Burg, C. J. & Lake, C. R. (1987).

Biochemical changes during clomipramine treatment of childhood obsessive–compulsive disorder. *Archives of General Psychiatry*, **44**, 219–55.

Foa, E. B., Steketee, G. S. & Ozarow, B. J. (1985). Behavior therapy with obsessive–compulsives: from theory to treatment. In *Obsessive–Compulsive Disorders*. eds M. Mavissakalian, S. Turner, L. Micheleson, pp. 49–129. New York: Plenum.

Frankel, M., Cummings, J. L., Robertson, Trimble, M. R., Hill, M. A. & Benson, D. F. (1986). Obsessions and compulsions in Gilles de la Tourette's syndrome. *Neurology*, **36**, 378–82.

Goodman, W. K., Price, L. H. & Rasmussen S. A., Delgado, P., Meninger, G. R. & Charney, D. S. (1989*a*). Efficacy of fluvoxamine in obsessive–compulsive disorder. *Archives of General Psychiatry*, **46**, 36–44.

Goodman, W. K., Price L. H., Rasmussen S. A. et al. (1989*b*). The Yale Brown Obsessive–Compulsive Scale (Y-BOCS) Part 1: development, use and reliability. *Archives of General Psychiatry*, **46**, 1006–11.

Goodman W. K., Price L. H., Rasmussen S. A. et al. (1989*c*). The Yale Brown Obsessive–Compulsive Scale (Y-BOCS), Part 2: Validity. *Archives of General Psychiatry*, **46**, 1012–16.

Goodwin, D. W., Guze, S. B. & Robins, E,. (1969). Follow-up studies in obsessional neurosis. *Archives of General Psychiatry*, **20**, 182–7.

Greist, J. H. (1991). Fluvoxamine treatment of obsessive–compulsive disorder. *Biological Psychiatry*, **29** (Supplement), 4385.

Greist, J. H. (1992). An integrated approach to treatment of obsessive–compulsive disorder. *Journal Clinical Psychiatry*, **53**, 4(suppl).

Insel, T. R., Mueller, E. A., Gillin, J. C., Siever, L. J. & Murphy, D. L. (1984). Biological markers in obsessive–compulsive and affective disorders. *Journal of Psychiatric Research*, **18**, 407–25.

Jenike, M. A. & Brandon, A. D. (1988). Obsessive–compulsive disorder and head trauma: a rare association. *Journal of Anxiety Disorders*, **2**, 353–9.

Lewis, A. J. (1936). Problems of obsessional illness. *Proceedings of the Royal Society of Medicine*, **29**, 194–8.

Luxenberg, J. S., Swedo, S. E., Flament, M. F., Friedland, R. P., Rapoport, J. & Rapoport, S. I. (1988). Neuroanatomical abnormalities in obsessive–compulsive disorder detected with quantitative X-ray computed tomography. *American Journal Psychiatry*, **145**, 1089–93.

Maguire, K. P., Schweitzer, I., Biddle, N., Bridge, S. & Tiller, J. W. G. (1987). The dexamethasone suppression test: importance of dexamethasone concentrations. *Biological Psychiatry*, **22**, 957–67.

Marks, I. M. (1981). *Cure and Care of Neuroses: Theory and Practice of Behavioral Psychotherapy*. New York: Wiley.

Meyer, V. (1966). Modification of expectations in cases with obsessional rituals. *Behavioral Research and Therapy*, **4**, 273–80.

Myers, J. K., Weissman, M. M., Tischler, et al. (1984). Six month prevalence of psychiatric disorders in three communities 1980 to 1982. *Archives of General Psychiatry*, **41**, 949–58.

Pato, M. T., Zohar-Kadouch, R., Zohar, J. & Murphy, D. L. (1988). Return of symptoms after discontinuation of clomipramine in patients with obsessive–compulsive disorder. *American Journal of Psychiatry*, **145**, 1521–25.

Pato, M. T., Hill J. L. & Murphy, D. L. (1990). A clomipramine dosage reduction in the course of long-term treatment of obsessive–compulsive disorder patients. *Psychopharmacology Bulletin*, **26**, 211–14.

Perse, T. (1988). Obsessive–compulsive disorder: a treatment review. *Journal of Clinical Psychiatry*, **49**, 48–55.

Pigott, T. A., Pato, M. T., Bernstein, S. E. et al. (1990). Controlled comparisons of clomipramine and fluoxetine in the treatment of obsessive–compulsive disorder. *Archives of General Psychiatry*, **47**, 926–32.

Pollitt, J. (1957). Natural history of obsessional states. *British Medical Journal*, **1**, 194–8.

Rachman, S. J. & Hodgson, R. J., (1980). *Obsessions and Compulsions*. Englewood Cliffs, N.J.: Prentice-Hall.

Rapoport, J. L. (1989). The biology of obsessions and compulsions. *Scientific American*, **260**, 62–9.

Rasmussen, S. A. & Tsuang, M. T. (1986). DSM-III Obsessive–compulsive disorder: clinical characteristics and family history. *American Journal of Psychiatry*, **143**, 317–22.

Rasmussen, S. A. & Eisen, J. L. (1988). Clinical and epidemiological findings of significance to neuropharmacologic trials in obsessive–compulsive disorder. *Psychopharmacology Bulletin*, **24**, 466–70.

Rasmussen, S. A. & Eisen, J. L. (1990). Epidemiology and clinical features of obsessive–compulsive disorder. In *Obsessive–Compulsive Disorder: Theory and Management*. Ed. M. A. Jenicke, L. Baer & W. E. Minichiello, pp. Chicago: Year Book Medical Publishers.

Rasmussen, S. A. & Eisen, J. L. (1992). Epidemiology and differential diagnosis of obsessive–compulsive disorder. *Journal of Clinical Psychiatry*, **53** (4), 2–10.

Ravenholdt, R. T. & Foege, W. H. (1982). 1918 Influenza, encephalitis lethargica, Parkinsonism. *Lancet*, **ii**, 860–3.

Robins, L. N., Helzer, J. E., Weissman, M. M. et al. (1984). Lifetime prevalence of specific psychiatric disorders in three sites. *Archives of General Psychiatry*, **41**, 958–67.

Schweitzer, I., Maguire, K. P., Gee, A., Tiller, J. W. G., Biddle, N. & Davies, B. (1987). Prediction of outcome in depressed patients by weekly monitoring with the dexamethasone suppression test. *British Journal of Psychiatry*, **151**, 780–4.

Tiller, J. W. G., Biddle, N., Maguire, K. P. & Davies, B. M. (1987). The dexamethasone suppression test and plasma dexamethasone in generalized anxiety disorder. *Biological Psychiatry*, **23**, 261–70.

Turner, S. M., Jacob, R. G., Beidel, D. C. & Himmelhoch, J. (1985). Fluoxetine treatment of obsessive–compulsive disorder. *Journal of Clinical Psychopharmacology*, **5**, 207–12.

Zohar, J. & Insel, T. R. (1987). Obsessive–compulsive disorder: psychobiological approaches to diagnosis, treatment and pathophysiology. *Biological Psychiatry*, **22**, 667–87.

Appendix: Yale-Brown obsessive-compulsive scale (Y-BOCS)

Adapted from Goodman et al. (1989b, c)

Patient name: **Date:**

Screening Questions For Obsessions:

'Do you have unwanted ideas, images or impulses that seem silly, nasty or horrible?'

More Detailed Questions to Elicit Specific Obsessions:

1. 'Do you worry excessively about dirt, germs or chemicals?'
2. 'Are you constantly concerned that harm will occur because you have left something important undone – like locking the door or windows or turning off appliances?'
3. 'Do you fear you will act or speak aggressively when you really don't want to?'
4. 'Are you always afraid you will lose something of importance?'

If some obsessions are evident, determine the severity by using the rating scale below and similarly rate compulsions on the reverse side of this page.

Obsession rating scale
Circle appropriate score

Item			None	Mild	Moderate	Severe	Extreme
1.	Time spent on Obsessions		0 hrs/day	0–1	1–3	3–8	> 8
		Score	0	1	2	3	4
2.	Interference from Obsessions		None	Mild	Manageable	Severe	Incapacitating
		Score	0	1	2	3	4
3.	Distress from Obsessions		None	Mild	Moderate	Severe	Disabling
		Score	0	1	2	3	4
4.	Resistance		Always resists	Much resistance	Some resistance	Often yields	Completely yields
		Score	0	1	2	3	4
5.	Control over Obsessions		Complete control	Much control	Moderate control	Little control	No control
		Score	0	1	2	3	4

Obsession subtotal (add items 1–5) ☐

Screening Questions for Compulsions/Rituals:
'Are there things you feel compelled to do to excess or thoughts you must think repeatedly, in order to feel comfortable?'
Questions to Elicit Specific Rituals:
1. 'Do you wash yourself or your environment excessively?'

2. 'Do you have to check things over and over again or repeat them numerous times to be sure they are done properly?'
3. 'Do you avoid situations or people you worry about harming by aggressive words or deeds?'
4. 'Do you feel you can't safely discard things so that you keep many useless objects?'

Obsession rating scale
Circle appropriate score

Item			None	Mild	Moderate	Severe	Extreme
6.	Time spent on Compulsions		0 hrs/day	0–1	1–3	3–8	> 8
		Score	0	1	2	3	4
7.	Interference from Compulsions		None	Mild	Manageable	Severe	Incapacitating
		Score	0	1	2	3	4
8.	Distress from Compulsions		None	Mild	Moderate	Severe	Disabling
		Score	0	1	2	3	4
9.	Resistance		Always resists	Much resistance	Some resistance	Often yields	Completely yields
		Score	0	1	2	3	4
10.	Control over Compulsions		Complete control	Much control	Moderate control	Little control	No control
		Score	0	1	2	3	4

Compulsion subtotal (add items 6–10) ☐
Y-BOCS total (add items 1–10) ☐

Total Y-BOCS score: range of Obsessive–Compulsive Disorder Severity
0 – None 10 – Mild 20 – Moderate 30 – Severe 40 – Extreme

6

Generalized anxiety and phobic disorders

JAMES LINDESAY SUBE BANERJEE

Introduction

Anxiety and fear are affective components of a large number of psychiatric disorders. It has been calculated that 54 of the 208 disorders in the American Psychiatric Association's DSM-III-R classification (1987) include anxiety or fear to some extent (Delprato & McGlynn, 1984). As well as being part of other syndromes however, they also form the core of their own set of disorders, namely the generalized anxiety, phobic and panic disorders. Panic disorders are discussed in Chapter 5; this chapter will focus on generalized anxiety disorder (GAD) and phobic disorders in the elderly.

While dementia and depression in the elderly have been extensively researched, it has not been until comparatively recently that anxiety disorders have received similar attention. The reasons for this are complex, and include the ideas that anxiety and fear are a normal and reasonable part of old age, that anxiety disorders are not important in the elderly, and also therapeutic nihilism on the part of clinicians. These preconceptions do not appear to be supported by research. For example, in the Epidemiologic Catchment Area (ECA) study, a 4.8% prevalence rate of phobic disorder in people over the age of 65 was identified in five areas of the United States (Regier et al., 1988). This is a small but significant minority of people who are high consumers of health and social services' resources, and there are therapeutic strategies which can effectively address their anxiety and phobias.

This chapter will outline the clinical syndromes of GAD and phobic disorder in the elderly. It will review their epidemiology, discuss etiological theories and address the problems of comorbidity with other clinical syndromes, differential diagnosis and management.

Clinical features

Phobic disorders

Phobia is defined as a persistent and irrational fear of a specific object, activity or situation that results in a compelling desire to avoid the dreaded object, activity or situation (the phobic stimulus) (DSM-III-R; American Psychiatric Association, 1987). Phobias generally are subdivided into agoraphobia, social phobia and simple or specific phobias. In agoraphobia the stimulus is a situation in which there might be difficulty or embarrassment in escaping; this includes being outside the home or travelling. Social phobia refers to fear of situations where the individual may act in a humiliating or embarrassing way such as eating or speaking in public. In simple or specific phobias, the stimulus may be any circumscribed object or situation, such as dogs or heights.

It appears that the types of phobia reported by the elderly are broadly similar to those found in younger populations. They include: going out alone, travelling, enclosed spaces, insects, being alone at home and animals (Lindesay, Briggs & Murphy, 1989). Some phobias such as social phobia appear to be less common in the elderly. The consequence of phobic avoidance in the elderly may be the affected person becoming housebound and therefore a drain on family or social services resources. Such behavior may also be reinforced by such support.

Generalized anxiety disorder

This is defined as generalized, persistent anxious mood with motor tension, autonomic symptoms, apprehensiveness and hypervigilance. There does not appear to be any difference between the form of GAD in the elderly and in younger individuals. The content of the worries is the same as those which normally concern elderly people, and include physical illness, money problems, the possibility of being a victim of crime and the health and safety of their families. The somatic symptoms of anxiety are the same as those found in younger age groups. However, in the elderly they may be misattributed to physical illness with the result that the affected individual receives unnecessary investigation and medication but does not receive effective treatment for his or her anxiety disorder. Conversely, Shamoian (1991) has suggested that the diagnosis of GAD may be wrongly attributed to elderly people because of their physical frailty and vulnerability. The difficulties associated with GAD as a diagnostic entity and with its diagnosis and differential diagnosis are discussed below.

Epidemiology

Low rates of anxiety disorders have been reported as primary psychiatric diagnoses in inpatient psychiatric settings and also in outpatient and casualty departments. Rates are higher, however, in primary care settings. There is an accumulation of chronic cases of psychiatric disorder with age (Shepherd et al., 1981) but a marked decrease in new consultations for anxiety disorders. This results in a decrease in primary care consultation rates for anxiety disorders. Consultation rates for ICD-9 anxiety disorder have been estimated to decrease from 43.7 per 1000 population at risk in the 45–65 age group to 36.6 in the 65–74 group and 30.4 in the over 75s. The equivalent figures for phobic disorders are 2.4, 1.5 and 0.8 per 1000 population at risk (OPCS, 1986).

Community prevalence studies have identified cases using standardized diagnostic systems such as the DSM-III (American Psychiatric Association, 1980) and the Geriatric Mental State (GMS)/AGECAT system (Copeland et al., 1976; Copeland, Dewey & Griffiths-Jones, 1986). These contain explicit diagnostic criteria and therefore increase the reliability of case definition, but their validity in relation to anxiety disorder in the elderly may be questioned on the grounds of their variable use of hierarchies and reasonableness criteria and also their differing ideas of what constitutes anxiety disorders.

The GMS/AGECAT system allots a diagnostic label on an hierarchical basis with anxiety disorders and other neuroses at the bottom; similarly, DSM-III has exclusion criteria so that a diagnosis of an anxiety disorder cannot be made if another condition such as a major depression is present. Given the comorbidity of anxiety disorders with other diagnoses, these systems may underestimate their true rate and obscure important associations (Lindesay & Banerjee, 1993). Inclusion of reasonableness criteria for fear and anxiety in a diagnostic system introduces a possible bias because of ageist assumptions on the part of the interviewer. Finally, the diagnostic algorithms of these systems are based on ideas of which symptoms should be considered morbid and which should not, and this may lead to an operationalized over- or underdiagnosis.

Phobic Disorder

In the ECA surveys, phobic disorders have been reported to be the most common psychiatric disorder in women and the second most common disorder (after cognitive impairment) in men over 65 years of age (Myers et al., 1984). Prevalence figures from the ECA surveys (Myers et al., 1984; Regier et al., 1988), the community studies of London, New York and Liverpool carried out by Copeland et al. (1987*a*, *b*) and a study of an urban community sample which used

Table 6.1. *Prevalence of cases of phobic disorders in subjects over 65 years of age*

	Area	System	Number	Period	Social phobia	Simple phobia	Agoraphobia	Total phobia
Myers et al., 1984	New Haven	DSM-III	611	6 months		4.7	2.8	5.9
	Baltimore	DSM-III	923	6 months	2.2	11.8	5.8	13.4
	St. Louis	DSM-III	576	6 months	1.2	4.5	2.7	5.4
Regier et al., 1988	5 Sites ECA	DSM-III	5702	1 month				4.8
Lindesay et al., 1989	London	PDS	890	1 month	1.3	2.1	7.8	10.0
Copeland et al., 1987*a*	Liverpool	GMS/AGECAT	1070	1 month				0.7
Copeland et al., 1987*b*	New York	GMS/AGECAT	445	1 month				0.0
	London	GMS/AGECAT	396	1 month				0.0

nonhierarchical and nonjudgmental criteria (Lindesay et al., 1989) are presented in Table 6.1. All figures refer to people over the age of 65.

The differences in the rates of phobic disorder reported may be due to the differences in the instruments used, discussed above. The highest rates (apart from the results from the Baltimore site of the ECA whose validity have been questioned) were found in the study which used a nonhierarchical and nonjudgmental system. The lowest rates were found in the studies using the GMS/AGECAT system at the diagnostic syndrome case level. Subcase level phobia was identified in 4.9% of the Liverpool sample which suggests that the very low reported levels of diagnostic syndrome cases may be due to higher severity criteria as well as the hierarchy.

Evidence on the incidence rates of phobic disorders in the elderly is still sparse. Eaton et al. (1989), however, reported the incidence of DSM-III phobic disorders as 2.66 per 100 person–years at risk for men, 5.52 for women and 4.29 in all people over 65 years of age. Larkin et al. (1992) in a three year follow-up study of a community sample using the GMS/AGECAT system made a minimum estimate of 4.4 new cases of neurosis (phobic, anxiety and obsessive compulsive disorders) per 1000 population at risk per year.

Generalized anxiety disorder

The number of people attracting the diagnosis of GAD has decreased as specific conditions such as panic disorder and post-traumatic stress disorder have been subtracted from it. Indeed, DSM-III-R states that 'when other disorders that could account for the anxiety symptoms are ruled out, the disorder is not commonly diagnosed in clinical samples'. Uhlenhuth et al. (1983, 1984) estimated a one-year prevalence rate of 7.1% of a DSM-III-like 'generalized anxiety syndrome' which increased with age and was more common in women. No data on GAD are available from the first wave of the ECA studies but the second wave has reported a 2.2% prevalence rate with no exclusions (Blazer, George & Hughes, 1991). Lindesay et al. (1989) found a one-month prevalence rate of 3.7% using a symptom scale with a validated cut-off point. The GMS/AGECAT surveys (Copeland et al., 1987*a, b*) found rates of 'anxiety neurosis' of 1.1% in Liverpool, 1.1% in London and 0.7% in New York. Subcase level 'anxiety neurosis' was much more common at 17.4% in Liverpool, 17.2% in London and 16.0% in New York.

Etiological factors

Reports of a lower level of anxiety disorders in the elderly compared to younger populations have prompted some to postulate an age-related difference in the psychological mechanisms leading to anxiety. Jarvik and Russell (1979) proposed that a 'freeze' reaction might replace the 'flight or fight' response. They described this novel method of responding to threat as 'acceptance, contemplation and reflection' and hypothesized that this might lead to the elderly developing psychosomatic rather than anxiety disorders. Kastenbaum (1984) suggested a different mechanism; that in old age novel stimuli may be treated as familiar so losing their salience and their capacity to provoke anxiety. However, the findings that the decrease in the prevalence of anxiety disorders with age in community populations is much less than that in clinical populations, and that the rate of self-reported anxiety symptoms increases with age call into question the basis of these hypotheses.

Other possible explanations for the changes in the rates of these disorders with age include differential survival of people who have anxiety disorders and those who are susceptible to them, with early death possibly mediated by factors such as physical illness, smoking and alcohol abuse. Another theory is that cognitive impairment may be incompatible with anxiety if the memory of anxiety-provoking stimuli is not recalled. Sampling bias in community surveys such as those mentioned above also may be a factor, either by failing to sample institutional settings where elderly people with anxiety disorders may be concentrated, or by failing to interview them since they may be less likely to answer their doors or consent to be interviewed by investigators because of their anxiety.

The relationship between socioeconomic status and anxiety disorders is not clear cut. Several studies (e.g. Bergman, 1971; Gurland & Cross, 1982; Lindesay, 1991) have found no evidence of association, while Himmelfarb and Murrell (1984) reported an association between low socioeconomic status and high self-reported rates of anxiety symptoms.

There seems to be little association between psychosocial factors such as retirement, bereavement and absence of confiding relationships and anxiety disorders in the elderly (Bergmann, 1971; Kay & Bergmann, 1980; Gurland and Cross, 1982; Lindesay, 1991). In a case-control study of phobic disorder in the elderly (Lindesay, 1991), however, an association was found between phobic disorder and parental loss before the age of 18 due to death or separation. It may be that childhood loss leads to the development of avoidant cognitive traits and therefore a vulnerability to develop phobic disorder in response to age-specific threats. If a combination of cognitive traits and age-specific threats are involved in the development of phobic disorders, then an important age-specific threat in the elderly appears to be episodes of physical illness. Lindesay (1991) found that cases of agoraphobia were predominantly of late onset and were most commonly attributed to physical illness events. Specific phobias were generally of early onset and had often been present in those who developed late-onset agoraphobias. The relationship between personality variables and anxiety disorders has not been widely investigated. Abnormal 'insecure/rigid' or 'anxious/hysterical' personality traits were found to be associated with late-onset neuroses by Bergmann (1971). He suggested that the development of neuroses in this age group was due to the interaction between episodes of physical illness and a vulnerable personality.

Anxiety disorders and physical illness

There is a complex relationship between physical illness and anxiety disorders in the elderly. Kay and Bergmann (1966) found anxiety disorders to be associated with increased mortality, while Larkin et al. (1992) found a death rate no higher than would have been expected in the general population at three-year follow-up. Also, greater levels of gastrointestinal, cardiovascular and respiratory complaints have been reported in elderly people with anxiety disorders (Bergmann, 1971; Lindesay, 1990).

Anxiety secondary to physical illness

Anxiety may be secondary to physical illness either by being a direct expression of the underlying pathology or as an emotional reaction to physical illness. A list of some of the more common physical disorders which may present with anxiety in old age is presented in Table 6.2. It is therefore important that assessment of the anxious elderly person should include a physical examination to exclude the possibility of a primary physical etiology.

Agoraphobic avoidance is one response to a traumatic physical health event; worry about physical illnesses and disability also may result in the development of generalized anxiety states in some cases. For example, Peach and Pathy (1979) reported that myocardial infarction in the elderly is often followed by the development of mild anxiety symptoms, and that rarely a severe, disabling 'cardiac neurosis' can develop.

Physical illness secondary to anxiety

Physical illness may develop in individuals with anxiety disorders because of the effects of palliative coping mechanisms such as smoking and alcohol abuse. Smoking may be a factor in the increased rates of cardiovascular and respiratory illnesses observed in the elderly who have anxiety disorders, although smoking did not account for the excess in ischemic heart disease found in 40 to 64 year old men with phobic disorders in the Northwick Park Heart Study (Haines, Imeson & Meade, 1987). They proposed that either hyperventilation caused by phobic anxiety might lead to coronary artery spasm or that there might be exaggerated hormonal responses to myocardial infarction in people with phobic disorders.

Table 6.2. *Physical disorders which may present with anxiety*

Cardiovascular
myocardial infarction
cardiac arrhythmias
orthostatic hypotension
Respiratory
pneumonia
pulmonary embolism
emphysema
asthma
hypoxia
chronic obstructive airways disease
Endocrine
hypo- and hyperthyroidism
hypo- and hypercalcaemia
Cushing's disease
carcinoid syndrome
insulinoma
phaeochromocytoma
Metabolic
hypo- and hypercalcemia
hyperkalemia
hypoglycemia
vitamin deficiency
Neurological
head injury
cerebral tumor
dementia
delirium
epilepsy
migraine
cerebral lupus erythematosis
demyelinating disorders
vestibular disturbances
subarachnoid hemorrhage
CNS infections
Drug-related
caffeine
sympathomimetics
dopamine agonists
corticosteroids
withdrawal syndromes
akathisia
digoxin toxicity

Anxiety disorders and other mental disorders

Depression

There is a high level of comorbidity between anxiety and depression at all ages. Boyd et al. (1984) found that agoraphobia was 15 times more common in those people with major depression using hierarchy-free DSM-III criteria, and using the GMS/AGECAT system anxiety disorders were 20 times more prevalent in depressed than in nondepressed subjects (Kay, 1988). Anxiety may be secondary to depression, or depression may develop because of anxiety, and the social impairment associated with it. It is also possible for anxiety and depression to arise together because of the same underlying disorder, such as hypothyroidism. Recently, Goldberg and Huxley (1992) have put forward a persuasive model of the common psychiatric disorders in which comorbidity between the symptomatic dimensions of anxiety and depression is explained in terms of latent trait analysis 'in which it is assumed that responses to a particular test instrument are all reflections of one or more underlying variables which cannot be observed directly'. They go on to suggest that traditional categories of what we used to call neurosis, such as hysteria, phobia and somatization, can be understood merely as different ways of responding to the basic experiences of anxiety and depression.

The clinical impression that late-onset anxiety is almost inevitably associated with depression may be due more to the characteristics of those who negotiate their way through the filters on the way to specialist psychiatric care rather than to the population of people with late-onset anxiety as a whole. Lindesay (1991) found that 19 out of 60 cases of phobia in the elderly were also depressed. In this study the idea that anxiety disorders are always secondary to depression was not confirmed; in only four cases were the phobic disorders assessed by the interviewing psychiatrist as being secondary to the depression, while the depression was judged to be secondary to the phobia in six cases. In this study there was also an increased past history of depression in people with phobic disorders, which is compatible with the hypothesis of Blazer, Hughes & Fowler, (1989) that in some cases anxiety may arise during episodes of depression and then persist afterwards.

Because of the high level of comorbidity between depression and anxiety, in clinical practice it is often not useful to attempt strictly to divide the two. It is usually more useful to look for the presence of the two sets of symptoms. Along with the 'biological' features of depression the presence of hypochondriasis, anhedonia, guilt, agitation, and panic attacks indicate the presence of an associated depressive disorder. An assessment of the temporal relationship of the anxiety and the depression should be made, with the use of a collateral informant history if possible, and then both the depressive and the anxiety elements may need to be treated in order to improve the problem as a whole.

Organic disorders

There does not appear to be a positive association between dementia and anxiety disorders (Eisdorfer, Cohen & Keckich, 1981; Lindesay et al., 1989), although the evidence from many large community studies is difficult to interpret because of their use of hierarchical systems with organic disorders at the top, and also because many do not include institutions where people with dementia may be concentrated.

Subjective complaints of memory impairment may be the primary presentation of anxiety disorders in the elderly; however, in these cases no objective evidence of cognitive impairment has been identified (Philpot & Levy, 1987). Use and abuse of anxiolytic medication may also complicate the assessment of cognition. Just as anxiety disorders may present as dementia, early dementia may present as anxiety. Cognitive testing may be difficult to interpret in these cases, especially if the subject is using anxiolytic medication, and a definitive diagnosis may only be able to be made with time as the cognitive impairment increases and becomes clear.

Delirium may present as anxiety in the elderly. This anxiety may be in response to hallucinations and delusions. In practice, diagnosis is not usually a problem if a full history and examination is performed and features of delirium such as fluctuating level of consciousness, attentional deficit and perceptual disturbances are identified.

Schizophrenia

As with delirium, the emotional responses to the frightening abnormal perceptual experiences of a paranoid psychosis may appear to be an anxiety disorder. Again with a full history and mental state examination the psychosis will usually be revealed.

Prognosis

There have been few studies of the course and outcome of anxiety disorders in the elderly, particularly late-onset cases. In their review of studies of general adult populations, Marks and Lader (1973) concluded that 41 to 59% of cases of anxiety neurosis (generalized anxiety and panic) were recovered or much improved at one to 20-year follow-up. Noyes and Clancy (1976) found that 33% of their patient sample was unchanged or worse at five-year follow-up, and that age of onset was a predictor of outcome in anxiety neurosis, with older men having a worse prognosis. In a recent three-year follow-up of neurotic disorder in an elderly community sample, Larkin et al. (1992) found that, while caseness did not persist over time, subjects did not recover fully and the predominant symptom tended to change. This supports the notion that specific anxiety and depressive syndromes may, in fact, be manifestations of a general neurotic syndrome with a chronic course and variable symptomatology.

Management

The basic principles of the management of anxiety disorders in the elderly are the same as for any psychiatric disorder. The presence of a problem needs to be recognized, then the nature and extent of that problem must be defined by taking a thorough history from the subject, and an informant if possible, and then by performing an examination of the person's mental and physical state. After further investigations an intervention needs to be planned and implemented.

Most anxiety disorders in the elderly go unrecognized and untreated in the community. When they are noticed, the general practitioner is most likely to prescribe a benzodiazepine hypnotic for associated insomnia rather than to address the underlying anxiety and depressive disorders. These disorders are concentrated in the community and need to be effectively managed by primary health care teams. The role of the specialist psychogeriatric service is probably best focused on passing expertise in assessment and effective intervention to the primary health care team rather than on managing these people directly.

As well as benefits for the patient, medical and social services may profit from treating elderly people with these disorders. Some are high users of health and social services and effective treatment may decrease their use by addressing problems leading to high levels of inappropriate attendance.

Psychological interventions

The psychological management of anxiety disorders in the elderly is essentially the same as in other age groups. While there have not been any large treatment evaluation studies, there are case studies of the successful use of systematic desensitization in elderly people with agoraphobia and specific phobias (Leng, 1985; Woods & Britton, 1985). It is important to ensure that treatment is accompanied by the withdrawal of unnecessary family and social domiciliary support since the continued presence of these reinforcers of the anxiety-related behaviors will undermine any intervention.

Anxiety management techniques for the elderly have been described by Garrison (1978) and Woods & Britton (1985). They can be carried out by any trained member of the primary health care team anywhere, and tape recordings can be used by the elderly people alone. As with systematic desensitization, this may be carried out individually or in groups. Cognitive therapy and cognitive behavioral therapy (McCarthy, Katy & Foa, 1991) can also be used as a component of anxiety management training in this age group.

Drug treatment

It is a general principle that drug treatment for anxiety cannot be recommended unless the disorder is severe, episodic, associated with a significant depressive disorder, or occurs in specific unavoidable circumstances. There are, however, differences between countries, with the use of anxiolytic medication being advocated more in the United States than in Britain. Among the drugs that have been used for anxiety in the elderly are: benzodiazepines, antidepressants, barbiturates, antipsychotics, beta blockers and newer compounds such as buspirone.

There has been much concern about the use of benzodiazepines because of problems such as dependence, tolerance and memory impairment (Tyrer, 1980; Curran, 1986). With the alteration in pharmacokinetics with age, elderly people are particulary prone to these problems and the long half-lives of many of these compounds lead to accumulation and consequently to drowsiness, falls, fractures, incontinence and even to delirium (Evans & Jarvis, 1972). These problems underline the importance of avoiding starting elderly people on long-term treatment and also of avoiding increasing the dose of benzodiazepines as tolerance to them develops. There is a place for these drugs in the short-term management of acute and severe anxiety in the elderly, when a short-acting benzodiazepine with no active metabolites such as oxazepam is to be preferred. Elderly people who have been long-term users of these drugs should, whenever possible, have the problem discussed with them and then be weaned off them (Higgitt, 1988).

Antidepressants are of value if there is depression associated with the anxiety. If they are used, then the same doses and administration as for the treatment of depression apply (see Chapters 12 and 25). The newer 5-HT reuptake inhibitors, such as fluoxetine and paroxetine, with their low level of side-effects are good drugs of first choice. The use of monoamine oxidase inhibitors, such as phenelzine, has been advocated; they are well tolerated by the elderly and are sometimes effective in phobic states associated with panic. Unless side-effects are intolerable, a trial of antidepressants should continue for at least six weeks before being abandoned.

Barbiturate use is associated with high levels of dependency, delirium and dangerous withdrawal states; they are also extremely toxic in overdose. They should never be started as a treatment for anxiety or insomnia and those patients who are found to be on these treatments should be carefully weaned off them if at all possible.

Propranolol has been used in an attempt to control the somatic symptoms of anxiety; however, its side-effects such as hypotension, bronchoconstriction, nightmares and insomnia limit its usefulness in the elderly. The side-effects of antipsychotics which are detailed elsewhere (Chapter 25) also mean that they cannot be recommended for the long-term management of anxiety disorders. It is also possible that drug-induced akathisia may mimic somatic symptoms of anxiety. The place of newer compounds such as buspirone in the management of anxiety disorders has yet to be established. While they have been reported to be well tolerated, and there seems to be no evidence of abuse or dependence, experience of their use in the elderly is limited, and the gradual onset of action makes them unsuitable for the treatment of acute anxiety states.

References

American Psychiatric Association (1980). *Diagnostic and Statistical Manual of Mental Disorders*, 3rd edition. Washington: American Psychiatric Association.

American Psychiatric Association (1987). *Diagnostic and Statistical Manual of Mental Disorders*, 3rd edition revised. Washington: American Psychiatric Association.

Bergmann, K. (1971). The neuroses of old age. In *Recent Developments in Psychogeriatrics*, ed. D. W. K. Kay and A. Walk, pp. 39–50. Kent: Headley Bros.

Blazer, D. G., Hughes, D. C. & Fowler, N. (1989). Anxiety as an outcome symptom of depression in elderly and middle-aged adults. *International Journal of Geriatric Psychiatry*, **4**, 273–8.

Blazer, D. G., George, L. K. & Hughes, D. (1991). The epidemiology of anxiety disorders: an age comparison. In *Anxiety in the Elderly*, ed. C. Salzman and B. D. Lebowitz. New York: Springer Pub. Co.

Boyd, J. H., Burke, J. D., Gruenberg, E., et al. (1984). Exclusion criteria of DSM-III: a study of co-occurrence of hierarchy-free syndromes. *Archives of General Psychiatry*, **41**, 983–9.

Copeland, J. R. M., Kelleher, M. J., Kellett, J. M., et al. (1976). A semi-structured clinical interview for the assessment of diagnosis and mental state in the elderly: the Geriatric Mental State Schedule: 1, development and reliability. *Psychological Medicine*, **6**, 439–59.

Copeland, J. R. M., Dewey, M. E. & Griffiths-Jones, H. M. (1986). Psychiatric case nomenclature and a computerized diagnostic system for elderly subjects: GMS and AGECAT. *Psychological Medicine*, **16**, 89–99.

Copeland, J. R. M., Dewey M. E., Wood, N., Searle, R., Davidson, I. A. & McWilliam, C. (1987*a*). Range of mental illness among the elderly in the community: prevalence in Liverpool using the GMS-AGECAT package. *British Journal of Psychiatry*, **150**, 815–23.

Copeland, J. R. M., Gurland, B. J., Dewey, M. E., Kelleher, M. J., Smith, A. M. R. & Davidson, I. A. (1987*b*). Is there more dementia, depression and neurosis in New York? A comparative study of the elderly in New York and London using the computer diagnosis AGECAT. *British Journal of Psychiatry*, **151**, 466–73.

Curran, H. V. (1986). Tranquillising memories: a review of the effects of benzodiazepines on human memory. *Biological Psychiatry*, **23**, 179–213.

Delprato, D. J. & McGlynn, F. D. (1984). Behavioral theories of anxiety disorders. In *Behavior Theories and Treatment of Anxiety*, ed. S. M. Turner. New York: Plenum Press.

Eaton, W. W., Kramer, M., Antony, J. C., Dryman, A., Shapiro, S. & Locke, B. Z. (1989). The incidence of specific DIS/DSM-III mental disorders: data from the NIMH Epidemiologic Catchment Area Program. *Acta Psychiatrica Scandinavica*, **79**, 163–178.

Eisdorfer, C., Cohen, D. & Keckich, W. (1981). Depression and anxiety in the cognitively impaired elderly. In *Anxiety: new research and changing concepts*, Ed. D. F. Klein, J. Rabkin, New York: Raven Press.

Evans, J. G. & Jarvis, E. H. (1972). Nitrazepam and the elderly. *British Medical Journal*, **iv**, 487.

Garrison, J. E. (1978). Stress management training in the elderly: a psychoeducational approach. *Journal of the American Geriatrics Society*, **26**, 397–403.

Goldberg, D. & Huxley, P. (1992) *Common Mental Disorders – A Bio-Social Model*. London: Routledge.

Gurland, B. J. & Cross, P. (1982). The epidemiology of mental disorders in old age: some clinical implications. *The Psychiatric Clinics of North America: Aging*, **5**, 11–26.

Haines, A. P., Imeson, J. D. & Meade, T. W. (1987). Phobic anxiety and ischaemic heart disease. *British Medical Journal*, **280**, 297–9.

Higgitt, A. (1988). Indications for benzodiazepine prescriptions in the elderly. *International Journal of Geriatric Psychiatry*, **3**, 239–49.

Himmelfarb, S. & Murrell, S. A. (1984). The prevalence and correlates of anxiety symptoms in older adults. *Journal of Psychology*, **116**, 159–67.

Jarvik, L. F. & Russell, D. (1979). Anxiety, aging and the third emergency reaction. *Journal of Gerontology*, **34**, 197–200.

Kastenbaum, R. J. (1984). Habituation as a model of human aging. *International Journal of Aging and Human Development*, **12**, 159–70.

Kay, D. W. K. & Bergmann, K. (1966). Physical disability and mental health in old age. *Journal of Psychosomatic Research*, **10**, 3–12.

Kay, D. W. K. & Bergmann, K. (1980). Epidemiology of mental disorders among the aged in the community. In *Handbook of Mental Health and Aging*, ed. J. E. Birren and R. B. Sloane, pp. 34–56. Englewood Cliffs: Prentice-Hall.

Kay, D. W. K. (1988). Anxiety in the elderly. In *Handbook of Anxiety, Vol. 2: Classification, Etiological factors, and Associated disturbance*, ed. R. Noyes, M. Roth, and G. D. Burrows, pp. 289–310. Englewood Cliffs: Prentice-Hall.

Larkin, B. A., Copeland, J. R. M., Dewey, M. E. et al., (1992). The natural history of neurotic disorder in an elderly urban population. Findings from the Liverpool longitudinal study of continuing health in the community. *British Journal of Psychiatry*, **160**, 681–6.

Leng, N. (1985). A brief review of cognitive–behavioral treatments in old age. *Age and Aging*, **14**, 257–63.

Lindesay, J., Briggs, C. & Murphy E. (1989). The Guy's/Age Concern survey: prevalence rates of cognitive impairment, depression and anxiety in an urban elderly community. *British Journal of Psychiatry*, **155**, 317–29.

Lindesay, J. (1990). The Guy's/Age Concern Survey: physical health and psychiatric disorder in an urban elderly community. *International Journal of Geriatric Psychiatry*, **5**, 171–8.

Lindesay, J. (1991). Phobic disorders in the elderly. *British Journal of Psychiatry*, **159**, 531–41.

Lindesay, J. & Banerjee, S. (1993). Phobic disorders in the elderly: A comparrison of three diagnostic systems. *International Journal of Geriatric Psychiatry*, **8**, 387–93.

Marks, I. & Lader, M. (1973). Anxiety states (anxiety neurosis): a review. *The Journal of Nervous and Mental Disease*, **156**, 3–18.

McCarthy, P. R., Katy, I. R. & Foa, E. B. (1991). Cognitive–behavioral treatment of anxiety in the elderly: a proposed model. In *Anxiety in the Elderly*, ed. C. Salzman and B. D. Lebowitz. New York: Springer Pub. Co.

Myers, J. K., Weissman, M. M., Tischler, G. L. et al. (1984). Six month prevalence of psychiatric disorders in three communities: 1980–1982. *Archives of General Psychiatry*, **41**, 959–67.

Noyes, R. & Clancey, J. (1976). Anxiety neurosis: a five-year follow-up. *Journal of Nervous and Mental Disease*, **162**, 200–205.

OPCS (Office of Population Censuses and Surveys) (1986). *Morbidity statistics from general practice: Third National Study 1981–82*. London: HMSO.

Peach, H. & Pathy, J. (1979). Disability of the elderly following myocardial infarction. *Journal of the Royal College of Physicians*, **13**, 154–7.

Philpot, M. & Levy, R. (1987). A memory clinic for the early diagnosis of dementia. *International Journal of Geriatric Psychiatry*, **2**, 195–200.

Regier, D. A., Boyd, J. H., Burke, J. D. et al. (1988). One-month prevalence of mental disorders in the United States. *Archives of General Psychiatry*, **45**, 997–86.

Shamoian, C. A. (1991). What is anxiety in the elderly? In *Anxiety in the Elderly*, ed. C. Salzman and B. D. Lebowitz. New York: Springer Pub. Co.

Shepherd, M., Cooper, B., Brown, A. C. & Kalton, G. (1981). *Psychiatric Illness in General Practice*. Oxford: Oxford University Press.

Tyrer, P. (1980). Dependence on benzodiazepines. *British Journal of Psychiatry*, **137**, 576–7.

Uhlenhuth, E. H., Mitchell, B. B., Mellinger, G. D., Cisin, I. H. & Clinthorne, J. (1983). Symptom checklist syndromes in the general population. *Archives of General Psychiatry*, **40**, 1167–73.

Uhlenhuth, E. H., Balter, M. B., Mellinger, G. D., Cisin, I. H. & Clinthorne, J. (1984). Anxiety disorders: prevalence and treatment. *Current Medical Research and Opinion*, **8**, 37–47.

Woods, R. T. & Britton, P. G. (1985). *Clinical Psychology with the Elderly*. London: Croom Helm.

Part 4

Affective disorders

7

The epidemiology of affective disorders in old age

JOHN SNOWDON

Introduction

Epidemiological studies can give information on the distribution of the various mood disorders (in time and place), and alert us to factors that appear to influence that distribution. Certain situations and changes may predispose individuals to develop depression or elevation of mood, precipitate it, prolong its course or alleviate it. Such knowledge may allow us to take a preventative approach, or may help in planning our clinical interventions.

Awareness of the prevalence and incidence of mood disorders is important when planning health services, but we need also to know how effective our various health services are. What do the outcome studies show? Of those who might benefit from our interventions, what proportion are referred to appropriate services?

In this chapter, attention will be given to the prevalence of depressive and bipolar disorders among elderly people in the community and in institutional settings. The importance of physical disorders in relation to depression in old age will be stressed, with particular mention of Parkinson's Disease, cerebrovascular disorders and organic brain disease.

More detailed discussion of depression in residential and primary care settings will be found in Chapters 10 and 11. The relationship between rates of suicide and depression will be reviewed in Chapter 14.

Perhaps the most important question to ask (before attempting to identify depressive disorders in the community, hospital or elsewhere) is this: if we find it, what can we do about it? Is it worth knowing? As will be shown, the prevalence of depressive symptoms and syndromes in old age is high, especially among the physically ill. Enough studies have shown us that. What we need now are studies of different strategies of management and how they affect outcome, to tell us where to concentrate resources. Recent outcome studies are reviewed in the following chapter.

What is a case of depression?

Before discussing prevalence rates of depression among elderly people living in the community, we need to know how the various researchers define depression. Those studies focusing on depressive symptoms show much higher rates than those requiring diagnostic criteria to be fulfilled in order to register subjects as depressed. Blazer (1989) drew attention to the different ways in which depression can be construed. If regarded as a unitary phenomenon, with the various manifestations of depression forming a continuum, checklists and self-rating scales may be appropriate in assessing severity. The percentage labelled as depressed will depend on the threshold considered to divide normal from pathological degrees of depression. If the same subjects are assessed during structured clinical interviews, using recognized criteria such as DSM-III-R to define cases of depression, it is possible to determine how well the threshold corresponds to a separation of subjects without clinical depression from those fulfilling criteria for one of the depressive disorders.

Another construct of depression depends on assessment of function. If depressive symptoms are severe enough to impair social function or life satisfaction, or to interfere with other functions, the case is worthy of clinical attention. Blazer (1989) emphasized that, although categorical approaches to diagnosis have been widely adopted, other constructs of depression should be used to complement that approach if it is to be useful in diagnosis, planning and assessing response to treatment. The DSM-III-R works 'for some, but not all, depressive syndromes in late life'. For example, long-lasting depressive symptoms in association with chronic ill health could be considered an adjustment disorder, but cannot be diagnosed as such if they last more than 6 months (Blazer et al., 1991).

Discussing their community study, Blazer & Williams (1980) commented that much of what is called 'depression' in the elderly may actually represent decreased life satisfaction and periodic episodes of grief secondary to the physical, social and economic difficulties encountered by ageing individuals in the community. However, Blazer et al. (1989), using grade-of-membership analysis, could not demonstrate that 'demoralization' (a cluster of symptoms including poor self-esteem, hopelessness and perceived poor physical health, as described by Dohrenwend et al., 1980) had clinical validity. The term 'minor depression' does not appear in DSM-III-R, but has been found useful in describing subjects displaying decreased energy, self-blame, worry, irritability, poor sleep, hopelessness, etc., often in association with physical illness, but not fulfilling all criteria for major depression. Such a syndrome is common in primary care settings (Oxman et al., 1990).

Gurland et al. (1983) used the label 'depression' as an umbrella term for conditions (including life dissatisfaction, demoralization syndromes and grief reactions) which have in common a tendency to depressed mood, worry, apathy, tension and pessimism. 'Clinical depression', however, refers to depressions which are sufficiently persistent, disruptive or severe to warrant evaluation and treatment by a health care professional.

The question, 'What is a case?' has been answered differently in different studies. For example, it is probable that researchers vary in the degree to which they believe that a case is not a case if there are associated physical problems. Some researchers measure severity on depression scales (some being weighted with somatic items) with arbitrary cut-off points, whereas others rely on interview schedules that allow testing of whether criteria for particular categories are fulfilled. The classification of mood disorders in old age is unsatisfactory and confusing; Murphy (1986) was unable to answer whether there are, indeed, different categories of depression, or whether subgroups merely reflect dimensions of severity. This confusion is reflected in the wide range of reported prevalence rates.

Prevalence of depression in the community

Table 7.1 summarizes a number of prevalence studies of depressive disorders among elderly people living in the community.

The Comprehensive Assessment and Referral Evaluation (CARE) was employed by Gurland et al. (1983) in lengthy interviews with 841 elderly persons in New York and London. About 20% were described as depressed, including 13% who were pervasively, i.e. clinically depressed. About 4% had vegetative symptoms and their depression could not be attributed to overwhelming stress, and half of these had an episodic history. These researchers found a strong and consistent relationship between the presence of depression and of physical illness (correlation coefficient = 0.4). Under the age of 75 years, depression was commoner among women; in the 80 to 84 years age group, men had a higher rate than women. Living alone or in isolation were not associated with depression.

Copeland et al. (1987) used AGECAT (a computerized diagnostic system) to reexamine the data of Gurland et al., and made DSM-III diagnoses where possible. Prevalence rates were: 4.6% major depression, 6.3% dysthymic disorder and 1.8% bereavement. In a later study, Copeland et al. (1992) reported an overall prevalence of 11.5% for diagnostic syndrome cases of depressive disorder among elderly people in Liverpool, UK; one-quarter of these depressed subjects displayed comorbid case or subcase levels of organic disorder. In Singapore, Kua (1992) assessed elderly Chinese people using AGECAT, and reported the prevalence of cases of depression was 5.7%.

Blazer and Williams (1980) also used a multidimensional instrument in their survey of 997 elderly Americans living in the community; a depression scale was abstracted from this. The prevalence of substantial depressive symptomatology

Table 7.1. *Selected studies of depression in community populations*

Authors	Population	*n*	Age (years)	Assessment strategy	Prevalence of depression
Blazer & Williams (1980)	Durham County	997	65+	OARS Depression Scale	3.7% major depression (DSM-III) but only 1.8% of these had 'primary depressive disorder' 6.5% dysphoric and physical health impairment 4.5% 'simply dysphoric'
Gurland et al. (1983)	New York	445	65+	CARE	13% pervasive
	London	396	65+	CARE	12.4% pervasive
Copeland et al. (1987)	London (same sample)	396	65+	AGECAT re-analysis	4.6% major depression (DSM-III) 6.3% dysthymic disorder 1.8% bereavement
Kay et al. (1985)	Hobart	274	70+	Modified CARE	16% pervasive 10.2% major depression (DSM-III) +19% with dysphoric symptoms
Kivelä et al. (1988)	Ahtari (Finland)	1529 (77 in institutions)	60+	Zung scale +interview with GP	3.7% major depression 20.6% dysthymic disorders 2.4% atypical depression

Weissman et al. (1988)	5 sites in US	5499	65+	DIS	1.0% major depression (DSM-III) 0.4% men (one year) 1.4% women (one year)
Weissman et al. (1988)	5 sites in US				1.0% lifetime dysthymia (men) 2.3% lifetime dysthymia (women)
Lindesay et al. (1989)	London	890	65+	Modified CARE	13.5% depression (CATEGO Index of Definition 4 or more)
Livingston et al. (1990)	London	779	Women 60+ Men 65+	Short CARE	15.9% pervasive without dementia 1.4% pervasive with dementia
Kua (1992)	Singapore Chinese	612	65+	GMS/AGECAT	5.7% 'cases' 3.6% 'subcases'
Copeland (1992)	Liverpool	1070	65+	GMS/AGECAT	11.5% 'cases' ($\frac{1}{4}$ with comorbid cognitive impairment)
Henderson et al. (1993)	Canberra	945	70+	CIE	0.4% major depression (DSM III-R) 0.6% dysthymia (DSM III-R) 2.9% ICD-10 depressive episode

was 14.7%. Making up the 14.7% were (1) 3.7% who met four or more of the symptom criteria for a DSM-III diagnosis of major depressive disorder; half of these subjects showed evidence of cognitive dysfunction and/or thought disorder, so that only 1.8% were regarded as having a 'primary depressive disorder'; (2) 4.5% who had substantial dysphoric symptoms but who met fewer than four of the above-mentioned DSM-III criteria, so were regarded as 'simply dysphoric'; (3) 6.5% who had 'substantial dysphoric symptoms associated with impairment in physical health'. The authors pointed out that 'masked depressions' (where substantial depressive symptomatology was manifested mainly by physiologic symptoms, and the subjects did not talk of themselves as depressed) were not registered among the cases of depression in the survey.

Both surveys demonstrated that a large percentage of older people have substantial depressive symptoms. Similar results were reported by Kay et al. (1985) who used a structured interview including items from the CARE schedule to assess 274 persons aged 70 years or more living in the community in Hobart, Australia. About 16% had pervasive depression. Applying DSM-III criteria, 10.2% of those aged 70 years or more had major depression (6.3% of 70 to 79 year olds and 15.5% of those aged 80 years or more); this did not include those who fulfilled the criteria but had been bereaved in the previous 12 months, nor the three subjects who had moderate or severe dementia as well. As well as the 10% with major depression, 19% of the 274 had dysphoric symptoms in the past month.

Lindesay, Briggs & Murphy (1989) in London used a structured interview schedule that incorporated items from the CARE schedule. The 890 subjects were aged 65 years or more, living at home. About 8% of the men and 17% of women were depressed, scoring above a defined cut point on the CARE depression scale. Generalized anxiety was shown by 3.7%, but only a small number of these subjects did not score as depressed. Elsewhere in London, Livingston et al. (1990) reported that 15.9% of elderly people were pervasively depressed without being demented, while a further 1.7% were depressed and dementing.

Kivela, Pahkala & Laippala (1988) included those in institutions when studying 1529 persons aged 60 years or more in one municipality in Finland. Using DSM-III criteria, prevalence rates were: major depression 3.7%, dysthymic disorder 20.6%, atypical depression 2.4%. Studies in other countries using comparable instruments report similar results; some earlier studies, e.g. Bollerup, 1975 reported lower rates.

The National Institute of Mental Health's Epidemiologic Catchment Area (ECA) Program's findings differed from those already discussed. Using the Diagnostic Interview Schedule (DIS), 5499 subjects aged 65 years or more in five sites were interviewed (Weissman et al., 1988), though one-quarter of the interviews were incomplete and/or were completed by informants. As noted by De Leo and Diekstra (1990), a surprising 89.5% were in excellent, good or fairly good physical health.

The one-year prevalence for major depression was 1.0% (0.4% for men, 1.4% for women), compared to 2.3% and 3.4% for the 45 to 64 and 18 to 44 years age groups, respectively. Additionally, lifetime prevalence rates of 2% for DSM-III dysthymia were about half those recorded for the two younger age groups. Using similar methodology, Bland, Newman & Orn (1988) obtained similar results in Edmonton (Canada).

If the ECA report of far lower rates of depression in old age were to be generally accepted, the implications would be considerable. Allocation of resources, availability of psychogeriatric treatment services, teaching of staff and students about the nature and meaning of symptoms could all be affected. The study's methodology, however, has been criticized (Kermis, 1986; Burvill, 1987; Snowdon, 1990). Use of the DIS led to an underestimate of depression due to exclusion of minor episodes and of depressions associated with physical disorders, and it is possible that phobia was diagnosed in some cases where both phobic and depressive symptoms were prominent. Diagnoses of atypical depression and adjustment disorder with depressed mood were not made, it seems, in the ECA study. Denial and somatization commonly cause difficulties in recognition of depressive illness in old age, and the DIS does not make it easier. Parker (1987) commented on the poor agreement obtained between lay interviewer-generated DIS diagnoses and psychiatrists' judgments at least for major depressive episodes.

Henderson et al. (1993) used the Canberra Interview for the Elderly (CIE) when assessing a community population aged 70 years or more; they pointed out that the CIE allows symptoms to be recorded as depressive even if they could be attributable to medical illness, medication, drugs or alcohol. In contrast to the Hobart findings, they reported that among elderly community residents in Canberra the point prevalence rates of DSM-III-R major depressive episode were even lower than those reported from North America: 0.2% of men and 0.6% of women. Another 0.6% had DSM-III-R dysthymia. Rates for ICD-10 moderate and severe depressive episodes were 0.6% among men and 1.5% among women; an additional 1.5% of men and 2.0% of women had ICD-10 *mild* depressive episodes. Only 0.3% had ICD-10 dysthymia. The researchers reported a much higher prevalence of depressive episodes among their instititutional sample.

It seems that mild ICD-10 depressive episodes lie at a lower threshold for 'caseness' than DSM-III-R major depression. Henderson et al. (1993) added that elderly people living in Canberra experience substantial levels of depressive symptoms but at a 'subthreshold' level; they recommended giving attention to the clinical significance of this finding. Blazer (1989), from the North Carolina site, admitted that many depressed elders fall through the diagnostic net, or are captured in the atypical or residual categories. 'Such elders suffering depression may not be atypical in frequency, but only in the lack of attention directed to their disorders by epidemiologists, phenomenologists and other clinical investigators'.

Risk factors for late life depression

Clearly, if selected populations are studied, bias may lead to variation in prevalence rates. Case registers depend on presentation of subjects to a service, and provide underestimates of prevalence rates because some depressed elderly people never attend health clinics, etc. Those attending general practitioner surgeries (MacDonald, 1986) and those in general hospital wards have higher rates of depression than would be found in a random sample of the general population; rates could be expected to be higher in areas of high unemployment, and in areas where physical ill-health and disability are more prevalent. The risk for clinically significant depression is considerably greater among elderly people with disabilities or persistent physical illnesses (Gurland, Wilder & Berkman, 1988).

Other factors associated with depression in old age have been discussed by Murphy (1982, 1986). She attributed the increased rate among those of low socio-economic status to their greater liability to suffer adverse events. She found that the most severely depressed group were just as likely to have predisposing social problems as the less severely depressed group and advised abandonment of the label 'endogenous'. Burvill et al. (1989), studying patients referred to psychiatrists, found that 44% of persons with a first ever episode of depression after the age of 60 years had a severe life event in the year before onset, compared to only 31% of those whose first depression occurred before 60 years of age. They and several others (see Brodaty et al., 1991) have reported lower rates of affective disorders in first-degree relatives of patients with late-onset (as compared with early-onset) depression.

Murphy (1982) and others have reported that elderly people with depression tend to lack close confiding relationships; Emmerson et al. (1989) found this to be the case with men but not women among severely depressed elderly patients. Henderson et al. (1986) noted a lowered level of interaction but questioned whether this was due to being depressed or whether the same personality traits had led to social isolation *and* depression. Blazer et al. (1991) demonstrated an association between depressive symptoms and lack of social support. Livingston et al. (1990) reported those living alone as more depressed; depression was highly associated with not being currently married.

The most consistent findings from the various studies are (1) that depression in old age is commonest among women, though the rates converge in the oldest age groups; (2) depression is commonly associated with physical ill-health.

Incidence of depression in old age

Prevalence rates largely depend on incidence and duration of the identified condition. Little has been written about incidence of depressive disorders in the community, perhaps because of the heterogeneity of such conditions. To be useful (for example, in planning services), studies of incidence should look at subtypes of depressive disorder and note factors associated with increased incidence rates.

Murphy (1982) found that, among 200 elderly people living in the community in London, 13 had had a psychiatric disorder for more than a year, and 19 (10%) of the remaining 187 had developed major depression during the last year. For those in good health with no major social problems and no severe events the risk was only 2.5% while in the presence of one of these factors the risk was 16%.

Copeland et al. (1992) estimated the annual incidence of depression among elderly people in Liverpool to be at least 2.37%; Snowdon and Lane (1994, unpublished observations) in an 8-year study in Sydney, found the annual incidence of DSM-III-R depressive disorders to be at least 1.6%. These figures do not allow for the unknown number of cases of depression which developed and recovered within the years (three and two, respectively) separating assessments.

Epidemiology of bipolar disorder in old age

Although bipolar disorder is relatively uncommon among cases of affective disorder in old age, it is usually clearly recognisable because of a history of manic episodes. According to the ECA study (Weissman et al., 1988), the one-year prevalence rate of bipolar disorder among persons aged 65 years or more living in the community was 0.1%, whereas for the age groups 18 to 44 years and 45 to 64 years the one-year prevalence rates were 1.4% and 0.4% respectively. The number of first admissions to psychiatric hospitals in Britain with mania was found to increase or stay steady with age (Spicer, Hare & Slater, 1973; Eagles & Whalley, 1985), though most studies report that the mean age of onset of bipolar disorder is around 30 years. Shulman and Post (1980) and Snowdon (1991*a*) remarked on the paucity of early-onset cases among admissions of elderly patients with bipolar disorder. There are several possible explanations for a lower prevalence in spite of there being no fall in first admission rate with age; it may be that patients with early-onset bipolar disorder cease to have episodes later on, or are better able to control episodes (and stay out of hospital) during later episodes, but another explanation is that mortality is considerably increased among those with bipolar disorder, so that many do not live to be old.

The incidence of episodes of bipolar disorder in old age has not been established. Snowdon (1991*a*) reported that at least 3 per 10 000 elderly persons were admitted to hospital once or more per year because of bipolar affective disorder. Several authors have demonstrated the importance of cerebral organic conditions as factors leading to the development of mania or bipolar disorder in old age (Shulman & Post, 1980; Stone, 1989; Broadhead & Jacoby, 1990; Snowdon, 1991*a*), the importance of genetic factors appearing correspondingly less. A small minority of such cases (in the published studies) might be regarded by some as having organic affective disorders. Shulman et al. (1992) considered that subtle cerebral changes due to ageing may have been responsible for the conversion to mania in 20 patients who experienced a long latency from first depression to onset of mania.

The literature concerning life events and mania is sparse, but there is evidence that inpatients whose first manic episode was in middle age were less likely to have experienced a significant life event in the four weeks prior to admission than those whose first manic episode was prior to age 35 years (Ambelas, 1987). Shulman (1989) suspects that later in life mania may be precipitated by events that are not so stressful, perhaps related to increased cerebral vulnerability.

Depression and dementia

Detailed discussion of the relationship between dementia and depression will be found in Chapter 9.

The prevalence of depressive disorders among persons with dementia is even more difficult to establish than it is for those without dementia. One of the difficulties is that many of the symptoms that are part of a depressive syndrome can also be features of dementia, for example, apathy, anhedonia and social withdrawal. For this reason, coexistent depression may not be diagnosed in cases of dementia, or may be diagnosed instead of dementia.

Depressive manifestations of various intensity occur in a large percentage of patients with dementia. Merriam et al. (1988) reported that 86% of a group of subjects with dementia fulfilled DSM-III criteria for major depressive episodes, based on reports from relatives, but they added that 90% of these depressed subjects were either always or frequently capable of being distracted or cheered by their caregivers. Burns, Jacoby & Levy (1990) found that 63% of patients with Alzheimer's disease reported at least one depressive symptom, 43% were considered depressed by relatives, and 24% were rated as depressed by a trained observer. None of their subjects fulfilled criteria for major depressive disorder, since this diagnosis and Alzheimer's disease were regarded as mutually exclusive in DSM-III-R.

Less commonly encountered in dementia is a sustained depressive syndrome. Greenwald et al. (1989) reported that 11% of their inpatients and outpatients with dementia had a major depression complicating a preexisting dementia. Reifler, Larson & Hanley (1982) reported that 23% of their patients with dementia fulfilled Research Diagnostic Criteria for depressive disorder; others provide similar figures. The prevalence of depression in Alzheimer's disease and multi-infarct dementia is probably similar, except that depression may be less prevalent among severe Alzheimer's cases (Burns, Jacoby & Levy, 1990); the mean depression score in severe multi-infarct dementia is about the same as for mild and moderate cases (Fisher, Simanyi & Danielczyk, 1990).

Depression among the physically ill

Detailed discussion of the relationship between mood disorders and cerebrovascular disorders will be found in Chapter 25, and much of Chapter 24 is concerned with depression in a general hospital setting.

The point prevalence of states approximating to major depression in general medical patients is said to be between 10 and 20%, e.g. Rodin & Voshart, 1986. Where lower rates are quoted, it may be that a larger proportion of patients were diagnosed as having 'adjustment disorder with depressed mood' rather than dysthymia or major depression. Moffic and Paykel (1975) in a study of younger patients found that 61% of those who were severely medically ill were depressed, compared with 21% of those who were mildly or moderately ill. In two-thirds of their subjects, depression appeared to be largely a consequence of physical illness. More than one-third of medical inpatients report moderate depressive symptoms, and 11% to 26% suffer from a depressive syndrome (Rodin & Voshart, 1986). Pitt (1991) quotes studies showing that 5% of elderly patients in general hospitals have major depression. At least 25% of cancer patients in hospital meet the criteria for major depression or adjustment disorder with depressed mood (Massie & Holland, 1990). The risk for clinically significant depression is said to be three times higher among disabled people than among the nondisabled, 35% versus 12% (see Gurland et al., 1988). The percentage of Parkinson's Disease patients reported to be depressed varies widely, probably due to differences in sampling and assessment techniques; Mayeux (1990), referring to several studies, reported that about 45% are depressed, most having major depression or dysthymia. Those with rigidity and bradykinesia have been reported as more likely to be depressed than those suffering from a predominance of tremor. Where a person with disability is depressed, it is likely that both biological factors and psychological stressors (in varying degrees) interact with personality and other factors to give rise to the depression.

House (1987) believes that depression following stroke is largely determined by social factors. Major depression has been reported immediately after stroke in 23% of patients, and in 34% six months later, with at least a further 20% having milder depression each time. There is controversy concerning the location of cerebral damage that is most likely to be associated with depressive disorders.

Summarizing, depression is especially common among those elderly people who have physical illnesses or disabilities, including strokes. It is therefore not surprising that the prevalence of depression in nursing homes and residential settings is high (see Chapter 10).

Use of health services

It is well recognized that elderly persons receive less attention for mental health problems than younger people (German, Shapiro & Skinner, 1985). In certain circumstances, mood disorder may be less responsive to treatment, and it may be that such circumstances are commoner in old age. A majority of elderly patients with mood disorder, however, respond well (see Chapter 9). There is therefore good reason for recognising such disorders, and for providing easily accessible mental health services for elderly people who are too disabled to visit doctors, or who cannot afford such visits, or who are in institutions (e.g. nursing homes) or who do not recognize that they could benefit from such services. Awareness of the prevalence and incidence of mental illnesses in old age in various situations and settings should lead to development of appropriate services. But will it? Referring to the prevalence and stability of depression in nursing homes, Katz et al. (1989) stated that their findings 'document the critical need for increasing the availability of mental health services within long-term care institutions'. It is disconcerting that in the United States this issue 'has been recognized but inadequately addressed for almost 30 years' (Drinka & Howell, 1991). In Britain, comprehensive psychogeriatric services have been developed in many areas; Pitt (1982) described one such service, where 34% of referred patients (mostly seen at home) were diagnosed as having mood disorders.

Comparable services in Canada, seeing similar proportions of depressed elderly, have been described (Harris, Marriott & Robertson, 1990).

Of elderly persons admitted to acute psychiatric inpatient facilities in Australia from defined catchment areas, about half had a depressive disorder (Gilchrist et al., 1985; Snowdon, 1991*b*). The length of stay of these patients in acute wards is greater than that of other diagnostic groups. The type and length of admissions varies between regions and countries, being affected by referral patterns, community resources available, etc.

Having regard to the heavy investment of acute inpatient resources in treating depression in old age, and recognizing the high prevalence of depression among elderly people in hospitals and other institutions, it is surprising that there have been so few clinical trials of treatments for depression in these settings and among depressed elderly people living at home. The epidemiological studies have demonstrated the problems and pointed to some of the contributory factors. Now we need to seek improved outcomes by an active approach, whatever the setting; sometimes a change of setting will be the key to improvement.

Conclusion

The following are significant correlates of depressive symptoms in old age: functional disability, chronic illness, lack of social support, lower income and cognitive impairment. Intervention to modify (where possible) risk factors among the elderly for depression could contribute substantially to more successful ageing (Blazer et al., 1991). This task devolves on governments and the community, not just on our psychogeriatric services.

References

Ambelas, A. (1987). Life events and mania: a special relationship? *British Journal of Psychiatry*, **150**, 235–40.

Bland, R. C., Newman, S. C. & Orn, H. (1988). Epidemiology of psychiatric disorders in Edmonton. *Acta Psychiatrica Scandinavica*, **77**, Supplement 338.

Blazer, D. G. (1989). Affective disorders in late life. In *Geriatric Psychiatry*, ed. E. W. Busse & D. G. Blazer, pp. 369–401. Washington: American Psychiatric Press.

Blazer, D., Burchett, B., Service, C. & George, L. K. (1991). The association of age and depression among the elderly: an epidemiologic exploration. *Journal of Gerontology*, **46**, M 210–15.

Blazer, D. & Williams, C. D. (1980). Epidemiology of dysphoria and depression in an elderly population. *American Journal of Psychiatry*, **137**, 439–44.

Blazer, D., Woodbury, M., Hughes, D. C., George, L. K., Manton, K. G., Bachar, J. R. & Fowler, N. (1989). A statistical analysis of the classification of depression in a mixed community and clinical sample. *Journal of Affective Disorders*, **16**, 11–20.

Bollerup, T. (1975). Prevalence of mental illness among 70 year-olds domiciled in nine Copenhagen suburbs. *Acta Psychiatrica Scandinavica*, **51**, 327–39.

Broadhead, J. & Jacoby, R. (1990). Mania in old age: a first prospective study. *International Journal of Geriatric Psychiatry*, **5**, 215–22.

Brodaty, H., Peters, K., Boyce, P. et al. (1991). Age and depression. *Journal of Affective Disorders*, **23**, 137–49.

Burns, A., Jacoby, R. & Levy, R. (1990). Psychiatric phenomena in Alzheimer's disease. III: disorders of mood. *British Journal of Psychiatry*, **157**, 81–6.

Burvill, P. W. (1987). An appraisal of the NIMH epidemiologic catchment area program. *Australian and New Zealand Journal of Psychiatry*, **21**, 175–84.

Burvill, P. W., Hall, W. D., Stampfer, H. G. & Emmerson, J. P. (1989). A comparison of early-onset and late-onset depressive illness in the elderly. *British Journal of Psychiatry*, **155**, 673–9.

Copeland, J. R. M., Gurland, B. J., Dewey, M. E., Kelleher, M. J., Smith, A. M. R. & Davidson, I. A. (1987). Is there more dementia, depression and neurosis in New York? A comparative study of the elderly in New York and London using the computer diagnosis AGECAT.*British Journal of Psychiatry*, **151**, 466–73.

Copeland, J. R. M., Davidson, I. A., Dewey, M. E. et al. (1992). Alzheimer's disease, other dementias, depression and pseudodementia: prevalence, incidence and three-year outcome in Liverpool. *British Journal of Psychiatry*, **161**, 230–9.

De Leo, D. & Diekstra, R. F. W. (1990). *Depression and Suicide in Late Life*, p.15. Toronto: Hogrefe & Huber.

Dohrenwend, B. P., Shrout, P. E., Egri, G. & Mendelsohn, F. S. (1980). Nonspecific psychological distress and other dimensions of psychopathology: measures for use in the general population. *Archives of General Psychiatry*, **37**, 1229–36.

Drinka, P. J. & Howell, T. (1991). The burden of mental disorders in the nursing home. *Journal of the American Geriatrics Society*, **39**, 730–1.

Eagles, J. M. & Whalley, L. J. (1985). Ageing and affective disorders: the age at first onset of affective disorders in Scotland, 1969–1978. *British Journal of Psychiatry*, **147**, 180–7.

Emmerson, J. P., Burvill, P. W., Finlay-Jones, R. & Hall, W. (1989). Life events, life difficulties and confiding relationships in the depressed elderly. *British Journal of Psychiatry*, **155**, 787–92.

Fischer, P., Simanyi, M. & Danielczyk, W. (1990). Depression in dementia of the Alzheimer type and in multi-infarct dementia. *American Journal of Psychiatry*, **147**, 1484–7.

German, P. S., Shapiro, S. & Skinner, E. A. (1985). Mental health of the elderly: use of health and mental health services. *Journal of the American Geriatrics Society*, **33**, 246–52.

Gilchrist, P. N., Rozenbilds, U. Y., Martin, E. & Connolly, H. (1985). A study of 100 consecutive admissions to a psychogeriatric unit. *Medical Journal of Australia*, **143**, 235–7.

Greenwald, B. S., Kramer-Ginsberg, E., Marin, D. B., Laitman, L. B., Hermann, C. K., Mohs, R. C. & Davis, K. L. (1989). Dementia with coexistent major depression. *American Journal of Psychiatry*, **146**, 1472–8.

Gurland, B., Copeland, J., Kuriansky, J., Kelleher, M., Sharpe, L. & Dean, L. L. (1983). *The Mind and Mood of Ageing*. London: Croom Helm.

Gurland, B. J., Wilder, D. E. & Berkman, C. (1988). Depression and disability in the elderly: reciprocal relations and changes with age. *International Journal of Geriatric Psychiatry*, **3**, 163–79.

Harris, A. G., Marriott, J. A. S. & Robertson, J. (1990). Issues in the evaluation of a community psychogeriatric service. *Canadian Journal of Psychiatry*, **35**, 215–22.

Henderson, A. S., Grayson, D. A., Scott, R., Wilson, J., Rickwood, D. & Kay, D. W. K. (1986). Social support, dementia and depression among the elderly living in the Hobart community. *Psychological Medicine*, **16**, 379–90.

Henderson, A. S., Jorm, A. F., MacKinnon, A. et al. (1993). The prevalence of depressive disorders and the distribution of depressive symptoms in later life: a survey using draft ICD-10 and DSM-III-R. *Psychological Medicine*, **23**, 719–29.

House, A. (1987). Depression after stroke. *British Medical Journal*, **294**, 76–8.

Katz, I. R., Lesher, E., Kleban, M., Jethanandani, V. & Parmelee, P. (1989). Clinical features of depression in the nursing home. *International Psychogeriatrics*, **1**, 5–15.

Kay, D. W. K., Henderson, A. S., Scott, R., Wilson, J., Rickwood, D. & Grayson, D. A. (1985). The prevalence of dementia and depression among the elderly living in the Hobart community: the effect of the diagnostic criteria on the prevalence rates. *Psychological Medicine*, **15**, 771–88.

Kermis, M. D. (1986). The epidemiology of mental disorder in the elderly: a response to the Senate/AARP report. *Gerontologist*, **26**, 482–7.

Kivela, S. L., Pahkala, K. & Laippala, P. (1988). Prevalence of depression in an elderly population in Finland. *Acta Psychiatrica Scandinavica*, **78**, 401–13.

Kua, E. H. (1992). A community study of mental disorders in elderly Singaporean Chinese using the GMS-AGECAT package. *Australian and New Zealand Journal of Psychiatry*, **26**, 502–6.

Lindesay, J., Briggs, K. & Murphy, E. (1989). The Guy's/Age Concern survey. Prevalence rates of cognitive impairment, depression and anxiety in an urban elderly community. *British Journal of Psychiatry*, **155**, 317–29.

Livingston, G., Hawkins, A., Graham, N., Blizard, B. & Mann, A. (1990). The Gospel Oak study: prevalence rates of dementia, depression and activity limitation among elderly residents in Inner London. *Psychological Medicine*, **20**, 137–46.

MacDonald, A. J. D. (1986). Do general practitioners 'miss' depression in elderly patients? *British Medical Journal*, **292**, 1365–7.

Massie, M. J. & Holland, J. C. (1990). Depression and the cancer patient. *Journal of Clinical Psychiatry*, **51**, 7 (Supplement), 12–7.

Mayeux, R. (1990). Depression in the patient with Parkinson's Disease. *Journal of Clinical Psychiatry*, **51**, 7 (Supplement), 20–3.

Merriam, A. E., Aronson, M. K., Gaston, P., Wey, S.-L. & Katz, I. (1988). The psychiatric symptoms of Alzheimer's Disease. *Journal of the American Geriatrics Society*, **36**, 7–12.

Moffic, H. & Paykel, E. (1975). Depression in medical in-patients. *British Journal of Psychiatry*, **126**, 346–53.

Murphy, E. (1982). Social origins of depression in old age. *British Journal of Psychiatry*, **141**, 135–42.

Murphy, E. (1986). *Affective Disorders in the Elderly*. Edinburgh: Churchill Livingstone.

Oxman, T. E., Barrett, J. E., Barrett, J., Gerber, T. (1990). Symptomatology of late-life minor depression among primary care patients. *Psychosomatics*, **31**, 174–80.

Parker, G. (1987). Are the lifetime prevalence estimates in the ECA study accurate? *Psychological Medicine*, **17**, 275–82.

Pitt, B. (1982). *Psychogeriatrics: An Introduction to the Psychiatry of Old Age*, 2nd edn. Edinburgh: Churchill Lingstone.

Pitt, B. (1991). Depression in the general hospital setting. *International Journal of Geriatric Psychiatry*, **6**, 363–70.

Reifler, B. V., Larson, E. & Hanley, R. (1982). Coexistence of cognitive impairment and depression in geriatric outpatients. *American Journal of Psychiatry*, **139**, 623–6.

Rodin, G. & Voshart, K. (1986). Depression in the medically ill: an overview. *American Journal of Psychiatry*, **143**, 696–705.

Shulman, K. I. (1989). The influence of age and ageing on manic disorder. *International Journal of Geriatric Psychiatry*, **4**, 63–5.

Shulman, K. & Post, F. (1980). Bipolar affective disorder in old age. *British Journal of Psychiatry*, **136**, 26–32.

Shulman, K. I., Tohen, M., Satlin, A., Mallya, G. & Kalunian, D. (1992). Mania compared with unipolar depression in old age. *American Journal of Psychiatry*, **149**, 341–5.

Snowdon, J. (1990). The prevalence of depression in old age. *International Journal of Geriatric Psychiatry*, **5**, 141–4.

Snowdon, J. (1991*a*). A retrospective case-note study of bipolar disorder in old age. *British Journal of Psychiatry*, **158**, 485–90.

Snowdon, J. (1991*b*). Bed requirements for an area psychogeriatric service. *Australian and New Zealand Journal of Psychiatry*, **25**, 56–62.

Spicer, C. C., Hare, E. H. & Slater, E. (1973). Neurotic and psychotic forms of depressive illness: evidence from age-incidence in a national sample. *British Journal of Psychiatry*, **123**, 535–41.

Stone, K. (1989). Mania in the elderly. *British Journal of Psychiatry*, **155**, 220–4.

Weissman, M. M., Leaf, P. L., Tischler, G. L., Blazer, D. G., Karno, M., Bruce, M. L. & Florio, L. P. (1988). Affective disorders in five United States communities. *Psychological Medicine*, **18**, 141–53.

8

The outcome of depressive illness in old age

PETER BURVILL

Historical

There is strong evidence that, in antiquity, physicians were well aware of senile depression as a condition apart from dotage (Post, 1986). In the eighteenth century, even nonmedical writers were conversant with recoverable senile depressions. In the nineteenth century, however, the flourishing of brain pathology generated the widespread belief that depressions occurring for the first time during old age were early indicators of cerebral deterioration and precursors of dementia. Post (1951) and Roth & Morrissey (1952) were the first to distinguish the comparatively hopeful outcome of depressed patients from the outcome of those suffering from organic disorders.

Landmark studies of the outcome of depressive illness in the elderly are the six-year follow-up study of Post (1962) and the later three-year follow-up by the same author (Post, 1972). He studied two cohorts of depressed elderly inpatients treated by himself: the first in 1950 when electroconvulsive treatment (ECT) and leucotomy were the only effective physical treatments available, and the second in the 1960s when tricyclic antidepressants had been added. He concluded that there had been no improvement in prognosis despite the advances in treatment. The disappointing result in the second cohort may, however, have been due to a larger number of socially disadvantaged patients in that series as well as the inclusion of patients who had failed to respond to pharmacotherapy (not available in 1950) prescribed by their family doctors or in the outpatient department (Post, 1986). Even before the introduction of specific antidepressive treatments, only 24% of depressived patients over the age of 60 years had remained continuously in a private mental hospital for 2–5 years after their admission (Post, 1944). The improved outcome of using ECT in older patients was shown by Roth (1955), comparing depressed patients aged over 60 years admitted between 1934 and 1936 with those admitted to the same area mental hospital in 1948 and 1949. Post found that permanent recovery was unusual, and most patients either continued ill or had relapses that were responsive to treatment. A series of follow-up studies (Post, 1962; Post, 1972; Kay, Roth & Hopkins, 1955; Kay, 1962; Murphy, 1983) have shown that the late appearance of symptoms and signs of dementia in depressed elderly is no more frequent than that found in the age-matched general population (Post, 1986). It has, however, been suggested that the small proportion with pseudodementia may have an increased risk of cognitive decline (Kral, 1983; Alexopoulos, 1989).

Recent outcome studies

The 12-month follow-up study of Murphy (1983) showed a high mortality during that year, and a poor overall prognosis with only 35% well at follow-up. This study led to the claim of Millard (1983) that, 'No matter what is done, a third get better, a third stay the same and a third get worse'.

In the past decade there have been a number of studies claiming a somewhat better outcome (Gordon, 1981; Godber, 1983; Godber et al., 1987; Baldwin & Jolley, 1986; Robinson, 1989; Burvill *et al.*, 1991*a*; Meats, Timol & Jolley, 1991). Table 8.1 outlines the four-month outcome of five studies of depressive illness in the elderly using the same outcome criteria as those of Murphy (1983). Although the range of the percentage well at the end of 12 months is considerable, from Murphy 35% to Meats et al. 68%, these studies show that, over the first 12 months, between 14% and 29% of elderly patients with major depressive disorders or a similar condition are continuously depressed and between 12% and 19% relapse.

Whereas most studies have been on inpatients, Kivela, Pahkala & Laippala (1991), in a study of patients living in the community in Finland, and treated by primary care physicians, showed a favorable outcome for patients with both major depressive illness and dysthymia. Two studies (Cole, 1985; Magni, Palazzolo & Bianchin, 1988) of elderly depressed patients attending psychiatric outpatients showed more than 60% of patients were 'more or less chronically' ill after a mean follow-up period of 48 and 15 months, respectively. Cole (1985) considered his findings on outpatients were comparable with similar follow-up studies of elderly depressed inpatients, including that of his own (Cole, 1983).

Table 8.2 outlines 3 three-year follow-up studies of elderly depressed patients (Post, 1962, 1972; Baldwin & Jolley, 1986), all using similar outcome criteria. Only 22–31% had lasting recovery over this period, and a very high proportion had further episodes with full recovery, or had depressive 'invalidism' during this time. Cole (1990) reviewed ten studies of the prognosis of depression in old age published between 1950 and mid-1989. When he analysed these studies as a group, the proportion of patients who remained well throughout dropped from 43.7% in those with a two-year follow-up to 27.4% of those followed up for a

Table 8.1. *Twelve month outcome of depressive illness in the elderly: five studies*

Study	*n*	Well	Relapse	Continuously depressed	Dementia	Death
Murphy (1983)	124	35	19	29	3	14
Baldwin & Jolley (1986)	98	58	15	18	—	8
Meats et al. (1991)	56	68	12.3	3.6	—	16
Burvill et al. (1991*a*)	103	47	18	24	—	11
Kivela et al. (1991)						
Major depression	42	45	12	14	14	14
Dysthymia	199	40	4	42	3	10

Table 8.2. *3 year follow-up of depressive illness in the elderly: three studies*

	Percentages		
	Post (1962) ($n = 81$)	Post (1972) ($n = 92$)	Baldwin & Jolley (1986) ($n = 96$)
Lasting recovery	31	26	22
Further episodes with full recovery	28	37	38
Depressive invalidism	23	25	32
Continuously ill	17	12	7

longer period. Thus available evidence from studies conducted over long periods, does not uphold the traditional teaching which has emphasized a relatively good prognosis for affective disorders. The same has been shown for younger adults by Kiloh, Andrews & Neilson, (1988) and Lee & Murray (1988), who found considerable morbidity and clearly showed that a large amount of depressive illness is recurrent over time. Depressive illness in old age is probably no worse an affliction than in young people (Post, 1986).

Range of outcomes

During the course of any follow-up study, a wide range of outcomes will be encountered. These include: complete recovery without further relapse, complete recovery with further relapses, varying degrees of depressive invalidism with or without further relapses of depressive illness, continual depression throughout the follow-up period, the development of dementia, and death. Obviously the longer the patients' follow-up period, the greater will be their chance of relapse, cognitive impairment and death. Baldwin & Jolley (1986) and Burvill, Stampfer & Hall (1991*b*) have discussed the complexities of these various categorizations of outcome of depressive illness in the elderly.

Invalidism

In the 12 months follow-up of 103 elderly depressed patients in Perth by Burvill et al. (1991*a*), 13 patients at follow-up had depressive symptoms far in excess of those classified by Murphy (1983) as having 'minor symptoms only', yet were not of sufficient severity to satisfy the DSM III criteria for depressive illness. The severity of their symptoms was much nearer the latter than the former. In all 13 patients these subclinical depressive symptoms had been present more or less continuously since discharge from the index admission. The range of severity of symptoms in such patients can be wide and fluctuate in severity during the follow-up period. These patients appeared akin to those classified by Post (1972) as 'invalidism', a classification also used by Baldwin & Jolley (1986) in their follow-up study. This is an important group of potentially chronic patients who have not been given adequate attention in previous studies, and Burvill et al. (1991*b*) accordingly advocated the inclusion of an 'invalidism' category in any follow-up clinical criteria.

Mortality

All the follow-up studies of depression in the elderly have shown an increase of 2–3 times mortality in the first 12 months, particularly in men, compared with general population groups of the same age. Murphy et al. (1988) found that, when the effect of physical illness was controlled, depressed elderly patients (particularly men) had a significantly higher four-year mortality, suggesting that the greater mortality in the depressed group was not due to differences of pre-depression physical health alone. Vascular disease (cardiovascular and cerebrovascular), respiratory disease and cancer were the principal causes of death, in that order. There is a well-documented relationship between depressive illness and certain types of cancer, for example, stomach, lungs and pancreas (Whitlock, 1978). Depression may precede the physical manifestations of the cancer by some time (Fran, Litin & Bartholomew, 1968). The finding that depression is specifically related to impaired t-lymphocyte function (Bartrop et al., 1977; Schliefer et al., 1985) suggests that compromised immune function secondary to depression may be the cause of the increased vulnerability to these diseases.

Meats et al. (1991) reported that patients judged to be *symptom-free at discharge* were significantly more likely to remain psychologically well over the next year and also were less likely to die. This effect on mortality of mental status at discharge was significantly stronger than that of physical status at discharge. Although it appears that depression can be a fatal disorder, particularly in the elderly, it has been shown that effective treatment significantly reduces subsequent mortality (Avery & Winokur, 1976). Thus it is of vital importance to improve the outcome of treatment and to prevent further relapse wherever possible (Murphy et al. 1988).

Most studies have shown that suicide is only a relatively minor cause of death; for example Burvill et al. (1991*a*) found that two of the 11 patients who died had committed suicide in the first 12 months, and Murphy et al. (1988) reported only one death by suicide in a four-year follow-up.

Dementia

The idea that depression in old age often marks the beginning of dementia tends to linger in spite of research carried out in the past 40 years (Post, 1986). Research has shown dementia and depression in the elderly to be associated with very different outcomes and death rates (Post, 1986). The rate of dementia after 12 months in Murphy's (1983) study was not significantly different from Kay's (1962) estimate of 2% annual average incidence.

Depressive personality change

It used to be taught that, whereas younger persons with affective disorders returned to their previous personality functioning after first and after recurrent attacks, elderly patients with depression tended to become chronic and to leave behind some form of enfeeblement (Post, 1986). This is not true and needs to be put into perspective. Following the work of Akiskal (1983) and his fellow workers, and long-term studies of younger depressed patients, it seems possible that the concept of a depressive personality change may be redundant, and that patients affected in this way are really chronic depressives shod of their major depressive symptoms (Post, 1986).

Prognostic indicators

A number of factors have been identified as possibly influencing prognosis of depressive illness in the elderly.

Age and sex

No studies of depressive illness in the elderly have shown any sex differences in outcome and any reported differences with age can be accounted for by there being more physical illness in older patients (Post, 1986). Although Baldwin & Jolley

(1986) found a poorer prognosis in men in their study, they attributed this to their male patients being more physically ill.

Severity of depression index

Murphy (1983) recorded a poor prognosis linked to severity of the depression index, but a number of other authors, did not find any such association (Baldwin & Jolley, 1986; Burvill et al., 1991*a*; Meats et al., 1991; Kivela et al., 1991; Copeland, 1988). Again, although Murphy (1983) found a particular association between poor prognosis and the presence of delusions and hallucinations, others failed to find such associations (Post, 1986; Post, 1972; Baldwin & Jolley, 1986; Burvill et al., 1991*a*; Meats et al., 1991). Baldwin and Jolley (1986) attributed the poor prognosis in those patients studied by Murphy (1983) as being due to their being given less vigorous treatment than in most psychogeriatric units and in particular to the relatively low proportion who were given ECT. Burvill, Stampfer & Hall (1986) hypothesized that less severe depressive illness, such as seen in outpatients or community settings, would have a better prognosis, but this is as yet unconfirmed by published work (Ames & Allen, 1991).

Duration of depressive illness

Post (1986) concluded, from his survey of available outcome studies, that duration of illness was the only unequivocal indicator of inferior outcome: unremitting depression for more than two years made a good response to treatment highly unlikely. There was a significant trend for patients who had been ill for less than one year to do better than those who had been depressed for one to two years. It is noteworthy that various studies over the past 30 years have reported progressive reductions in the duration of illness before admission, probably reflecting improved early detection and treatment of depression by general practitioners, and the earlier referral of more severe, difficult patients to psychiatrists, as well as a more widespread use of tricyclic antidepressants and other treatments.

Physical illness

There are contradictory reports in the literature about the association of physical illness and prognosis of depression in the elderly. The association is complex. A number of authors have reported a positive association between poor outcome and chronic health problems (Post, 1972; Murphy, 1983; Baldwin & Jolley, 1986; Cole, 1985; Roth & Kay, 1956; Kay & Bergman, 1966) but others (Post, 1962; Burvill et al., 1991*a*; Meats et al., 1991) found no such association. Meats et al. (1991) specified a poor physical status at the time of discharge as being significantly associated with poor psychiatric outcome. Kivela et al., (1991) found a significant association only in women who had diabetes mellitus, this being the only report linking outcome with a specific physical illness.

Post (1986) expressed the opinion that once a depressive illness had become established it seemed to run its course uninfluenced by improvement in physical health. Burvill et al. (1991*a*) considered that in chronic depressive disorders, factors other than physical health were more important to outcome, but they found a very positive association between acute physical illness at the onset of the depressive illness and 12 months prognosis. Most of the acute physical illnesses were noncerebral. Baldwin & Jolley (1986) found that the presence of active, e.g. effort angina physical, but not inactive, e.g. old myocardial infarct, health problems at entry was associated with poor outcomes.

Biological aging factors

Post (1972) observed that, in his clinical experience with depressed elderly patients whom he had seen for many years, those patients who previously had recovered satisfactorily with treatment but who, in an episode of depressive disorder in later life, had had a much poorer response with similar treatment, were often found to have developed a certain degree of cerebral organic deterioration in the interim. The poor prognosis of depression in those with central nervous system pathology has been noted by other authors (Cole, 1985; Magni et al., 1988; Jacoby, 1981). Jacoby (1981), in a review of the relationship between dementia, depression and CT-scan findings, concluded that the latter may prove to be a useful prognostic indicator in affective disorder of the elderly. He and his coworkers found enlarged cerebral ventricles in a subgroup of hospitalized elderly depressed patients, and reported, in a two-year follow-up of 40 such patients, that 5 of the 9 patients with enlarged ventricles had died. Death had occurred in only 4 of the remaining 31 with normal ventricles. Only 6% of normal elderly controls had died during the same time (Jacoby et al., 1983). These depressed patients with enlarged ventricles did not appear to have developed dementia. All deaths were due to noncerebral causes. Philpot (1986), after reviewing several relevant studies, concluded that the ventricular enlargement was probably present before the onset of depression and may have increased vulnerability to it.

Personality

The place of personality in the etiology and prognosis of depressive illness in old age has yet to be satisfactorily explored. Post (1962, 1972) found a strong trend, just failing to reach statistical significance, for favorable outcome to be associated with a previously normal mood, and for patients with longstanding dysthymic tendencies to have a greater likelihood of remaining continuously depressed. Burvill et al. (1991*a*) found no difference in the personality, as measured by the Eysenck Personality Inventory (EPI), between those with a good and poor 12 months prognosis. They noted, however, that measurement of personality by questionnaire when a patient is depressed may give spurious results, as follow-up data showed that the EPI scores can change in many patients once the depression has lifted.

Age of onset

Some authors have drawn a distinction between early-onset depression, (the first ever episode before the age of 60 years) and late-onset depression. Post (1986) declared that all studies agreed that there was no difference in outcome between early- and late-onset depression, a finding confirmed in the Perth study by Burvill et al. (1989). Roth (1955), Cole (1983) and Magni et al. (1988), however, found a better prognosis in late-onset cases. Post (1978) had noted that patients with a lifelong history of recurrent depression suffer more severe episodes as they grow older, the attacks of depression becoming more frequent, more protracted and more difficult to treat.

Social factors

Finnish studies, in which the majority of patients were suffering from dysthymic rather than depressive illness, showed that clinical outcome of depression in the elderly was not associated with educational level, occupation or earlier occupation, marital status, participating in work, amount of hobbies, intimacy of relationships with neighbours or spouse, or the occurrence of social or life stress factors before the onset of depression (Kivela et al., 1991; Kivela & Pahkala, 1989). In men, poor outcome was associated with low social participation and with low frequency of visiting contacts and, in women, with not living alone and with low social participation. Murphy (1983) and Burvill et al. (1991*a*) found no significant difference in outcome between those depressed elderly living alone and those not alone. Kivela et al. (1991) suggested that, in females, family dynamics and the dependent female role play a certain part in the continuation of symptoms of depression.

Surtees (1980) suggested that a reciprocally confiding relationship conferred partial immunity to adverse life events in those recovering from a depressive illness, whereas a more diffuse social network, such as might be provided by neighbours, social services or clubs, did not. Murphy (1983), however, found no evidence that an intimate relationship protected against relapse in the face of continuing life stress in elderly depressives. She had found severe life events in the 12-month follow-up period to be associated with poor prognosis, although Burvill et al. (1991*a*) found no such relationship. The social class differences found in outcome in Murphy's (1983) study were thought to be due to class differences in the experience of severe life events, the lower socioeconomic patients being at increased risk for severe life events.

Two findings raise serious doubts about the reliability of self-ratings about the presence or absence of confidants in depressed patients, and theories based upon such measurements. Murphy (1983) found 13 of 77 patients from whom relative information was available at follow-up, changed their rating about the presence or absence of a good confidant between the index admission and 12-month follow-up. A similar change in responses to EPI of elderly depressed patients who were no longer depressed at 12-month follow-up was reported by Burvill et al. (1991*a*). These findings suggest that some depressed patients are likely to view their immediate social environment rather more negatively than when not depressed.

Treatment

The bulk of current outcome literature deals with naturalistic studies in which depressive disorder has been treated, and such studies assume that the treatment given is both orthodox and adequate (Burvill et al. 1991*b*). Outcome cannot be separated from adequacy of treatment, both in the acute stage and over longer periods, and treatment adequacy cannot be assumed. In any follow-up study the amount, duration and type of treatment given vary markedly from patient to patient and with the treatment setting from which the patients were derived. Most follow-up studies to date have not taken this into account. Treatment variables include: the use of ECT, the dosage type and duration of antidepressants used, the use of supplementary medication such as lithium carbonate or L-tryptophan in more recalcitrant patients, the use of maintenance chemotherapy, and the rigor of both initial and follow-up treatment. Godber et al. (1987) argued strongly for more effective use of ECT in elderly depressed patients, claiming it had an important and generally underestimated place in the treatment of depression in the elderly. Benbow has reviewed this important topic in Chapter 26.

Aftercare

Most outcome studies of depressive illness in the elderly have not addressed the question of aftercare treatment. In fact, the prophylaxis and aftercare of depression in old age has yet to be systematically evaluated (Baldwin, 1988). Godber et al. (1987) and Baldwin (1988) have argued strongly for the permanent aftercare of elderly depressed patients, based on their higher known relapse rate, pointing out that these relapses are often undetected without planned aftercare, and that further treatment is often successful. Cole (1985) listed long-term follow-up and maintenance of antidepressant therapy as good prognostic factors. Meats et al.

(1991) attributed their findings of an excellent prognosis to a dynamic service, which provided support to the vulnerable and was able to detect early and treat any relapses. A prospective study of the role of maintenance antidepressant therapy in the aftercare of such patients would be very valuable (Murphy, 1983).

Issues in outcome studies

Burvill et al. (1991*b*) have made a number of concluding recommendations regarding future outcome studies of depression in the elderly, relating to research design, outcome assessment and statistical analysis. They advocated that researchers should recruit a wide range of patient severity by including outpatients as well as inpatients, and that follow-up assessment should be done at regular intervals. Cole (1990) and Ames & Allen (1991) have drawn attention to the six evaluation criteria for the prognosis of disease propounded by the Department of Clinical Epidemiology and Biostatistics at McMaster University Health Sciences Centre (1981). These include: adequate description of referral pattern to avoid sample bias, an inception cohort designed to identify depression at an early and uniform point in its course, a clear definition of relapse and blind outcome assessment. All ten studies reviewed by Cole (1990) had multiple serious flaws when subjected to these evaluation criteria.

Outcome criteria

A major problem in comparing outcome studies is the great variability and imprecision of outcome criteria used. It is highly desirable that the outcome criteria be defined precisely and unambiguously to enable use by other researchers in comparison studies.

A composite picture of the course pursued by the patient may be obtained by combining two sets of data, firstly the status of the patient at follow-up and secondly the patient's psychiatric health during the follow-up period.

Whereas most outcome studies have used only clinical criteria, a comprehensive outcome assessment of the elderly should include psychiatric, physical and psychosocial factors. Post (1962) considered that often the quality of life led by the patient after an affective illness may be of more importance than clinical outcome, as the latter often gave a too pessimistic outlook. He combined his four clinical outcome groups with the patients' level of social and interpersonal adjustment. Tsuang, Woolson & Fleming (1979) used four outcome variables, marital, residential, occupational and psychiatric symptomatology, each of which was categorized on a some/more incapacitating basis. Katschnig & Nutzinger (1988) suggested evaluating clinical outcome criteria and social adjustment separately by use of a multivariant data collection system.

Keller et al. (1987) have devised a somewhat different approach to the assessment of outcome, namely the Longitudinal Interval Follow-up Evaluation (LIFE). This is a comprehensive method of assessing outcome in prospective longitudinal studies and gives:

(i) a concurrent record of the course of each illness initially diagnosed,
(ii) a concurrent record of the course of each illness developing during the follow-up:
(iii) psychosocial information: and
(iv) treatment information.

Such a scheme has a number of major attractions, namely:

(a) its comprehensiveness in measuring clinical, treatment and psychosocial variables, with clearly defined and graded criteria of clinical status according to accepted, stringent research criteria;
(b) the ability to chart the course of the illness and of any new developments during that course; and
(c) the ability to link all these data temporally.

Tohen, Waternaux & Tsuang (1989) pointed to the problems in defining 'chronicity'. They identified four possible methods: presence of interepisode symptoms, psychosocial dysfunction, multiple relapses and hospitalization, and continuous hospitalization due to presence of severe symptoms and psychosocial dysfunction. Others have used two measures of chronicity, namely the length of single episodes and the cumulative length of time spent in all episodes during the follow-up period. Copeland (1983) advocated incorporation of both cumulative lengths of hospitalization and time in relapse, irrespective of hospitalization, in any outcome criteria.

Statistical analysis

There have been several new approaches in recent years to assessing outcome and analysing the results. These include survival analysis (or time-to-event analysis), the Cox Regression Model (Allgulander & Fisher, 1986), the Proportional Hazard Methods (Kalbfleish & Prentice, 1980), and the Kaplan–Meir Method (Allgulander & Fisher, 1986). These statistical methods introduce two other variables of outcome, namely, the probability of remaining in remission once recovery has occurred, and the length of time of remission after recovery. Both are of practical use and interest in any potentially recurrent illness such as depression. More attention needs to be paid to ensuring that outcome studies have sufficient statistical power to provide a reasonable chance of detecting relationships between patient characteristics and outcome. Burvill et al. (1991*b*) suggested a minimum sample size of 200. To date, all published outcome studies of depression in the elderly have had less than this number.

Conclusion

Varying opinions have been expressed about the prognosis of depression in the elderly, from marked optimism (Meats et al. 1991) to pessimism (Millard, 1983). However available evidence indicates that a high proportion of depressive illness in the elderly, as in the young, either proceeds to varying degrees of chronicity or is recurrent, and carries a higher than expected mortality rate. Review of the literature would indicate that early treatment and vigorous treatment of presenting depressive illness, including the use of ECT, together with close attention to aftercare, offer the best prospects for improving the prognosis of affective illness (Burvill et al., 1991*a*). Further advances in knowledge will necessitate more sophisticated approaches to research methodology than in past studies.

References

Akiskal, H. S. (1983). Dysthymic disorders: psychopathology of proposed chronic depressive symptoms. *American Journal of Psychiatry*, **149**, 11–20.

Alexopoulous, G. S. (1989). Late-life depression and neurological brain disease. *International Journal of Geriatric Psychiatry*, **4**, 187–90.

Allgulander, C. & Fisher, L. D. (1986). Survival analysis (or time to an event analysis), and the Cox regression model – methods for longitudinal psychiatric research. *Acta Psychiatrica Scandinavica*, **74**, 529–35.

Ames, D. & Allen, N. (1991). Editorial. The prognosis of depression in old age: good, bad or indifferent? *International Journal of Geriatric Psychiatry*, **6**, 477–81.

Avery, D. & Winokur, G. (1976). Mortality in depressed patients treated with electroconvulsive therapy and antidepressants. *Archives of General Psychiatry*, **33**, 1029–37.

Baldwin, R. E. (1988). Late life depression: undertreated? *British Medical Journal*, **269**, 519.

Baldwin, R. E. & Jolley, D. J. (1986). The prognosis of depression in old age. *British Journal of Psychiatry*, **149**, 574–83.

Bartrop, R. W., Lazarus, L., Luckhurst et al. (1977). Depressed lymphocyte function after bereavement. *The Lancet*, **i**, 834–6.

Burvill, P. W., Hall, W. D., Stampfer, H. G. & Emmerson, J. P. (1989). A comparison of early-onset and late-onset depressive illness in the elderly. *British Journal of Psychiatry*, **155**, 673–9.

Burvill, P. W., Hall, W. D., Stampfer, H. G. & Emmerson, J. P. (1991*a*). The prognosis of depression in old age. *British Journal of Psychiatry*, **158**, 64–71.

Burvill, P. W., Stampfer, H. G. & Hall, W. (1986). Does depressive illness in the elderly have a poor prognosis? *Australian & New Zealand Journal of Psychiatry*, **20**, 422–7.

Burvill, P. W., Stampfer, H. G. & Hall, W. D. (1991*b*). Issues in the assessment of outcome in depressive illness in the elderly. *International Journal of Geriatric Psychiatry*, **6**, 269–77.

Cole, M. G. (1983). Age, age of onset and course of primary depressive illness in the elderly. *Canadian Journal of Psychiatry*, **28**, 102–4.
Cole, M. G. (1985). The course of elderly depressed out-patients. *Canadian Journal of Psychiatry*, **30**, 217–20.
Cole, M. G. (1990). The prognosis of depression in the elderly. *Canadian Medical Association Journal*, **143**, 633–9.
Copeland, J. R. M. (1983). Psychotic and neurotic depression: Discriminant function analysis and five-year outcome. *Psychological Medicine*, **13**, 373–83.
Copeland, J. R. M. (1988). Physical ill-health, age and depression. In *Depressive Illness: Prediction of Course and Outcome*, ed. T. Helgason & R. J. Daly, Berlin: Springer-Verlag.
Department of Clinical Epidemiology and Biostatistics, McMaster University Health Sciences Centre (1981). How to read clinical journals: 3. To learn the clinical course and prognosis of disease. *Canadian Medical Association Journal*, **124**, 869–72.
Fran, I., Litin, E. M. & Bartholomew, L. G. (1968). Mental symptoms as an aid in the early diagnosis of carcinoma of the pancreas. *Gastroenterology*, **55**, 191–8.
Godber, C. (1983). Depression in old age. *British Medical Journal*, **237**, 758.
Godber, C., Rosenvinge, H., Wilkinson, E. et al. (1987). Depression in old age: prognosis after E. C. T. *International Journal of Psychiatry*, **2**, 19–24.
Gordon, W. F. (1981). Elderly depressives: treatment and follow-up. *Canadian Journal of Psychiatry*, **26**, 110–13.
Jacoby, R. J. (1981). Depression in the elderly. *British Journal of Hospital Medicine*, **25**, 40–7.
Jacoby, R. J., Dolan, R. J., Levy, R. & Baldy, R. (1983). Quantitative computed tomography in elderly depressed patients. *British Journal of Psychiatry*, **143**, 124–7.
Kalbfleish, J. D. & Prentice, R. L. (1980). *The Statistical Analysis of Failure Time Data*. New York: Wiley.
Katschnig, H. & Nutzinger, D. O. (1988). Psychosocial aspects of course and outcome in depressive illness. In *Depressive Illness: Prediction of Course and Outcome*, ed T. Helgason and R. J. Daly, Berlin: Springer-Verlag.
Kay, D. W. K. (1962). Outcome and cause of death in mental disorders of old age: a long-term follow-up of functional and organic psychosis. *Acta Psychiatrica Scandinavica*, **38**, 249–76.
Kay, D. W. K. & Bergmann, K. (1966). A follow-up of a random sample of elderly people seen at home. *Journal of Psychosomatic Research*, **13**, 3–12.
Kay, D. W. K., Roth, M. & Hopkins, B. (1955). Affective disorders in the senium: 1 their association with organic cerebral degeneration. *Journal of Mental Science*, **101**, 302–18.
Keller, M. B., Lavari, P. W., Friedman, B. et al. (1987). The longitudinal interval follow-up evaluation. *Archives of General Psychiatry*, **44**, 540–8.
Kiloh, L. G., Andrews, G. & Neilson, M. (1988). The long-term outcome of depressive illness. *British Journal of Psychiatry*, **153**, 752–7.
Kivela, S-L. & Pahkala, K. (1989). The prognosis of depression in old age. *International Psychogeriatrics*, **1**, 119–33.
Kivela, S-L., Pahkala, K. & Laippala, P. (1991). A one-year prognosis of dysthymic

disorder and major depression in old age. *International Journal of Geriatric Psychiatry*, **6**, 81–87.

Kral, V. (1983). The relationship between senile dementia (Alzheimer type) and depression. *Canadian Journal of Psychiatry*, **28**, 304–6.

Lee, A. S. & Murray, R. M. (1988). The long-term outcome of Maudsley depressives. *British Journal of Psychiatry*, **153**, 741–51.

Magni, G., Palozzolo, O. & Bianchin, G. (1988). The course of depression in elderly outpatients. *Canadian Journal of Psychiatry*, **33**, 21–4.

Meats, P., Timol, M. & Jolley, D. (1991). Prognosis of depression in the elderly. *British Journal of Psychiatry*, **159**, 659–63.

Millard, P. H. (1983). Depression in old age. *British Medical Journal*, **287**, 375–6.

Murphy, E. (1983). The prognosis of depression in old age. *British Journal of Psychiatry*, **142**, 111–19.

Murphy, E., Smith, R., Lindsay, J. et al. (1988). Increased mortality rates in late-life depression. *British Journal of Psychiatry*, **152**, 347–53.

Philpot, M. P. (1986). Biological factors in depression in the elderly. In *Affective Disorders in the Elderly*, ed. E. Murphy, Edinburgh: Churchill Livingstone.

Post, F. (1944). Some problems arising from a study of patients over the age of sixty years. *Journal of Mental Science*, **90**, 554–65.

Post, F. (1951). The outcome of mental breakdown in old age. *British Medical Journal*, **1**, 436–48.

Post, F. (1962). *The Significance of Affective Symptoms in Old Age*. Maudsley Monograph no. 10, London: Oxford University Press.

Post, F. (1972). The management and nature of depressive illness in late life: a follow-through study. *British Journal of Psychiatry*, **121**, 393–404.

Post, F. (1978). The functional psychoses. In *Studies in Geriatric Psychiatry*, ed. A. D. Isaacs & F. Post, Chichester: John Wiley.

Post, F. (1986). Course and outcome of depression in the elderly. In *Affective Disorders in the Elderly*, ed. E. Murphy, Edinburgh: Churchill Livingstone.

Robinson, J. R. (1989). The natural history of mental disorder in old age: a long-term study. *British Journal of Psychiatry*, **154**, 783–9.

Roth, M. (1955). The natural history of mental disorders in old age. *Journal of Mental Science*, **101**, 281–301.

Roth, M. & Kay, D. W. K. (1956). Affective disorder arising in the senium: II Physical disability as an etiological factor. *Journal of Mental Science*, **102**, 141–50.

Roth, M. & Morrissey, J. D. (1952). Problems in the diagnosis and classification of mental disorder in old age. *Journal of Mental Science*, **98**, 66–88.

Schliefer, S. J., Keller, S. E., Sivis, S. G. et al. (1985). Depression and Immunity. *Archives of General Psychiatry*, **42**, 129–33.

Surtees, P. P. G. (1980). Social support, residual adversity and depressive outcome. *Social Psychiatry*, **15**, 71–80.

Tohen, M., Waternaux, C. M. & Tsuang, M. T. (1989). Outcome in mania: II. Predictors of relapse utilising survival analysis. Department of Psychiatry and Epidemiology,

Harvard Program in Psychiatric Epidemiology, Harvard School of Medicine and Public Health, 1–28.

Tsuang, M. T., Woolson, R. F. & Fleming, J. A. (1979). Long-term outcome of major psychoses. *Archives of General Psychiatry*, **39**, 1295–301.

Whitlock, F. A. (1978). Suicide, cancer and depression. *British Journal of Psychiatry*, **132**, 269–74.

9

Pseudodementia in geriatric depression

ROTIMI BAJULAIYE GEORGE S. ALEXOPOULOS

Introduction

The term pseudodementia has been used to describe a dementia syndrome that develops in the context of a psychiatric disorder and subsides when the psychiatric symptomatology is ameliorated. The term was first used by Madden, Luban & Kaplan (1952) to describe patients with psychiatric disorders accompanied by defects in recent memory, calculation, and judgment that improved upon alleviation of their psychiatric condition. Pseudodementia was observed in 10% of patients in the series of Madden et al. (1952). Since then, the term pseudodementia has been associated with a reversible dementia syndrome resulting from a psychiatric illness. The concept of pseudodementia generated further interest when Kiloh (1961) reported ten cases of pseudodementia associated with hysteria, malingering, Ganser syndrome, paraphrenia, depression and mixed mood disorders. Kiloh emphasized that failure to identify cases with reversible dementia due to psychiatric disorders may promote therapeutic nihilism and abandonment of treatable cases or lead to unnecessarily invasive diagnostic studies.

The term pseudodementia has been questioned by authors who emphasized the role of brain dysfunction in such cases. Folstein & McHugh (1978) argued that depression can give rise to a dementia syndrome which, although reversible, has a biological basis and should not be viewed as a false dementia. Conceptualization of pseudodementia as a nondementia, may hinder the search for underlying biologic mechanisms. Given the high frequency of pseudodementia in the elderly, Folstein & McHugh (1978) hypothesized that pseudodementia develops when the neurobiological disturbances of affective disorders are superimposed on a compromised aging brain. Based upon this concept they proposed the term 'dementia syndrome of depression'. Reifler, Larson & Hanley (1982), diagnosed depression in 23% of cognitively impaired geriatric outpatients; 20% only had depression, and 85% had depression superimposed on an underlying dementia. They suggested that the term pseudodementia should be avoided, because it fosters an unnecessary organic–functional dichotomy especially in patients who have depression as well as a neurological dementing disorder. McAllister (1983) reviewed 34 cases of pseudodementia and noted that they had at least two clinical presentations. The first consisted of impairment in memory and other high intellectual functions and mainly occurred in depressed elderly patients with evidence of coarse brain disease. The other clinical subtype of pseudodementia presented as a caricature of dementia with exaggerated memory complaints and was primarily observed in patients with personality disorders.

In this chapter, the clinical presentation, neuropsychological findings, course of illness and biological findings of patients with pseudodementia syndromes will be reviewed. We will specifically focus on the pseudodementia of depressed elderly patients and argue that this is a heterogeneous syndrome that results from a spectrum of interacting disorders that lead to memory impairment.

Clinical presentation

The clinical presentation of patients with pseudodementia varies widely. Some of the reasons may be age, setting and underlying psychiatric disorder. Wells (1979) described a syndrome of pseudodementia in ten essentially middle-aged patients who were treated in a general hospital for a variety of psychiatric disorders. He observed that patients with dementia developing as part of their psychiatric disorders expressed excessive complaints and distress about their cognitive loss. These patients were able to identify precisely the onset of illness and describe its course. However, when faced with cognitive tests, they refused to answer even when the task was obviously within their capabilities. It is likely that the excessive memory complaints and the inability to respond to cognitive tasks were in part a catastrophic reaction in patients who mainly suffered from neurotic, post-traumatic or personality disorders. While specific studies are lacking the existing studies do not report excessive cognitive complaints in elderly depressives (McAllister, 1983). A study of hospitalized patients (Young, Manley & Alexopoulos, 1985)) showed that depressed and demented elderly patients offer similar numbers of 'I don't know' responses when confronted with standardized cognitive tasks.

In a mixed sample of elderly depressed inpatients and outpatients, those with reversible pseudodementia had significantly more psychic and somatic anxiety, early morning awakening, and reduction in libido than patients with primary degenerative dementia (Reynolds et al., 1986). The affective symptomatology of elderly hospitalized depressed patients with pseudodementia may be characterized by more motor retardation, delusions, hopelessness and helplessness than that of depressed patients with irreversible dementia or of cognitively intact geriatric depressive patients (Alexopoulos & Abrams, 1990, 1991). Pseudodementia therefore is not a homogeneous clinical syndrome, its presentation varies depending on age, setting and underlying disease.

The clinical differentiation of the pseudodementia syndrome from syndromes of irreversible dementia is difficult. An important reason is that the symptoms and signs of irreversible dementia overlap with those of depression and thus interfere with clinical diagnosis. Miller (1980) compared symptomatology of elderly depressed with that of demented patients in a community residing population. She observed a rather broad overlap of clinical manifestations, especially decreased libido, insomnia, weight loss and fatigue. Feinberg & Goodman (1984) noted that dementing disorders may masquerade as depression (pseudodepression) and warned of the risk of missing the diagnosis of a potentially treatable dementing disorder.

Depression is frequent in patients with irreversible dementia. Reifler et al. (1986) reported that 19–30% of psychiatric patients with dementia due to neurological disorders have major depression. Lazarus et al. (1987) emphasized psychic rather than vegetative features in demented patients with depression; they observed that patients with probable Alzheimer's disease scored higher on Hamilton Depression Rating Scale items such as depressed mood, anxiety, hopelessness and worthlessness than did age-matched elderly patients. Patients themselves appear to report less depressive symptomatology than what is reported by their relatives or elicited by trained interviewers using structured interviews (Miller, 1980; Burke et al. 1988; Teri & Wagner, 1991). These observations suggest that multiple sources of information should be used in evaluating the depression of irreversibly demented patients.

In conclusion, it appears that elderly patients with pseudodementia normally have a severe depressive syndrome frequently accompanied by anxiety, retardation, hopelessness, helplessness and delusions. In contrast, depression occurring in patients with irreversible demented syndrome have a wide range of severity and result in marked subjective discomfort that is easily communicated by patients and their relatives. Despite these differences, the clinical presentation of depression by itself does not offer sufficient information for the identification of pseudodementia.

Neuropsychological findings

The overall severity of cognitive disturbance of pseudodementia of elderly depressives is usually of mild intensity. This observation has been confirmed in both inpatient and outpatient populations (Rabins, Merchant & Nestadt 1984; Alexopoulos, Young & Mattis, 1989). Attention and free recall appear to be mainly affected, while spatial functions are less impaired (Alexopoulos et al., 1989). Impairment in various aspects of learning have been observed in both non-demented depressives and in patients with mild degenerative dementia (Hart et al.,

1987). The demented patients, however, forgot the learned material at a more rapid rate than the depressed patients (Hart et al., 1987). Depressives with pseudodementia appear to have more impairment in delayed recall than nondemented depressives; the scores of pseudodemented patients were comparable to those of patients with primary degenerative dementia (Emery, 1988). Ron et al. (1979) noted that unlike irreversibly demented patients, pseudodemented patients did not have significant differences between verbal and performance tests on the Wechsler Adult Intelligence Scale. Another study showed that patients with pseudodementia occurring in the context of depression do not have severe problems in object naming (Nott & Fleminger, 1975). A series of 17 elderly patients with depressive pseudodementia showed that the most impaired functions were attention, motor speed, spontaneous elaboration and analysis of detail. In contrast repetition, reading comprehension, naming, verbal delayed recall and recognition, calculation, finger tapping and motor praxis were relatively preserved. Based on these observations, Caine (1981) argued that pseudodementia of elderly depressives is a subcortical dementia syndrome.

While the above findings suggest that cortical functions are relatively preserved in depressive pseudodementia, more recent studies demonstrated a variety of language disturbances. Language tests of low complexity, involving naming and meta-naming tasks were most useful in differentiating depressive pseudodementia from Alzheimer's disease, while more complex tests, of word fluency and syntactic complexity showed similar impairments in those groups of patients (Emery 1988). Calculation tasks were helpful in differentiating Alzheimer's patients and depressive pseudodementia from normal controls or nondemented depressed patients, while tests of apraxia discriminated depressive pseudodementia from Alzheimer's patients (Emery, 1988).

The wide spectrum of cognitive disturbances identified in depressed pseudodemented elderly patients may be explained by the heterogeneous biological background of this syndrome. Pseudodementia may result from the interaction of depression with early stage neurological dementing disorders resulting in a wide range of cognitive impairment.

Cognitive dysfunction occurring as part of the depressive syndrome includes decreased attention, speed of cognitive response, problem solving, memory, and learning (Weingartner et al., 1981). Weingartner & Silberman (1982) proposed that depressed mood creates an informational context that determines how information is processed, encoded, and organized in memory. Weingartner et al. (1981) reported that depressed patients use weak encoding strategies to organize and transform events that they need to remember, thereby making the events less memorable. McAllister (1981) reported that depressed patients have poor memory for nonemotionally charged material. Elderly depressives sometimes perform as poorly in memory tests as patients with neurologically based dementia (Miller &

Lewis, 1977). It has been reported that the severity of depression is directly related to long-term and short-term memory impairment (Weingartner & Silberman, 1982; Sternberg & Jarvik, 1976). Alleviation of memory deficits has been found to correlate directly with the clinical improvement of depression (Sternberg & Jarvik, 1976). However, L-dopa and L-tryptophan have been found to improve memory in depressives without reducing the severity of depressive symptomatology (Henry, Weingartner & Murphy, 1973). These observations suggest that memory disturbance is part of the depressive syndrome and not merely a clinical byproduct of affective symptomatology. Cognitive dysfunction may originate from biological mechanisms that are related to the mechanism underlying the affective syndrome but are not identical to them.

The cognitive impairment of depressed patients appears to be qualitatively and quantitatively different from that of patients with neurologically based dementias. Alzheimer's patients exhibit deficits in semantic encoding and retrieval in automatic processes while the deficits of depressed patients are essentially limited to a dysfunction of effortless processes (Cohen et al. 1982; Hasher & Zacks, 1979). Elderly depressives were reported to have less impairment in visuospatial paired-associate learning compared to patients with early stage Alzheimer's disease patients (Abas, Sahakian & Levy, 1990). Albert (1984) reported that severe impairments in naming have not been thought to result from depression.

Despite differences in the cognitive impairment of depression from that of neurologically based dementias, identification of the precise contribution of each is difficult in patients suffering from both conditions. This may be due to an additive effect or even a dynamic interaction of the two conditions; neuropsychological tests in pseudodementia patients may exaggerate the part of the intellectual disturbance that results from the coarse dementing disorder and predict a rather poor cognitive recovery.

Course of illness

The course of cognitive symptomatology in elderly patients with depression and dementia sometimes is difficult to predict. Several studies observed that patients who initially were considered to have a progressive dementing disorder on follow-up received different diagnoses. This was exemplified in the report by Marsden & Harrison (1972) who reported changes in diagnoses from dementia to depression in 7.8% of their patients. A diagnostic change from dementia to depression was found in 8.2% of patients studied by Kendell (1974). Smith & Kiloh (1981) reported that 10 out of 200 patients admitted with the diagnosis of dementia were later reclassified as depressive pseudodementia since their cognitive functions improved after antidepressant treatment. A study of 52 patients admitted with the diagnosis of presenile dementia showed that 31% were rediagnosed during hospitalization as having a nondementing disorder. History of a mood disorder and presence of depressed mood during the initial evaluation were more common in patients whose diagnosis changed into a nondementing disorder (Ron et al., 1979). There is evidence suggesting that elderly patients with memory complaints often develop dementia on follow-up. Approximately 57% of depressed elderly patients evaluated in a dementia clinic developed irreversible dementia during a three-year follow-up. However, a considerable number of these patients had signs of neurological disease during the initial evaluation (Reding, Haycox & Blass, 1985).

While some authors viewed pseudodementia as an entity distinct from irreversible dementia (Kiloh, 1961; Wells, 1979) there is evidence that amelioration of depression often leads only to a partial improvement of cognition (Reifler, 1982; Abas et al., 1990). The persistence of mild cognitive impairment suggests that depressive pseudodementia frequently develops in patients with early stage dementing diseases.

Few longitudinal studies examined the long-term outcome of geriatric depressive pseudodementia. Most of these studies were uncontrolled and used dissimilar definitions of the syndrome. However, they all suggest that elderly patients with pseudodementia are at high risk for developing irreversible dementia. In a study of 23 hospitalized elderly patients with major depression and reversible dementia, 39% developed irreversible dementia during a follow-up period of 30 months (Alexopoulos et al., 1987*b*). Reynolds et al. (1986) observed that 50% of depressed elderly patients with an initially reversible dementia syndrome developed irreversible dementia within two years. Two other studies showed that irreversible dementia developed in 9–11% of patients per year (Rabins et al., 1984; Pearlson et al. 1989). The longest follow-up study to date, evaluated its subjects over an eight year period. In this series, 89% of pseudodemented geriatric depressives developed irreversible dementia (Kral & Emery 1989). A considerable number of these patients had a long symptom-free interval between the remission of the pseudodementia syndrome and the time at which the irreversible dementia became clinically evident.

Despite various methodological problems the existing studies suggest that elderly patients with depressive pseudodementia develop irreversible dementia at the rate of 9–25% per year. Most of these patients are left with some degree of cognitive impairment when the depression subsides, while others may have a more or less complete cognitive recovery. While controlled studies are needed, the presence of pseudodementia in a depressed elderly patient should be viewed as a potential harbinger of a progressive dementing disorder rather than as a benign clinical syndrome.

Neurobiological findings

Neuroimaging

Structural brain abnormalities have been identified in both geriatric depression and dementia. Brain computerized tomography (CT) studies showed that elderly depressives have dilatation of lateral ventricles and attenuation of brain tissue greater than that of similarly aged controls (Jacob & Levy, 1980; Jeste, Lohr & Goodwin, 1988). Late-onset depressives have greater size of lateral ventricles than same age early-onset depressives (Jacoby & Levy, 1980), and similar to that of Alzheimer's patients (Alexopoulos et al., 1987*b*). A negative correlation has been reported between depressive symptomatology and the size of the third and of the lateral ventricles in Alzheimer's patients (Burns, Jacoby & Levy, 1990). It is possible that depression was easier to identify in Alzheimer's patients at an early stage of the disease before the ventricular enlargement progressed. Another explanation may be that periventricular structures are required for the development of depression and destruction of these areas does not permit depression to occur.

Only one brain CT study to our knowledge focused on geriatric depression with pseudodementia. This study observed that ventricular dilatation and brain tissue attenuation in pseudodementia patients had intermediate values between non-demented depressives and Alzheimer's patients (Pearlson et al., 1989). It is noteworthy that most of the pseudodementia patients in this study did not develop dementia on follow-up. It is possible, therefore, that structural brain abnormalities are associated with predisposition to depressive pseudodementia even in patients who do not have an early stage dementing disease.

Magnetic resonance imaging (MRI) studies have shown that elderly depressed patients and demented patients have white matter hyperintensity more frequently than normal persons (Coffey et al., 1990; Rabins et al., 1991). The clinical and biological significance of these findings remains unclear. Studies of postmortem brains suggest that white matter hyperintensity areas correspond to sites of demyelization, infraction or dilatation of periventricular spaces (Braffman et al., 1988 *a,b*; Marshall et al., 1988; Awad et al., 1986). White matter hyperintensity does not appear to correlate with neuropsychological impairment in normal elderly persons (Hunt et al., 1989). Some findings on younger adults, however, suggest that, white matter hyperintensity may be a meaningful biological finding in mood disorders. Dupont et al. (1990) reported that a rather large percentage (47%) of nongeriatric patients with bipolar disorders have subcortical white matter hyperintensities while none of the controls had such lesions. It should be noted that bipolar patients appear to have long-term memory deficits similar to those of patients with subcortical dementia (Dupont et al., 1990). These findings suggest the need for studies that will examine whether white matter hyperintensity can be used to predict the course of specific memory disturbances in elderly depressives with pseudodementia.

Functional neuroimaging has identified several abnormalities in irreversible dementia and in depressive syndromes without severe cognitive impairment. In positron emission tomography (PET) studies, patients with Alzheimer's disease were reported to have a temporoparietal pattern of glucose hypometabolism which distinguishes them from patients with depression and from normal subjects (Small et al., 1989; Friedland, 1989). Depressed patients appear to have a small anteroposterior gradient in glucose metabolism compared to normal subjects. Buchsbaum et al. (1984) reported a relative hypofrontality in bipolar depressed patients and observed that bipolars were distinguished from unipolar patients and normal subjects by their anterior/posterior gradients of cortical glucose metabolism. Other abnormalities in depressed patients include low metabolic rate of the caudate, the left frontal regions (Baxter et al., 1985) and the inferior-orbital regions of the frontal lobe (Post et al., 1987), low metabolic ratio of dorsal anterolateral prefrontal cortex to hemisphere (Baxter et al., 1989), and decreased left prefrontal metabolic activity compared to right (Martinot et al., 1990).

In summary, these findings suggest that depression is associated with hypometabolism in the caudate and hypofrontality that appears more prominent in the left prefrontal cortex. Extensive antidepressant treatment leads to partial reversal of most of these abnormalities. Although promising, the few available and mostly uncontrolled studies have not contributed significantly to the pathogenetic understanding of depressive pseudodementia.

Neuropathology and biochemistry

The high comorbidity of depression and dementia raise the question of a biological relationship between the two syndromes. Some investigators suggested that depressive disorders may predispose to dementing diseases. Agbayewa (1986) noted that 18% of patients with Alzheimer's disease had been depressed or paranoid at an earlier age. Others observed that Alzheimer's disease or vascular dementias occur more frequently in depressed than in schizophrenic patients (Brown et al., 1986). However, prospective studies of cognitively unimpaired elderly depressives show that the probability of developing progressive dementia is only slightly higher then that of the general population (Murphy, 1983). Based on the limited available information one has to conclude that if depressive disorders are associated with vulnerability to progressive dementias, they account for only a small percentage of demented patients.

While it is uncertain whether and to what extend mood disorders predispose to progressive dementias, there is evidence that some brain changes of Alzheimer's disease may promote depression. Depressed Alzheimer's patients were observed to have a greater number of neurofibrillary tangles in the locus ceruleus, substantia nigra and central superior raphe nucleus compared to Alzheimer's patients without a disturbance of mood (Zubenko & Moossy, 1988; Zweig et al., 1988). These brain areas contain the cell bodies of norepinephrine, dopamine and serotonin pathways; abnormalities in monoaminergic neurotransmitter systems have been implicated in mood disorders. A related finding is that depressed Alzheimer's patients have a 10 to 20 fold reduction in the cortical levels of norepinephrine and a relative preservation of choline acetyltransferase activity in subcortical regions compared to nondepressed Alzheimer's patients (Zubenko, Moossy & Kopp, 1990). These findings suggest that patients with Alzheimer's disease can present a spectrum of depressive and cognitive manifestations that depend on the site of the lesions and perhaps the stage of the disease.

Peripheral tissue studies suggest that at least a subgroup of patients with depressive pseudodementia may have an Alzheimer's disease process. Geriatric depressives with pseudodementia were found to have platelet monoamine oxidase (MAO) activity higher than cognitively unimpaired depressives and comparable to that of Alzheimer's with and without depression (Alexopoulos et al., 1987*a*). Increased MAO activity in the brain (Adolfsson et al., 1980) and the platelets (Adolfsson et al., 1978, 1987*a*) have been found in Alzheimer's disease compared to controls. These findings raise the question whether increased platelet MAO activity in depressive pseudodementia reflects an early stage Alzheimer's disease that is still not clinically evident.

Neuroendocrine tests have been used in the study of depression since they can reflect neurotransmitter abnormalities. Early escape of plasma cortisol from dexamethasone suppression (DST test) was proposed as a procedure useful for the identification of depressive pseudodementia (Jenike & Albert, 1984). However, controlled studies showed that patients with depressive pseudodementia have abnormal DST at a frequency similar with that of depressed Alzheimer's patients and of cognitively unimpaired geriatric depressives, while nondepressed Alzheimer's patients have an abnormal DST at a lower frequency (Alexopoulos et al., 1985). These findings suggest that some biological abnormalities are common in primary depression and in dementing disorders.

Electrophysiology

The electroencephalogram (EEG) may aid to some extent the differential diagnosis of Alzheimer's disease from depressive pseudodementia (Ron et al., 1979). Approximately one-third of Alzheimer's patients have significant EEG abnormalities (Brenner, Reynolds & Ulrich, 1989). Patients with depressive pseudodementia have more EEG abnormalities than similarly aged normal persons; these abnormalities mainly consist of slowing of EEG activity in the posterior dominant areas (Brenner et al., 1989). Despite these differences, the overlap of EEG abnormalities among the various diagnostic groups does not permit the use of this procedure for the diagnosis of an individual patient.

Sleep electroencephalography appears to distinguish patients with pseudodementia from depressed Alzheimer's patients. Higher rapid eye movement (REM) percentage and phasic REM activity/intensity were observed in pseudodemented compared to depressed patients who also had irreversible dementia (Buysse et al., 1988). After sleep deprivation leading to improvement of depression, a greater first REM period duration was observed in pseudodemented patients, while both groups had comparable increases in sleep efficiency, sleep maintenance and slow wave sleep. These findings were thought to reflect differences in the cholinergic and monoaminergic regulation of REM sleep between depressed and Alzheimer's patients.

Conclusions

Pseudodementia was a term developed to describe a transient dementia syndrome that occurs in patients with a variety of psychiatric disorders. An explicit purpose of some of the early clinical reports was to identify pseudodemented patients through clinical criteria and thus avoid invasive diagnostic procedures or therapeutic neglect that may have resulted if these patients were thought to be irreversibly demented. Therefore, early literature on pseudodementia was motivated by clinical concerns and constructed an approximately utilitarian definition rather than a conceptually or empirically based entity. Review of recent investigations suggests that pseudodementia is not a single entity but rather a heterogeneous clinical syndrome that can develop in patients with a variety of psychiatric disorders and a wide spectrum of neurological brain diseases.

Personality disorders, neurotic disorders and post-traumatic stress disorders may be the psychiatric background for a considerable number of middle-aged patients with pseudodementia. In contrast, elderly patients usually present a pseudodementia syndrome as part of a severe depressive disorder often accompanied by retardation, depressive delusions, anxiety, hopelessness and helplessness.

Unlike the depressive symptomatology which as a rule is severe, the cognitive disturbance of pseudodemented patients is rather mild. Cognitive disturbances usually consist of impairment in attention, free recall of verbal information, spontaneous elaboration and analysis of detail, and in low complexity naming and meta-naming tasks. Cognitive disturbances vary widely from patient to patient probably due to the heterogeneous background of the pseudodementia syndrome. Despite recent clarification of the behavioral and cognitive manifestations of pseudodementia, in some cases the only way to identify whether the cognitive dysfunction is reversible and to what extent is by providing antidepressant treatment until the depressive syndrome subsides.

Early literature emphasized the benign outcome of pseudodemented patients. More recent evidence suggests, however, that a large percentage of pseudo-demented depressed elderly patients have only a partial cognitive improvement after remission of depression. While these patients no longer meet criteria for dementia, the remaining cognitive disturbance suggests an underlying brain disease. Long-term follow-up studies show that depressed elderly patients with the initial diagnosis of pseudodementia proceed to develop progressive dementia at a rate of 9–25% per year. Although controlled studies are not yet available this percentage is higher then the incidence of dementia in the general population of the same age. It appears, therefore, that pseudodementia occuring in the context of geriatric depression is a predictor of eventual development of irreversible dementia. This may be true even in patients with a long period of relatively unimpaired cognition after the remission of the pseudodementia syndrome. Given the high risk for irreversible dementia, clinicans should pursue a thorough work-up in pseudodemented patients aiming to identify treatable neurological disorders.

Biological studies have demonstrated that the syndromes of depression and dementia share abnormalities of brain structure and function. Limited findings in pseudodementia show that these patients have ventricular dilatation and brain tissue attenuation even if they do not develop irreversible dementia on follow-up. Elderly patients with depressive pseudodementia appear to have high MAO similar to that of Alzheimer's patients.

Taken together the above findings suggest that pseudodementia of depressed elderly patients may result from the interaction of depression with neurological disorders. Pseudodementia cases may be ordered along a continuum depending on the contribution of the underlying condition. On one end of the continuum, are cases in whom the cognitive disturbance is mostly due to the depressive syndrome itself with minimal contribution by a neurological brain disease. On the other end of the continuum, are cases in whom the intellectual impairment originates mainly from a coarse brain disease with rather mild contribution by the depressive syndrome. Most cases of pseudodementia are due to an additive or dynamic interaction between the cognitive disturbance of depression and of a variety of neurological brain diseases.

Acknowledgement

This paper was supported by NIMH grants ROI-MH-42819, T32 MH-19132, P20MH-49762, and by the Xerox Foundation.

References

Abas, M. D., Sahakian, B. J. & Levy R. (1990). Neuropsychological deficits and CT scan changes in elderly depressives. *Psychological Medicine*, **20**, 507–20.

Adolfsson, R., Gottfries, C. G, Oreland, L., Wilberg, A. & Winblad, B. (1980). Increased activity in brain and platelet monoamine oxidase in dementia of Alzheimer's type. *Life Science*, **27**, 1029–34.

Adolfsson, R. Gottfries, C. G., Oreland, L., Roos, B. E. & Winblad, B. (1978). Reduced levels of catecholamines in the brain and increased activity of monoamine oxidase in platelets in Alzheimer's disease. Therapeutic implications. In *Alzheimer's Disease*. ed. R. Katzman, R. D. Terr & K. L. Bick, p. 441 New York: Raven Press.

Agbayewa, M. O. (1986). Earlier psychiatric morbidity in patients with Alzheimer's disease. *Journal of the American Geriatric Society*, **34**, 561–4.

Albert, M. (1984). Assessment of cognitive function in the elderly. *Psychosomatics*, **25**, 310–17.

Alexopoulos, G. S. & Abrams, R. C. (1991). Depression in Alzheimer's disease. *Psychiatric Clinics of North America*, **14**, (2), 327–40.

Alexopoulos, G. S. & Abrams, R. C. (1990). Clinical presentation and outcome of geriatric depressive pseudodementia [abstract]. Presented at the meeting of the Royal College of Psychiatrists, London.

Alexopoulos, G. S., Young, R. C. & Mattis, S. (1989). Cognitive disturbances in geriatric depression with reversible dementia. Unpublished paper presented at the annual meeting of the American Association for Geriatric Psychiatry, Orlando, Florida.

Alexopoulos, G. S., Young, R. C., Meyers, B. S., Abrams, R. C. & Shamoian, C. A. (1988). Late-onset depression. *Psychiatric Clinics of North America*, **11** (1), 101–15.

Alexopoulos, G. S., Young, R. C., Lieberman, K. W. & Shamoian, C. A. (1987*a*). Platelet MAO activity in geriatric patients with depression and dementia. *American Journal of Psychiatry*, **144**, 1480–3.

Alexopoulos, G. S., Abrams, R. C., Young, R. C. & Shamoian, C. A. (1987*b*). Late life depression and dementing disorders. Abstract, Puerto Rico, American College of Neuropsychopharmacology.

Alexopoulos, G. S., Young, R. C., Haycox, J. A., Shamoian, C. A. & Blass, J. P. (1985). Dexamethasone suppression test in depression with reversible dementia. *Psychiatry Research*, **16**, 277–85.

Awad, I. A., Johnson, P. C., Spetzler, R. F. & Hodak, J. A. (1986). Incidental subcortical lesions identified on magnetic resonance imaging in the elderly. II. Post mortem pathological correlation. *Stroke*, **17** (6), 1090–7.

Baxter, L. R. Jr., Schwartz, J. M., Phelps, M. E. et al. (1989). Reduction of prefrontal cortex glucose metabolism common to three types of depression. *Archives of General Psychiatry*, **46**, 243–50.

Baxter, L. R., Phelps, M. E., Mazziotta, J. C. et al. (1985). Cerebral metabolism rates for glucose in mood disorders: Studies with positron emission tomography and fluorodeoxyglucose F18. *Archives of General Psychiatry*, **42**, 441–7.

Braffman, B. H., Zimmerman, R. A., Trojanowski, J. Q., Gonatas, N. K., Hickley, W. F. &

Schlaepfer, W. W. (1988*a*). Brain MR pathologic correlation with gross and histopathology.1. Lacunar infarction and Virchow-Robin spaces. *American Journal of Radiology*, **151** (3), 551–8.

Braffman, B. H., Zimmerman, R. A., Trojanowski, J. Q., Gonatas, N. K., Hickley, W. F. & Schlaepfer, W. W. (1988*b*). Brain MR pathologic correlation with gross and histopathology.2. Hyperintense white-matter foci in the elderly. *American Journal of Radiology*, **151** (3), 559–66.

Brenner, R., Reynolds, C. & Ulrich, R. (1989). EEG findings in depressive pseudodementia and dementia with secondary depression. *Electroencephalography and Clinical Neurophysiology*, **72**, 298–304.

Brown, R., Colter, N., Corsellis, J. N. et al. (1986). Postmortem evidence of structural brain changes in schizophrenia. *Archives of General Psychiatry*, **43**, 36–42.

Buchsbaum, M. S., DeLisi, L. E., Holocomb, H. H. et al. (1984). Antero-posterior gradients in cerebral glucose use in schizophrenia and affective disorders. *Archives of General Psychiatry*, **41**, 1159–66.

Burke, W., Rubin, E., Morris, J., et al. (1988). Symptoms of 'depression' in dementia of the Alzheimer's type. *Alzheimer Disease and Associated Disorders*, **2**, 356–62.

Burns, A., Jacoby, R. & Levy, R. (1990). Psychiatric phenomena in Alzheimer's disease. III. Disorders of mood. *British Journal of Psychiatry*, **157**, 81–6.

Buysse, D. J., Reynolds, C. F., Kupfer, D. J. et al. (1988). Electroencephalographic sleep in depressive pseudodementia. *Archives of General Psychiatry*, **45**, 568–76.

Caine, E. D. (1981). Pseudodementia. *Archives of General Psychiatry*, **38**, 1359–64.

Coffey, C. E., Figiel, C. S., Djang, W. T. & Weiner, R. D. (1990). Subcortical hyperintensity on magnetic resonance imaging: a comparison of normal and depressed elderly subjects. *American Journal of Psychiatry*, **147**, 187–9.

Cohen, R. M., Weingartner, H., Smallberg, S. A., Pickar, D. & Murphy, D. L. (1982). Effort and cognition in depression. *Archives of General Psychiatry*, **39**, 593–7.

Dupont, R., Jernigan, R., Butters, N., Delis, D., Hesselink, J. R., Heindel, W. & Gillin, J. C. (1990). Subcortical abnormalities detected in bipolar affective disorder using magnetic resonance imaging. *Archives of General Psychiatry*, **47**, 55–9.

Emery, O. B. (1988). *Pseudodementia: A Theoretical and Empirical Discussion.* ed. R. W. Hubbard & J. Kowal. Cleveland Western Reserve Geriatric Education Center Interdisciplinary Monograph series. Case Western Reserve University School of Medicine.

Feinberg, T., Goodman, B. (1984). Affective illness, dementia, and pseudodementia. *Journal of Clinical Psychiatry*, **45**, 88–103.

Folstein, M. F. & McHugh, P. R. (1978). Dementia syndrome of depression. In *Alzheimer's Disease: Senile Dementia and Related Disorders.* ed. R. Katzman, R. D. Terry & K. L. Bick, New York: Raven Press.

Friedland, R. (1989). 'Normal'-pressure hydrocephalus and the saga of the treatable dementias. *Journal of the American Medical Association*, **262**, 2577–81.

Hart, R. P., Kwentus, J. A., Taylor, J. R. & Harkins, S. W. (1987). Rate of forgetting in dementia and depression. *Journal of Consulting and Clinical Psychology*, **55**, 101–5.

Hasher, L. & Zacks, R. T. (1979). Automatic and effortful processes in memory. *Journal of Experimental Psychology General*, **108**, 356–88.
Henry, G. M., Weingartner, H. & Murphy, D. L. (1973). Influence of affective states and psychoactive drugs on verbal learning and memory. *American Journal of Psychiatry*, **130**, 996–71.
Hunt, A. L., Orrison, W. W., Yeo, R. W. et al. (1989). Clinical significance of MRI white matter lesions in the elderly. *Neurology*, **39**, 1470–4.
Jacoby, R. & Levy, R. (1980). Computed tomography in the elderly, 3. Affective disorder. *British Journal of Psychiatry*, **136**, 270–5.
Jenike, M. A. & Albert, M. S. (1984). The dexamethasone suppression test in patients with presenile and senile dementia of the Alzheimer's type. *Journal of the American Geriatric Society*, **32**, (6) 441–4.
Jeste, D., Lohr, J. & Goodwin, F. (1988). Neuroanatomical studies of major depression; a review and suggestions for future research. *British Journal of Psychiatry*, **153**, 444–59.
Kendell, R. E. (1974). The stability of psychiatric diagnosis. *British Journal of Psychiatry*, **124**, 352–6.
Kiloh, L. (1961). Pseudodementia. *Acta Psychiatrica Scandinavica*, **37**, 336–51.
Kral, V. A. & Emery, O. B. (1989). Long term follow-up of depressive pseudodementia of the aged. *Canadian Journal of Psychiatry*, **34**, 445–6.
Lazarus, L., Newton, N., Cohler, B., Lesser, J. & Schweon, C. (1987). Frequency and presentation of depressive symptom in patients with primary degenerative dementia. *American Journal of Psychiatry*, **144**, 41–5.
Madden, J., Luban, J. & Kaplan, L. (1952). Nondementing psychosis in older persons. *Journal of the American Medical Association*, **150**, 1567–72.
Marsden, C. D. & Harrison, M. J. (1972). Outcome of investigation of patients with presenile dementia. *British Medical Journal*, **2**, 249–52.
Marshall, V. G., Bradley, W. G., Marshal C. E., Bhoopat, T. & Rhodes, R. H. (1988). Deep white matter infarction: correlation of MR imaging and histopathologic finding. *Radiology*, **167** (2), 517–22.
Martinot, J. L., Hardy, P., Feline, A. et al. (1990). Left prefrontal glucose hypometabolism in depressed state: a confirmation. *American Journal of Psychiatry*, **147**, (10), 1313–7.
McAllister, T. W. (1983). Overview: pseudodementia. *American Journal of Psychiatry*, **140**, 528–33.
McAllister, T. W. (1981). Cognitive functioning in the affective disorders. *Comprehensive Psychiatry*, **22**, 572–86.
Miller, N. E. (1980). The measurement of mood in senile brain disease: Examiner ratings and self-reports. In *Psychopathology of the Aged*. ed. J. O. Cole & J. E. Barrett, New York: Raven Press.
Miller, P. & Lewis, P. (1977). Recognition memory in elderly patients with depression and dementia: a signal detection analysis. *Journal of Abnormal Psychology*, **86**, 84–6.
Murphy, E. (1983). The prognosis of depression in old age. *British Journal of Psychiatry*, **142**, 111–19.

Nott, P. N. & Fleminger, J. J. (1975). Presenile dementia: the difficulties of early diagnosis. *Acta Psychiatrica Scandanavica*, **51**, 210–17.

Pearlson, G. D., Rabins, P. V., Kim, W. S. et al. (1989). Structural brain CT changes and cognitive deficits in elderly depressives with and without reversible dementia (Pseudodementia). *Psychological Medicine*, **19**, 573–84.

Post, F. (1975). Dementia, depression and pseudodementia. In *Psychiatric Aspects of Neurological Disease*. ed. F. Benson, & D. Blumer, New York: Grune and Stratton.

Post, R. M., DeLisi, L. E., Holcomb, H. H. Unde, Cohen, R. & Buchsbaum, M. S. (1987). Glucose utilization in the temporal cortex of affectively ill patients: positron emission tomography. *Biological Psychiatry*, **22**, 545–53.

Rabins, P. V., Merchant, A. & Nestadt, G. (1984). Criteria for diagnosing reversible dementia caused by depression: validation by 2-year follow-up. *British Journal of Psychiatry*, **144**, 488–92.

Rabins, P. V., Pearlson, G. C., Aylward, E., Kumar, A. J. & Dowell, K. (1991). Cortical magnetic resonance imaging changes in elderly inpatients with major depression. *American Journal of Psychiatry*, **148**, 617–20.

Reding, M., Haycox, J. & Blass, J. (1985). Depression in patients referred to a dementia clinic: a 3-year prospective study. *Archives of Neurology*, **42**, 894–6.

Reifler, B. V., Larson, E., Teri, L. & Poulsen, M. (1986). Dementia of the Alzheimer's type and depression. *Journal of the American Geriatric Society*, **34**, 855–9.

Reifler, B. V. (1982). Arguments for abandoning the term Pseudodementia. *Journal of the American Geriatric Society*, **30**, 665–8.

Reifler, B. V., Larson, E. & Hanley, R. (1982). Coexistence of cognitive impairment and depression in geriatric outpatients. *American Journal of Psychiatry*, **139**, 623–6.

Reynolds, C. F., Kupfer, D. J., Hoch, C. C., Stack, J. A., Houck, P. R. & Sewitch, D. E. (1986). Two year follow-up of elderly patients with mixed depression and dementia. Clinical and electroencephalographic sleep findings. *Journal of the American Geriatric Society*, **34**, 793–9.

Ron M. A., Toone B. K., Garralda, M. E. & Lishman, W. A. (1979). Diagnostic accuracy in presenile dementia. *British Journal of Psychiatry*, **134**, 161–8.

Small, G. W., Kuhl, D. F., Riege, W., Fujikawa, D. W., Ashford, J. W., Metter, E. J. & Mazziotta, J. C. (1989). Cerebral glucose metabolic patterns in Alzheimer's disease: effect of gender and age at dementia onset. *Archives of General Psychiatry*, **46**, 527–32.

Smith, J. S. & Kiloh, L. A. (1981). The investigation of dementia, results in 200 consecutive admissions. *Lancet*, **i**, 824–7.

Sternberg, D. E. & Jarvik, M. E. (1976). Memory function in depression improvement with antidepressant medication. *Archives of General Psychiatry*, **33**, 219–24.

Teri, L. & Wagner, A. W. (1991). Assessment of depression in patients with Alzheimer's disease: concordance among informants. *Psychology and Aging*, **6** (2), 280–5.

Weingartner, H., Cohen, R., Murphy, D., Martello, J & Gerdt. C. (1981). Cognitive process in depression. *Archives of General Psychiatry*, **38**, 42–7.

Weingartner, H. & Silberman, E. (1982). Models of cognitive impairment: cognitive changes in depression. *Psychopharmacology Bulletin* **18**, 27–42.

Wells, C. (1979). Pseudodementia. *American Journal of Psychiatry*, **38**, 42–7.

Young, R. C., Manley, M. W. & Alexopoulos, G. S. (1985). 'I don't know' responses in elderly depressives and in dementia. *Journal of the American Geriatric Society*, **33**, 253–7.

Zubenko, G. S., Moossy, J & Kopp. U. (1990). Neurochemical correlates of major depression in primary dementia. *Archives of Neurology*, **47**, 209–14.

Zubenko, G. S. & Moossy, J. (1988). Major depression in primary dementia – clinical and neuropathologic correlates. *Archives of Neurology*, **45**, 1182–6.

Zweig, R., Ross, C., Hedreen, J. et al. (1988). The neuropathology of aminergic nuclei in Alzheimer's disease. *Annals of Neurology*, **24**, 233–42.

10

Depression in nursing and residential homes

DAVID AMES

Introduction

It has been estimated that 43% of Americans turning 65 in 1990 will enter a 'nursing home before death (Kemper & Murtaugh, 1991) and that 55% will stay in such a home for over one year. Although the extent and type of residential and nursing home provision vary extensively between developed countries, increased longevity and rising social mobility mean that in those places where community services to support the old in their own homes do not improve, the demand for places in long-term care is likely to rise. It is probable that factors leading to admission (Loebel et al., 1991*b*; Ames, 1992*a*) and the characteristics of the institutions themselves (Godlove, Richard & Rodwell, 1982; Rodwell, 1982; Mann, Graham & Ashby, 1984*a*; Vousden, 1987; Ames, 1992*a*) play a significant role in determining rates of mental disorder among inmates of nursing and residential homes. Thus it is appropriate that research on the mental health of the elderly in such homes should be a matter of concern to psychiatrists and others involved with the prevention of disability and the delivery of health care. The rapid growth of the research literature in this field indicates a dawning awareness of these realities.

Although dementia is the commonest psychiatric disorder reported in residential and nursing homes worldwide (Spagnoli et al., 1986; Ineichen, 1990; Jorm & Henderson, 1990; Rovner et al., 1991) depression is common in long-term care institutions for the old too. Other psychiatric disorders have been little studied in these settings. This chapter summarizes current knowledge regarding the prevalence, associations, incidence, treatment and outcome of depression among residents of nursing and residential homes for the aged. It concludes with some suggestions for future action and research.

The essential difference between nursing and residential homes relates to the full-time provision of skilled nursing care. For the purposes of this chapter, papers' descriptions of institutions as nursing or residential homes have been taken at face

Table 10.1. *Prevalence of depression among residents of nursing homes*

Study	Country City/Area Setting	Number fully assessed	Instrument	Diagnostic criteria	Findings	Remarks
Kay et al., 1964	UK Newcastle Geriatric and Psychiatric long-stay wards	83	Interview by psychiatrist	Roth 1955	7% Manic-depressive 11% neurosis (mainly depressive)	Cross-sectional study. Rate in community for MDP and neurosis combined was 26%
Teeter et al., 1976	USA Midwest 2 homes	74	Interview by psychiatrist	Idiosyncratic	26% Primary 24% Secondary depression	Cross-sectional. Only 16% had no psychiatric diagnosis. 74% response
Hyer & Blazer, 1982	USA N. Carolina 5 homes	149	Clinical interview checklist	DSM-III	25% Major depression	Cross-sectional. Only best 1/3 assessed
Kay & Holding, 1983	AUSTRALIA Hobart N Homes and long-term hospital wards	119	GMS6	Operationalized ICD-9	37% depressed	Cross-sectional. Further 80 too cognitively impaired to rate Additional 4% anxiety diagnosis
Mann et al., 1984*b*	USA New York	82	6 items from CARE DEP scale	score 2+	53% depressed	Cross-sectional stratified city-wide random sample of women in long-term nursing care
	UK London	49			83% depressed	
	GERMANY Mannheim	71			55% depressed	

Table 10.1. (*cont.*)

Study	Country City/Area Setting	Number fully assessed	Instrument	Diagnostic criteria	Findings	Remarks
Rovner et al., 1986	USA Baltimore 1 home	50	GMS and MMSE	DSM-III	6% Major depression alone +18% Dementia with depressed mood	Cross-sectional. Only 6% had no psychiatric diagnosis. 74% had dementia
Snowdon & Donnelly, 1986	AUSTRALIA Sydney 6 homes	206	GDS	score 11–13 score 14+	13% possibly depressed 26% probably depressed	Cross-sectional. Further 133 not able/willing to do GDS
Snowdon, 1986	AUSTRALIA Sydney 12 homes	217	Gilleard depression questionnaire	score 15+	18% prob. DSM-III Major depression	Cross-sectional. 68% response. 74% probably demented
Burns et al., 1988	USA 4 cities 112 homes	526	Report from nurse and chart review	Not stated	8% Depression diagnosis	Cross-sectional. 39% Organic brain syndrome diagnosis
Katz et al., 1989	USA Philadelphia Geriatric center	51	MSQ, GDS and structured interview	GDS 11+ DSM-III	43% possibly depressed 20% major depression	Cross-sectional. Further 51 too demented to rate for depression
Parmalee et al., 1989	USA Philadelphia NH wards in one large geriatric institution	116 new and 161 long-term residents	SADS and GDS screen followed by clinical evaluation	DSM-III-R	Maj D 10% new 9% LT Minor D 14% and 17% cog imp't+ Maj D 21% and 8% CI+ Min D 22% and 21%	Both admission and cross-sectional samples. 34% and 25% had cognitive impairment without dep'n. Only 11% and 18% normal. Only 59% and 41% response

Harrison et al., 1990	UK London Geriatric and Psychiatric long-term wards	36 Geriatric 33 Psychiatric	BAS	Score 7+ on DEP scale	44% Geriatric depressed 42% Psych. depressed	Cross-sectional. Further 61 in Geriatric and 90 in Psychiatric wards too demented to rate. Similar depression rates in sheltered housing and home care
Rovner et al., 1991	USA Baltimore 8 homes	454	Modified PSE	DSM-III-R	13% had DSM-III-R 'Depressive disorder' plus 18% 'depressive symptoms'	Admission study. 81% response. 67% dementia. Excluding dementia patients, 15% depressive disorder, 25% depressive symptoms
Phillips & Henderson, 1991	AUSTRALIA Melbourne 24 homes	165	CIE Depression Items after MMSE	DSM-III-R ICD-10	10% Major Depression 19% ICD-10 Depressive Episode	Cross-sectional. 405 subjects selected, 82 excluded (ill/no English), 19 refused, 139 had MMSE < 18 so not assessed by CIE
Horiguchi & Inami, 1991	JAPAN Ehime prefecture 32 homes	920	Zung	Score 50+	61% depressed	Cross-sectional. 36% depressed among community comparison group
Henderson et al., 1993	AUSTRALIA Canberra Goulburn 6 N homes and sheltered accommodations	59	CIE	DSM-III-R ICD-10	6% Major Depression 6% Depressive Episode 3% Dysthymia	Cross-sectional. Community rate for DSM-III-R Major Dep+ Dysthymia 1% ICD-10 D Ep 3%, Dysthymia 0.3%

value and surveys of patients in long-term hospital wards have been included with those conducted in nursing homes. Where papers have reported overall rates for nursing and residential homes combined, the data have been considered as nursing home data.

Epidemiology of depression in nursing and residential homes

History and methodology

After a few pioneering reports in the 1960s (Kay, Beamish & Roth, 1964; Jensen, 1966) and 1970s (Lowther & McLeod, 1974; Teeter et al., 1976) studies of the epidemiology of psychiatric disorder in long-term care facilities for the elderly burgeoned in the 1980s. An important distinction may be drawn between cross-sectional point-prevalence studies and those that have examined an admission cohort (Wayne & Rhyne, 1991). A further contrast exists between studies which report rates of depressive symptoms and those which have attempted to make discrete psychiatric diagnoses. Of the latter, some early diagnostic surveys used idiosyncratic criteria which are difficult to replicate (Kay et al., 1964; Jensen, 1966; Teeter et al., 1976). The advent of internationally accepted criteria (American Psychiatric Association, 1980; 1987) and the development of computerized diagnostic algorithms (Copeland, Dewey & Griffiths-Jones, 1986) should permit the conduct of investigations whose results easily may be compared with those performed elsewhere.

Studies which have reported depression rates in nursing and residential homes are summarized in tables 10.1 and 10.2. Surveys which report on dementia alone are excluded from consideration.

Nursing homes

Rates for depressive symptoms in cross-sectional nursing home studies vary from 39% to 83%, with the highest levels found in London's long-stay hospital wards (Mann et al., 1984*b*) and the lowest in Sydney's nursing homes (Snowdon & Donnelly, 1986). Many studies which made discrete psychiatric diagnoses report only one diagnosis per subject and rates for depressive disorders are very much influenced by the prevalence of conditions such as dementia which rank higher in most diagnostic hierarchies. Using DSM-III and DSM-III-R criteria (APA, 1980, 1987), rates for major depression range from 6% to 20%, though when other diagnostic criteria, dual diagnoses and milder depressive disorders are taken into account, rates for depressive disorders from all studies vary from 6% (Henderson et al., 1993) to 50% (Teeter et al., 1976).

Two admission studies were traced for this review. Parmalee, Katz & Lawton (1989) found little difference between the rates of DSM-III-R depressive disorder detected in newly admitted and long-standing residents of a large geriatric facility, though the new admissions were more likely to have major depression. The study of Rovner et al. (1991) found DSM-III depressive disorders (usually co-morbid with dementia) in 13% of 454 admissions. Among the 33% free of dementia, 15% had depression on admission.

Some nursing home studies have been able to compare rates of disorder with those found in other settings using the same methodology. Generally higher rates of depression have been found in the nursing homes. In an early study, rates of affective disorder and neurosis in Newcastle-upon-Tyne were reported to be *lower* in both nursing and residential home groups of elderly than among the old living at home (Kay et al., 1964), but this is likely to have been an artefact produced by the higher rates of organic mental impairment (these diagnoses took precedence) found among those in hospital wards and welfare homes. A later study by Kay and Holding (1983) compared residents of Hobart, Australia who were in receipt of domiciliary nursing, residential and nursing home care with those who lived independently at home. Rates in nursing home residents were comparable to those found among the domiciliary nursing sample. For those in residential care depression rates were intermediate between the two physically dependent samples and the well elderly at home who were least likely to be depressed. Harrison, Savla & Kafetz (1990) studied six separate groups of dependent elderly in one London borough using the Brief Assessment Scale (BAS – Mann et al., 1989). Rates of dementia varied widely but among those who could be assessed for depression, percentages classed as depressed varied in a narrow band between 42% and 52%. In Finland those in long-term institutional care together with those in receipt of home nursing or help were 1.7 times more likely to have a diagnosis of DSM-III depression than those living independently at home (Kivelä, Pakhala & Laippala, 1988). A large study in Japan (Horiguchi & Inami, 1991) found nursing home residents to be nearly twice as likely to have depressive symptoms as were old people living in the local community. In Australia, Henderson et al. (1993) found DSM-III-R depressions to be over six times more prevalent among institutional residents than among the old at home, though ICD-10 depressions were only three times more common. A cross-national comparative study (Mann et al., 1984*b*) was flawed by the brevity of the depression screen employed, but is noteworthy for its consistent finding of higher depression rates for females living in nursing care in London as compared with those in New York and Mannheim.

From work published to date it may be concluded that depressive symptoms are extremely common among residents of nursing homes. Depressive disorders diagnosed by psychiatrists are found between two and six times more frequently in nursing homes than among old people living in the general community.

Table 10.2. *Prevalence of depression in residential homes for the aged*

Study	Country City/Area setting	Number fully assessed	Instrument	Diagnostic criteria	Findings	Remarks
Kay et al., 1964	UK Newcastle LAHs	125	Interview by psychiatrist	Roth, 1955	6% neurosis (mainly depressive)	Cross sectional sample. Community rate 26%
Jensen, 1966	DENMARK One county 4 homes	126	Staff and patient interview	Idiosyncratic psychiatric diagnosis	4% endogenous, 2% reactive Depression	Cross-sectional. 1% of 546 old in local parish had depression
Lowther & McLeod, 1974	UK Edinburgh 1 LAH	100	Interview by psychiatrist	Psychiatrist's diagnosis	9% had depression diagnosis	Admission sample 47.5% had other psych. diagnoses (mainly dementia)
Gillis et al., 1982	S. Africa Cape Town 30 homes	100	400 item protocol	ICD-9	8% had affective disorder	Admission sample. 'Depression' led to referral to the home for 23%
Kay & Holding, 1983	AUSTRALIA Hobart Hostel and 'hospital welfare'	113	GMS6	Operationalized ICD-9	26% depressed	Cross-sectional. Further 8% had anxiety diagnosis
Mann et al., 1984*a*	UK London 12 LAHs	289	BAS	Score 7+ on DEP scale	38% depressed	Cross-sectional Additional 134 too demented for DEP screen, 112 refused/not interviewable

Mann et al., 1984*b*	USA New York	36	6 items from CARE DEP scale items	Score 2+	33% depressed	Cross-sectional stratified city-wide random *sample of women* in residential care
	UK *London*	70			75% depressed	
	GERMANY Mannheim	68			50% depressed	
Spagnoli et al., 1986	ITALY Milan 13 Homes	278	IPG (Adapted CARE) OBS and DEP scales	Feighner criteria based on DEP score 11+	33% Feighner Depression	Cross-sectional. 76% response to DEP scale
Lau-Ting et al., 1987	SINGAPORE 5 non-govt old age homes	356	6 item interview	Positive response	30% depressed	Cross-sectional. 67% response
Ames et al., 1988; Ames, 1990	UK London 12 LAHs	271	BAS DEP scale screen then GMS and chart review	score 7+ AGECAT DSM-III	34% dep'd. 41/86 were AGECAT Depression cases 25/92 Major Depression. 20/92 had other DSM-III Depression	Cross-sectional 2-stage study. 86/93 who were Depressed at screen rated by GMS. 92/93 could be given DSM-III dx. Further 119 too demented for DEP screen and 49 refused/not interviewable
Snowdon & Mackintosh, 1989	AUSTRALIA Sydney 3 hostels	100	GDS BAS DEP scale	score 11–13 score 14+ score 7+ DSM-III	9% ?depressed 15% depressed 20% depressed 12% DSM-III affective disorder alone + 3% with both aff. disorder and dementia	20% of 140 elderly in local community classed as depressed byBAS

Table 10.2. (*cont.*)

Study	Country City/Area setting	Number fully assessed	Instrument	Diagnostic criteria	Findings	Remarks
Steel, 1989	AUSTRALIA Melbourne 5 Special accommodation Houses (SAHs)	84	BAS	score 7+ on DEP scale	29% depressed	Cross-sectional. Further 16 residents refused interview and 9 too demented for DEP screen
Livingston et al., 1990	UK London 1 LAH	34	Short CARE	Depression diagnostic scale	35% depressed	Cross-sectional. 17% local community elderly were depressed
Harrison et al., 1990	UK 1 London borough all LAHs and PRHs	195 in LAHs 117 in PRHs	BAS	Score 7+ on DEP scale	51% LAHs depressed 52% PRHs depressed	Cross-sectional. Further 160 in LAHs and 55 in PRHs too demented to rate
Weyerer et al., 1990	GERMANY Mannheim 16 homes	376	BAS	Score 7+ on DEP scale	32% depressed	Cross-sectional. Further 13 too demented for DEP screen and 153 not inter-viewable/refused
Lobo et al., 1990	SPAIN Soria 1 home	101	CIS	ICD-9	14% depressed	Cross-sectional. 7% had other psych. diagnoses 96% response

Rosewarne et al., 1991	AUSTRALIA Victoria 64 Hostels	584	GDS	Score 11–13 14+	13% poss. depressed 27% prob. depressed	Cross-sectional. Includes demented residents.
Clark, 1992	UK Fife 4 LAHs	32	SADS, BDI and GHQ	RDC	22% Major Depression 13% Minor Depression	Admission study Of 32 matched controls 1 had Minor Depression Further 4 residents too demented for affective assessment. Only 45% response
Flicker et al., 1992	AUSTRALIA Melbourne 5 SAHs	94	GDS	Score 14+	28% prob. depressed	Cross-sectional. 81% response
Weyerer et al., 1994	UK London 15 LAH/PRHs	48	BAS	Score 7+ on DEP scale	48% depressed	Comparative admission and follow-up study
	GERMANY Mannheim 14 r. homes	52	BAS	Score 7+ on DEP scale	35% depressed	Rates not significantly different

Residential homes

Cross-sectional studies of depression in residential homes have been more likely to assess symptoms alone and the BAS has proved a popular screening instrument. Findings using the depression scale (DEP) of this interview have pointed consistently to depression rates being higher in London's local authority homes (LAHs) than among the less dependent residents of hostel accommodation in Australia (Mann et al., 1984*a*; Ames et al., 1988; Snowdon & MacKintosh, 1989; Steel, 1989), while the cross-national study referred to in the previous section (Mann et al, 1984*b*) again found Londoners in residential care to be more often depressed than their American and German counterparts, though this was not the case for those who lived at home in London and New York (Gurland et al., 1983). Rates for depression in one London residential home were double those in the surrounding community (Livingston et al, 1990).

The frequency of depressive disorder diagnosed by a psychiatrist in cross-sectional studies of residential homes has ranged from 6% (Jensen, 1966) to 26% (Kay & Holding, 1983) but there has been less consistency of diagnostic practice than in the predominantly American nursing home studies.

Two admission studies in very different cultures (Lowther & McLeod, 1974; Gillis et al., 1982) found similarly low rates of depressive disorder in their cohorts, but a tiny study in Fife found much higher rates (Clark, 1992). Weyerer and colleagues (1994) found higher rates of depressive symptomatology among those newly admitted to private and voluntary residential homes (PRHs) and LAHs in London than was the case in similar institutions in Mannheim, though because of small numbers the difference was not quite significant in statistical terms.

As is the case with nursing homes, depressive symptoms are highly prevalent in residential populations, and there is some evidence to suggest that rates in British homes exceed those in the USA, Germany and Australia.

Associations with depression in homes

What factors account for high rates of depression in nursing and residential homes and why are there differences in rates between institution types and between different countries? Depression which predates admission, the association of physical illness with depression, cultural factors, the quality of the home environment and the treatments provided to depressed residents all may play a part in determining prevalence rates, but it is likely that methodological factors account for some of the variations between different studies.

In their study of dependent elderly in North London, Harrison et al. (1990) found that a reported past history of depression was a strong predictor of current depressive symptoms. The study of Weyerer et al. (1994) indicated that one plausible reason for depression rates being higher in London in earlier comparative institutional prevalence studies (Mann et al., 1984*b*) was that more Londoners admitted to homes were depressed on arrival. The question remains as to whether they were selected for admission because they were depressed, whether knowledge of their impending institutionalization made them miserable or whether the depression was secondary to some other factor (such as physical dependency) which prompted their entry to a home. One worrying American study (Loebel et al., 1991*b*) indicated that notes left by some elderly suicide victims cited anticipation of nursing home placement as a reason for taking their own lives.

It is well known that depression has a high correlation with physical illness (Gurland et al., 1983) and that physical disability and illness worsen the outcome for those with depression (see Chapter 8). Most people who enter long-term care do so because they can no longer cope at home, and physical ill health is a major determinant of such breakdown. Complaints of pain were associated with depression in one study, and this effect persisted when functional disability and health status were controlled (Parmalee, Katz & Lawton, 1991). The facts that depression rates appear higher in homes with more physically dependent elderly (Weyerer et al., 1990; 1994) and that physical dependency seems to be a more robust predictor of depression than residence in a particular location (Kay & Holding, 1983; Spagnoli et al., 1986; Harrison et al., 1990) point to the conclusion that physical factors are a key determinant of depression prevalence.

It has been suggested that some older people enter residential care in the hope of finding company, but in British LAHs its quality has been described as 'the same sort of company that they would have at a bus stop or in a public launderette' (Rodwell, 1982). The typical LAH also lacks privacy (Counsel and Care, 1991) and often fails to meet the nursing needs of its residents (Royal College of Nursing, 1992). Nevertheless, attempts to correlate environmental factors with depression rates have yielded less convincing associations than might have been expected (Ames, 1990; Phillips & Henderson, 1991), though lack of autonomy appears to be linked to depression (Saup, 1986) and it is hard to believe that environments where most of the day is spent doing absolutely nothing (Godlove et al., 1982) or where frank abuse occurs (Vousden, 1987) are not perpetuating or causing depression. The fact that rates of depression which are high at admission do not rise further afterwards (Katz et al., 1989; Weyerer et al., 1994) is hardly a tribute to the success of homes in managing the depressed elderly. Depression is a treatable condition and it is not unreasonable to expect that where treatment and care are optimal, rates of depression among new arrivals ought to show a clear decline in the months following admission. The effect of treatment on rates of depression is addressed below.

Incidence of depression in nursing and residential homes

Studies of depression incidence should be more useful in pointing to causative associations than studies of mere prevalence, but only four such investigations in nursing or residential homes have been reported. All had relatively small numbers of subjects and high attrition rates. Thus they cast disappointingly little light on the question of etiology.

The largest and lengthiest incidence study to date (Ames et al., 1988) reassessed 73 residents of Camden's LAHs who were not rated as depressed when interviewed with the BAS DEP in 1982, remained in the homes for 3.6 years and could be rerated for depression with the BAS in 1985/6. Eleven (15%) had become depressed (BAS DEP score $\geqslant 7$). A prospective study of 60 admissions to ten Camden LAHs, 5 Camden PRHs and 14 old people's homes in Mannheim (Weyerer et al., 1994) showed an eight month incidence rate for BAS rated depression (BAS DEP $\geqslant 7$) of 30% in Mannheim and 33% in Camden, but only 20 individuals who were neither depressed nor severely cognitively impaired at admission formed the denominator for this result in Mannheim while in London there were only 15 eligible subjects for this aspect of the study. In Camden, but not Mannheim, lack of visits by friends and relatives seemed to be a risk factor for the development of depression.

Katz et al. (1989) enrolled 51 nursing home residents in a prospective study of depression and were able to reassess 45 of them six months later. Of the 22 or 23 residents with an initial Geriatric Depression Scale (GDS) score below 11 (the paper is imprecise on this point) six (26%–27%) had developed GDS scores above 10 at follow-up. The incidence rate for DSM-III major depression was 14%, though as most of these cases had some depressive symptoms at study entry the authors speculated that they might suffer from chronic fluctuating depression rather than being truly new incident cases of major depression.

Foster, Cataldo & Boksay (1991) screened a large number of new admissions to a New York medical long-term facility and tried to follow for one year 104 who were free of depression (GDS < 10, Hamilton Depression Rating Scale (HDRS) $<$ 15, no DSM-III affective disorder detected) on admission. There was a cumulative incidence rate for Research Diagnostic Criteria (RDC) defined depression of between 14% and 15% depending on the statistical methodology employed. Minor depression appeared twice as often as major depression. It should be noted that there was a high attrition rate (25 subjects completed 12 months of study) and that the average age at intake was only 49 years, indicating that these subjects were different to most residents of nursing homes. This may limit the generalizability of the results to other long-term care facilities for the young chronic sick.

There is a need for large-scale prospective studies of depression incidence in nursing and residential homes. Such studies must be carefully planned to take into account high rates of cognitive impairment and depression at entry and high rates of attrition throughout. In addition to social variables such as visiting, changes in physical illness levels and disability, alterations in medication and adverse life events and difficulties previously shown to be associated with depression (Murphy, 1982) will require prospective assessment.

Treatment of depression in homes

There is evidence that assessment, recognition and management of depression by attending medical staff and nursing staff at long-term care facilities often is inadequate (Teeter et al., 1976; Gillis et al., 1982; Ames, 1990; Lavizzo-Mourey, Mezey & Taylor, 1991). Although antidepressants are prescribed relatively infrequently to residents (Mann et al., 1984*c*; Mann, Graham & Ashby, 1986) there is liberal dispensation of neuroleptics and benzodiazepines in these environments, and often these prescriptions continue unreviewed indefinitely for dubious indications (Mann et al., 1984*c*, Mann, Graham & Ashby, 1986; Weedle, Poston & Parish, 1988; Avorn et al., 1989; Ames, 1992*a*). Where antidepressants are prescribed with greater frequency, their administration correlates poorly with the presence of a depressive disorder (Phillips & Henderson, 1991). In North America, physical restraints are employed with a cavalier enthusiasm that is nothing short of scandalous (Tinetti et al., 1991). Psychiatric referral rates are low for nursing home residents in the United States (Borson et al., 1987) and are more likely to be made for disturbed behavior than for depression (Loebel et al., 1991*a*). In London depressed residents of LAHs were unlikely to be in contact with psychiatric help despite a high likelihood of having received psychiatric inpatient treatment in the past (Ames, 1990).

These findings beg the question as to whether the types of depression found in nursing and residential homes will respond to standard therapies. Five studies which shed some light on this issue have been performed.

In an original and inspiring study, Rodin (1986) found that enhancing responsibility and a sense of control for residents was associated with an improvement in general health and survival, though depressed residents were not the specific focus of the interventions.

At the other end of the treatment spectrum, another American study (Katz et al., 1990) of 30 depressed nursing home residents found a response rate of 58% in patients given nortriptyline opposed to a 9% response rate in a placebo treated group.

A more broad-ranging study by Ames (1990) attempted to assess the efficacy of a psychiatrist's recommendations in alleviating depressive symptoms among 90 LAH residents in London. No positive effect was demonstrated for the intervention group, but the results may reflect the frequency with which the psychiatrist's recommendations were ignored or could not be implemented.

An anecdotal study of interventions advised by a consultation–liaison nurse specialist reported that antidepressant medication was indicated for 13 of 100 referred residents (Santmyer & Roca, 1991). Separate results for depressed residents were not reported, but 68/100 residents referred for a variety of reasons were said to improve in longitudinal follow-up. If these results could be replicated in a controlled study, they would have important implications for the provision to residents of effective psychiatric help at reasonable cost.

The most recent study with implications for the treatment of depression in long-term care examined the effect of exercise on residents of LAHs in Dundee, Scotland (McMurdo & Rennie, 1993) and found that a small but significant ($P < 0.01$) fall in GDS score occurred in the exercise group.

In contrast to the copious literature on depression prevalence, investigators have barely scratched the surface of the issue of treating depression in long-term care. There is an urgent need for studies which assess the efficacy of antidepressants, psychotherapies, environmental enhancement and staff education about depression. It is fair to say that no future prevalence study should be funded unless it forms part of a treatment evaluation program.

Outcome for depressed residents of homes

Given the frail nature of those likely to seek nursing or residential care it is hardly surprising that death rates are raised even in the latter class of institution (Smith & Lowther, 1976; Booth et al., 1983). However, few researchers have followed their study participants to relate outcome to psychiatric variables. There is some evidence that depression may have an independent effect on mortality (see Chapter 8) and at least three research groups have addressed this issue as it applies to residents of long-term care facilities.

In the Camden studies of two LAH cohorts examined in 1982 and 1985/6 (Mann et al., 1984*a*; Ames et al., 1988; Ames, 1992*b*; Ashby et al., 1991) detailed long term follow-up was undertaken. With regard to depression the key findings were that only 20% of residents rated as depressed in 1982 who did not dement or die had recovered nearly four years later. In the second cohort the recovery rate was 28% (17/60) at one year. Among 45 who were AGECAT depression cases, 59% died, 15% demented, 20% remained depression cases, 2% developed schizophrenia and 5% became subcases after a four year period (Ames, 1992*b*). Depressed residents were three times more likely to die than those who were cognitively intact at screening (Ashby et al., 1991) but the available data could not refute the possibility that this higher death rate may have been due to preexisting physical factors.

Rovner et al. (1991) found that major depression among nursing home entrants raised the likelihood of death at one year by 59% independent of selected health measures. Parmalee, Katz and Lawton (1992) reported residents with major depression to have raised death rates over a 30-month period, but this association seemed to be completely explained by the association of depression with ill health.

The cross-national study of Weyerer et al. (1994) was designed to test the assumption that higher rates of depression in London might be caused by an apparently more impoverished environment, but although London's depression rates were higher at admission (see above) at neither centre did rates diverge further nor show statistically significant rises or falls over eight months.

The studies performed to date do not resolve the question of whether depression has an independent effect in raising death rates, but they do establish that depression is more likely to be chronic than to recover. This reinforces the importance of prevention and early treatment, as the longer patients have been depressed, the less likely they are to get better (see Chapter 8).

Conclusions

According to Arie (1992) long-stay care is the 'Achilles heel of care of the aged'. Research to date has been of variable quality, but has succeeded in drawing attention to the high prevalence and relative chronicity of depression and depressive symptoms in residents of nursing and residential homes. It is clear that depression may be missed by staff and is undertreated in many centres. The challenges for researchers in the 1990s are to determine what preventable factors lead to high rates of depression at admission, how best to help residents who are depressed, and how to prevent new depressive syndromes arising. Future studies should be longitudinal rather than cross-sectional and should examine incidence of depressive disorders as well as the response of these syndromes to controlled biological, psychological and social treatments.

Although much of the delivery of care in long-term facilities is substandard, clear guidelines for its improvement have been spelt out (Royal College of Physicians and the British Geriatrics Society, 1991). Doctors have a professional responsibility to take a leading role in seeking to improve the quality of care in nursing and residential homes (Snowdon, 1991). Those who work with the elderly should not be satisfied until the quality of care in residential institutions is such that they would have no hesitation in living there themselves if the need arose (Murphy, 1992). Given the high lifetime risk of nursing home use in at least one developed country (Kemper & Murtaugh, 1991) there exists the strong motivation that some researchers may reap the benefits of their work in the long run!

References

American Psychiatric Association (1980). *Diagnostic and Statistical Manual of Mental Disorders*, 3rd edition. Washington: American Psychiatric Association.

American Psychiatric Association (1987). *Diagnostic and Statistical Manual of Mental Disorders*, 3rd edition revised. Washington: American Psychiatric Association.

Ames, D., Ashby, D., Mann, A. H. & Graham, N. (1988). Psychiatric illness in elderly residents of Part III homes in one London borough: prognosis and review. *Age and Ageing*, **17**, 249–56.

Ames, D. (1990). Depression among elderly residents of local-authority residential homes: its nature and the efficacy of intervention. *British Journal of Psychiatry*, **156**, 667–75.

Ames, D. (1992*a*). Residential care. *Current Opinion in Psychiatry*, **5**, 575–9.

Ames, D. (1992*b*). Psychiatric diagnoses made by the AGECAT system in residents of local authority homes for the elderly: outcome and diagnostic stability after four years. *International Journal of Geriatric Psychiatry*, **7**, 83–7.

Arie, T. (1992). The old old and the sick old. *BJP Review of Books*, **3**, 6–8.

Ashby, D., Ames, D., West, C. R., MacDonald, A. J. D., Graham, N. & Mann, A. H. (1991). Psychiatric morbidity as predictor of mortality for residents of local authority homes for the elderly. *International Journal of Geriatric Psychiatry*, **6**, 567–75.

Avorn, J., Dreyer, P., Connelly, K. & Soumerai, S. B. (1989). Use of psychoactive medications and the quality of care in rest homes: findings and policy implications of a statewide study. *New England Journal of Medicine*, **320**, 227–32.

Booth, T., Phillips, D., Barrit, A., Berry, S., Martin, D. & Melotte, C. (1983). Patterns of mortality in homes for the elderly. *Age and Ageing*, **12**, 240–4.

Borson, S., Liptzin, B., Nininger, J. & Rabins, P. (1987). Psychiatry and the nursing home. *American Journal of Psychiatry*, **144**, 1412–18.

Burns, B. J., Larson, I. D., Goldstrom, W. E., Johnson, C. A., Taube, C. A., Miller, N. E. & Mathis, E. S. (1988). Mental disorder among nursing home patients: preliminary findings from the national nursing home survey pretest. *International Journal of Geriatric Psychiatry*, **3**, 27–35.

Clark, S. A. (1992). Mental illness among new residents to residential care. *International Journal of Geriatric Psychiatry*, **7**, 59–64.

Copeland, J. R. M., Dewey, M. & Griffiths-Jones, H. (1986). Computerized psychiatric diagnostic system and case nomenclature for elderly subjects: GMS and AGECAT. *Psychological Medicine*, **16**, 89–99.

Counsel and Care. (1991). *Not Such Private Places*. London: Counsel and Care.

Flicker, L., Keppich-Arnold, S., Chiu, E., Calder, R., & Theisinger, J. (1992). The prevalence of depressive symptoms and cognitive impairment in supported residential services in Victoria: a pilot study. *Australian Journal on Ageing*, **11**, 16–18.

Foster, J. R., Cataldo, J. K. & Boksay, I. J. E. (1991). Incidence of depression in a medical long-term facility: findings from a restricted sample of new admissions. *International Journal of Geriatric Psychiatry*, **6**, 13–20.

Gillis, L. S., Elk, R., Trichard, L., Le Fevre, K., Zabow, A., Joffe, H. & van Schalwyk, D. J.

(1982). The admission of the elderly to places of care: a socio-psychiatric survey. *Psychological Medicine*, **12**, 159–68.

Godlove, C., Richard, L. & Rodwell, G. (1982). *Time for Action: an Observation Study of Elderly People in Four Different Care Environments*. Sheffield: University of Sheffield.

Gurland, B., Copeland, J. R. M., Kuriansky, J., Kelleher, M., Sharpe, L. & Dean, L. (1983). *The Mind and Mood of Aging*. New York: Haworth Press.

Harrison, R., Savla, N. & Kafetz, K. (1990). Dementia, depression and physical disability in a London borough: a survey of elderly people in and out of residential care and implications for future developments. *Age and Ageing*, **19**, 97–103.

Henderson, A. S., Jorm, A. F., Mackinnon, A., Christensen, H., Scott, L. R., Korten, A. E. & Doyle, C. (1993). The prevalence of depressive disorders and the distribution of depressive symptoms in later life: a survey using draft ICD-10 and DSM-III-R. *Psychological Medicine*, **23**, 719–29.

Horiguchi, J. & Inami, Y. A. (1991). A survey of living conditions and psychological states of elderly people admitted to nursing homes in Japan. *Acta Psychiatrica Scandinavica*, **83**, 338–41.

Hyer, L. & Blazer, D. (1982). Depression in long-term care facilities. In *Depression in Late Life*, ed. D. G. Blazer, pp. 268–295. St. Louis: Mosby.

Ineichen, B. (1990). The extent of dementia among old people in residential care. *International Journal of Geriatric Psychiatry*, **5**, 327–35.

Jensen, K. (1966). Psychiatric problems in four Danish old age homes. *Acta Psychiatrica Scandinavica*, Suppl. **169**, 411–19.

Jorm, A. F. & Henderson, A. S. (1990). *The Problem of Dementia in Australia*. Canberra: Australian Government Publishing Service.

Katz, I. R., Lesher, E., Kleban, M., Jethanandi, V. & Parmalee, P. (1989). Clinical features of depression in the nursing home. *International Psychogeriatrics*, **1**, 5–15.

Katz, I. R., Simpson, G. M., Curlik, S. M. & Muhly, C. (1990). Pharmacological treatment of major depression for elderly patients in residential care settings. *Journal of Clinical Psychiatry*, **51** (Suppl.), 41–8.

Kay, D., Beamish, P. & Roth, M. (1964). Old age mental disorders in Newcastle-upon-Tyne. Part 1. A study of prevalence. *British Journal of Psychiatry*, **110**, 146–58.

Kay, D. W. K. & Holding, T. A. (1983). *The Dependent Aged in Hobart*. Hobart: University of Tasmania.

Kemper, P. & Murtaugh, C. M. (1991). Lifetime use of nursing home care. *New England Journal of Medicine*, **324**, 595–600.

Kivelä, S.-L., Pahkala, K. & Laippala, P. (1988). Prevalence of depression in an elderly population in Finland. *Acta Psychiatrica Scandinavica*, **78**, 401–13.

Lau-Ting, C., Ting, T. & Phoon, W. O. (1987). Mental status of residents in old people's homes. *Annals of the Academy of Medicine of Singapore*, **16**, 118–21.

Lavizzo-Mourey, R., Mezey, M. & Taylor, L. (1991). Completeness of admission of residents assessments in teaching nursing homes. *Journal of the American Geriatrics Society*, **39**, 676–82.

Livingston, G., Hawkins, A., Graham, N., Blizard, B. & Mann, A. (1990). The Gospel Oak study: prevalence rates of dementia, depression and activity limitation among elderly residents in inner London. *Psychological Medicine*, **20**, 137–46.

Lobo, A., Ventura, T. & Marco, C. (1990). Psychiatric morbidity among residents in a home for the elderly in Spain: prevalence of disorder and validity of screening. *International Journal of Geriatric Psychiatry*, **5**, 83–91.

Loebel, J. P., Borson, S., Hyde, T., Donaldson, D., Van Tuinen, C., Rabbitt, T. M. & Boyko, E. J. (1991*a*). Relationships between requests for psychiatric consultations and psychiatric diagnoses in long-term care facilities. *American Journal of Psychiatry*, **148**, 898–903.

Loebel, J. P., Loebel, J. S., Dager, S. R., Centerwall, B. S. & Reay, D. T. (1991*b*). Anticipation of nursing home placement may be a predictor of suicide among the elderly. *Journal of the American Geriatrics Society*, **39**, 407–8.

Lowther, C. P. & McLeod, H. M. (1974). Admissions to a welfare home. *Health Bulletin*, **32** (1), 14–18.

McMurdo, M. E. T. & Rennie, L. (1993). A controlled trial of exercise by residents of old people's homes. *Age and Ageing*, **22**, 11–15.

Mann, A. H., Graham, N. & Ashby, D. (1984*a*). Psychiatric illness in residential homes for the elderly: a survey in one London borough. *Age and Ageing*, **13**, 257–65.

Mann, A. H., Wood, K., Cross, P., Gurland, B., Schieber, P. & Häfner, H. (1984*b*). Institutional care of the elderly: a comparison of the cities of New York, London and Mannheim. *Social Psychiatry*, **19**, 97–102.

Mann, A. H., Jenkins, R., Cross, P. & Gurland, B. (1984*c*). A comparison of the prescriptions received by the elderly in long-term care in New York and London. *Psychological Medicine*, **14**, 891–7.

Mann, A. H., Graham, N. & Ashby, D. (1986). The prescription of psychotropic medication in local authority old people's homes. *International Journal of Geriatric Psychiatry*, **1**, 25–9.

Mann, A. H., Ames, D., Graham, N. et al. (1989). The reliability of the Brief Assessment Schedule. *International Journal of Geriatric Psychiatry*, **4**, 221–5.

Murphy, E. (1982). Social origins of depression in old age. *British Journal of Psychiatry*, **141**, 135–42.

Murphy, E. (1992). A more ambitious vision for residential long-term care. *International Journal of Geriatric Psychiatry*, **7**, 851–2.

Parmalee, P. A., Katz, I. R. & Lawton, M. P. (1989). Depression among institutionalized aged: assessment and prevalence estimation. *Journal of Gerontology*, **44**, M22–9.

Parmalee, P. A., Katz, I. R. & Lawton, M. P. (1991). The relationship of pain to depression among institutionalized aged. *Journal of Gerontology*, **46**, P15–21.

Parmalee, P. A., Katz, I. R. & Lawton, M. P. (1992). Depression and mortality among institutionalized aged. *Journal of Gerontology*, **47**, P3–10.

Phillips, C. & Henderson, A. S. (1991). The prevalence of depression among Australian nursing home residents: results using draft ICD-10 and DSM-III-R criteria. *Psychological Medicine*, **21**, 739–48.

Rodin, J. (1986). Aging and health: effects of the sense of control. *Science*, **233**, 1271–6.

Rodwell, G. (1982). Busy doing nothing. *Community Care*, **427**, 16–18.

Rosewarne, R., Carter, M. & Bruce, A. (1991). *Hostel Dementia Care: Survey of Programs and Participants (Victoria).* Melbourne: Aged Care Research Group.

Rovner, B. W., Kafonek, S., Filipp, L., Lucas, M. J. & Folstein, M. F. (1986). Prevalence of mental illness in a community nursing home. *American Journal of Psychiatry*, **143**, 1446–9.

Rovner, B. W., German, P. S., Brant, L., J., Clark, R., Burton, L. & Folstein, M. F. (1991). Depression and mortality in nursing homes. *Journal of the American Medical Association*, **265**, 993–6.

Royal College of Nursing. (1992). *A Scandal Waiting to Happen?* London: Royal College of Nursing.

Royal College of Physicians and the British Geriatrics Society. (1991). *High Quality Care for Elderly People: a Joint Report.* London: Royal College of Physicians.

Santmyer, K. S. & Roca, R. P. (1991). Geropsychiatry in long-term care: a nurse centered approach. *Journal of the American Geriatric Society*, **39**, 156–9.

Saup, W. (1986). *Lack of Autonomy in Old-Age Homes: a Stress and Coping Study. Augsburger Berichte zur Entwicklungpsychologie und Paedogogischen Psychologie, Nr. 5.* Augsburg: University of Augsburg.

Smith R. & Lowther, C. (1976). Follow up study of two hundred admissions to a residential home. *Age and Ageing*, **5**, 176–80.

Snowdon, J. (1986). Dementia, depression and life satisfaction in nursing homes. *International Journal of Geriatric Psychiatry*, **1**, 85–91.

Snowdon, J. & Donnelly, N. (1986). A study of depression in nursing homes. *Journal of Psychiatric Research*, **20**, 327–33.

Snowdon, J. & Mackintosh, S. (1989). Depression and dementia in three Sydney hostels. *Australian Journal on Ageing*, **8** (4), 24–8.

Snowdon, J. (1991). Our nursing homes. *Medical Journal of Australia*, **155**, 120–1.

Spagnoli, A., Foresti, G., MacDonald, A. & Williams, P. (1986). Dementia and depression in Italian geriatric institutions. *International Journal of Geriatric Psychiatry*, **1**, 15–23.

Steel, J. (1989). *Depression in the Elderly (Dissertation for Part II of Fellowship of RANZCP)*, Melbourne: Royal Australian and New Zealand College of Psychiatrists.

Teeter, R. B., Garetz, F. K., Miller, W. R. & Heiland, W. F. (1976). Psychiatric disturbances of aged patients in skilled nursing homes. *American Journal of Psychiatry*, **133**, 1430–4.

Tinetti, M. E., Wen-Liang Liu, Marottoli, R. A. & Ginter, S. F. (1991). Mechanical restraint use among residents of skilled nursing facilities: prevalence, patterns and predictors. *Journal of the American Medical Association*, **65**, 468–71.

Vousden, M. (1987). Nye Bevan would turn in his grave. *Nursing Times*, **83** (32), 18–19.

Wayne, S. J. & Rhyne, R. L. (1991). Sampling issues in nursing home research. *Journal of the American Geriatrics Society*, **39**, 308–11.

Weedle, P., Poston, J. & Parish, P. (1988). Use of hypnotic medicines by elderly people in residential homes. *Journal of the Royal College of General Practitioners*, **38**, 156–8.

Weyerer, S., Häfner, H., Denzinger, R. et al. (1990). *Prävalenz und Verlauf von Depression und Demenz bei Altenheimbewohnern. Ergebnisse einer Querschnitts- und Longitudinalstudie in Mannheim und Camden (London)*. Mannheim: Zentralinstitut für Seelische Gesundheit.

Weyerer, S., Häfner, H., Mann, A. H., Ames, D. & Graham, N. (1994). Prevalence and course of depression among consecutive admissions to residential homes in Mannheim and Camden (London). Submitted to *International Psychogeriatrics*.

11

Depression in primary care settings

MARTIN BLANCHARD ANTHONY MANN

Introduction

It is unacceptable that treatable illnesses should mar any enjoyment that retirement may bring to an older person, or increase any burden from isolation and loss that occurs at that age. The primary care team is in an ideal position to identify and alleviate depression, a widespread and treatable disorder. This chapter addresses that task, demonstrating both the extent of the problem and possible solutions. Throughout, reference will be made to a series of studies carried out in the North London area of Gospel Oak. These studies were set up to describe mental illnesses amongst older people identified by household enumeration in an electoral ward, the use by these people of the local Health and Social Services and the outcome of interventions for treatment of mental illnesses (Livingston et al., 1990*a,b*).

The prevalence and nature of depression in primary care

Prevalence surveys of depression in older people have measured morbidity at three levels: Community, Primary Care and Hospital Clinic. The results are not comparable because of the large hidden morbidity in the older population that will be discovered in a community sample, the large number of cases that never reach specialist mental health resources from primary care, and the severe and resistant cases which tend to accumulate in clinics (Shepherd et al., 1966; Goldberg & Huxley, 1992). In addition, all published prevalence studies have their own idiosyncracies of case definition, sample frame and means of assessment that make differences between results hard to interpret.

Prevalence data from primary care surveys is sparsest of the three levels. Samples taken here will differ from community samples in that attenders have decided to consult their doctor, thus passing the first filter in the pathway to care (Goldberg & Huxley, 1992). The first filter will be determined by the individual's illness behavior, in turn affected by upbringing, culture and personal experience. Women are more likely to consult than men. Consultation may well be for a physical condition, so recognition of an accompanying depression will be dependent on general practitioner diagnosis; those recognized being part of the conspicuous morbidity in primary care, while those not recognized constitute part of the hidden morbidity. General practice surveys therefore are of a self-selected group, likely to have increased physical morbidity by dint of their consultation. Surveys may report on total morbidity if the survey used a screening procedure or on conspicuous morbidity alone if the prevalence data is drawn from general practitioner records.

Within primary care, the Third National Morbidity Survey (of conspicuous morbidity) 1981–82 of Great Britain (RCGP/OPCS/DHSS, 1986) discovered episode rates per 1000 people aged 65 or over at risk of 4.0 for affective psychosis and 40.7 for depression. Illiffe et al. (1991) examined a random sample of patients aged 75 years registered with London general practitioners, and utilising the short-CARE (Gurland et al., 1984), found evidence of depression in 22% of subjects. The majority of these cases of depression, representing total morbidity were mild in nature. A study from the USA (Borson et al., 1986) measured depression in attenders of Veterans Primary Care facilities. Using the Zung self-report depression scale (Zung et al., 1983) they classed 24.4% of these men over 60 years as cases, with an estimated 10% prevalence of DSM-III-R major depression. Only 1% of the depressed reported the use of mental health services.

Blazer (1989) claims that the majority of depressed older adults do not fit DSM-III-R criteria for depression but rather have depressive symptoms associated with physical illness and/or adjustment to life stress. Even if this proves to be true, as Kennedy et al. (1989) state:

> any health policy based on the prevalence of major depressive disorders will be ineffective if the loss of social, emotional, physiological, and cognitive function is associated with depressive symptoms that are substantial and widespread but not congruent with a diagnosis of a major disorder.

The burden for primary care

Depression in older people is associated with an increased burden on the primary care services. Using the Zung depression scale, Waxman, Carner & Blum (1983) demonstrated that older patients with the greatest measure of depressive symptoms averaged four times as many visits to their general practitioner each year than the less depressed, but the more depressed patients were no more likely to be referred to specialist mental health facilities. This study also discovered a general relationship between affective state and feelings of physical ill-health in the community and in particular a correlation between complaints of cardiovascular symptoms and depression. Widner and Cadoret (1978), in a study of adults of all ages, compared depressed primary care attenders retrospectively with age, sex and season of attendance matched controls. They found that depressed patients increased their attendance rate to the general practitioner's surgery in the seven months prior to a diagnosis of depression. Depressed patients presented 'functional' physical symptoms such as pain, fatigue and dizziness for which no organic etiology was evident. There was also an increase in psychological complaints relating to mood change such as tension, inability to relax and worrying about inconsequential things.

An analysis of prescribing may be used as an indicator of general practitioner activity, and three studies indicate further the large burden that psychological complaints in older people place on the primary care facility. Williams (1980) surveyed 6000 community residents aged over 65 years in London to determine their psychotropic drug use. Fourteen per cent of men and 22% of women were taking either antidepressants, and/or tranquillizers, and/or hypnotics. More recently the Consumers' Association (1990) analysed 805 general practice patients aged over 65 years and found that 15% were taking hypnotics, sedatives or anxiolytics of which 90% had been started outside hospital – remarkably similar results a decade apart.

That this activity becomes longstanding has been demonstrated by a study from Liverpool (Sullivan et al., 1988) where over half the patients prescribed benzodiazepines three years previously were found still to be in receipt of them.

Livingston et al. (1990*b*) examined the use of health and social services by older people in an Inner London community and discovered that those described as cases of 'probable pervasive depression', in contrast to those that were not, were more likely to have seen their general practitioner in the previous month (48% versus 37%). They were also more likely to have visited a hospital (39% versus 24%), require a district nurse (18% versus 9%), a home help (30% versus 19%), and be more frequent users of local day centre facilities (21% versus 11%). It would seem logical to assume that if depression in older people does increase the work load to this extent, then extra efforts and resources required to manage this condition effectively could well be cost-effective.

The outcome of depression in primary care

There have been few studies examining the outcome of depression in older people within the community setting (see Chapter 8), but even fewer specifically in the primary care setting. In a general practice population, Mann, Jenkins & Belsey (1981) followed up 100 patients aged between 18 and 85 with neurosis after one year and found a good outcome in 49%. Lesser severity of illness and good quality of social life at follow-up were the only factors which significantly predicted this good outcome. It was noted that there was a trend for persistent morbidity to occur among the older members of the cohort with significant physical illness.

Burvill, Stampfer & Hall (1986) suggested that the classification of primary and secondary depression is of major importance to the prognosis in older people and that the relationships of both demoralization and of bereavement to depressive illness are still unclear. Cole (1983) holds that in the absence of organic signs and physical illness, age is not related to prognosis in depression. He studied 55 older outpatients with a primary depressive illness for 24–63 months and found that 38 (69%) remained well for more than 60% of their follow-up period and 17 (32%) remained chronically ill. Good outcome was related to treatment compliance, maintenance therapy and the absence of physical disability.

There has been dispute about the place of standard antidepressant treatments in the management of depression in older people, but in two recent reviews (Gerson, Plotkin & Jarvik, 1988; Rockwell, Lam & Zisook, 1988) antidepressants have been found to be effective treatments compared to placebo controls, and limiting side-effects were comparable with those seen in younger populations. Baldwin (1991) suggested that, based on hospital studies with standard treatment 75–80% of older people would recover from an individual episode of depression. Also it is now believed that relapses may be reduced by treating for at least four months after the disappearance of all depressive symptoms (Priern & Kupfer 1986), and lithium is as effective as a prophylactic in older depressives as it is in younger ones (Abou-Saleh & Coppen, 1983). These findings may not be applicable for all cases of depression found in primary care, but a recent study of younger adults (Hollyman et al., 1988) indicated that more primary care cases of depression may respond to correct pharmacotherapy than was previously expected. Indeed Ames and Allen (1991) state 'the reported poor prognosis of depressive illness in the elderly could be due to inadequate levels of antidepressant medication'.

The role of the primary care service

The general practitioner, by nature of his provision of primary care to a population, is well placed to monitor psychiatric disorder in the community as a whole and to identify those patients serious enough to warrant treatment.
(Shepherd et al., 1966)

This quotation, taken from the first major investigation of psychiatric morbidity in primary care, is particularly relevant for older people who contact their general practitioners in large numbers. As noted above, the depressed among them are high users (Livingston et al., 1990*b*) and it is important now to review the role of the primary care staff in the recognition and management of depression. It is also important to emphasise that the findings are relevant for all primary care workers – practice nurses, health visitors or counsellors – as well as for family doctors.

Recognition

An early and often quoted study (Williamson et al., 1964) indicated that general practitioners were unaware of three-quarters of the depressions amongst their patients. A similar observation was made more recently in an Australian setting in which 11 participating general practitioners failed to identify 12 out of 15 patients, meeting criteria for depression using a standard interview (Bowers et al., 1990). MacDonald (1986), comparing general practitioners' identification of depression amongst 235 consecutive attenders in a general practice in London with an independent psychiatric assessment, surprisingly found that the general practitioners only 'missed' 9% of depressions. They were, in fact, overidentifying depression, labelling a large number of older people as depressed who did not meet research criteria. Thus, MacDonald claimed, a more important problem was that lack of diagnostic precision led to no active management. Whether the error is inaccurate overidentification or underidentification, it is necessary to explore possible reasons why these consultations do not produce a diagnosis of depression and what strategies may be introduced to improve matters.

A diagnostic consultation may be adversely affected by characteristics of the doctor and of the patient. Butler (1969) wrote of ageism among health care professionals: '*an attitude implying that old people are in a state of decline*'. Complaints, therefore, do not reflect features of treatable illnesses. The doctor may have mixed feelings about treating older patients, based upon fears of the doctor's own old age or ambivalent feelings towards his or her parents. In addition to this there could be anxiety over the side-effects of treatment, particularly in the case of antidepressant medication. Recognition of depression may lead to a treatment dilemma for some doctors, which can be avoided by simply raising the threshold for diagnosis. Research in this area has been handicapped by lack of an objective measure of attitudes for use among primary care staff. The Depression Attitude Questionnaire [DAQ] (Botega et al., 1993) has been developed to meet this need. One proposition to be rated in the questionnaire is '*depression is an inevitable part of old age*'. The DAQ has been piloted amongst a sample of 98 general practitioners in the United Kingdom and, happily, most respondents disagreed with this proposition. However, the old age item did appear in one of the four factors found to underlie the data – a component summarized as 'Inevitability'. A high score on this factor implied belief that depression was a natural component of life stages and little could be done about it. Subsequent cluster analysis showed that the participating doctors could be subgrouped into three approximately equally sized groups according to their scores on the four factors, one of which indicated that they found depressed patients unrewarding and the condition inevitable. However, the most important finding from this preliminary work was to demonstrate the variability amongst family doctors in their attitudes to depressed patients. Thus, if educational initiatives are to be introduced to improve recognition of depression, it needs to be remembered that although there are some who do have negative attitudes, at least two thirds of such a sample would resent any implications that their work with depressed older patients was affected by such attitudes.

The other partner to the consultation is the older patient. Such a patient may well belong to a generation for which mental illness carries a stigma, being associated with treatment in asylums. Confession to depression or anxiety would be guarded, even if the patient were aware of such feelings. The latter may not be the case, for depression in older people may be experienced as subjective malaise, or excessive self-concern over health or actual somatic symptoms. These complaints may take up the consultation. Little research has been done on whether and why older patients declare a depressed mood to their doctor. However, Blanchard, Waterreus & Mann, (1993), in a detailed study of 90 depressed older people from the community screening of the Gospel Oak population of North London, did discover that only 38% of cases stated that they had declared their current psychological symptoms to their general practitioner. Declaration appeared to be associated with previous contact for emotional problems, and in 'neurotic' cases, with knowledge of a relative with depression and younger age. The evidence, therefore, is that older patients do not present their depression to the doctor, although they may show these feelings to a less intimidating primary care worker with whom they are in contact, such as a health visitor or practice nurse. These workers need to be sensitive to the condition.

As recognition is the necessary first phase to accurate assessment and management, the current situation would seem to be in need of improvement. Some change may occur as a result of social evolution. Mental illness and depression are more openly discussed, so the younger old may be more likely to present such difficulties in a consultation. Education of primary care practitioners in recent years has contained much more teaching on mental illness, both in the undergraduate and postgraduate curricula. Nevertheless, specific strategies to improve recognition are being researched, leading to the possibility of practical interventions.

Training of practitioners in better interview techniques (Gask, 1992)

Research into the verbal and nonverbal behaviors of doctors and patients in consultation has identified those features associated with an interchange in which depression is recognized and one where it is not. Nonverbal cues and the style of questioning from the doctor can facilitate or suppress the patient's production of statements with emotional content. Once these features were defined, then training packages could be designed for doctors. Although this research has not focused specifically on older people, there is no reason to suppose that such findings do not apply.

Screening questionnaires and computerized diagnostic assessments for use in primary care settings

To be relevant in day-to-day use in primary care, rather than as a research tool, such instruments have to be brief, be able to be administered by those not trained in psychiatry and be acceptable to respondents who do not necessarily see themselves as mentally ill. Examples of screening scales for depression, which can be used in general practice patients, are the SELFCARE (D) (Bird et al., 1987) and the Geriatric Depression Scale (GDS) (Yesavage, Rose & Lum, 1983). Of the computerized assessments, the GMS-AGECAT program (Copeland, Dewey & Griffiths-Jones, 1986) is now being modified to act as a brief screen both for dementia and depression for use by primary care staff. These measures will be capable of indicating rapidly to a general practitioner or other staff member which of their older patients are depressed.

Education of all practice staff

Practice staff who are in regular contact with older patients, such as district nurses and health visitors, should be made aware both of the forms of presentation of depression and of who may be at risk. Training of these staff to be at ease with a series of questions that probe for depression, and in their interpretation, would identify patients who could then be referred to a general practitioner for further examination.

Assessment

Management of most cases of depression ought to be carried out entirely within primary care. For a few, depression may be a continuity of a longstanding manic depressive disorder, usually associated with a positive family history. These patients are best supervized by the psychiatric services. For the remainder, the patient is likely to be unknown to psychiatric services (only 4% of those with depression in the community in North London were currently in contact with the old age psychiatry services, compared with 38% declared to the general practitioner). The general practitioner may, therefore, need to assess a depressed patient de novo. Not only must the severity be assessed, but the relative contribution of physical, social and psychological factors to the illness explored. After assessment, decisions should be made as to whether pharmacotherapy is appropriate, and/or whether physical, social or psychological help is feasible. Exploration of relevant contributory factors may suggest specific interventions to mitigate against their causative influence, or their role in the persistence of the depressed state.

Such a detailed assessment by the general practitioner will be greatly limited by lack of time. A screening questionnaire or computerized assessment may give a satisfactory indication of severity of depression, but a fuller assessment of its context will be necessary for sensible management. The use of another practice staff member, who may have more time to spend with the patient, could be considered. To evaluate this approach, a research study of practice nurses, who have been trained in a specially devised assessment interview for depression, is underway. This study, supported by the United Kingdom Department of Health, aims to determine whether the nurse's assessment of depression is accurate and useful and whether she can act as a monitor of the progress of primary care treatment. It includes adult patients up to the age of 74, and pilot results are promising (Wilkinson et al., 1993).

Management

In a study examining the effect of increased recognition on levels of management, German et al. (1987) interviewed 1242 people in a primary care setting using the General Health Questionnaire (GHQ) (Goldberg & Hiller, 1978) and divided them into two age groups with the division at 65 years. They then 'fed-back' the GHQ scores to the general practitioners for a random half of the patients in each group. Feedback led to an increase in identification of depression, especially in the older group, but actual management only increased from 32% to 42%, and only 1% of the depressed aged over 65 saw a mental health specialist. Also, those aged over 65 years were treated less with both medication and counselling – an indicator of the present bias against treating older patients.

Once an assessment has been carried out and diagnosis made, it is important to follow this through with appropriate management. In primary care this should include pharmacotherapy, but with specific attention to correction of adverse social factors, psychological stresses or accompanying physical ill health. These factors, so far as they affect older depressed people in general, are dealt with in other chapters, but there are some specific observations relevant to primary care.

Pharmacotherapy

The particular problem with the use of antidepressant medication in older patients by general practitioners stems from anxiety about dose and side-effects. Specific educational material on the regimes that benefit older people will help here. Secondly, as with all primary care prescriptions, compliance may be an issue. This is highlighted by the recent Consumers' Association (1990) study discussed above, which discovered that 40% of patients prescribed psychotropics had not discussed their medication with a doctor for at least six months. Also, 28% of the prescribed medicines identified by general practitioners were not reported by patients to the interviewers while 36% were reported by the patient but not by the general practitioner. Depressed older patients may not understand why they are being offered a pill, unless the link between their current complaints and the antidepressant is made plain. With the delayed therapeutic action of antidepressants, minor side-effects, such as dry mouth or dizziness, may well become intolerable if they are unexplained and occur in an anxious patient already suffering from excessive somatic self-concern. For these reasons compliance can be poor.

Psychological factors

The primary care team is likely to be aware of bereavement amongst their patients. While many of the bereaved will overcome their loss without long-term ill-effects, others do not and move into a state of chronic depression. Of the depressed cases found in Gospel Oak, 27/96 (28%) started in the six months following a significant bereavement, and of these 23/96 (24%) had a duration of greater than two years. The patient, and his or her family, may well regard this continuing depression as 'understandable' and to be endured. It is important that practice staff do not share this belief and are aware of those at risk of delayed bereavement reactions. An advantage for primary care management would be the availability of skilled counselling. Other groups for which practice-based counselling may be of help are for those whose depression seems to reflect lack of adjustment to life changes, associated with ageing – retirement or the onset of physical limitations – and those with marital or filial difficulties. The general practitioner has the advantage of knowing the patient over the longer term, thus having an idea of the patient's personality structure and value system. Such knowledge would be helpful in counselling these patients.

Physical health

Poor physical health bears adversely on the prognosis of depression (Murphy, 1983, Kennedy, Kelman & Thomas, 1990). The effect may be mediated through the experience of constant pain, through limitation of activity, through increasing dependence, or through its significance to the individual, each of which will lower self-esteem. It is also possible that depression may be part of the symptom state of the physical illness or a side-effect of the treatment for it. Kinzie et al. (1986) used Research Diagnostic Criteria (RDC) (Spitzer, Endicott & Robbins, 1975) to examine depression in 50 older community residents and found that it was associated (by independent determination, duration and temporal association) with medical illness or medication in half of them. Likewise Murrell, Himmelfarb & Wright (1983) used the Center for Epidemiologic Studies Depression Scale (CES-D) (Radloff, 1977) (cut-off > 20) and found half of their depressed cases reported taking medication and half had seen a physician in the previous six months. They estimated that one quarter of men and one third of women reporting a physical illness had a concomitant depression.

Whatever the cause, the general practitioner has a unique opportunity to see this interaction and thus minimize its impact. Symptoms of physical illness, therefore, need vigorous attention amongst depressed people; small improvements may well have large psychological benefit. A gain in exercise tolerance of 100 yards may make shopping possible, while strengthening the quadriceps may allow greater mobility and, therefore, independence around the home. Improvement in vision or hearing may enhance social activity; Mulrow et al. (1990) studied the effect of treating hearing impairment on the quality of life in 95 older people compared to a waiting-list control. At a four months follow-up significant positive changes were seen in treated patients for communication function, social and emotional function and depression scores. But the most important point for the doctor, is not to collude with any depressive cognitions of the patient in the belief that deterioration and pain are inevitable in old age.

Social factors

Once again, the primary care team are most able to be aware of the facilities in a community to help those depressed older people facing adverse social factors such as loss of role through retirement, isolation through bereavement or children moving away. The effect of reestablishing social interaction has been demonstrated by Schonfield, Garcia & Streuber (1985) who examined two groups ($n = 42$, $n = 47$) aged 55–91 years. They followed one group through a mental health treatment program which emphasized the strengthening of social networks, and the other through a nutrition program. Initially the mental health program group scored significantly higher on the Beck Depression Inventory and had fewer friends as measured on the Social Support Network Inventory. 'Graduates' of the mental health program improved significantly in their Beck scores with a concomitant increase in friends. The investigators concluded that continued socialization in later years may serve to allay depression.

The social facilities required may be provided either by statutory social services or through voluntary agencies, but it is usually the primary care staff who are the point of contact and who should be making referrals.

Coordination of approach

Most assessments of depressed older people indicate that the management is multifaceted. It is likely that the primary care physician's orientation will be towards prescription of medication. Without adequate follow-up, however, even this treatment may be fruitless. Other interventions may be limited by lack of time or by lack of familiarity by the doctor. Other practice staff, such as community psychiatric nurses, counsellors or social services ought to be included in the management. But then coordination between various agents and adequate meetings to monitor progress become new hurdles. The possibility of a nurse acting as 'case manager' for depressed older patients has been considered, and an evaluative study of this role is being undertaken in North London. The study has been as follows. All short-CARE (Gurland et al., 1984) screened depression diagnostic cases were interviewed in detail and then, with their and their general practitioner's agreement, randomized to either community psychiatric nurse (CPN) addition or current primary care, for a three-month period. The CPN worked alongside the general practitioners and in liaison with a hospital-based multidisciplinary old-age psychiatry team. Management plans were generated for all the cases but only implemented during the study period for those randomized to the CPN and included pharmacological, physical, psychological and social elements. After the three month period, all cases were reinterviewed, interventions documented, and comparisons made. The management plans were then sent to all the general practitioners involved.

Preliminary results indicate a reluctance amongst general practitioners and patients to prescribe and take antidepressants. Despite that, it was possible to bring about a significant improvement in mental state over a short period of time by addition of the community nurse. This improvement appears to have stemmed from the specific personal contacts with certain patients, the effect being most demonstrable in subjects with marked nonhealth difficulties (Blanchard et al., 1993). A longer-term follow-up is under way.

Conclusions

Depression is a common problem amongst older people which ruins lives and creates an added burden to the primary care team. It is important to recognize it and manage it specifically but by taking a multifaceted approach. An exploration of the context of a depression is fundamentally important to management but may be difficult and time consuming. Thus a way forward may be to employ members of the primary care team other than the general practitioner to develop skills for this purpose.

References

Abou-Saleh, M. & Coppen, A. (1983). The prognosis of depression in old age: The case for lithium therapy. *British Journal of Psychiatry*, **143**, 527–8.

Ames, D. & Allen, N (1991). The prognosis of depression in old age: good, bad or indifferent? *International Journal of Geriatric Psychiatry*, **6**, 477–82.

Baldwin, R. (1991). The outcome of depression in old age. *International Journal of Geriatric Psychiatry*, **6**, 395–400.

Bird, A., MacDonald, A., Mann, A. & Philpot, M. (1987). Preliminary experience with the SELFCARE (D): a self-rating depression questionnaire for use in elderly, noninstitutionalized subjects. *International Journal of Geriatric Psychiatry*, **2**, 31–8.

Blanchard, M., Waterreus, A. & Mann, A. (1994). The nature of depression amongst older people in inner London, and the contact with primary care. *British Journal of Psychiatry*, in press.

Blazer, D. (1989). Depression in the elderly. *New England Journal of Medicine*, **320**, 164–6.

Borson, S., Barnes, R. A., Kukull, W. A. et al. (1986). Symptomatic depression in elderly medical outpatients. I. Prevalence, demography and health service utilization. *Journal of the American Geriatrics Society*, **34**, 341–7.

Bowers, J., Jorm, A. F., Henderson, A. S. & Harris, P. (1990). General practitioners' detection of depression and dementia in elderly patients. *The Medical Journal of Australia*, **153**, 192–6.

Botega, N., Blizard, R., Wilkinson, G. & Mann A. (1993). General practitioners' and depression: first use of the Depression Attitude Questionnaire. *International Journal of Methods in Psychiatric Research*, in press.

Burvill, P., Stampfer, H. & Hall, W. (1986). Does depressive illness in the elderly have a poor prognosis? *Australian and New Zealand Journal of Psychiatry*, **20**, 422–7.

Butler, R. N. (1969). Ageism: another form of bigotry. *The Gerontologist*, **9**, 243–6.

Cole, M. (1983). Age, age of onset and course of primary depressive illness in the elderly. *Canadian Journal of Psychiatry*, **28**, 102–4.

Consumer Association Limited (1990). Elderly people: their medicines and their doctors. *Drugs and Therapeutics Bulletin*, **28** (20), 77–9.

Copeland, J. R. M., Dewey, M. E. 7 Griffiths-Jones, H. (1986). Computerized psychiatric diagnostic system and case nomenclature for elderly subjects: GMS and AGECAT. *Psychological Medicine*, **16**, 89–99.

Gask, L. (1992). Training general practitioners to detect and manage emotional disorders. *International Review of Psychiatry*, **4**, 293–300.

German, P., Shapiro, S., Skinner, E. et al. (1987). Detection and management of mental health problems of older patients by primary care providers. *Journal of the American Medical Association*, **257** 489–93.

Gerson, S., Plotkin, D. & Jarvik, L. (1988). Antidepressant drug studies, 1964 to 1986: empirical evidence for ageing patients. *Journal of Clinical Psychopharmacology*, **8**, 311–22.

Goldberg, D. & Hiller, V. (1978). A scaled version of the General Health Questionnaire. *Psychological Medicine*, **9**, 139–45.

Goldberg, D. & Huxley, P. (1992). *Common Mental Disorders – A Biosocial Model.* London: Routledge.

Gurland, B., Golden, R., Teresi, J. & Challop, J. (1984). The SHORT-CARE: an efficient instrument for the assessment of depression, dementia and disability. *Journal of Gerontology*, **39**, 166–9.

Hollyman, J., Freeling, P., Paykel, E., Bhat, A. & Sedgwick, P. (1988). Double-blind placebo trial of amitriptyline among depressed patients. *British Journal of Psychiatry*, **148**, 642–7.

Illiffe, S., Haines, A., Gallivan, S., Booroff, A., Goldenberg, E. & Morgan, P. (1991). Assessment of elderly people in general practice: 1. Social circumstances and mental state. *British Journal of General Practice*, **41**, 9–12

Kennedy, G., Kelman, H., Thomas, C. et al. (1989). Hierarchy of characteristics associated with depressive symptoms in an urban elderly sample. *American Journal of Psychiatry*, **146**, 220–5.

Kennedy, G., Kelman, H. & Thomas, C. (1990). Persistence and remission of depressive symptoms in late life. *American Journal of Psychiatry*, **148**, 174–8.

Kinzie, D., Lewinsohn, P., Maricle, R. & Teri, L. (1986). The relationship of depression to medical illness in an older community population. *Comprehensive Psychiatry*, **27**, 241–6.

Livingston, G., Hawkins, A., Graham, N., Blizard, R. & Mann, A. (1990*a*). The Gospel Oak Study: prevalence rates of dementia, depression and activity limitation among elderly residents in inner London. *Psychological Medicine*, **20**, 137–46.

Livingston, G., Thomas, A., Graham, N., Blizard, R. & Mann, A. (1990*b*). The Gospel Oak Project: the use of health and social services by dependent elderly people in the community. *Health Trends*, **2**, 70–3.

MacDonald, A. (1986). Do general practitioners 'miss' depression in elderly patients? *British Medical Journal*, **292**, 1365–7.

Mann, A., Jenkins, R & Belsey, E. (1981). The twelve month outcome of patients with neurotic illness in general practice. *Psychological Medicine*, **11**, 535–50.

Mulrow, C., Aguilar, C., Endicott, J. et al. (1990). Quality of life changes and hearing inpairment. A randomized trial. *Annals of Internal Medicine*, **113**, (3), 188–94.

Murphy, E. (1983). The prognosis of depression in old age. *British Journal of Psychiatry*, **142**, 111–19.

Murrell, S., Himmelfarb, S & Wright, K. (1983). Prevalence of depression and its correlates in older adults. *American Journal of Epidemiology*, **117**, (2), 173–85.

Priern, R. & Kupfer, D. (1986). Continuation therapy for major depressive episodes: how long should it be maintained? *American Journal of Psychiatry*, **143**, 18–23.

Radloff, L. S. (1977). The CES-D scale: a self-report depression scale for research in the general population. *Applied Psychological Measurement*, **1**, 385–401.

Rockwell, E., Lam, R. & Zisook, S. (1988). Antidepressant drug studies in the elderly. *Psychiatric Clinics of North America*, **11** (1), 215–33.

Schonfield, L., Garcia, J. & Streuber,P. (1985). Factors contributing to mental health treatment of the elderly. *Journal of Applied Gerontology*, **4** (2), 30–9.

Shepherd, M., Cooper, B., Brown, A. & Kalton, G. (1966). *Psychiatric Illness in General Practice*. Oxford: Oxford University Press.

Spitzer, R. L., Endicott, J. & Robins, E. (1975). *Research Diagnostic Criteria. Biometrics Research*, New York State Department of Mental Hygiene.

Sullivan, C. F., Copeland, J. R. M., Dewey, M. E. et al. (1988). Benzodiazepine usage amongst the elderly: findings of the Liverpool Community Survey. *International Journal of Geriatric Psychiatry*, **3**, 289–92.

Third National Study 1981–82 RCGP/OPCS/DHSS (1986). *Morbidity Statistics from General Practice*. London: Her Majesty's Stationery Office.

Waxman, H., Carner, E. & Blum, P. (1983). Depressive symptoms and health service utilization among the community elderly. *Journal of the American Geriatrics Society*, **31**, 417–20.

Widner, R. & Cadoret, R. (1978). Depression in primary care: changes in pattern of patient visits and complaints during developing depression. *The Journal of Family Practice*, **7**, 293–302.

Wilkinson, G., Allen, P., Marshall, E., Walker, J., Browne, W. & Mann, A. (1993). A pilot study of the effect of practice nurse intervention on compliance with antidepressant medication in general practice. *Psychological Medicine*, **23**, 229–37.

Williams, P. (1980). Prescribing antidepressants, hypnotics and tranquillizers. *Geriatric Medicine*, **10**, 50–5.

Williamson, J., Stokoe, I., Gray, S., Fisher, M., Smith, A., McGhee, A. (1964). Old people at home: their unreported needs. *Lancet*, **i**, 1117–20.

Yesavage, J., Rose, T. & Lum, O. (1983). Development and validation of a geriatric depression screening scale: a preliminary report. *Journal of Psychiatric Research*, 17, 37–49.

Zung, W. W. K., Magill, M., Moore, J. T. et al. (1983). Recognition and treatment of depression in a family medicine practice. *Journal of Clinical Psychiatry*, **44**, 3–9.

12

Treatment of depression in the elderly

HENRY BRODATY KAARIN ANSTEY

Why treatment of depression in the elderly is different

Age is associated with differences in response to, and side-effects from, treatment. Pharmacokinetics alter with age (see Chapter 25), rates of pharmacologic side-effects increase (see Chapter 25), issues of concern for psychotherapy are qualitatively distinct (see Chapters 27, 28, 29) and the outcome of electro-convulsive therapy (ECT) (see Chapter 26), even allowing for diagnosis, may be better in late life (Benbow, 1991).

Secondly, treatment differs in old age because of diagnostic variations. Depression in the elderly may appear phenomenologically similar to that in younger patients but have a different etiology. The reverse may hold too; a depression of putatively similar etiology is more likely to be psychotic and to be associated with psychomotor agitation in an older than in a younger person. Even within the elderly depressive population, there is heterogeneity. Depression with first onset in late life (late-onset depression) is more likely to have an organic basis than depression with first onset early in life and recurrence or persistence into later years (early-onset depression), which is more likely to be associated with a family history of affective disorder (Brodaty et al., 1991). Further, patients with depression of organic etiology or depression and concurrent physical morbidity are likely to have a poorer outcome.

Thirdly, the general health of the older depressed patient must also be considered in setting realistic goals for therapy. Elderly patients with depression are far more likely than younger ones to suffer from medical problems which may be a cause of or concomitant with their depression (Rothblum et al., 1982). The clinical presentation of the depression is likely to be colored by somatic symptoms, even though depressed elderly are not necessarily more hypochondriacal (Costa & Macrae, 1985; Brodaty et al., 1991), and treatment possibilities may be limited by the priorities of physical illness.

Fourthly, depression in the elderly is frequently associated with bereavement

(Bruce et al., 1990; Zisook & Schuchter, 1991: Horne & Blazer, 1992), including loss of intimates, robust health and job. Other stresses associated with older age may include assumption of a care-giver role, interpersonal disputes or interpersonal deficiency unmasked by a narrowing world (Rothblum et al., 1982).

Finally, there are differences in access to assessment and treatment. Older people are less likely to acknowledge depressive symptoms as having a psychological basis or are less likely to seek treatment because of negative bias or ignorance. The older person may not acknowledge the possibility of depression. For example, if an older person believes he is more tired because he is just getting old, or because he is sick, he will not identify these symptoms as depressive and will feel resigned to them continuing. When older people do present themselves to doctors, they are less likely to have their depression identified, to be referred for psychiatric treatment and, if referred, to receive psychological rather than somatic therapies (Brodaty et al., 1993).

Psychotherapy for depression

General approach to psychotherapy with older persons

In adapting cognitive, behavioral and other psychotherapies to the older adult, there must be consideration of the person's cultural background, education and prior exposure to therapy (Morris & Morris, 1991).

Older patients often expect to be treated according to a more medical model and may not be accustomed to the idea of 'talking therapies'. Older people therefore require more information so that they, as well as the therapist, clearly understand what to expect from treatment (Morris & Morris, 1991).

Account must be taken of changes which may occur with increasing age, such as decline in memory, sensory deficits, decreased flexibility of thinking and a decline in the ability to learn new information. Creative means of successfully circumventing these changes may include patients taking notes during sessions or audiotaping them. Additional treatment sessions may be required where progress is slower, and follow-up sessions can be scheduled to allow the patient to review progress. Structure and goal setting are also important with older people so as to prevent confusion about the purpose and length of therapy (Chaisson-Stewart, 1985). The therapist must also be aware of the potential for countertransference to interfere with the therapeutic process.

Cognitive and behavioral therapies

There are several reasons why cognitive and behavioral therapies are especially suited to treating the elderly. Rather than concentrating on the patient's past history and aiming for personality change such therapies emphasize skill acquisition and current concerns. These aspects are especially relevant where the patient resists dynamic psychotherapy because of obstructive beliefs that he or she is too old to change. Cognitive and behavior therapies also encourage engagement in activities which counteract tendencies toward apathy. Moreover, the behavioral aspects of the therapy are especially useful for those with difficulties in abstract thinking (Steuer & Hammen, 1983). Cognitive elements of therapy challenge ageist beliefs and stereotypes which contribute to poor self-efficacy in the elderly.

Cognitive behavior therapy (CBT) (Beck et al., 1979) is highly structured, collaborative and time-limited with an empirical hypothesis testing approach. As well as encompassing behavior therapy, it involves identifying, evaluating and challenging negative cognitions and substituting these with more realistic, positive responses and attitudes. Behavior therapy for depression, originating from Lewinsohn (1974), emphasizes the role of reduced positive reinforcement in the origin and maintenance of depression. Therapy aims to break patterns of inertia and increase the frequency of positive experiences in a person's life. Goal-directed graded tasks are set which when accomplished give the patient a sense of achievement. Behavior therapy may involve relaxation training, social skills training and assertiveness training.

Cognitive and behavioral therapies may be adapted for the elderly by concentrating on concrete rather than abstract concepts, and by considering life changes specific to old people such as changes in role and social status, illness and loss of friends and spouse. Individual differences in cognitive functioning and cultural background lead to marked variability in the way older patients cope with and respond to treatment. A treatment program for CBT with the elderly has been outlined by Teri (1991).

There are few well-controlled studies which have evaluated the efficacy of psychotherapies for depression in the elderly. Gallagher and Thompson (1983), comparing cognitive therapy, behavioral therapy and brief insight-orientated therapy, found no significant differences between them at the immediate conclusion of 12 weeks of treatment, although patients receiving cognitive and behavioral therapies had fewer relapses and their depression scores were lower than patients receiving insight-orientated therapy. Those with nonendogenous depression showed an earlier and greater degree of improvement in response to psychotherapy. Their result was replicated in a study of 120 patients diagnosed with Research Diagnostic Criteria (RDC)-defined major depressive disorder randomly assigned to cognitive, behavioral, psychodynamic and control conditions of whom 91 completed the 16–20 week course of treatment (Thompson, Gallagher & Breckenridge, 1987). Of patients in the three treatment groups, 70% achieved significant improvement or complete remission by the end of treatment, with no difference in efficacy being found between groups.

Group therapy

One of the major benefits of group psychotherapy in the elderly is its potential to overcome social isolation. However, group psychotherapy in the elderly may become dominated by depressive affect (Leszcz, 1990) and when unchecked, the process of exploring and understanding may lead to an increase in feelings of helplessness and demoralization. The efficacy of group psychotherapy in the elderly for depression has been reported in controlled (Beutler et al., 1987; Gallagher, 1981) and uncontrolled (Steuer et al., 1984) outcome studies. Group therapies have been found to be equally effective in comparisons of group behavior therapy and group supportive psychotherapy (Gallagher, 1981); and cognitive-behavior therapy (CBT) and psychodynamic group psychotherapy (Steuer et al., 1984). The only difference found has been a greater reduction in self-reported Beck Depression Inventory (BDI) scores for subjects receiving CBT (Beutler et al., 1987; Steuer et al., 1984). This result must be interpreted with caution because the BDI is loaded with items which measure negativistic cognitions and so CBT may 'teach the scale'. Moreover, the result has not been validated by scores on other outcome measures used in the same studies such as the Zung Depression Scale (Steuer et al., 1984) or the Hamilton Rating Scale for Depression (Beutler et al., 1987; Steuer et al., 1984).

Reminiscence therapy

Reminiscence or life review aims to promote continuity between past states of the self and the present. It uses the natural process of review, organization and evaluation of the individual's past to reintegrate the self (Butler, 1963; Leszcz, 1990). Techniques such as examining photographs from the past, and writing and taping autobiographies facilitate the life review process (Chaisson-Stewart, 1985). When used appropriately, reminiscence may restore feelings of worth and competence through the articulation of past successes and may also facilitate appropriate grieving and conflict resolution. It is important to be aware that reminiscence may also lead to fixation on past events, guilt over irreparable errors and a morbid self-absorption resulting in social isolation (Leszcz, 1990). Reminiscence can be incorporated into cognitive therapy and used to demonstrate cognitive biases and selective attention to negative past events which can then be challenged. When elderly depressed patients are instructed on how to deal with negative memories resulting from reminiscence, they have shown greater reduction in depressive symptoms and an increase in self-confidence compared with patients in an unstructured reminiscence group and an 'activity' control group (Fry, 1983, cited by Morris & Morris, 1991).

Problem solving

Problem solving involves the learning of skills which reduce the probability of a problem recurring or increase the probability of an adaptive solution. Hussian and Lawrence (1981) found that depression was reduced at two-week follow-up in an elderly group receiving problem solving orientated treatment compared with a group receiving social reinforcement and a wait-list control. However, no treatment effects were found at three-months suggesting follow-up treatment may be necessary.

Family therapy and interpersonal therapy

As with any psychiatric illness, there is an interaction between the depression, the patient and the family (Bloch et al., in press). It is important to ensure that the spouse or other close family is consulted and included in the plan of management. No studies of the efficacy of family therapy for depression in the elderly could be located for this review.

Interpersonal therapy (IPT), which has demonstrable efficacy in younger patients (Weissman et al., 1981), requires further evaluation with the elderly. One study has shown IPT to be partially more effective than nortriptyline (Sloane, Staples & Schneider, 1985) in reducing depressive symptoms in elderly patients. A more comprehensive maintenance trial of IPT, modified for specific use with elderly patients suffering recurrent, late-life depression is underway at the University of Pittsburgh (Klerman & Weissman, 1992).

Summary

Individual and group psychotherapies are effective treatments for depression in the elderly. As with younger adults (Robinson, Berman & Neimeyer, 1990; Elkin et al., 1991) there appears to be no difference in the efficacy of the various types of psychotherapy with the elderly. Problem-solving and reminiscence techniques are appealing but require further empirical evaluation. Family therapy and interpersonal therapy have proved effective in younger populations but remain to be evaluated as treatments for depression in the elderly.

Somatic therapies

Antidepressants

Starting an antidepressant

Identification of suitable patients for antidepressants, alterations in pharmacokinetics with age, and the adage to start low and go slow with medication are discussed in Chapter 25. The efficacy of particular antidepressants is also reviewed there. Few, if any, psychogeriatricians would now prescribe tertiary amine tricyclics such as amitriptyline, imipramine or doxepin as their first line of treatment for a depressed patient, unless there was a past history of success with that drug in that individual or his family. The secondary amine tricyclics, selective serotonin reuptake inhibitors, reversible monoamine oxidase inhibitors and other newer agents are preferred as they have fewer side-effects with equivalent efficacy. Recommended psychopharmacological screening criteria, contraindications, dosages and durations of treatment are provided elsewhere (American Psychiatric Association Committee on Quality Assurance, 1992; RANZCP Committee on Psychotropic Drugs and Other Physical Treatments, in press). Dosages required to achieve therapeutic levels in the elderly are usually lower; sometimes less than half those required in younger adults.

Treatment of side-effects

Side-effects of antidepressants (see list in table 12.1), seem to occur more frequently with age and to have a more deleterious impact. Sometimes they can be avoided by careful monitoring of drug blood levels. Plasma level monitoring may also indicate compliance and whether the dose of medication is within the therapeutic range.

Forewarning the patient, and often the family, about possible side-effects will allow early attention to them and importantly can improve compliance, as may clear instructions (in large writing) about dosage. Bulk and high fibre in the diet can help prevent constipation. Use of pilocarpine 1% eyedrops can alleviate difficulties with reading, and when added to water (5 drops to 10–20 ml) can be used as a mouthwash to relieve anticholinergic-induced dry mouth, especially if there are difficulties with eating. Particular attention needs to be paid to oral hygiene in older patients, as lack of saliva predisposes to infection and ill-fitting dentures which cause abrasions. On occasions, urinary outflow pathology requires surgical correction before suitable antidepressant medication can be commenced. Postural hypotension, which increases the risk of falls and fractures in the elderly, usually requires a reduction in dose or change in antidepressant type (nortriptyline being the least hypotensive tricyclic). On the other hand, side-effects can sometimes be used to advantage by allowing the treatment of two conditions simultaneously. For example, the hypotensive action of monoamine oxidase inhibitors (MAOIs) may allow the cessation of antihypertensives (which in any case may be having a depressogenic effect), and the anticholinergic actions of tricyclics may lessen dyspeptic symptoms.

Cyclic antidepressants

The efficacy of cyclic antidepressants is well established in geriatric major depression and unless contraindicated should be considered when antidepressant medication is required (Alexopoulos, 1992). Side-effects will generally determine

Table 12.1. *Relative side-effects of cyclic and atypical antidepressants in the elderly patient* according to different sources*

Drug	Sedation	Hypotension	Anticholinergic	Altered cardiac rate and rhythm
Tertiary amines				
Imipramine	+ ++ +++	++ +++	++(+) ++ ++++	++
Doxepin	++(+) ++++ ++++	++ ++++	+++ ++ ++	++
Amitriptyline	+++ +++ +++++	++ ++++	++++ +++ ++++	+++
Trimipramine	+++ ++++	++	+++ ++++	+++
Secondary amines				
Despiramine	+ + +	+(+) ++	+ + +	+
Nortriptyline	+ ++ ++	+ +	++ + +++	+
Amoxapine	+ ++	++	++ ++	++
Protriptyline	+	++	+++	++
Maptrotiline	++(+) ++++	++	++ ++	+
Atypical				
Trazodone	++ ++++	++	+ ++	+(+)
Fluoxetine	+/- +/-	0 +/-	0	0

0 = nil.
\+ = mild.
+(+) = mild–moderate.
++ = moderate.
++(+) = moderate–strong.
+++ = strong.
++++ = very strong.
+/- = some patients stimulated, others sedated.
\+ = Salzman, 1990*a*.
\+ = Dewan et al., 1992.
\+ = Bernstein, 1984.
* Table adapted from Dewan et al., 1992; Salzman, 1990*a*; Bernstein, 1984
Legend follows that of Dewan et al., 1992 and Salzman, 1990*a*.

which cyclic is chosen (see above). They are contraindicated, however, in elderly patients with recent myocardial infarction, heart block, or in those receiving a cardiac depressant such as quinidine, and should be prescribed with caution to patients with narrow angle glaucoma and prostatic hypertrophy (Salzman & van der Kolk, 1984).

Tertiary amines

Tertiary amines such as amitriptyline, imipramine, trimipramine, maprotiline and doxepin are more likely to cause hypotension than secondary amines such as nortriptyline, desipramine and protriptyline. The former drugs also have antihistaminic side-effects which may produce sedation and weight gain (Davidson, 1989). Their marked anticholinergic side-effects can cause impaired memory and concentration, confusion, delirium, urinary retention, erectile impairment, constipation, paralytic ileus and tachycardia in the elderly. Tertiary amines are therefore not recommended as a first line of treatment for patients susceptible to these side-effects, though claims have been made that dothiepin causes fewer intolerate side-effects and less cardiotoxicity and that it is particularly helpful for elderly depressed patients with anxiety (Zusky et al., 1986). Amitriptyline is the least desirable tricyclic for treatment of depression in the elderly because of its notable anticholinergic activity and its associated risk of hypotension (Gerson, Plotkin & Jarvik, 1988). Monitoring of plasma levels may help prevent side-effects by ensuring the lowest dose of drug necessary. However, as many of these drugs have multiple metabolites, plasma levels may be unreliable guides to therapeutic efficacy.

Secondary amines

Secondary amines generally have much weaker anticholinergic side-effects than tertiary amines. In particular, nortriptyline and desipramine have the fewest toxic side-effects of the secondary amines (Salzman, 1990*a*) and have the added advantage that plasma levels are reasonably useful gauges of therapeutic efficacy. Of all the cyclic antidepressants, nortriptyline produces the least frequent and least severe hypotension (Davidson, 1989).

Irreversible mono amine oxidase inhibitors (MAOIs)

Irreversible MAOIs are usually reserved as a second or third line of treatment for typical depression in the elderly. Until recently, MAOIs were thought to reduce depression by decreasing the metabolism of norepinephrine and serotonin (Salzman & van de Kolk, 1984), but evidence now suggests that they have complex effects on monoamine receptors, including down-regulation of the beta and alpha 2-noradrenergic receptors as well as the serotonin 1 and serotonin 2 receptors (Alexopoulos, 1992). As with the cyclic antidepressants, there is no strong evidence for the therapeutic superiority of one MAOI over another, and the choice of drug depends more on its known side-effects and the clinical features of the patient.

Irreversible MAOIs may be used as a first line treatment in atypical depressions characterized by reverse vegetative features (increased sleep, appetite and weight, and interpersonal sensitivity); by predominant anxiety and phobias; or by apathy and anergia. For the latter, tranylcypromine in particular may be helpful in view of its stimulant properties.

Common side-effects of irreversible MAOIs are weight-gain and hypotension, as well as dry mucous membranes, insomnia, overstimulation, sexual dysfunction and peripheral oedema. As with most antidepressants, irreversible MAOIs may exacerbate memory loss, confusion, restlessness, agitation, paranoia and insomnia.

New generation drugs

Trazodone is an atypical antidepressant which is as effective as classical tricyclics, and has been recommended as a second choice antidepressant for those elderly patients who have not responded to desipramine or nortriptyline (Salzman, 1990*a*). Trazodone is markedly sedating and has been associated in the elderly with cardiac arrhythmias, hypotension, priapism and confusion. It produces fewer side-effects in a geriatric population than traditional antidepressants though it may cause gastric irritation (Altamura et al., 1989*a*). There is evidence of a linear relationship between steady-state plasma trazodone levels and clinical response (Monteleone & Gnocchi, 1990).

Fluoxetine, a selective serotonin reuptake inhibitor, has no affinity for dopaminergic, noradrenergic or muscarinic receptors (Small, 1991). Common side-effects of fluoxetine include insomnia, anxiety and nausea, particularly anorexia and weight loss in the elderly (Brymer & Winograd, 1992). Its major disadvantage in the elderly is its long elimination half-life, which for young adults is 70 hours, and that of its active metabolite which is 330 hours (Small, 1991) and even longer in the elderly. Although fluoxetine has not yet been systematically studied in patients with heart disease, both animal and clinical studies indicate minimal cardiac effects at both therapeutic doses and at overdose. However, there have been case studies reported of unexpected deaths in medical patients receiving fluoxetine (Spier & Frontera, 1991), as well as of bradycardia and dysrhythmia (Buff et al., 1991).

Sertraline lacks the cardiovascular, anticholinergic, antihistaminergic and antidopaminergic effects associated with other classes of antidepressants (Cohn et al., 1990). Sertraline has a 25-hour half-life, which is long enough to allow for daily administration and yet compares favorably with the longer half life of fluoxetine. In a recent double-blind study examining the effects of sertraline compared with mianserin on psychomotor performance of elderly volunteers, it was found that single or multiple doses of up to 200 mg/day did not affect

Table 12.2. *Summary of double-blind antidepressant trials in the elderly (1987–1991)*

Study	Number of pts. entered/ completed	Mean age (range)	Diagnostic criteria	Drug(s)	Dose	Design	Duration	Outcome and comments
Georgotas et al. (1987*a*, *b*)	90/90 (75 in data analysis)	> 54 years	RDC MDD outpatients	Nortriptyline (NOR) Phenelzine (PHEN) Placebo(PLB)	25–125 mg 15–75 mg	Double-blind Placebo controlled	7 weeks	(*a*) Both drugs effective vs PLB. NOR more effective in reducing mid/late insomnia (*b*) Both drugs caused equal orthostatic hypotension, with mean drop in systolic pressure 9–10 mm Hg, persisting through 7 weeks
Altamura et al. (1988)	75/75	66.05 (60–83)	DSM-III	Amitriptyline (AMI) Mianserin (MIAN) Trazodone (TRA)	75 mg 60 mg 150 mg	Double-blind	5 weeks	3 drugs equally effective. TRA had fewest S. E.
Altamura et al. (1989*b*)	28/22	68.5	DSM-III MDE inpatients	Fluoxetine (FLU) AMI	20 mg 75 mg	Double-blind	5 weeks	Both drugs effective. AMI > anti-cholinergic S. E. and weight gain.
Altamura et al. (1989*a*)	106/92	65.83	DSM-III MDE inpatients	TRA MIAN AMI	150 mg 60 mg 75 mg	Double-blind multicentre	5 weeks	3 drugs equally effective. TRA had fewest S. E., AMI was quickest acting
Fairbairn et al. (1989)	62/48	77 (65–85)	DSM-III MDE in and outpatients	Lofepramine (LOF) Dothiepin (DOTH)	70–140 mg 50–100 mg	Double-blind Two-centre	6 weeks	Both drugs equally effective. LOF produced quicker improvement. LOF produced fewer anticholinergic S. E. and less sedation.

Guillibert et al. (1989)	79/58	68.7	DSM-III MDD	Paroxetine (PAR) Clomipramine (CLOM)	20–30 mg 25–75 mg	Double-blind Double-dummy	6 weeks	CLOM and PAR equally effective and safe. 65% PAR and 72% CLOM responded. PAR was better tolerated and had fewer S. E.
Hostmaelingen et al. (1989)	51/47	(65–88)	No criteria General practice	Flupenthixol (FLUP) AMI	0.5–1 mg 25–50 mg	Double-blind Double-dummy	4 weeks	80% of patients on FLUP and AMI improved. FLUP group responded more quickly and had milder and fewer S. E.
Bohm et al. (1990)	40/37	72 (65–77)	ICD-9 ND or anxiety state. Primary care practice	Buspirone (BUS) PLB	15–30 mg	Double-blind placebo controlled	4 weeks	BUS equally effective for anxiety and neurotic depression and well tolerated by those with chronic medical conditions.
De Vanna et al. (1990)	80/80	(60–80)	DSM-III MDE	Moclobemide (MOCL) MIAN	300–500 mg 75–125 mg	Double-blind multicentre	4 weeks	Overall efficacy good or very good for over 60% of patients in each group. MOCL S. E. included headache, agitation and nausea. MIAN S. E. included sleepiness, agitation and anxiety
De Vanna et al. (1990)	39/39	> 60 years	ICD-9 ED, ND or depressive disorder not caused by brief reactive states, hospital inpatients	MOCL Maprotiline (MAPR)	150–300 mg 75–150 mg	Double-blind	6 weeks	Overall efficacy good or very good for over 90% of patients in each group. MOCL S. E. included restlessness, nervousness and insomnia. MAPR S. E. included tiredness and 1 patient developed delirium

Table 12.2. (*cont.*)

Study	Number of pts. entered/ completed	Mean age (range)	Diagnostic criteria	Drug(s)	Dose	Design	Duration	Outcome and comments
Cohn et al. (1990)	241/121	70.2 (63–85)	DSM-III MDE, BD-D outpatients	Sertraline (SER) AMI	50–200 mg 50–150 mg	Double-blind multicentre	8 weeks	SER and AMI equally effective. 69.5% SER and 62.5% AMI responded. SER had few anticholinergic S. E. and more gastrointestinal S. E.
Schifano et al. (1990)	48/35	75	DSM-III MDE, DD mentally ill inpatients	MIAN MAPR	45–90 mg 75–150 mg	Double-blind	4 weeks	40% of patients in each group considered improved or much improved
Feighner et al. (1990)	30/15	68.2 (60–85)	DSM-III MDE outpatients	Adinazolam (ADIN) Desipramine (DES)	10–60 mg 25–150 mg	Double-blind	8 weeks	ADIN had 57% response rate and S. E. were drowsiness, lightheadedness. DES had 27% response rate and S. E. were dry mouth, constipation, nervousness. ADIN group responded more rapidly
Katz et al. (1990)	30/23	84	DSM-III institutionalized frail elderly	NOR PLB	65.2 mg	Double-blind Placebo controlled	7 weeks	$\frac{1}{3}$ of patients withdrew due to adverse medical events. NOR group showed significant improvement on HRSD and CGI but not GDS

Phanjoo et al. (1991)	57/31	> 65	DSM-III MDE hospital inpatients or outpatients	Fluvoxamine (FLUV) MIAN	100–200 mg 40–80 mg	Double-blind multicentre	6 weeks	Significant but not large improvement with both drugs. MIAN S. E. included agitation, dizziness and backpain. FLUV S. E. included agitation, dizziness, ataxia and tension
Rahman et al. (1991)	52/36	74 (61–86)	DSM-III MDE hospital patients	FLUV DOTH	50–200 mg 50–200 mg	Double-blind multicentre	6 weeks	Both drugs equally effective and well tolerated with no serious adverse effects. DOTH produced more anticholinergic S. E. than FLUV

S. E. = Side-effects.
'Responders' are classified as patients with at least 50% reduction of symptoms on the Hamilton Rating Scale for Depression (HRSD).
MDD = Major depressive disorder.
MDE = Major depressive episode.
DD = Dysthymic disorder.
BD-D = Bipolar disorder-depressed.
ND = Neurotic depression.
ED = Endogenous depression.
CGI = Clinical global improvement.
GDS = Geriatric depression scale.
NB: Studies on maintenance therapy, continuation therapy, adjunctive therapy and studies with the cognitively impaired are excluded.

performance, and that mianserin was tolerated much more poorly than sertraline (Hindmarch, Shillingford & Shillingford, 1990).

Moclobemide, a new reversible inhibitor of monoamine oxidase-A, has been found to be tolerated far better than the tricyclic antidepressants (Versiani et al., 1990) and is equally well tolerated by older and younger adult patients. Moclobemide is free from cardiotoxicity, is not sedative, does not induce dry mouth, constipation or blurred vision, and has a good safety profile in long-term treatment (Versiani et al., 1990). Moclobemide has been shown to be as effective as the tricyclics, mianserin and maprotiline (De Vanna et al., 1990) and to have minimal or no interaction with alcohol, even in the elderly (Tiller, 1990; Zimmer et al., 1990).

Mianserin is a tetracyclic compound which enhances noradrenergic transmission by blocking presynaptic autoreceptors. It has a weak anticholinergic effect whereas its antihistaminic effect is more important. Mianserin produces some sedation, a weak hypotensive effect and, in rare cases, blood dyscrasias. Serum mianserin concentrations have been shown to be unaffected by age, although concurrent neuroleptic treatment may increase serum mianserin levels (Leinonen, 1991).

Choosing an antidepressant: outcome studies

The range of antidepressants available for depression is continually expanding. The potential of newer drugs for equivalent (though not greater) efficacy with fewer side-effects is particularly important for older patients. However, caution is required in extrapolating the results of drug trials from younger adult subjects to the elderly population. Very few studies actually include older subjects or, if they do, they fail to specify their particular outcome (Gerson et al., 1988). Even in studies limited to older patients with depression, subjects are unlikely to be typical as they have to satisfy many exclusion criteria before being considered eligible to participate.

This deficiency in the literature is now being redressed by a growing number of outcome studies which allow for evaluation of the efficacy of particular antidepressants for the elderly. In 1986 there had only been 24 double-blind drug studies with 189 subjects older than 55 years in controlled outcome studies (excluding amitriptyline and imipramine because of side-effects; Gerson et al., 1988) but, since then, a further 15 controlled trials reported between 1987 and 1991 inclusive, completed by 791 subjects 55 years or older can be identified (see Table 12.2). These data do not point to any antidepressant having obvious superiority. In choosing an antidepressant, the clinician is forced to rely on side-effect profile and individual responsiveness.

Lithium

Particular caution is required with the use of lithium in older patients. The initial dose should be low and increased gradually. Lithium is excreted through the kidneys and since renal clearance takes longer in the elderly (about 36 hours), it may take up to 180 hours to reach a steady-state (Davidson, 1989). Lithium has weak antidepressant action by itself but may be used as augmentation for patients who fail to respond to a cyclic alone (Small, 1991). However, in a recent trial of lithium augmentation, the four elderly patients in the study all developed severe side-effects requiring discontinuation of treatment (Austin, Arana & Melvin, 1990). As toxicity may occur even at recommended plasma levels, monitoring of red blood cell lithium levels has been suggested (Abou-Saleh, 1992).

Carbamazepine

Post (Post et al., 1986; Post, 1992) reported that carbamazepine was an effective treatment for one third of 54 cases of mixed-age depression unresponsive to other medications. While no studies have yet looked at carbamazepine in an elderly population, one report of its use in treatment resistant melancholia is relevant (Cullen et al., 1991). Of 16 patients, 13 were 60 years of age or older (range = 60–88). Five of these (38.5%) had moderate or marked improvement with carbamazepine despite the chronicity of the depression (mean 31 months, range = 3–70), psychotic nature (in one improved subject) and coexisting cerebral infarcts (in two improved subjects), although many had to discontinue the drug because of adverse effects.

Psychostimulants

Methylphenidate has been reported to improve depressive symptoms in withdrawn, medically ill elderly patients with depression who do not tolerate tricyclics (Salzman, 1990*b*), with the most common side-effects being tachycardia and mild increases in blood pressure. Psychosis and confusion may be exacerbated or precipitated by methylphenidate, especially in patients with dementia.

Unfortunately, there are few conclusive, well controlled studies on the effectiveness of stimulants in the treatment of depression in the elderly. In a recent review of the use of stimulants in the treatment of depression in general, Satel and Nelson (1989) concluded from the ten placebo controlled studies of stimulant drugs in primary depression, that, with one exception, these agents had little advantage over placebo. Whilst controlled studies with geriatric patients tended to be more positive, outcome only demonstrated partial improvement.

Benzodiazepines

The efficacy of benzodiazepines in treating depression is controversial and yet to be fully evaluated. Recent studies have shown the elderly to have reduced capacity to metabolize benzodiazapines and a reduced capacity to inhibit adverse drug effects, one of which may be depression itself (Nikaido et al., 1990; Kroboth, McAuley & Smith, 1990).

Electroconvulsive therapy

Electroconvulsive therapy (ECT), usually not the initial treatment of choice for major depression in the elderly, may be prescribed after other treatments have been ineffective (Blazer, 1989) or in certain cases of depression. ECT has been demonstrated to be particularly effective in major depression associated with melancholia and psychomotor agitation or retardation, and in psychotic depression (Buchan et al., 1992; Hickie, Parsonage & Parker, 1990). Suicidal or self-destructive behavior and life-threatening malnutrition may indicate the need for urgent ECT (Blazer, 1989; Coffey & Weiner, 1990). ECT should also be considered when the side-effects of other drug therapy, such as heart block, are potentially worse than those of ECT. Indications for ECT in late life, its safety and efficacy and other aspects of its use are considered in Chapter 26.

Poor response to ECT has been reported to be related to the previous nonresponse to tricyclics (Prudic, Sackheim & Devanaud, 1990) and to the onset of physical illness during the index episode (Murphy, 1983; Baldwin & Jolley, 1986). Bilateral ECT appears more effective than unilateral but may cause more side-effects, especially in older patients. Supra-threshold ($>$ 2.5 $\times$ threshold) unilateral ECT seems more effective than threshold unilateral ECT, i.e. just enough electrical energy to cause a fit, and may (Abrams, Swartz & Vedak, 1991) or may not (Sackheim, Devandand & Prudic, 1991) be equivalent in efficacy to bilateral ECT. The high relapse rate within a year of ECT ($>$ 30–60%; Prudic et al., 1990) indicates a need for maintenance antidepressant medication after completion of a course of ECT.

Patients whose depression has responded to ECT should be placed on continuation anti-depressants after the depression has abated. For some patients, a single ECT treatment every 4–6 weeks may prevent depressive recurrence (Salzman 1990*b*; Thienhaus, Marletta & Bennett, 1990; Benbow, 1991).

Cognitive outcome of ECT

A recent naturalistic uncontrolled study of 55 patients older than 55 years examined the cognitive outcome six months after treatment with ECT plus antidepressants (Stoudmire et al., 1991). ECT was administered thrice weekly, unilaterally to the nondominant hemisphere and treatment was continued with TCAs. Among the 19 patients with pretreatment cognitive impairment, ($<$ 130 on the Mattis Dementia Scale), four had complete reversal of cognitive dysfunction, seven had remission of depressive symptoms but remained cognitively impaired and the remainder had minimal improvement in cognition and depression.

Psychosurgery

Psychosurgery is rarely recommended nowadays and almost never for older patients. The presence of organic brain disease or serious physical illness usually contraindicates this treatment, though old age per se is not a barrier to psychosurgery (Baldwin, 1991).

Continuation and maintenance treatment

Treatment of major depression is commonly divided into three phases:

(i) acute, aiming for remission of an episode;
(ii) continuation, aiming to prevent relapse of an episode after its resolution;
(iii) maintenance, attempting to prevent recurrences or new episodes occurring (Prien, Carpenter & Kupfer, 1991). As the average duration of an untreated episode in later life is 12–48 months (compared with the 5–6 months in younger adults), continuation therapy needs to be longer than the usual period of six months recommended for younger depressives (Prien & Kupfer, 1986; Flint, 1992).

The elderly appear to be at greater risk of recurrence than younger adults (Grof, Angst & Haines, 1974; Zis et al., 1980), and with each recurrence the risk of further recurrences and chronicity increases (Keller et al., 1983; Scott, 1988). Flint (1992), in an excellent review, argued that a first episode of depression occurring after the age of 60 years should be treated in the same way as a recurrent episode of early-onset depression. This implies a need to continue to be quite assertive in treating elderly patients after they have recovered from an episode.

It is not easy to predict which patients are at risk for relapse or recurrence (see Frank et al., 1991 for definitions), as factors determining prognosis remain to be elucidated (see Chapter 8). Also, the ideal duration and dose for continuation and maintenance therapies are unclear (Flint, 1992). The limited, sometimes contradictory, available data on older patients with depression provide limited assistance to the psychogeriatrician in making these decisions. Georgotas et al. (1988) found that the cumulative percentage of patients remaining well during 4–8 months continuation therapy was 86% with nortriptyline and 83% with phenelzine. Recurrence rates in the subsequent 12 months maintenance phase were 13% with phenelzine, 54% with nortriptyline and 65% with placebo (Georgotas, McCue & Cooper, 1989). The poor result with nortriptyline is puzzling and contradicts an open-study finding that 82% of patients remained recurrence-free over 18 months (Reynolds et al., 1989).

In younger adults with a history of recurrent major depression, Frank et al. (1990) found that maintenance therapy using acute treatment doses of antidepressants provided superior protection against recurrence (60% survival over three years) than previous studies using lower doses (20–48% survival over 1–5 years). Interpersonal therapy was superior to placebo as maintenance treatment but did not add significantly to the efficacy of high maintenance dose (200 mg/day) imipramine.

The roles of high dose antidepressant medication and of psychological therapies in continuation and maintenance phases of treatment have not been investigated in older patients with depression. Assertive follow-up is recommended for at least 18 months (the period of maximal risk for recurrence) and perhaps permanently (Baldwin, 1988). Flint (1992) suggested that newer antidepressants with fewer side-effects may be more acceptable for long-term maintenance treatment. Carbamazepine and lithium may also be effective maintenance therapies (Murphy & MacDonald, 1992).

Special problems in the treatment of depression in the eldery

Failure to respond

Treatment resistance, initially characterized as failure to respond to a standard course of antidepressant, embodies several concepts (Wilhelm et al., in press, *a*). It may indicate a 'true' resistance to appropriate treatment, be it somatic or psychological, given in appropriate dosage and for sufficient duration. It may also reflect treatment intolerance where side-effects, patient reluctance or non-compliance prevent an adequate trial of treatment.

Treatment resistance may appear more common than it really is because patients who are treatment resistant may have had many consultations although studies have included mainly younger adults. Rates of 8–16% of 'true' treatment resistance have been reported amongst attenders at specialist mood disorder clinics (MacEwan & Remick, 1988; Wilhelm et al., in press, *b*). These compare with rates of 20% for chronicity in long-term (15–18 years) follow-up studies of depressed patients (Lee & Murray, 1988; Kiloh, Andrews & Neilson, 1988). In the elderly chronicity, but not treatment resistance, has been investigated (see below).

Principles of managing treatment-resistant depression are similar in older and younger patients. Re-evaluation of diagnosis, reconsideration of appropriateness of treatment strategies, checking of compliance and questioning about perpetuating factors – biological or psychosocial – are always necessary in managing patients whose depression has failed to resolve. Concurrent thyroid disease, which may be subclinical, and minor organic cerebral changes as evidenced by hyperintensities on MRI scan, may portend resistance to treatment, especially in older patients

(Hickie et al., 1992; Coffey et al., 1990). The latency period for response to antidepressant medication may be longer in older patients, averaging six weeks (range 2–12) (Georgotas et al., 1986, 1987*a*, 1989).

Subsequent treatment strategies for refractory cases include increasing dosage of antidepressant, changing medication, adding psychological therapy or augmenting one medication with another. Lithium may be used as augmentation for patients who fail to respond to a cyclic alone (Small, 1991), although there is a lack of empirical research to establish its safety and efficacy in older people.

Other drugs which can be added to cyclic antidepressants include triiodothyronine 25 mg daily and L-tryptophan at doses of 1 to 4 daily. Methylphenidate can be added but this brings with it a risk of agitation, insomnia and occasionally psychosis. Augmentation with a MAOI requires management by an experienced psychopharmacologist (Blazer, 1989). Other types of combination therapies, e.g. fluoxetine and cyclics, have usually been described in younger patients only.

Even so, about 15–20% of patients with depression in mixed-aged samples (Kiloh et al., 1988; Lee & Murray, 1988) and 20% in older populations (Cole, 1990; Brodaty et al., 1993) remain chronically depressed. A difficulty facing the clinician is when to desist with further trials of yet another antidepressant or another combination of drugs. Patient, family and doctor may need to realign their thinking to an impaired model and learn to live with a handicap rather than clinging to a model of seeking a cure for an illness. The burden of chronic depression on family carers can be considerable and support for them, including respite care, may sometimes be required.

Depression in residential care settings (see Chapter 10)

The prevalence of depression in the residential care setting is high (Katz et al., 1990; Ames, 1991) and its diagnosis and treatment is often complicated by concurrent illness and dementia. Ames (1990) reported that a psychogeriatric team was more likely to recommend social rather than specific psychiatric interventions and that medical attention for pain or untreated illness was often required. The negative results of the study may have reflected the chronicity of the conditions, the negative effects of the residential setting and substantial non-compliance with recommended interventions. Nortriptyline has proved effective in treating depression in the residential care setting in a double-blind, placebo-controlled trial (Katz et al., 1990), although 35% of subjects required early termination of treatment owing to adverse medical events. High levels of self-care disability and low levels of serum albumin were associated with poor outcome of the depression but good outcome was not associated with an improvement in self-care. There is a pressing need for the development of effective treatment strategies for depressed residents in nursing homes.

Depression and dementia

Between 0 and 86% of Alzheimer patients have been reported to have a comorbid DSM-III or RDC-defined major depressive disorder (Wragg & Jeste, 1989; Alexopoulos & Abrams, 1991; Burns, 1991) with 25% being the modal frequency (e.g. Reifler, Larson & Hanley, 1982). Whatever the true prevalence, the presence of a coexisting depression increases the risk of nursing home admission and represents excess of disability which is potentially treatable. Environmental and psychological approaches to treating depression in dementing patients should always be considered. Specific techniques such as CBT are not necessarily precluded by impairment in short-term memory. Teri and Gallagher-Thompson (1991) provide guidelines for the use of both CBT in mildly demented patients with co-existing depression and behavioral techniques for moderately advanced cases. Teri and Logsdon (1991) have also developed the Pleasant Events Schedule-AD specifically for patients with Alzheimer's disease or other dementias. Outcome studies are still needed, however, to evaluate psychological interventions for depression coexisting with dementia.

There is more evidence for the efficacy of antidepressant medication. Tricyclic antidepressants have been shown to improve mood, neurovegetative symptoms and activities of daily living, but have not been shown to improve cognition in patients with depression and dementia (Reifler et al., 1989). Irreversible MAOIs may have specific efficacy because of the exaggerated age-related rise of MAO levels in dementia (Ashford & Ford, 1979; Jenike, 1985). There may, however be practical difficulties in dementing patients adhering to dietary restrictions required while taking irreversible MAOIs. Newer antidepressants such as fluoxetine, moclobemide, trazodone and bupropion hold promise (Alexopoulos & Abrams, 1991). Two open studies reported L-deprenyl (selegiline) in low doses (10 mg/day) improved depression scores as well as lowering agitation, tension and excitement (Tariot et al., 1987; Schneider et al., 1988).

In their review of the literature on ECT in the treatment of depression in dementia, Price and McAllister (1989) noted the lack of well-controlled studies using strict diagnostic criteria and specifying the technical details of treatment. In spite of this, it appeared that there was generally a significant reduction in depressive symptoms with the use of ECT in dementia. Nelson and Rosenberg (1991) also reported that the outcome for ECT in patients with depression and dementia was encouraging – almost as good as for patients with depression alone. The overall 86% response rate reported by Price and McAllister (1989) is probably inflated owing to the tendency to report successful treatment. Of particular importance is the finding that improvement in cognitive functioning occurred after ECT in nearly half of the patients. This was especially the case for patients with dementias of unknown cause, multi-infarct dementia, normal pressure hydrocephalus and the primary degenerative cortical dementias. Only 21% of patients experienced cognitive and memory disturbances or delirium. Nelson & Rosenberg (1991) reported more confusion after ECT in patients with dementia and depression than in patients with 'pure' depression but no greater incidence of cardiac side-effects. In older patients, especially those with organic mental disorders, unilateral ECT may have an advantage over bilateral ECT as it is associated with less memory impairment (Alexopoulos, Young & Abrams, 1989). The decision to administer ECT depends on the presence of a severe depression in patients who are not able to tolerate, or are unresponsive to, drug treatment (Alexopoulos & Abrams, 1991; Nelson & Rosenberg, 1991).

Depression and stroke

Depression occurs commonly after stroke (see Chapter 24). When untreated, poststroke depression increases morbidity from the stroke – indicating a particular need for assertive treatment in this population. The role of the caregiver cannot be underestimated in poststroke depression, and may be the single most important factor predicting independence (Clothier & Grotta, 1991). Tricyclic antidepressants, particularly nortriptyline, as well as ECT, have been reported to be effective in the treatment of depression complicating stroke (Lipsey et al., 1984; Fedoroff & Robinson, 1989; Murray, Shea & Conn, 1987).

At present, there have been too few trials of antidepressants in patients with poststroke depression to enable the relative efficacy of medications to be established, although nortriptyline tends to be favored. The choice of drug therefore depends mainly on side-effects, especially orthostasis, as well as the clinical status of the patient. Since an important aspect of recovery after stroke is new learning, optimal pharmacological treatments should have minimal effects on memory. For this reason benzodiazepines and sedating tricyclics are not recommended.

Depression in Parkinson's disease (PD) and other neurological disorders.

Depression occurs in 40% of patients with PD and is distinguished by higher levels of concurrent anxiety and less self-reproach than depression in patients without PD (Cummings, 1992). About one in five PD patients experiences a first depressive illness before the onset of any neurological symptoms. Depression in PD is associated with lower CSF levels of 5-hydroxyindole acetic acid, and greater involvement of dopaminergic and noradrenergic systems than in depression in other patients. Lower levels of serotonin may predispose the PD patient to depression. Against this background, it is not surprising that more than half of the depressed PD patients meet criteria for a major depressive disorder and that a variety of antidepressants have been found to be effective.

Four double-blind trials of antidepressants: imipramine 150–200 mg/day, desipramine 100 mg/day, bupropion 450 mg/day and nortriptyline 150 mg/day, in a total of 101 subjects have been published. Subjects demonstrated moderate improvement with response rates of 42–60%. Nortriptyline excepted, the other three antidepressants were also associated with improvement in motor symptoms. Open studies have suggested that bupropion, 5-hydroxytryptophan, L-deprenyl and bromocriptine may be helpful (for reviews see Cummings, 1992; Fava, 1992), but that l-dopa, sergyline and methylphenidate had no effect or a negative effect. ECT has also proved efficacious in relieving depression in PD and, temporarily, motor disorder. Response to standard treatments is variable (Fava, 1992) and current preoccupations with somatic therapies should not obscure the need for assisting the patient and family with psychological and social aspects of PD.

Other neurological disorders such as cerebral tumor, multiple sclerosis, Huntington's disease and normal pressure hydrocephalus are often associated with the depressive illness which again may precede neurological symptoms.

Conjugal bereavement

Conjugal bereavement, which is considered one of the most stressful life events, occurs most often in the elderly population (Horne & Blazer, 1992). Therefore, the elderly are most at risk for developing depression from death of a spouse. About a third of a newly widowed population have a symptom profile of major depression (Bruce et al., 1990). Far fewer, however, meet sufficient criteria to qualify as DSM-III-R defined major depression, i.e. self-depreciation, functional impairment, psychomotor retardation, guilt and suicidality (Bruce et al., 1990). Zisook and Schuchter (1991) found that 24% of 350 widows met DSM-III-R criteria for depression two months after bereavement, 23% at seven months and 16% at 13 months, which was significantly greater on each occasion than the 4% rate of depression in a control group. Factors predictive of depression in widows include depression at two and/or seven months postbereavement, past history of major depression, younger age when bereaved, poor interpersonal supports, poor physical health, low socio-economic status, absence of a confidant and mode of death (Nuss & Zubenko, 1992; Horne & Blazer, 1992; Tweed, 1993 in press, cited by Horne & Blazer).

Strategies to prevent depression developing in this population have had mixed results in studies of widows across a wide but predominantly older age range. Gerber et al. (1975) reported that regular therapy – in the home, office or over the telephone – was effective in reducing the number of visits to physicians, minor illnesses and medications taken at three months follow-up. Raphael (1977) found that widows receiving nondirective psychotherapy, with a focus on support of relevant bereavement processes in the widow's home in sessions of two or more hours per session, had fewer hospitalizations for depression during 13 months follow-up than widows receiving no intervention. Results from another intervention study (Vachon et al., 1980) involving a self-help program, Widow-to-Widow, in which widows received limited training and contact with other widows, suggested that a 'high-distress' group receiving intervention followed the same course of bereavement as controls but adapted to their situation more rapidly and reported better physical health and more new relationships. Marmar et al. (1988), comparing brief dynamic psychotherapy and mutual self-help groups, found both interventions resulted in equal reductions in stress-specific and general symptoms, as well as improvements in social and work functioning.

There are few empirical trials evaluating antidepressant treatment for depression associated with pathological bereavement. In a small ($n = 13$) open trial for a median of 6.4 weeks, nortriptyline (mean dose 49.2 mg/day) reduced Hamilton Rating Scale for Depression scores without affecting the intensity of the grief (Pasternak et al., 1991). An even smaller study reported that desipramine was effective in relieving depressive symptoms in seven out of ten bereaved middle-aged (average age = 55 years) depressed spouses (Jacobs et al., 1987).

In summary, conjugal bereavement in old age does increase the risk for depression. Psychosocial interventions directed at those at risk have the potential to prevent the occurrence of conditions associated with pathological grief, including depression. Antidepressant medication may be indicated in those with major depression complicating bereavement.

Caregivers and depression

Caregivers of cognitively impaired dependents are at risk of depression. Particularly at risk are socially isolated wives whose dementing husbands exhibit problem behaviors, and who have a deteriorating marital relationship and a lack of perceived social support (Brodaty & Hadzi-Pavlovic, 1990). Moritz, Kasl & Berkman (1989) reported that caregiving husbands were more likely to have depressive symptoms if they perceived their financial support to be inadequate. While most studies have concentrated on dementia caregivers, similar levels of psychological morbidity have been reported in caregivers of stroke victims (Draper et al., 1992).

When depression occurs in caregivers it is more likely to be nonendogenous, minor or intermittent. Even conceding that many studies appear to have overinterpreted their data (Brodaty, 1990), there probably is a real increased risk of caregivers developing RDC-defined major depression (Gallagher et al., 1989), which usually is neither severe nor melancholic.

Interventions with caregivers have the potential to reduce psychological morbidity and, by implication, rates and levels of depressive symptoms or depression. However, most studies have failed to find effects on psychological morbidity (for review see Brodaty, 1992). Kahan et al. (1985) reported that eight, weekly, two-hour meetings consisting of education and problem-solving techniques decreased the level of depression compared to a control group. Brodaty and Gresham (1989) found no effect on Zung Depression Scale scores for their intensive 10-day intervention program comprising educational, psychological and problem-solving techniques, even though General Health Questionnaire scores were significantly improved and time to institutionalization was delayed. Mohide et al (1990) reported that an intervention comprising education, assistance with problem-solving, in-home respite and group support improved quality of life without influencing care-givers' depression or anxiety scores.

Neither residential respite care nor day care programs have been shown to influence measures of psychological morbidity in caregivers (Brodaty & Gresham, 1992; Wells et al., 1990) although placement of dementia sufferers (many with problem behaviors) in a special nursing home resulted in significant improvement in psychological symptoms of caregivers compared to a control group of caregivers whose dependents had not been placed (Wells & Jorm, 1987).

In summary, there is the potential for educational and psychosocial programs to decrease depression in caregivers but more careful targeting of interventions is required.

Prevention of depressive disorders

Primary prevention

Primary prevention is the preclusion of a condition from ever beginning. It results in a decrease in incidence (defined as the number of new cases developing per unit time). Rabins' (1992) assertion that there were no proven primary prevention strategies for any of the three primary categories of depression: major depression, dysthymic disorder, or adjustment disorder with depressed mood, remains largely correct, but there are two studies which point to promising interventions.

First, Raphael (1977) demonstrated that psychological intervention for recently bereaved widows at high risk of psychiatric morbidity prevented hospitalization for depression. Secondly, the results of a large two-wave epidemiological study have implications for intervention. Oxman et al. (1992) found that loss of a spouse, functional disability, increase in functional disability, decreased social support, decreased tangible support adequacy (particularly for males), loss of a confidant and fewer children making weekly visits were significant predictors of depressive symptoms occurring over a three year period. Few elderly subjects with depressive symptoms met criteria for a major depressive disorder. This lends confirmation to a previous report that lack of perceived social support interacts with life events to increase the risk of psychological symptoms developing in the general population

(Henderson, Byrne & Duncan-Jones, 1981). Oxman's group suggested that primary care physicians might consider the following preventative strategies: more frequent follow-up, more contact by older people with their offspring, and even trials of antidepressants in older persons with functional disability who perceive their emotional support to be inadequate and have few children making weekly visits.

Secondary prevention

Secondary prevention aims to decrease morbidity associated with a disorder by either limiting the length of a disorder or by reducing the disability it causes. It includes early identification of the disorder, prompt initiation of treatment and timely attention to social and psychological concomitants of disease. Secondary prevention leads to a decreasing prevalence, i.e. the number of cases present in a population during a specific time interval.

Screening persons at high risk for development of depression may lead to early and successful treatment. Conditions associated with high risk include caring for a cognitively impaired person, stroke, Parkinson's disease (Ehmann et al., 1990), Alzheimer's disease, Huntington's disease (Folstein et al., 1983), other dementias, severe medical illness (Harris et al., 1988; Koenig et al., 1988), alcoholism, drug dependence, chronic pain and bereavement (Rabins, 1992). Also, residency in a nursing home or hostel (Snowdon & Donnelly, 1986; Ames et al., 1988; Ames, 1991, 1992) and certain medications such as antihypertensives are associated with a propensity to depression.

The early recognition of depression is an opportunity for secondary prevention. Delayed intervention in the treatment of depression may be associated with more recalcitrant illness. Furthermore, major depression in an older person can result in immobility, poor medical compliance and self-neglect and may exacerbate coexisting medical illness and frailty (Rabins, 1992). Early recognition and adequate treatment of major depression could decrease suicide rates amongst this high risk group (Hagnell, Lanke & Rorsman, 1981; Conwell & Caine, 1991).

Evidence presented above suggests that medication has a definite place as a secondary preventative treatment for depression following bereavement (Jacobs et al., 1987; Pasternak et al., 1991) and stroke (Fedoroff & Robinson, 1989). Also comprehensive psychosocial interventions have the capacity to reduce psychological morbidity in caregivers of people with dementia (Brodaty, 1992).

Tertiary prevention

Tertiary prevention is the avoidance or diminution of long-term sequelae of illness. It includes preventing or delaying recurrence and lessening the morbidity caused by a chronic condition. Recurrence, which occurs in the majority of depressed patients, is less likely with maintenance therapy (see above), though research examining the prevention of depressive recurrence specifically in the elderly is in its infancy (Old Age Depression Interest Group, 1993).

The prevention of suicide, known to be highest in elderly white males should be a major focus for tertiary prevention. Other important foci include rehabilitation of the chronically depressed patient, educating the family about depression as well as helping them understand and live with the condition.

Conclusions

There are both qualitative and quantitative differences in the treatment of depression in older people. Overall, as the prognosis for depression in later life is not worse than for younger patients (Baldwin & Jolley, 1986; Brodaty et al., 1993), ageist and nihilistic attitudes to intervention should be abandoned. Response may take longer, treatment may be complicated and residual disabilities in other bodily functions may continue, but the clinician needs to remain assertive, optimistic and assiduous. Skill and knowledge are required in matching treatment to depressive subtype and in managing side-effects in the individual patient. The family can be a useful ally or can perpetuate depression and the environment must be considered in planning management. For the minority of cases who remain resistant to treatment, a model of living with impairment is more appropriate than ceaseless trials of new drugs. In those cases, management is aimed at containing symptoms, education and support of both patient and family.

References

Abou-Saleh, M. (1992). Lithium. In *Handbook of Affective Disorders*. 2nd edition. ed. E. S. Paykel. Edinburgh: Churchill Livingstone.

Abrams, R., Swartz, C. M. & Vedak, C. (1991). Antidepressant effects of high-dose right unilateral electroconvulsive therapy. *Archives of General Psychiatry*, **48**, 746–8.

Alexopoulos, G. S. (1992). Treatment of depression. In *Clinical Geriatric Psychopharmacology*. ed. C. Salzman. Baltimore: Williams and Wilkins.

Alexopoulos, G. S. & Abrams, R. C. (1991). Depression in Alzheimer's disease. *Psychiatric Clinics of North America*, **14**, 327–40.

Alexopoulos, G. S., Young, R. C. & Abrams, R. C. (1989) ECT in the high-risk geriatric patient. *Convulsive Therapy*, **4**, 75–87.

Altamura, A. C., Mauri, M. C., Colacurcio, F. et al. (1988) Trazodone in late life depressive states: a double-blind multicenter study versus amitriptyline and mianserin. *Psychopharmacology*, **95**, S34–6.

Altamura, A. C., Mauri, M. D., Rudas, N. et al. (1989*a*). Clinical activity and tolerability of trazodone, mianserin and amitriptyline in elderly subjects with major depression: a controlled multicenter trial. *Clinical Neuropharmacology*, **12**, S25–33.

Altamura, A. C., Percudani, M., Guercetti, G. & Invernizzi, G. (1989*b*). Efficacy and tolerability of fluoxetine in the elderly: a double-blind study versus amitriptyline. *International Journal of Clinical Psychopharmacology*, **4**, 103–6.

American Psychiatric Association Committee on Quality Assurance. (1992). *Manual of Psychiatric Quality Assurance*. Washington, DC: American Psychiatric Association.

Ames, D. (1990). Depression among elderly residents of local-authority residential homes: its nature and the efficacy of intervention. *British Journal of Psychiatry*, **156**, 667–75.

Ames, D. (1991). Epidemiological studies of depression among the elderly in residential and nursing homes. *International Journal of Geriatric Psychiatry*, **6**, 347–54.

Ames, D. (1992). Residential care. *Current Opinion in Psychiatry*, **5**, 575–9.

Ames, D., Ashby, D., Mann, A. H. & Graham, N. (1988). Psychiatric illness in elderly residents of part III homes in one London borough: prognosis and review. *Age and Ageing*, **17**, 249–56.

Ashford, J. W. & Ford, C. V. (1979). Use of MAO inhibitors in elderly patients. *American Journal of Psychiatry*, **136**, 1466–7.

Austin, L. A., Arana, G. W. & Melvin, J. A. (1990). Toxicity resulting from lithium augmentation of antidepressant treatment in elderly patients. *Journal of Clinical Psychiatry*, **51**, 344–5.

Baldwin, R. (1988). Depression in later life: a fresh challenge to an old problem. In *Symposium on Affective Disorders in the Elderly*. Southampton: Duphar Medical Relations.

Baldwin, R. & Jolley, D. (1986). The prognosis of depression in old age. *British Journal of Psychiatry*, **149**, 574–83.

Baldwin, R. C. (1992). Depressive illness. In *Psychiatry in the Elderly*. ed. R. Jacoby & C. Oppenheimer. Oxford: Oxford University Press.

Beck, A. T., Rush, J., Shaw, B. & Emery, G. (1979). *Cognitive Therapy of Depression*. New York: Guildford.

Benbow, S. M. (1991). ECT in late life. *International Journal of Geriatric Psychiatry*, **6**, 401–6.

Bernstein, J. G. (1984). Pharmacotherapy of geriatric depression. *Clinical Psychiatry*, **45**, 30–4.

Beutler, L. E., Scogin, F., Kirkish, P. et al. (1987). Group cognitive therapy and alprazolam in the treatment of depression of older adults. *Journal of Consulting and Clinical Psychology*, **55**, 550–6.

Blazer, D. (1989). Affective disorders in late life. In *Geriatric Psychiatry*. ed. E. Busse & D. Blazer. Cambridge University Press: Cambridge.

Bloch, S., Harari, E., Hafner, J. & Szmukler, G. *The Family and Psychiatry*. Oxford: Oxford University Press, in press.

Bohm, C., Robinson, D. S., Gammans, R. E., Shrotriya, R. C., Alms, D. R., Leroy, A., Placchi, M. (1990). Buspirone therapy in anxious elderly patients: a controlled clinical trial. *Journal of Clinical Psychopharmacology*, **10**, 47S–51S.

Brodaty, H. (1990). Resilience in the face of dementia. *6th Alzheimer's Disease International Conference*. Mexico City, Keynote address, 25/9/1990.

Brodaty, H. (1992). Carers: training informal carers. In *Recent Advances in Psychogeriatrics II*. ed. T. Arie. London: Churchill Livingstone.

Brodaty, H. & Gresham, M. (1989). Effect of a training program to reduce stress in carers of patients with dementia. *British Medical Journal*, **299**, 1375–9.

Brodaty, H. & Gresham, M. (1992). Prescribing residential respite care for dementia – effects, side-effects, indications and dosage. *International Journal of Geriatric Psychiatry*, **7**, 357–62.

Brodaty, H. & Hadzi-Pavlovic, D. (1990). Psychosocial effects on carers living with persons with dementia. *Australian and New Zealand Journal of Psychiatry*, **24**, 351–61.

Brodaty, H., Harris, L., Peters, K. et al. (1993) Prognosis of depression in the elderly: a comparison with younger patients. *British Journal of Psychiatry*, **163**, 589–96.

Brodaty, H., Peters, K., Boyce, P. et al. (1991) Age and depression. *Journal of Affective Disorders*, **23**, 137–49.

Bruce, M. L., Kim, K., Leaf, P. J. & Jacobs, S. (1990). Depressive episodes and dysphoria resulting from conjugal bereavement in a prospective community sample. *American Journal of Psychiatry*, **147**, 608–11.

Brymer, C. & Winograd, C. H. (1992). Fluoxetine in elderly patients: is there cause for concern? *Journal of the American Geriatric Society*, **40**, 902–5.

Buchan, H., Johnstone, E., McPherson, K., Palmer, R. L., Crow, T. J., Brandon, S. (1992). Who benefits from electroconvulsive therapy? *British Journal of Psychiatry*, **160**, 355–9.

Buff, D. D., Brenner, R., Kirtane, S. S. & Gilboa, R. (1991). Dysrhythmia associated with fluoxetine treatment in an elderly patient with cardiac disease. *Journal of Clinical Psychiatry*, **52**, 174–6.

Burns, A. (1991). Affective symptoms in Alzheimer's disease. *International Journal of Geriatric Psychiatry*, **6**, 371–6.

Butler, R. N. (1963). The life review: an interpretation of reminiscence. *Psychiatry*, **26**, 65–76.

Chaisson-Stewart, G. M. (1985). *Depression in the Elderly: An Interdisciplinary Approach*. New York: John Wiley & Sons.

Clothier, J. & Grotta, J. (1991). Recognition and management of poststroke depression in the elderly. *Clinical Geriatric Medicine*, **7**, 493–506.

Coffey, C. E., Figiel, G. S., Djang, W. T. & Weiner, R. D. (1990). Subcortical hyperintensity on magnetic resonance imaging: a comparison of normal and depressed elderly subjects. *American Journal of Psychiatry*, **147**, 187–9.

Coffey, C. E. & Weiner, R. D. (1990). Electroconvulsive therapy: an update. *Hospital and Community Psychiatry*, **41**, 515–21.

Cohn, C. K., Shrivastava, R., Mendels, J. et al. (1990). Double-blind, multicenter comparison of sertraline and amitriptyline in elderly depressed patients. *Journal of Clinical Psychiatry*, **51**, 28–33.

Cole, M. G. (1990). The prognosis of depression in the elderly. *Canadian Journal of Psychiatry*, **30**, 217–20.

Conwell, Y. & Caine, E. D. (1991). Rational suicide and the right to die; reality and myth. *New England Journal of Medicine*, **325**, 1100–2.

Costa, P. T. & Macrae, R. R. (1985). Hypochondriasis, neuroticism and aging: When are somatic complaints unfounded? *American Journal of Psychology*, **40**, 19–28.

Cullen, M., Mitchell, P., Brodaty, H. et al. (1991). Carbamazepine for treatment-resistant melancholia. *Journal of Clinical Psychiatry*, **52**, 472–6.

Cummings, J. L. (1992). Depression and Parkinson's disease: a review. *American Journal of Psychiatry*, **149**, 443–54.

Davidson, J. (1989). The pharmacologic treatment of psychiatric disorders in the elderly. In *Geriatric Psychiatry*. ed. E. Busse & D. Blazer. Cambridge: Cambridge University Press.

De Vanna, M., Kummer, J., Agnoli, A. et al. (1990). Moclobemide compared with second-generation antidepressants in elderly people. *Acta Psychiatrica Scandinavica*, **360**, 64–6.

Dewan, M. J., Huszonek, J., Marvin, K., Hardoby, W. & Ispahani, A. (1992). The use of antidepressants in the elderly: 1986 and 1989. *Journal of Geriatric Psychiatry and Neurology*, **5**, 40–4.

Draper, B. M., Poulos, C. J., Cole A. M. D., Poulos, R. G. & Ehrlich, F. (1992). A comparison of caregivers for elderly stroke and dementia victims. *Journal of American Geriatric Society*, **40**, 896–901.

Ehmann, T. S., Beninger, R. J., Gawel, M. J. & Riopelle, R. J. (1990). Depressive symptoms in Parkinson's disease. A comparison with disabled control subjects. *Journal of Geriatric Psychiatry and Neurology*, **3**, 3–9.

Elkin, J., Shea, M. T., Watkins, J. T. et al. (1991). National Institute of Mental Health Treatment of Depression Collaborative Research Program: general effectiveness of treatment. *Archives of General Psychiatry*, **46**, 971–83.

Fairbairn, A. F., George, K. & Dorman, T. (1989). Lofepramine versus dothiepin in the treatment of depression in elderly patients. *British Journal of Clinical Practice*, **43**, 55–60.

Fava, G. A. (1992). Depression in medical settings: In *Handbook of Affective Disorders*. 2nd edition. ed. E. S. Paykel. Edinburgh: Churchill Livingstone.

Fedoroff, J. P. & Robinson, R. G. (1989). Tricyclic antidepressants in the treatment of poststroke depression. *Journal of Clinical Psychiatry*, **50**, 18–23.

Feighner, J. P., Boyer, W. F., Hendrickson, G. G., Pambakian, R. A. & Doroski, V. S. (1990). A controlled trial of adinazolam versus desipramine in geriatric depression. *International Journal of Clinical Psychopharmacology*, **5**, 227–32.

Flint, A. J. (1992). The optimum duration of antidepressant treatment in the elderly. *International Journal of Geriatric Psychiatry*, **7**, 617–19.

Folstein, S. E., Abbott, H. H., Chase, G. A., Jensen, G. A. Folstein, M. F. (1983). The association of affective disorder with Huntington's disease in a case series and in families. *Psychological Medicine*, **13**, 537–42.

Frank, E., Kupfer, D. J., Perel, J. M. et al. (1990). Three-year outcome for maintenance therapies in recurrent depression. *Archives of General Psychiatry*, **47**, 1093–9.

Frank, E., Prien, R. F., Jarret, R. B. et al. (1991). Conceptualization and rationale for consensus definitions of terms in major depressive disorder. *Archives of General Psychiatry*, **48**, 851–5.

Fry, P. S. (1983). Structured and unstructured reminiscence training and depression among the elderly. *Clinical Gerontology*, **1**, 15–37.

Gallagher, D., Rose, J., Rivera, P., Lovett, S. & Thompson, L. W. (1989). Prevalence of depression in family caregivers. *The Gerontologist*, **29**, 449–56.

Gallagher, D. & Thompson, L. W. (1983) Effectiveness of psychotherapy for both endogenous and nonendogenous depression in older adult outpatients. *Journal of Gerontology*, **38**, 707–12.

Gallagher, D. E. (1981). Behavioral group therapy with elderly depressives: an experimental study. In *Behavioral Group Therapy*. ed. D. Upper and S. Ross, Champaign, Illinois: Research Press.

Georgotas, A., McCue, R. E. & Cooper, T. (1989). A placebo-controlled comparison of nortriptyline and phenelzine in maintenance therapy of elderly depressed patients. *Archives of General Psychiatry*, **46**, 783–6.

Georgotas, A., McCue, R. E., Cooper, T., Chang, E., Mir, P. & Welkowitz, J. (1987). Clinical predictors of response to antidepressants in elderly patients. *Biological Psychiatry*, **22**, 733–40.

Georgotas, A., McCue, R. E., Cooper, T. B., Nagachandran, H. & Chang, I. (1988). How effective and safe is continuation therapy in elderly depressed patients? Factors affecting relapse rate. *Archives of General Psychiatry*, **45**, 929–32.

Georgotas, A., McCue, R. E., Friedman, E. & Cooper, T. B. (1987*a*). Response of depressive symptoms to nortriptyline, phenelzine and placebo. *British Journal of Psychiatry*, **151**, 102–6.

Georgotas, A., McCue, R. E., Friedman, E. & Cooper, T. B. (1987*b*). A placebo-controlled comparison of the effect of nortriptyline and phenelzine on orthostatic hypotension in elderly depressed patients. *Journal of Clinical Psychopharmacology*, **7**, 413–16.

Georgotas, A., McCue, R. E., Hapworth, W. et al. (1986) Comparison efficacy and safety of MAOIs versus TCAs in treating depressed elderly. *Biological Psychiatry*, **21**, 115.

Georgotas, A. & McCue, R. (1989). The additional benefit of extending an antidepressant trial past seven weeks in the depressed elderly. *International Journal of Geriatric Psychiatry*, **4**, 191–5.

Gerber, I., Weiner, A., Battin, D. & Arkin, A. M. (1975). Brief therapy to the aged bereaved. In *Bereavement, its Psychosocial Aspects*. ed. G. Schenberg, I. Gerber, A. Weiner et al. New York: Columbia University Press.

Gerson, S. C., Plotkin, D. A. & Jarvik, L. F. (1988). Antidepressant drug studies, 1964 to 1986: empirical evidence for ageing patients. *Journal of Clinical Psychopharmacology*, **8**, 311–22.

Grof, P., Angst, J. & Haines, T. (1974). The clinical course of depression: practical issues. In *Classification and Prediction of Outcome of Depression*. ed. J. Angst, Stuttgart–New York: F. K. Schattauer Verlag.

Guillibert, E., Pelicier, Y., Archambault, J. C. et al. (1989). A double-blind, multicentre study of paroxetine versus clomipramine in depressed elderly patients. *Acta Psychiatrica Scandinavica*, **80**, 132–4.

Hagnell, O., Lanke, J. & Rorsman, B. (1981). Suicide rates in the Lundby Study: mental illness as a risk factor for suicide. *Neuropsychobiology*, **7**, 248–53.

Harris, R. E., Mion, L. C., Patterson, M. B. & Frengley, J. D. (1988). Severe illness in older patients. The association between depressive disorders and functional dependency during the recovery phase. *Journal of American Geriatric Society*, **36**, 890–6.

Henderson, S., Byrne, D. G. & Duncan-Jones, P. (1981). *Neurosis and the Social Environment*. Sydney: Academic Press.

Hickie, I., Parsonage, B. & Parker, G. (1990). Prediction of response to ECT: preliminary validation of a sign-based typology of depression. *British Journal of Psychiatry*, **157**, 65–71.

Hickie, I., Scott, E., Mitchell, P., Wilhelm, K., Austin, M. P. & Bennett, B. (1992). Subcortical hyperintensities on magnetic resonance imaging: clinical correlates and prognostic significance in patients with severe depression. *Presentation at The Australian Society of Psychiatric Research*, Adelaide: Australia.

Hindmarch, I., Shillingford, J. & Shillingford, C. (1990). The effects of sertraline on psychomotor performance in elderly volunteers. *Journal of Clinical Psychiatry*, **51**, 34–6.

Horne, A. & Blazer, D. G. (1992). The prevention of major depression in the elderly. *Health Promotion and Disease Prevention*, **8**, 159–72.

Hostmaelingen, H. J., Asskilt, O., Austad, S. G. et al. (1989). Primary care treatment of depression in the elderly: a double-blind, multi-centre study of flupenthixol ('Fluanxol') and sustained-release amitriptyline. *Current Medical Research and Opinion*, **11**, 593–9.

Hussian, R. A. & Lawrence, P. S. (1981). Social reinforcement of activity and problem-solving training in the treatment of depressed institutionalized elderly patients. *Cognitive Therapy and Research*, **5**, 57–69.

Jacobs, M., Frank, E., Kupfer, D. & Carpenter, L. L. (1987). Recurrent depression: an assessment of family burden and family attitudes. *Journal of Clinical Psychiatry*, **48**, 395–400.

Jenike, M. (1985). Monoamine oxidase inhibitors as treatment for depressed patients with primary degenerative dementia (Alzheimer's disease). *American Journal of Psychiatry*, **142**, 763–4.

Kahan, J., Kemp, B., Staples, F. & Brummel-Smith, K. (1985). Decreasing the burden in families caring for a relative with a dementing illness. A controlled study. *Journal of American Geriatric Society*, **33**, 664–70.

Katz, I. R., Simpson, G. M., Curlik, S. M., Parmelee, P. A. & Muhly, C. (1990). Pharmacological treatment of major depression for elderly patients in residential care settings. *Journal of Clinical Psychiatry*, **5**, 41–7.

Keller, M. B., Lavori, P. W., Lewis, C. E. & Klerman, G. L. (1983). Predictors of relapse in major depressive disorder. *Journal of the American Medical Association*, **250**, 3299–304.

Kiloh, L. G., Andrews, G. & Neilson, M. (1988). The long-term outcome of depressive illness. *British Journal of Psychiatry*, **153**, 752–7.

Klerman, G.L & Weissman, M. M. (1992). Interpersonal psychotherapy. In *Handbook of Affective Disorders*. 2nd Edition. ed. E. S.Paykel, Edinburgh: Churchill Livingstone.

Koenig, H. G., Meador, K. G., Cohen, H. J. & Blazer, D. G. (1988). Depression in elderly hospitalized patients with medical illness. *Archives of Internal Medicine*, **148**, 1929–36.

Kroboth, P. D., McAuley, J. W. & Smith, R. B. (1990). Alprazolam in the elderly: pharmacokinetics and pharmacodynamics during multiple dosing. *Psychopharmacology*, **100**, 477–84.

Lee, A. S. & Murray, R. M. (1988). The long-term outcome of Maudsley depressives. *British Journal of Psychiatry*, **153**, 741–51.

Leinonen, E. (1991). Serum mianserin concentrations in psychiatric inpatients of different ages. *Acta Psychiatrica Scandinavica*. **83**, 278–82.

Leszcz, M. (1990). Towards an integrated model of group psychotherapy with the elderly. *International Journal of Group Psychotherapy*, **40**, 379–99.

Lewinsohn, P. (1974). A behavioral approach to depression. In *The Psychology of Depression: Contemporary Theory and Research*, ed. R. Friedman and M. Katz, New York: Wiley.

Lipsey, J. R., Robinson, R. G., Pearlson, G. D., Rao, K. & Price, T. R. (1984). Nortriptyline treatment of post-stroke depression: a double-blind study. *Lancet*, **ii**, 297–300.

MacEwan, G. W. & Remick, R. A. (1988). Treatment resistant depression: a clinical perspective. *Canadian Journal of Psychiatry*, **33**, 788–92.

Marmar, C. R., Horowitz, M. J., Weiss, D. S., Wilner, N. R. & Kaltreider, N. B. (1988). A controlled trial of brief psychotherapy and mutual-help group treatment of conjugal bereavement. *American Journal of Psychiatry*, **145**, 203–9.

Mohide, E. A., Pringle, D. M., Streiner, D. L., Gilbert, J. R., Muir, G. & Tew, M. (1990). A randomized trial of family caregiver support in the home management of dementia. *Journal of the American Geriatrics Society*, **38**, 446–545.

Monteleone, P. & Gnocchi, G. (1990). Evidence for a linear relationship between plasma trazodone levels and clinical response in depression in the elderly. *Clinical Neuropharmacology*, **13**, 84–9.

Moritz, D. J., Kasl, S. V. & Berkman, L. F. (1989). The health impact of living with a cognitively impaired elderly spouse: depressive symptoms and social functioning. *Journal of Gerontology*, **44**, S17–27.

Morris, R. G. & Morris, L. W. (1991). Cognitive and behavioral approaches with the depressed elderly. *International Journal of Geriatric Psychiatry*, **6**, 407–13.

Murphy, E. (1983). The prognosis of depression in old age. *British Journal of Psychiatry*, **142**, 111–19.

Murphy, E. & MacDonald, A. (1992). Affective disorders in old age. In *Handbook of Affective Disorders*. 2nd edition. ed. E. S. Paykel, Edinburgh: Churchill Livingstone.

Murray, G. B., Shea, V. & Conn, D. K. (1987). Electroconvulsive therapy for post-stroke depression. *Journal of Clinical Psychiatry*, **47**, 258–60.

Nelson, J. P. & Rosenberg, D. R. (1991). ECT treatment of demented elderly patients with major depression: a retrospective study of efficacy and safety. *Convulsive Therapy*, **7**, 157–65.

Nikaido, A. M., Ellinwood, E. H., Heatherly, D. G. & Gupta, S. K. (1990). Age-related increase in CNS sensitivity to benzodiazepines as assessed by task difficulty. *Psychopharmacology*, **100**, 90–7.

Nuss, W. S. & Zubenko, G. S. (1992). Correlates of persistent depressive symptoms in widows. *American Journal of Psychiatry*, **149**, 346–51.

Old Age Depression Interest Group (1993). How long should the elderly take antidepressants? A double-blind placebo controlled study of continuation/prophylaxis therapy with dothiepin. *British Journal of Psychiatry*, **162**, 175–82.

Oxman, T. E., Berkman, L. F., Kasi, S., Freeman, D. H., Jr., & Barrett, J. (1992). Social support and depressive symptoms in the elderly. *American Journal of Epidemiology*, **135**, 356–68.

Pasternak, R. E., Reynolds, III, C. F., Schlernitzauer, M. et al. (1991). Acute open-trial nortriptyline therapy of bereavement-related depression in late life. *Journal of Clinical Psychiatry*, **52**, 307–10.

Phanjoo, A. L., Wonnacott, S. & Hodgson, A. (1991). Double-blind comparative multicentre study of fluvoxamine and mianserin in the treatment of major depressive episode in elderly people. *Acta Psychiatrica Scandinavica*. **83**, 476–79.

Post, R. M. (1992). Anticonvulsant and novel drugs. In *Handbook of Affective Disorders*. 2nd edn. ed. E. S. Paykel, Edinburgh: Churchill Livingstone.

Post, R. M., Uhde, T. W., Roy-Byrne, P. P. & Joffe, R. T. (1986). Antidepressant effects of carbamazepine. *American Journal of Psychiatry*, **143**, 29–34.

Price, T. R. P. & McAllister, T. W. (1989). Safety and efficacy of ECT in depressed patients with dementia: a review of clinical experience. *Convulsive Therapy*, **5**, 61–74.

Prien, R. F., Carpenter, L. L. & Kupfer, D. J. (1991). The definition and operational criteria for treatment outcome of major depressive disorder: a review of the current research literature. *Archives of General Psychiatry*, **48**, 796–800.

Prien, R. F. & Kupfer, D. J. (1986). Continuation drug therapy for major depressive episodes: how long should it be maintained? *American Journal of Psychiatry*, **143**, 18–23.

Prudic, J., Sackeim, H. A. & Devanaud, D. P. (1990). Medication resistance and clinical response to electro-convulsive therapy. *Psychiatry Research*. **31**, 287–96.

Rabins, P. V. (1992). Prevention of mental disorder in the elderly: current perspectives and future prospects. *Journal of the American Geriatrics Society*, **40**, 727–33.

Rahman, M. K., Akhtar, M. J., Savla, N. C., Kellett, J. M. & Ashford, J. J. (1991). A double-blind, randomized comparison of fluvoxamine and dothiepin in the treatment of depression in elderly patients. *British Journal of Clinical Practice*, **45**, 255–8.

RANZCP Committee on Psychotropic Drugs and Other Physical Treatments (in press). *RANZCP Quality Assurance Guidelines for Psychotropic Drugs*. Melbourne: Royal Australian and New Zealand College of Psychiatrists.

Raphael, B. (1977). Preventive intervention with the recently bereaved. *Archives of General Psychiatry*, **34**, 1450–4.

Reifler, B. V., Larson E. & Hanley, R. (1982). Coexistence of cognitive impairment and depression in geriatric outpatients. *American Journal of Psychiatry*, **139**, 623–36.

Reifler, B. V., Teri, L, Raskind, M., Veith, R., Barnes, R., White, E. & McLean, P. (1989). Double-blind trial of imipramine in Alzheimer's disease patients with and without depression. *American Journal of Psychiatry*, **146**, 45–9.

Reynolds, C. F., Perel, J. M., Frank, E. et al. (1989). Open, trial maintenance pharmacotherapy in late-life depression: survival analysis. *Psychiatry Research*, **27**, 225–31.

Robinson, L. A., Berman, J. S. & Neimeyer, A. (1990). Psychotherapy for the treatment of depression: a comprehensive review of controlled outcome research. *Psychological Bulletin*, **108**, 30–49.

Robinson, R. G., Kubos, K. L., Starr, L. B., Rao, K. & Price, R. R. (1984). Mood disorders in stroke patients. Importance of location of lesion. *Brain*, **107**, 81–93.

Rothblum, E. D., Sholomskas, A. J., Berry, C. & Prusoff, B. A. (1982). Issues in clinical trials with the depressed elderly. *Journal of the American Geriatrics Society*, **30**, 694–9.

Sackeim, H. A., Devandand, D. P. & Prudic, J. (1991). Stimulus intensity, seizure threshold, and seizure duration: impact on the efficacy and safety of electroconvulsive therapy. *Psychiatric Clinics of North America*, **14**, 803–43.

Salzman, C. (1990*a*). Antidepressants. *Clinics in Geriatric Medicine*, **6**, 399–410.

Salzman, C. (1990*b*). Practical considerations in the pharmacologic treatment of depression and anxiety in the elderly. *Journal of Clinical Psychiatry*, **51**, 40–3.

Salzman, C. & van der Kolk, B. (1984). Treatment of depression. In *Clinical Geriatric Psychopharmacology*, ed. C. Salzman, New York: McGraw-Hill.

Satel, S. L. & Nelson, J. C. (1989). Stimulants in the treatment of depression: a critical overview. *Journal of Clinical Psychiatry*, **50**, 241–9.

Schifano, F., Garbin, A., Renesto, V. et al. (1990). A double-blind comparison of mianserin and maprotiline in depressed medically ill elderly people. *Acta Psychiatrica Scandinavica*. **81**, 289–94.

Schneider, L. S., Gleason, R., Zemonsky, M. F., Pollock, V. E., Sevenson, J. A. & Sloane, R. B. (1988). Deprenyl in the treatment of Alzheimer's disease. Gerontological Society of America. 41st Annual Scientific Meeting. November, 1988. *Gerontologist*, **28** (10), 2A.

Scott, J. (1988). Chronic depression. *British Journal of Psychiatry*, **153**, 287–97.

Sloane, R. B., Staples, F. R., Schneider, L. S. (1985). Interpersonal therapy versus nortriptyline for depression in the elderly. In *Clinical and Pharmacological Studies in Psychiatric Disorders*. ed. G. D. Burrows, T. R. Norman & L. Dennerstein, pp.344–346, London: John Libbey.

Small, G. W. (1991). Recognition and treatment of depression in the elderly. *Journal of Clinical Psychiatry*, **52**, 11–12.

Snowdon, J. & Donnelly, N. (1986). A study of depression in nursing homes. *Journal of Psychiatric Research*, **20**, 327–33.

Spier, S. A. & Frontera, M. A. (1991). Unexpected deaths in depressed medical inpatients treated with fluoxetine. *Journal of Clinical Psychiatry*, **52**, 377–82.

Steuer, J. L. & Hammen, C. L. (1983). Cognitive–behavioral group therapy for the depressed elderly: issues and adaptations. *Cognitive Therapy and Research*, **7**, 285–96.

Steuer, J. L., Mintz, J., Hammen, C. L. et al. (1984) Cognitive–behavioral and psychodynamic group psychotherapy in treatment of geriatric depression. *Journal of Consulting and Clinical Psychology*, **52**, 180–9.

Stoudmire, A., Hill, C. D., Morris, R., Martino-Saltzman, D., Markwalter, H. & Lewison, B. (1991). Cognitive outcome following tricyclic and electroconvulsive treatment of major depression in the elderly. *American Journal of Psychiatry*, **148**, 1336–40.

Tariot, P. N., Cohen, R. M., Sunderland, T. et al. (1987). L-deprenyl in Alzheimer's disease. Preliminary evidence for behavioral change with monoamine oxidase B inhibition. *Archives General Psychiatry*, **44**, 427–33.

Teri, L. (1991). Behavioral assessment and treatment of depression in older adults. In *Handbook of Clinical Behavior Therapy with the Elderly Client*. ed. P. A. Wisocki, New York: Plenum Press.

Teri, L. & Gallagher-Thompson, D. (1991). Cognitive–behavioral interventions for treatment of depression in Alzheimer's disease. *The Gerontologist*, **31**, 413–16.

Teri, L. & Logsdon, R. G. (1991). Identifying pleasant activities for Alzheimer's disease patients: the Pleasant Events Schedule-AD. *The Gerontologist*, **31**, 124–7.

Thienhaus, O. J., Marletta, S. & Bennett, J. A. (1990). A study of the clinical efficacy of maintenance ECT. *Journal of Clinical Psychiatry*, **51**, 141–4.

Thompson, L. W., Gallagher, D. & Breckenridge, J. S. (1987). Comparative effectiveness of psychotherapies for depressed elders. *Journal of Consulting Clinical and Psychology*, **53**, 385–90.

Tiller, J. W. G. (1990). Antidepressants, alcohol and psychomotor performance. *Acta Psychiatrica Scandinavica*, **360**, 13–17.

Tweed, D. (1993). Identification of illness for care finding studies. In *The Psychiatry of Old Age: An International Handbook*, ed. J. Copeland, M. Abou-Sellah, D. Blazer, New York: John Wiley & Son, in press.

Vachon, M. L.S, Lyall, W. A. L., Rogers, J., Freedman-Letofsky, K. & Freeman, S. J. J. (1980). A controlled study of self-help intervention for widows. *American Journal of Psychiatry*, **137**, 1380–4.

Versiani, M., Nardi, A. E., Figueira, I. L. V. & Stabl, M. (1990). Tolerability of moclobemide, a new reversible inhibitor of monoamine oxidase-A, compared with other antidepressants and placebo. *Acta Psychiatrica Scandinavica*. **360**, 24–8.

Weissman, M. M., Klerman, G.L, Prusoff, B. A., Sholomskas, D. & Padian, N. (1981). Depressed outpatients. Results one year after treatment with drugs and/or interpersonal psychotherapy. *Archives of General Psychiatry*, **38**, 51–5.

Wells, Y. & Jorm, A. F. (1987). Evaluation of a special nursing home for dementia sufferers: a randomized controlled comparison with community care. *Australian and New Zealand Journal of Psychiatry*, **21**, 524–31.

Wells, Y. D., Jorm, A. F., Jordan, F., Lefroy, R. (1990). Effects on care-givers of special day care programs for dementia sufferers. *Australian and New Zealand Journal of Psychiatry*, **24**, 82–90.

Wilhelm, K., Mitchell, P., Boyce, P. et al. (in press *a*). Treatment resistant depression in an Australian context. I. The utility of the term and approaches to management. *Australian and New Zealand Journal of Psychiatry*, in press.

Wilhelm, K., Mitchell, P., Sengoz, A., Hickie, I., Brodaty, H. & Boyce, P. (in press *b*) Treatment resistant depression in an Australian context. II. Outcome of a series of patients. *Australian and New Zealand Journal of Psychiatry*, in press.

Wragg, R. E. & Jeste, D. V. (1989). Overview of depression and psychosis in Alzheimer's disease. *American Journal of Psychiatry*, **146**, 577–89.

Zimmer, R., Gieschke, R., Fischbach, R. & Gasic, S. (1990). Interaction studies with moclobemide. *Acta Psychiatrica Scandinavica*, **360**, 84–6.

Zis, A. P., Grof, P., Webster, M. & Goodwin, F. K. (1980). Prediction of relapse in recurrent affective disorder. *Psychopharmacology Bulletin*, **16**, 47–9.

Zisook, S. & Schuchter, S. R. (1991). Depression through the first year after the death of a spouse. *American Journal of Psychiatry*, **148**, 1346–52.

Zusky, P., Manschreck, T. C., Blanchard, E., Rosenbaum, J., Elliot, C. & Lou, P. (1986). Dothiepin hydrochloride: treatment efficacy and safety. *Journal of Clinical Psychiatry*, **47**, 504–7.

13

Mania in late life: conceptual and clinical issues

KENNETH I. SHULMAN

Conceptual issues and the classification of affective disorders

The investigation of mania in old age invites a reconsideration of the fundamental nature of affective illness. Studying an elderly cohort offers the opportunity to examine a prolonged longitudinal course of the illness as well as focusing attention on the role of cerebral-organic factors. Recent studies of mania in old age have questioned the legitimacy of separating unipolar from bipolar disorders (Shulman & Post, 1980; Snowdon, 1991). Many unipolar depressives are apparently 'converted' into bipolars in old age after a latency of many years and numerous depressive episodes (Stone, 1989; Snowdon, 1991). This is also true of many young unipolar patients. Akiskal et al. (1983) found that 20% of young depressed patients with no prior history of mania became manic after an average 3-year prospective follow-up. Indeed, most clinicians are aware of subtle hypomanic shifts in 'unipolar' depressed and dysthymic patients. Because the study of the elderly lends itself to a retrospective cohort analysis, the longitudinal course of affective disorders is more readily revealed.

The notion of a spectrum of affective disorder as described by Akiskal (1983) is appealing. Milder expressions of the disorder include temperaments such as dysthymic, or hyperthymic. The range of expression continues from unipolar single episode to recurrent unipolar, bipolar II with mild hypomania to bipolar I with full-blown manic episodes. In this conceptual framework, mania is considered a more severe form of the disorder. Tsuang, Faraone and Fleming (1985) have proposed a 'threshold hypothesis' in which a manic predisposition requires lower levels of stress to elicit a decompensation.

Kraepelin (1921) had linked the manic and depressive expressions of affective disorder in an inextricable way by using the term Manic-Depressive Psychosis. Moreover, he subclassified six types of mixed states including: depressive/anxious mania; excited depression; mania with poverty of thought; manic stupor; depression with flight of ideas; and inhibited mania. To add to these subtypes,

Clothier, Swann and Freeman (1992) described dysphoric mania. Thus, both on cross-sectional and longitudinal views, the blurring of manic and depressive states is highlighted.

As will be described below, the notion of functional versus organic disorders also blurs when studying affective disorders in old age. Neurological and subtle cerebral-organic changes appear to be significant contributing factors to the manifestation of mania in the elderly. Thus geriatric psychiatry has a great deal to offer the investigation and understanding of so-called 'mood' disorders. Indeed, the primacy of mood as the fundamental disturbance in these illnesses in old age has been challenged (Shulman, 1989).

Epidemiology and age of onset

Snowdon (1991) has highlighted the fact that the incidence of mania as determined by first hospitalization does not diminish with age. Indeed, there is a trend for a rise in incidence after age 70. The one-year prevalence of mania in the recent Epidemiologic Catchment Area project however, shows a decrease with age from 1.4% prevalence in 18–44 year olds to 0.4% in those 45–64 years of age, finally diminishing to 0.1% in over 65s (Weissman et al., 1988). Where have all the young bipolars gone?

Shulman & Post (1980) found that only 8% of their sample of elderly bipolar subjects had become manic before the age of 40. This was replicated by Snowdon (1991) who noted that only 4 out of 75 elderly bipolar patients in his sample had been manic before the age of 40 and all had suffered from mania as their first affective episode. Snowdon (1991) has speculated about the potential causes of the fall in prevalence with ageing. Likely causes include an increase in mortality over time, better control of the disorder after many years of treatment and the possibility of eventual burnout with time.

Long-term follow-up of young sufferers from bipolar disorder has shown a mortality rate twice that of the general population (Goodwin & Jamison, 1984). Indeed, half of these bipolar patients died before the age of 70 and this certainly could contribute to the decreased prevalence of the disorder in old age. Moreover, other long-term studies have shown an excess mortality (Weeke & Vaeth, 1986) and significantly higher suicide rates among younger bipolar subjects (Tsuang, 1978). The reasons however, for the discrepancy in prevalence between the young and old remain murky and require further investigation.

Mania is not an uncommon condition on psychogeriatric inpatient units (Shulman, Tohen & Satlin, 1992*a*). A review of the treated prevalence of mania in old age reveals an average rate of eight cases per year and a female preponderance of roughly 2:1. Snowdon (1991) found that 0.03% of local area residents over the age of 65 had been admitted at least once to an inpatient unit because of bipolar disorder. Thus the issues of management of mania in late life are clinically important and will be reviewed later in this chapter.

We have virtually no information on the treated prevalence of hypomania and mania in outpatient or community components of comprehensive geriatric psychiatry services. With better information systems, these statistics should be forthcoming and help to shed light on the impact of these conditions on specialized geriatric psychiatry services.

Familial predisposition

A significant genetic predisposition to psychiatric disorder in first degree relatives has been noted in numerous studies of affective disorder (Goodwin & Jamison, 1984). While bipolar disorders appear to have a stronger genetic component (Gershon, Baron & Leckman, 1975), Tsuang et al. (1985) could find no difference in risk for affective disorder between the relatives of young bipolar and unipolar probands. This suggests that both phenotypes (unipolar and bipolar) may share a pool of predisposing factors which include environmental, psychological, biological and genetic components.

The study of familial predisposition to affective disorder in the first-degree relatives of elderly manic probands reveals a range from 24 to 50% (Glasser & Rabins, 1984; Stone, 1989; Broadhead & Jacoby, 1990; Snowdon, 1991; Shulman et al., 1992*b*). The elderly, of course, are well suited to the study of familial predisposition as they allow for much longer periods of exposure in siblings and children as well as grandchildren.

Stone (1989) has demonstrated that a positive family history for affective disorder in elderly manic probands is associated with an earlier age of onset. Conversely, secondary mania associated with coarse neurological disorders carries a significantly lower genetic predisposition than elderly manic patients without a concomitant cerebral-organic disorder (Snowdon, 1991; Shulman et al., 1992*b*). In the study by Shulman et al. (1992*b*) the prevalence of affective illness in first-degree relatives of patients with neurological disorders was still in the order of 30%, comparable to elderly patients with unipolar affective disorders. Even though genetics may play a lesser role in this subgroup, the familial predisposition is still high and helps to explain why these individuals with neurological disorder are different than the vast majority of elderly people who suffer a wide variety of cerebral insults.

Clinical sub-groups

Recent studies of mania in old age consistently show an age of onset of affective illness in middle age ranging from 45 to 55 years depending on whether the age of index is established at 60 or 65 years and over (Shulman & Post, 1980; Broadhead & Jacoby, 1990; Snowdon, 1991). In about half of these cases, the first affective episode is depression with a mean latency of 15 years prior to the manifestation of mania (Broadhead & Jacoby, 1990; Snowdon, 1991). This first manic episode tends to occur very late in life, on average in the late fifties. When associated with a long latency period, mania generally does not occur in the context of coarse cerebral-organic disorders (Shulman et al., 1992*b*). When mania is the first affective episode in late life, however, it is significantly associated with heterogeneous neurological disorders (Shulman et al., 1992*b*; Snowdon, 1991). This is consistent with Krauthammer and Klerman's (1978) concept of secondary mania associated with a lower genetic predisposition, where mania tends to be the first-ever affective episode. Snowdon (1991) showed that 13 out of 75 elderly bipolar patients had experienced a frank neurologic disorder before their first manic episode. This subgroup also had a significantly lower family history of affective illness in first degree relatives. Shulman & Post (1980) using retrospective data have suggested that those with a unipolar manic course may also form a distinct subgroup. In their sample, 8% of elderly bipolar subjects pursued a manic-only clinical course and in all six cases mania first occurred before the age of 40. Moreover, these were the only individuals who experienced a manic episode prior to the age of 40. Similarly, Snowdon (1991) found only 4 of 75 elderly bipolar patients to have experienced mania before the age of 40. Only two of these cases pursued a unipolar mania course. Recent efforts to substantiate the distinctiveness of unipolar mania in younger patients have failed to differentiate this group from the larger sample of bipolar patients (Abrams & Taylor, 1974; Nurnberger, Roose & Dunner, 1970; Pfohl, Vasquez & Nasrallah, 1982). Concerns persist that retrospective recall of past depressive episodes may be unreliable.

Thus, only two distinct subgroups of elderly manics emerge. The first whose affective illness begins with a depressive pattern in middle age and after a very long latency and repeated depressive episodes eventually 'converts' to mania late in life. This could be accounted for by normal ageing of the brain in a genetically or psychologically vulnerable individual. The second subgroup is consistent with the notion of secondary mania. Here, mania is the first affective episode often associated with a coarse neurological disorder and a relatively lower genetic predisposition but with a definite affective vulnerability.

Recently, Charron, Fortin & Paquette (1991) described six cases of 'de novo' mania in old age ranging from age 66 to 77 years. These authors did not find coarse cerebral organic disorders or any prior history of affective illness. 'De novo' mania contrasts with secondary mania where coarse systemic or neurologic disorders are evident. All of the cases that Charron et al. described were treated with psychotropics and apparently resolved without residual cognitive dysfunction. This still does not rule out the possibility however, that subtle cerebral changes resulting in a 'manic delirium' might have been responsible for this subgroup. Advances in neuroimaging technology may help to elucidate the underlying pathophysiology in cases where neurologic disorder is not obvious (Rabins et al. 1991).

The clinical presentation of mania in old age is not fundamentally different than in the young (Glasser & Rabins, 1984). Broadhead & Jacoby (1990) did a direct comparison of old and young manic patients and could not find significant differences other than severity of mania as measured by a standardized rating scale. The symptoms most prominent in old age mania were: decreased sleep, physical hyperactivity, flight of ideas or thought disorder, overspending, grandiose delusions, irritability and hypersexuality (Glasser & Rabins, 1984).

Outcome

Only two studies have examined the longterm outcome of mania in old age (Dhingra & Rabins, 1991; Shulman et al., 1992*b*). Both used a retrospective cohort method for an average follow-up of 6 years. Dhingra & Rabins (1991) tracked 38 of an original cohort of 42 manic subjects who were 60 years and over at index. At follow-up, 13 of 38 (34%) were dead. This compares to a 50% mortality found by Shulman et al. (1992*b*). This difference may be accounted for by two factors. First, if one assumes that the four subjects who were not traced had in fact died, the mortality rate rises to 40% in the Dhingra & Rabins' study. Furthermore, Shulman et al., (1992*b*) had a longer maximum range of follow-up to ten years whereas Dhingra & Rabins had a seven year maximum. The additional three years at risk produced a significant increase in mortality. Interestingly, only one patient in the cohort of 100 subjects followed by Shulman et al. died by suicide.

When compared to an age and sex-matched group of unipolar depressives, the mortality rates are significantly higher for the manic patients. This is consistent with the thesis that mania represents a more severe form of the disorder and in old age translates into a more severe disruption of central nervous system function. Dhingra & Rabins (1991) examined cognitive function at follow-up and found that 32% of manic patients experienced a significant decline as measured by a score of less than 24 on the Mini-Mental State Examination. A frank dementia however, does not appear to be an outcome that occurs with any greater frequency than expected in a general population. Indeed, Dhingra & Rabins (1991) showed that 72% of subjects who were still alive at follow-up were symptom-free and 80% were still living independently in the community. Compared to the earlier report by Roth (1955), it would appear that the prognosis for mania in old age is much improved. This may be due in large measure to developments in psychopharmacological management.

Drug management

Most of what we know about the treatment of mania in old age comes from anecdotal reports or extrapolations from studies in younger manic patients. In a number of retrospective studies, lithium is reported to have had a favorable effect on the course of bipolar disorder in old age (Shulman & Post, 1980; Stone, 1989). Lithium continues to be the mainstay of drug therapy for mania but is associated with a high incidence of neurotoxicity in the elderly (Himmelhoch et al., 1980; Stone, 1989). Differences in volume of distribution and creatinine clearance result in altered pharmacokinetics and a prolonged half-life (Hardy et al. 1987). Shulman, MacKenzie & Hardy (1987) call for dramatically lower dosages as well as blood levels for the elderly. In their sample of geriatric clinic patients, an average dose of 400 mg per day (150–600 mg) achieved a mean 12 hour blood level of 0.5 mmol/l. A single night-time dosage regimen appears to be safe and practical (Hardy et al. 1987). Maximum blood levels at two hours were only in the range of 0.8 mmol/l.

Charron et al. (1991) noted that five of their six cases of 'de novo' mania were successfully managed with lithium although no dosages or blood levels were reported. More systematic naturalistic studies will be extremely valuable in confirming these early clinical impressions.

A recent literature review by Chou (1991) suggests that caution should be exercised in using lithium–neuroleptic combinations. The combination appears to confer little advantage with respect to rapidity of resolution of mania and yet significantly increases the cost in terms of side-effects such as acute extrapyramidal symptoms, tardive dyskinesia and neuroleptic malignant syndrome. In light of the increased incidence of neurotoxicity in old age reported with lithium alone, combination treatment should be used only with great caution and in much lower dosages.

Anticonvulsants (mood stabilisers)

For lithium nonresponders, the mood stabilizing drugs carbamazepine and valproic acid are viable alternative therapies (Chou, 1991). The encouraging results with carbamazepine (Post et al., 1987) and more recently with valproic acid (McElroy et al., 1992) suggest that similar effects in the elderly can be expected with appropriate reductions in dosage. The antimanic armamentarium is now extensive and includes benzodiazepines such as clonazepam (Chouinard, 1988) and lorazepam (Modell, Lenox & Weiner, 1985) as well as calcium channel blockers such as Verapamil (Dubovsky et al., 1986). Little is known about their use in old age. An anecdotal report by McFarland, Miller & Straumfjord (1990) describes the successful use of valproate as an adjunct to lithium. Once again, concerns about increased susceptibility to neurotoxicity call for a very cautious approach.

Finally, one should always consider electroconvulsive therapy (ECT) as a treatment option in those cases of drug refractory mania where significant physical risks to the elderly patient exist from the excessive excitement and overactivity associated with the manic condition (Black, Winokur & Nasrrallah, 1987; Small et al., 1988). Indeed, bilateral ECT may be a safer and faster method for control of the severely agitated and overactive manic patient (Small et al., 1985).

Future research directions

The exciting frontier represented by the study of mania in late life offers unique opportunities to those interested in the elderly. Comparisons between early- and late-onset mania should continue to bear fruit. Prospective comparisons of elderly manic and elderly depressive patients should help to elucidate underlying brain pathophysiology. In this regard, the recent developments in neuroimaging technologies such as MRI and PET scanning and the more practical SPECT scanners offer considerable hope for progress in this important clinical arena.

Some strategies that are likely to yield more information include prospective multicentre studies involving several specialized psychogeriatric services. Increasingly, in North America and for a long time in the United Kingdom, specialized psychiatric services for the elderly have offered a critical mass of subjects for investigation. Furthermore, the prospective follow-up of middle-aged bipolars and unipolar depressed subjects into old age may answer many questions regarding outcome and factors that 'convert' depressives into bipolars late in life.

Naturalistic prospective drug studies are also more likely to be generalizable and yield practical information about the management of affective disorders in old age. While double-blind randomized controlled studies have a role to play, practical and ethical considerations preclude a great deal of progress from this methodology. One particularly important area of psychopharmacological research includes questions about the discontinuation of maintenance medications. Given the recurrent nature of affective disorder as well as the cost–benefit issues of drug treatment, the issue of prophylaxis remains an important and yet unanswered clinical issue.

References

Abrams, R. & Taylor, M. A. (1974). Unipolar mania, a preliminary report. *Archives of General Psychiatry*, **30**, 441–3.

Akiskal, H. (1983). Diagnosis and classification of affective disorders: new insights from clinical and laboratory approaches. *Psychiatric Developments*, **2**, 123–60.

Akiskal, H., Walker, P., Puzantian V. R. et al. (1983). Bipolar outcome in the course of depressive illness. *Journal of Affective Disorders*, **5**, 115–28.

Black, D. W., Winokur, G. & Nasrallah, A. (1987). Treatment of mania: a naturalistic study of electroconvulsive therapy in 438 patients. *Journal of Clinical Psychiatry*, **48**, 132–9.

Broadhead, J. & Jacoby, R. (1990). Mania in old age: a first prospective study. *International Journal of Geriatric Psychiatry*, **5**, 215–22.

Charron, M., Fortin, L. & Paquette, I. (1991). De novo mania among elderly people. *Acta Psychiatrica Scandinavica*, **84**, 503–7.

Chou, J. C. Y. (1991). Recent advances in treatment of acute mania. *Journal of Clinical Psychopharmacology*, **11**, 3–21.

Chouinard, G. (1988). The use of benzodiazepines in the treatment of manic-depressive illness. *Journal of Clinical Psychiatry*, **49** (suppl. Nov), 15–19.

Clothier, J., Swann, A. C. & Freeman, T. (1992). Dysphoric mania. *Journal of Clinical Psychopharmacology*, **12** (suppl.), 13S-16S.

Dhingra, U. & Rabins, P. V. (1991). Mania in the elderly: A 5–7 year follow-up. *Journal of the American Geriatrics Society*, **39**, 591–83.

Dubovsky, S. L., Franks, R. D., Allen, S. et al. (1986). Calcium antagonists in mania: a double-blind study of verapamil. *Psychiatry Research*, **18**, 309–20.

Gershon, E. S., Baron, M. & Leckman, J. F. (1975). Genetic models of the transmission of affective disorders. *Journal of Psychiatric Research*, **12**, 301–17.

Glasser, M. & Rabins, P. (1984). Mania in the elderly. *Age & Ageing*, **13**, 210–13.

Goodwin, F. K. & Jamison, K. R. (1984). The natural course of manic-depressive illness. In *Neurobiology of Mood Disorders*, ed. R. M. Post & J. C. Ballenger. Edinburgh: Williams & Wilkins.

Hardy, B., Shulman, K., MacKenzie, S. et al. (1987). Pharmacokinetics of lithium in the elderly. Journal of *Clinical Psychopharmacology*, **7**, 153–58.

Himmelhoch, J. M., Neil, M. F., May, S. J. et al. (1980). Age, dementia, dyskinesias and lithium response. *American Journal of Psychiatry*, **137**, 941–5.

Kraepelin, E. (1921). *Manic Depressive, Insanity and Paranoia*. Edinburgh: Livingston. Reprinted New York: Ages Company Publishers, 1976.

Krauthammer, C. & Klerman, G. L. (1978). Secondary mania. Manic syndromes associated with antecedent physical illness or drugs. *Archives of General Psychiatry*, **35**, 1333–9.

McElroy, S., Keck, P., Pope, H. et al. (1992). Valproate in the treatment of bipolar disorder: literature review and clinical guidelines. *Journal of Clinical Psychopharmacology*, **12** (suppl. 1), 42S-52S.

McFarland, B. H., Miller, M. R. & Straumfjord, A. A. (1990). Valproate use in the older manic patient. *Journal of Clinical Psychiatry*, **51**(11), 479–81.

Modell, J. G., Lenox, R. H. & Weiner, S. (1985). Inpatient clinical trial of lorazepam for the management of manic agitation. *Journal of Clinical Psychopharmacology*, **71**, 79–82.

Nurnberger, J. Jr., Roose, S. P. & Dunner, D. L. (1970). Unipolar mania: a distinct clinical entity? *American Journal of Psychiatry*, **136**, 1420–3.

Pfohl, B., Vasquez, N. & Nasrallah, H. (1982). Unipolar vs. bipolar mania: a review of 247 patients. *British Journal of Psychiatry*, **141**, 453–8.

Post, R. M., Uhde, T. W., Roy-Byrne, P. O. et al. (1987). Correlates of antimanic response to carbamazepine. *Psychiatry Research*, **21**, 71–83.

Rabins, P. V. & Pearlson, G. D., Aylward, E. et al. (1991). Cortical magnetic resonance imaging changes in elderly inpatients with major depression. *American Journal of Psychiatry*, **148**, 617–20.

Roth, M. (1955). The natural history of mental disorder in old age. *Journal of Mental Science*, **101**, 281–301.

Shulman, K. & Post, F. (1980). Bipolar affective disorder in old age. *British Journal of Psychiatry*, **136**, 26–32.

Shulman, K., MacKenzie, S. & Hardy, B. (1987). The clinical use of lithium carbonate in old age: a review. *Progress in Neuro-Psychopharmacology*, **11**, 159–64.

Shulman, I. I. (1989). Conceptual problems in the assessment of depression in old age. *The Psychiatric Journal of the University of Ottawa*, **14**, 364–366.

Shulman, K. I., Tohen, M. & Satlin, A. (1992*a*). Mania revisited. In *Recent Advances in Psychogeriatrics (II)*, ed. T. Arie, pp. 71–79. London: Churchill-Livingstone.

Shulman, K. I., Tohen, M., Satlin, A. et al. (1992*b*). Mania compared with unipolar depression in old age. *American Journal of Psychiatry*, **149**(3), 341–5.

Small, J. G., Small, I. F. Milstein, V. et al. (1985). Manic symptoms: an indication for bilateral ECT. *Biological Psychiatry*, **20**, 125–34.

Small, J. G., Klapper, M. H., Kellams, J. J. et al. (1988). Electroconvulsive treatment compared with lithium in the management of manic states. *Archives of General Psychiatry*, **45**, 727–32.

Snowdon, J. (1991). A retrospective case-note study of bipolar disorder in old age. *British Journal of Psychiatry*, **158**, 485–90.

Stone, K. (1989). Mania in the elderly. *British Journal of Psychiatry*, **155**, 220–4.

Tsuang, M. T. (1978). Suicide in schizophrenics, manics, depressives and surgical controls. *Archives of General Psychiatry*, **35**, 153–5.

Tsuang, M. T., Faraone, S. V. & Fleming, J. A. (1985). Familial transmission of major affective disorders: is there evidence supporting the distinction between unipolar and bipolar disorders? *British Journal of Psychiatry*, **146**, 268–71.

Weeke, A. & Vaeth, M. (1986). Excess mortality of bipolar and unipolar manic-depressive patients. *Journal of Affective Disorders*, **11**, 227–34.

Weissman, M. M., Leaf, P. J., Tichler, G. L. et al. (1988). Affective disorders in five United States communities. *Psychological Medicine*, **18**, 141–53.

14

Suicide in the elderly

AJIT SHAH THIRUNAVUKARASU GANESVARAN

Introduction

Suicides are of considerable social and medical significance. The identification of patients who are likely to commit suicide is an important component of psychiatric practice, yet psychiatrists are poor at predicting suicides (Pokorny, 1983). Suicide rates among the elderly continue to be higher than in any other age group in most countries (McClure, 1987; World Health Organization (WHO), 1992). Suicide has powerful emotive qualities and causes considerable distress to relatives and professional carers (Shah, 1992*a*). However, suicides in older age groups have been sparsely studied (Hendon, 1982; Cattell, 1988). Furthermore, Lindesay (1991) suggests that there have been no major advances in the understanding of suicides in the elderly in recent years.

Theories of suicide are based on sociological and psychological models. Durkheim (1951) argued that suicide was an individual's response to certain social circumstances and divided suicides into three categories: egoistic, anomic and altruistic. Freud (1949) postulated a psychoanalytic formulation of suicide where a love–hate relationship with the lost love object incorporated into the ego leads to attack on the self. Stengel (1977) was among the first to collect systematic data to develop clinical concepts of suicide and attempted suicide. A variety of psychological factors, including presence of mental illness, have been suggested to be important in suicides. These and other related factors in the elderly may have a special and peculiar interaction with suicides.

In this chapter the literature on suicide in the elderly is reviewed with particular emphasis on methodology, cross-national rates and trends, correlates, means of suicide, overlap with attempted suicide and prevention.

Research methodology

Definition

Suicide can be defined as an individual taking his or her own life. Yet, there is no generally accepted definition of suicide. Most studies and statistics are based on the legal definition of suicide (Sainsbury, 1955; Barraclough, 1971; Cattell, 1988; Modestin, 1989; Conwell et al., 1991). In England and Wales and Australia, this is based upon verdicts reached in the coroner's court. Comparable legal institutions provide similar data in other countries. These 'verdicts' however, depend upon the stringency of the legal criteria in different countries. In England and Wales, suicides must be proved beyond reasonable doubt; if there is doubt then an open or an accidental verdict must be returned. The legal definition rests on evidence of intention to kill oneself. Intention is a difficult concept in suicide. Stengel (1977) points out that victims neither want to live or die, but to do both at the same time, usually one more than the other. Moreover, intention is not a static phenomenon as it can rapidly change (Ganesvaran & Rajarajeswaran, 1988). Thus, it is likely that the official statistics are underestimates of the true rate of elderly suicides (Adelstein & Marden, 1975). It has been suggested that underreporting of suicides is highest in old age because suicidal behavior such as refusal to eat, medication non-compliance and overdose go unrecognized (Shulman, 1978; Zarit, 1980). These have been variously described as 'subintentional death', 'hidden suicide' and 'indirect self-destructive behavior' (Nelson & Farberow, 1980). Therefore, it has been suggested that studies of suicide should include deaths due to accidental poisoning and undetermined causes in addition to those due to official suicides. This strategy, however, has not yet been employed in studies of elderly suicides.

Design

A number of different study designs have been adopted. By their very nature studies of suicide must be retrospective and the most important witness is not available for direct examination. Studies among the elderly have been descriptive (Barraclough, 1971; Alexopoulos, 1991; Conwell et al., 1991) or analytic (Cattell, 1988; Modestin, 1989).

Descriptive studies have either been an in-depth case analysis (Alexopoulos, 1991) or a relatively small series of up to 30 suicides (Barraclough, 1971; Conwell et al., 1991). Analytic studies have used a comparison group of younger suicides (Gardiner, Bahn & Mack, 1964; Modestin, 1989), comparison with the general population (Barraclough, 1971; Cattell, 1988), a control group of accidental deaths (Cattell, 1988), and, for inpatient suicides, a control group of alive inpatients (Modestin, 1989). Comparison with younger suicides is fraught with difficulties as it makes no allowance for the interaction between age, cohort and period effects on suicide (Murphy, Lindesay & Grundy, 1986; Surtees & Duffy, 1989). Comparison with national figures for the general population (Cattell, 1988) is not sufficiently exact to permit statistical evaluation (Shah, Fineberg & James, 1991; Shah, 1992*b*). It would be more appropriate to use the general population from the same geographical area as the suicides for comparison rather than the national population. The use of accidental deaths as a control group is problematic (Cattell, 1988) because verdicts of accidental deaths contain a number of concealed suicides (Holding & Barraclough, 1975). If data are collected from the coroner's inquest, however, the use of accidental deaths as a control group would have the advantage of the same retrospective data collecting procedure, thus reducing any bias due to data collection (Cattell, 1988). The main drawback of using 'alive' inpatients as a control group is that this group may be a self-selected group of severely ill patients (Harkey & Hyer, 1986).

Methods of data collection include psychological autopsies (Alexopoulos, 1991; Barraclough, 1971; Conwell et al., 1991), coroner's inquests (Cattell, 1988), case-notes (Modestin, 1989) and case-registers (Gardiner et al., 1964). The technique of psychological autopsy involves collection of standardized data on completed suicides by interviewing informants familiar with the individuals' psychological, social and medical characteristics prior to death (Ebert, 1987).

This method has been widely used to study suicides among younger adults (Dorpat & Ripley, 1960; Barraclough et al., 1974; Robins et al., 1959; Chynoweth, Tonge & Armstrong, 1980; Rich, Young & Fowler, 1986), adolescents (Brent et al., 1988; Shafii et al., 1985) and to a lesser extent the elderly (Barraclough, 1971; Conwell et al., 1991). Shortcomings of this technique include absence of control or comparison groups (Conwell et al., 1991) and the lack of reliability and validity data on this method of data collection (Conwell et al., 1991). The latter is particularly important in the elderly as more remote lifetime histories make the data subject to variations in recall, particularly during the emotive period after death (Cattell, 1988). Despite these shortcomings, this technique can be used to collect qualitative and quantitative data on psychological and psychopathological precursors of suicide (Conwell et al., 1991). Data from the coroner's inquest have been widely used in studies of younger suicides (Sainsbury, 1955; Capstick, 1960; Seagar & Flood, 1965; Overstone & Kreitman, 1974) and to a lesser extent the elderly (Cattell, 1988). This method has obvious limitations (Barraclough, 1971) as the purpose of the inquest is legal rather than medical or research oriented. It allows study, however, of a large and specific population with the use of accidental death as a control group (Cattell, 1988). Data collected from case-notes are difficult to interpret unless there is evidence of good reliability and validity with regard to information recorded therein (Modestin, 1989). Case-register data only identify suicides previously known to the register.

Several studies (Pierce, 1987; Hawton & Fagg, 1990) have reported on attempted suicides in the elderly. It has been suggested that, among the aged, this group of patients is very similar to those who commit suicide (Lindesay & Murphy, 1987) and that survival was fortuitous. Thus, information gathered by direct interview with those who have attempted suicide is thought to provide insight into those who succeed in killing themselves.

Suicide trends over time have been studied in the elderly (McIntosh, 1984; Murphy et al., 1986; Surtees & Duffy, 1989; Diekstra, 1989). Difficulties with this approach arises where the legal criteria for the verdict of suicide have been altered during the study period and where age, cohort and period effects on suicide have not been addressed. More sophisticated studies have addressed the latter variables (Murphy et al., 1986; Surtees & Duffy, 1989). One study reported cross-national comparison in suicide rates for the elderly using the national figures produced in the WHO Statistics Annual (WHO, 1992) and the WHO data bank as part of a larger cross-national comparison of all suicides (Diekstra, 1989). Such cross-national comparisons, however, need to be viewed with caution as data are not available from all countries and the validity of this data is unclear (Diekstra, 1989). Legal criteria for proof of suicide vary across countries. This is particularly important when there are difficulties in differentiating between suicides, homicides and accidental deaths. There may be underreporting of suicides in some countries due to religious stigma attached to suicide. Some countries have poorly developed registration procedures.

Suicide rates and recent trends

As discussed in the previous section all the cross-national comparisons in this section should be viewed with considerable caution.

International variation in suicide rates in the elderly

There are large variations in suicide rates for the elderly (Table 14.1) when cross-national comparisons are made using the most recent WHO data (WHO, 1992). Elderly suicide rates range from zero in Malta to very high levels in Hungary, Singapore and Sri Lanka. Southern European countries such as Greece and Malta have low elderly suicide rates. Other European countries tend to have higher rates. Data for only a few Asian countries are available and here elderly suicide rates are high. Latin American countries have variable rates (WHO, 1992).

International variation in elderly suicide rates versus younger suicide rates

As shown in Table 14.1, with a few exceptions, suicide rates in the elderly tend to be higher than the average suicide rate for both sexes (WHO, 1992). It therefore

Table 14.1. *Cross-national comparison of suicide rates: overall and the elderly*

Country	Overall rate per 100 000 population			*Elderly rate per 100 000 population		
	Males	Females	Total	Males	Females	Total
Argentina	10.0	4.4	7.4	40.0	11.3	23.7
Austria	34.8	13.4	23.6	84.2	28.6	48.0
Bulgaria	20.7	8.8	14.7	62.4	29.2	43.7
Canada	20.9	6.0	13.3	26.8	6.0	14.8
Cz'slovakia	27.3	8.9	17.9	70.5	20.0	36.4
Denmark	32.2	16.3	24.1	58.9	31.0	42.5
Finland	46.4	11.5	28.5	66.7	14.1	32.6
France	30.5	11.7	20.9	76.4	23.2	44.1
Greece	5.6	2.1	3.8	3.9	12.1	7.5
Hong Kong	11.8	9.1	10.5	46.4	31.5	38.0
Hungary	59.9	21.4	31.1	134.2	54.0	84.6
Iceland	27.4	3.9	15.7	33.3	0	14.8
Ireland	27.4	3.7	7.9	19.2	7.5	12.6
Israel	9.7	4.0	6.8	26.3	12.6	18.9
Japan	20.4	12.4	16.4	46.4	35.1	42.4
Malta	4.6	0	1.3	0	0	0
Netherlands	13.0	7.5	10.2	24.0	12.2	18.0
Norway	23.0	8.4	15.6	31.7	10.7	19.2
Poland	22.0	4.5	13.0	27.7	7.3	14.9
Portugal	13.5	4.5	8.8	40.3	11.6	23.3
Puerto Rico	16.4	1.9	8.9	4.0	2.5	3.0
Singapore	15.4	13.2	14.3	47.0	63.2	54.3
Spain	10.6	4.0	7.2	33.0	9.9	19.4
Sri Lanka	46.9	18.9	33.2	93.7	15.4	56.8
Sweden	26.4	11.5	18.9	40.6	14.6	25.7
Switzerland	31.5	17.7	21.8	65.9	23.3	40.3
Trinidad	19.0	7.4	13.3	51.7	5.5	26.2
Uruguay	18.1	4.4	11.1	55.6	9.9	29.3
USSR	34.4	9.1	21.1	62.9	23.3	34.6
UK	12.6	3.8	8.1	16.1	6.1	10.1
Yugoslavia	23.2	9.9	16.5	74.3	29.7	47.5

Derived from the *WHO Statistics Annual 1992*. Most figures are for 1989 or 1990 and these are the latest available at the time of writing.
*Elderly = > 65 years.

follows that rates are higher in the elderly than the younger generations. The exceptions are countries like Jordan (Daradkeh, 1989) and India (Adiyanjee, 1986; Bhatia, Khan & Mediratta, 1987) and Indian immigrants in the United Kingdom (Raleigh, Busulu & Balarajan, 1990) for both sexes, Greece, Malta and

Puerto Rico for males and Iceland, Trinidad and Sri Lanka for females. In the United States the suicide rate increases with age in white males but decreases in nonwhite males with age (Seiden, 1981). Among American women, the suicide rate increases with age, peaking at menopause and declining thereafter (Woodbury, Manton & Blazer, 1988).

International variation in recent trends in elderly suicides

Rates of suicide in the elderly for both sexes have declined over recent years in most countries (Diekstra, 1989; WHO, 1992). The exceptions are Ireland, where the suicide rate for both sexes has increased, and Denmark, where the rate for women has increased.

Age, period and cohort effects

A major advance in recent years has been the development of techniques to study age, period and cohort effects on suicide rates (Murphy et al., 1986; Surtees & Duffy, 1989). This concept is based on the assumption that the suicide rate for any given age at a given time is a result of risk factors attributable to age, period and cohort membership. Thus, individuals born in a particular cohort will have suicide rates peculiar to that cohort, i.e. cohort effect. Moreover, the individual's age at any given time within the cohort will further influence the suicide rate, i.e. age effect. Furthermore, environmental effects related to the period of study will further influence the suicide rate, i.e. period effect. As each of these variables is a function of the other two, independent effects of each of these three variables are difficult to separate and each is examined in turn.

Cohort effect

Several studies have demonstrated a cohort effect on suicide rates (Soloman & Hellon, 1977; Murphy & Wetzel, 1980; Blazer, Bachar & Manton, 1986; Manton, Blazer & Woodbury, 1987; Surtees & Duffy, 1989). Surprisingly, only a few studies have addressed cohort effects in groups older than 50 years. Murphy et al. (1986) studied suicides in successive cohorts between 1921 and 1980 in England and Wales. They found a fall in suicide rates in successive older cohorts. Moreover, they were able to demonstrate a more prolonged cohort effect on suicide rates of the middle-aged and the elderly associated with the period effects of World War II and the detoxification of domestic gas. Surtees and Duffy (1989), essentially studying the same cohorts, using a more sophisticated statistical technique to partial out the independent effects of age, period and cohort showed a decline in male rates for ten cohorts born from 1871 to 1916. Suicide rates in subsequent male cohorts increased and decreased in female cohorts.

How do cohort effects work? The suggestion that early experiences of a cohort sustain an enduring effect on suicide rates (Murphy & Wetzel, 1980; Hellon & Solomon, 1980) lacks evidence (Murphy et al., 1986; Wetzel et al., 1987). It has been suggested that the overall cohort size may influence the suicide rates (Lindesay, 1991). This hypothesis is based on Durkheim's (1951) sociological model of suicide. Traditionally, suicide rates tend to be higher in those age groups that constitute the larger proportion of the population. Moreover, this may be a result of competition for scarce resources (Lindesay, 1991). Using this model, Lindesay (1991) predicts that suicide rates will increase in the 'baby boom generation' (as they age and as the numbers of the very elderly will increase) unless health, social service and welfare resources are also increased appropriately.

Age effects

Surtees and Duffy (1989) showed that in England and Wales suicide rates are independently affected by age. They showed that rates increase with age and peak at age 65–79 years for both sexes. This pattern was consistent throughout each of the 8 five year periods (1946–1985) studied. For males aged 65–79, there had been a decline in rates over the first five periods and an increase for the last three periods. In females, the decline in rates over the first five periods was matched and continued for the last three periods. Other studies have shown that suicide rates increase with age in males, but in females rates first increase with age, peaking at menopause and then decline thereafter (Woodbury et al., 1988).

Inpatient studies do not show any increase in suicide rates with age (Modestin, 1989; Copas & Robin, 1982). Several reasons have been advanced to explain this (Copas & Robin, 1982; Modestin, 1989). Inpatient psychogeriatric populations have significant numbers of demented patients who are unlikely to commit suicide. Due to poor identification of depression among the old in the community relatively few elderly with suicide risk find their way into hospital. Protective measures in psychiatric hospitals may have good efficacy.

How do age effects work? Lindesay (1991) divided age effects into two categories: those related to the experience of ageing at any given time and those inherent to the ageing process. Lindesay (1991) has suggested a vulnerability hypothesis to explain the relationship between suicide and age. Physical illness, bereavement, loss of income and loss of status are associated with suicide in the elderly. These factors are particularly prevalent in late life. As only a small number of individuals with these factors commit suicide it was suggested that other vulnerability factors may operate (Lindesay, 1991). Personality traits including incapacity for close relationships (Murphy, 1982), a tendency to be helpless and hopeless (Sendbuehler, 1977) and an inability to tolerate change and loss of control (Wolff, 1969) are thought to be vulnerabilty factors predisposing to elderly suicides (Lindesay,

1991). As this evidence is drawn from studies of depression and attempted suicides its applicabilty to suicides is unclear. Retirement is considered as a further vulnerabilty factor as it contributes to socioeconomic decline. Social decline has been shown to be associated with increased elderly suicide rates in the United States (Marshall, 1978). In the same society, however, elderly blacks and native Americans, who are socioeconomically less prosperous, have lower suicide rates (McIntosh, 1984). In order to explain this paradoxical finding, a model of lifelong adversity has been argued (Lindesay, 1991). Individuals with life long adversity are better able to tolerate hardships (Seiden, 1981). Moreover, those with little previous experience of adversity will tolerate it less well. Shimizu (1990) has suggested a similar model for Japanese elderly suicides.

Cultural factors need to be considered in the vulnerability hypothesis. Among Arabs (Daradekh, 1989), Indians (Bhatia et al., 1987), Indian immigrants in Britain (Raleigh et al., 1990) and non-white Americans (Seiden, 1981) suicide rates decline with age. Traditionally, the elderly in these societies are respected, held in high esteem and live in a closely knit extended family. This persists in India (Bhatia et al., 1987; Raleigh et al., 1990), the middle east and among non-white Americans, offering protection towards suicide. Similar hypotheses have been suggested to explain the increasing suicide rates in elderly Japanese and Hong Kong women who have lost their traditional role in the family (Shimizu, 1990) and Singapore's three ethnic groups (Kua & Ko, 1992). Physical proximity (living under the same roof) of the extended family is not important. Emotional proximity (respect and high esteem) is the main factor.

There is no clear evidence to link increasing suicide rates with age and factors related to the ageing process.

Period effects

Murphy et al. (1986) demonstrated a period effect of World War II and detoxification of domestic gas on suicide rates in their cohorts. Before the 1960s, in the UK, domestic gas contained carbon monoxide and was a popular method of commiting suicide for the elderly. Elderly suicide rates declined after the detoxification of gas. Moreover, this decline was sustained and not replaced by other methods of suicide. In addition, there was a more prolonged effect on suicide within these period events (Murphy et al., 1986). Surtees and Duffy (1989), using statistical techniques to partial out independent effect, confirmed this, particularly for men.

Other correlates of elderly suicides

Sex

In general, suicide rates are greater among elderly males than females (Gardiner et al., 1964; Diekstra, 1989; Lindesay, 1991; WHO, 1992). As discussed earlier, suicide rates continue to increase with age among white American men, whereas in women they increase with age until menopause and decline thereafter (Gardiner et al., 1964; Woodbury et al., 1989). This has not been shown in other countries. In studies of suicides with comparison or control groups, however, no sex difference has been identified (Cattell, 1988; Modestin, 1989).

Social factors

Social factors are important in the genesis of elderly suicides. Elderly people who kill themselves often live alone (Barraclough, 1971; Cattell, 1988; Conwell et al., 1991), and this holds even when comparisons are made with population norms (Cattell, 1988; Barraclough, 1971). Cattell (1988) reported that 18% of his suicides had no contact with family or friends. About a quarter live alone for a prolonged period through choice (Barraclough, 1971). Widowed, single or divorced individuals are over-represented among elderly suicides (Sainsbury, 1955; Gardiner et al., 1964; Cattell, 1988; Modestin, 1991; Conwell et al., 1991). Thus, it may be that many of these elderly suicides were isolated through circumstances rather than choice. Those isolated through choice may have adverse physical factors and depressive illness (Cattell, 1988). In either scenario, social isolation by depriving individuals of emotional support and reducing the opportunity for therapeutic intervention may aggravate suicidal intent (Barraclough, 1971).

Psychological factors

The majority of elderly suicides have suffered from depressive illness at the time of death with prevalences ranging from 55% to 87% (Sainsbury, 1955; Gardiner et al., 1964; Barraclough, 1971; Cattell, 1988; Modestin, 1989; Conwell et al., 1991). Other than Cattell's (1988) study, sample sizes were small (30 or less), indicating possible sources of error. Cattell's sample size was 104, but information on depressive symptoms from coroner's inquest data was limited. Nevertheless, 79% were judged to have significant depressive symptoms and 32% to be true cases of depressive illness (Cattell, 1988). These prevalences are significantly higher than prevalences of 11.3% to 15.9% observed in the general population (Lindesay, Briggs & Murphy, 1989; Copeland et al., 1987; Livingston et al., 1990). There was, however, no difference in the prevalence of depression between suicides and a control/comparison group in the inpatient study (Modestin, 1989).

Symptoms of agitation, anergia, anhedonia, dysphoria, guilt, somatic preoccupations and insomnia are commonly associated with suicides in the depressed elderly (Barraclough, 1971; Conwell et al., 1991). The severity of depression ranges from mild to severe (Barraclough, 1971; Cattell, 1988; Conwell et al., 1991). The duration of depressive illness prior to suicide is usually prolonged. Over 60% of Cattell's series had depression for more than six months and the mean duration of depressive episode in the study by Conwell et al. (1991) was 11.4 months. In Barraclough's (1971) series, however, almost 50% had depression for less than six months, although 23% had depression for over a year. First episode of depression is a particularly vulnerable time for committing suicide. Of suicides, 25–35% occur during a first episode of depression (Cattell, 1988; Conwell et al., 1991). Of suicides 43% have been reported to have had a previous depressive episode (Cattell, 1988).

Of elderly suicides, 10–44% have alcohol or substance abuse or dependence (Cattell, 1988; Conwell et al., 1991). These figures are considerably higher than the single figure prevalences reported in community surveys (Carraci & Miller, 1991). There were no differences, however, in the prevalence of alcoholism between suicides and a comparison group of accidental deaths (Cattell, 1988). Nearly 30% of Cattell's (1988) series had alcohol in their blood. Alcohol may be the predominant intoxicating agent (Cattell, 1988), may potentiate other poisonous agents like barbiturates (Cattell, 1988) or may be taken for 'dutch courage', leading to disinhibition.

A smaller, but, a significant proportion of elderly suicides have suffered from schizophrenia or paraphrenia with prevalences of 6–14% (Cattell, 1988; Modestin, 1989). These prevalences are significantly higher than 0.1% reported in the general population (Copeland et al., 1987). There was no difference, however, in the prevalence of schizophrenia between the suicide group and the control group in the inpatient study (Modestin, 1989).

Dementia hardly features on the diagnostic list of suicides. Sainsbury (1955) reported that suicide rates among the mildly demented were higher than the general population but were lower in the severely demented. Sendbuehler and Goldstein (1977) speculate that the presence of confusion may explain some elderly suicide attempts. The relationship with neurotic disorders and personality disorders is unclear. More significantly, up to 13% of elderly suicides have been judged to have no mental illness (Barraclough, 1971; Cattell, 1988; Conwell et al., 1991). Cattell (1988) suggest that a number of these were 'rational suicides'. It is possible that retrospective study designs are not sufficiently sensitive to identify mental illness in such suicides. The implications of these findings are unclear and merit further investigation.

Physical factors

The relationship between elderly suicides and serious physical illness is well established (Sainsbury, 1955; Gardiner et al., 1964; Barraclough, 1971; Barraclough et al., 1974; Stewart, 1960; Cattell, 1988; Conwell, Rotenberg & Caine, 1990; Conwell et al., 1991). Moreover, the prevalence of physical illness in elderly suicides is higher than in younger suicides (Sainsbury, 1955). In Cattell's (1988) study, general practitioners assessed 53% of suicides to have had physical illness sufficiently severe to cause discomfort or interfere with daily living.

How does physical illness influence suicide? The relationship between physical factors and suicide is complex. Cattell (1988) has developed a model to explain this. Two important factors in the equation are the meaning of the physical disability to the individual and the actual objective disability. Using this approach, Cattell (1988) identified four overlapping scenarios. Firstly, suicide may be adopted, in the absence of any other factors, to relieve continued physical problems, the undoubted poor prognosis of which is known to the individual. Affective illness secondary to physical illness may be present. This scenario appears to be uncommon (O'Neal, Robins & Schmidt, 1956; Cattell, 1988). Secondly, physical illness may interact with other psychological and social variables to promote suicide. Thus a mild to moderate physical illness of a recurrent chronic nature, may interact with depression to encourage suicide. Thirdly, it is well recognized that physical illness in the elderly is important in the development of depression and its prognosis (Murphy, 1983; Baldwin & Jolley, 1986; Murphy et al., 1988). Relapses may lead to despair and hopelessness which may precipitate suicide. Finally, physical symptoms may be hypochondriacal symptoms of depression, which in turn may lead to suicide.

Pain is not an uncommon accompaniment of suicide in the elderly. Cattell (1988) reported the presence of significant pain in 21% of his series. Pain associated with suicides can be divided into three groups: severe pain associated with definite organic pathology such as ischemic cardiac disease, less severe but chronic pain associated with the musculoskeletal system, and pain as a hypochondriacal symptom. Postherpetic neuralgia has been shown to precede suicide (Cattell, 1988). Pain may act as a precipitant for suicides by altering self perceptions, impairing capacity for enjoyment and fostering dependence (Cattell, 1988).

Postmortem data provide further evidence of a link between physical illness and elderly suicides. An association between carcinoma and elderly suicides has been speculated (Barraclough, 1971; Cattell, 1988). A significant number of elderly suicides have an occult carcinoma (Cattell, 1988). All these patients also had depression and this concurs with the traditional observation that neoplasms may be heralded by depression prior to their clinical appearance.

Barraclough (1971) suggests that both metastatic and nonmetastatic effects of carcinoma (Brain, 1963) can precipitate mental illness, which in turn leads to suicide.

Cattell (1988) reported abnormal cerebral pathology in 22% of his sample. This included postmortem evidence of strokes, cerebral ventricular dilatation and cortical atrophy. The latter two variables however, were not different from the comparison group of accidental deaths. Benign cerebral tumors including meningiomas and pituitary adenomas are over represented in elderly suicides (Whitlock, 1978). The significance of cerebral pathology in elderly suicides has been poorly studied and is, therefore, unclear.

Precipitating factors

Complex interactions between a variety of factors may result in suicides. Some factors may create situations conducive to suicides and others may precipitate suicides. Some of these factors have been discussed above. Bereavement is another important precipitant of suicide (MacMohan & Pugh, 1965; Cattell, 1988). Suicide rates are higher in the first few years after loss of spouse and the rates are higher in men then women (MacMohan & Pugh, 1965). As the majority of bereaved spouses do not commit suicide, the quality and nature of the marital relationship is considered an important factor. Depressive illness associated with the bereavement process may be important. Data on this are, however, limited. Cattell (1988), reviewing suicide notes, concluded that the relationship was likely to be of a dependent nature. Marital and family discord has been suggested as another precipitant (Conwell et al., 1991).

Recent hospital discharge and paradoxically the suggestion of hospitalization have been shown to be important suicide precipitants (Cattell, 1988). Discharge may be associated with hopelessness in patients who perceive persistent physical or psychological illness despite inpatient care. They may feel angry with discharge and may return to social isolation – both promoting suicides (Cattell, 1988). It is unclear why the thought of hospitalization could precipitate suicide. It may act by increasing any existing feelings of hopelessness and helplessness. Anticipation of placement in a nursing home has been shown to be associated with elderly suicides, particularly in married couples (Loebel et al., 1991). For married couples, this may represent a life event in the form of seperation and severance of mutual support (Loebel et al., 1991).

It is of note that up to a third of cases have no recognisable precipitants (Cattell, 1988). There are no studies of independent life events in elderly suicides.

Medical contact

Elderly suicides often make contact with their doctors prior to death (Barraclough, 1971; Cattell, 1988; Conwell et al., 1991). Up to 90% are reported to have seen their general practitioner in the preceding three months and up to 50% in the preceding week (Barraclough, 1971; Cattell, 1988; Conwell et al., 1991). In Barraclough's series very few had seen a psychiatrist. This contrasts with Cattell's (1988) series where 20% had seen a psychiatrist in the preceding month. This may simply reflect changes in psychiatric service delivery between 1971 and 1988. Data on the nature of doctor/patient contact are not available. Only a small number of suicides were on antidepressants (12%–39%) (Barraclough, 1971; Cattell, 1988; Conwell et al., 1991), usually on inadequate doses (Barraclough, 1971), despite depression being the most prevalent diagnosis. A significant number of suicides, however, were on sedatives or hypnotics (Conwell et al., 1991).

Methods and location

With increasing age violent methods are more frequently used (McIntosh & Santos, 1985–1986; Conwell et al., 1990). Elderly men use violent methods more often then women (Cattell, 1988; Crombie, 1990). Hanging, jumping from a height, drowning and suffocation are not uncommon means of suicide among the old in the United Kingdom (Lindesay, 1991), Japan (Shimuzu, 1990) and Singapore (Kua & Ko, 1992). In contrast to the United States, however, (McIntosh & Santos, 1985–1986; Conwell et al., 1991), presumably due to tighter firearm regulations, in these three countries shooting is uncommon (Shimuzu, 1990; Kua & Ko, 1992). In Sri Lanka, self-poisoning with agricultural organophosphates is a common method among the elderly (Ganesvaran, Subramaniam & Mahadevan, 1984). In the United Kingdom, there has been a reduction in elderly suicides by self-poisoning, largely due to reduction in barbiturate poisoning (Lindesay, 1991). Elderly suicides due to benzodiazepines and analgesics, however, have increased in recent years (Nowers & Irish, 1988). Moreover, analgesics are the commonest drugs taken in overdoses. Over 90% of such deaths are due to asprin, paracetamol or dextropropoxiphene (Lindesay, 1991). Tricyclic antidepressants are rarely used (Cattell, 1988; Lindesay, 1991; Conwell et al., 1991). Suicide by the inhalation of car exhaust fumes is on the increase (Lindesay, 1991).

Suicide notes are usually a marker of severity of the attempt and provide valuable insight into the victim's thinking. Fewer elderly suicides however, leave notes then their younger counterparts (Shimuzu, 1990) and thus absence of suicide note must not be considered as an indicator of less serious suicide attempt. When notes are left, they are brief (Shimuzu, 1990). The content is usually self reproachful, suggestive of their depressive thought content (Shimuzu, 1990). Shimuzu (1990) suggests that fewer old people leave notes because many are isolated and have no one to write to, while others have lost the ability to express themselves.

The majority of suicides occur at the individual's home, usually when alone (Cattell, 1988). Up to a fifth of suicides occur when the individual is away from home. A smaller number occur in hospitals – both psychiatric and others. Individual locations include rivers, large open spaces and anonymous hotel rooms (Cattell, 1988).

Overlap with attempted suicide

A significant overlap between elderly populations of attempted suicides and completed suicides has been suggested (Shulman, 1978; Lindesay & Murphy, 1987). The pattern of behavior variously described as nonfatal deliberate self-harm, parasuicide or attempted suicide is relatively less common in the elderly. For example, the elderly account for up to 11% of all attempted suicides (Kreitman, 1976; Morgan et al., 1975; Pierce, 1987; Sendbuehler & Goldstein, 1977; Hawton & Fagg, 1990). Conversly, as discussed above, the elderly are over-represented in most populations of completed suicides. This has led to the suggestion that attempted suicides in the elderly are unsuccessful suicides where the individual survives fortuitously.

Evidence for the seriousness of these attempted suicides in the elderly comes from several sources. Social isolation is thought to be important with an association with not being married (Pierce, 1987; Hawton & Fagg, 1990) and living alone (Pierce, 1987). Prevalence of depression is very high (> 90%) (Pierce, 1987). Many of the earlier studies showed a significant prevalence of dementia (Batchelor & Napier, 1953; O'Neal et al., 1965; Sendbuehler & Goldstein, 1977). A more recent study, however, using a standardized interview technique, reported a very low prevalence for dementia (Pierce, 1987). Pierce (1987) explained this discrepancy by suggesting that his sample was different from that of Sendbuehler and Goldstein (1977) due to selection bias. Alcoholism and alcohol consumption before attempted suicide are common (Kreitman, 1976; Hawton & Fagg, 1990), particularly in men. Serious physical illness and pain leading to demoralization and attempted suicides are not uncommon (Pierce, 1987). Sendbeuhler and Goldstein (1977) suggested that many attempted suicides in late life are serious bids which have failed due to confusion from physical illness, overmedication and alcohol misuse. However, in contrast, Pierce (1987) reported that individuals with organic brain disease tended to make impulsive and hazardous attempts, often with more than one means, in the context of confusion, depression and cerebral disinhibition.

Violent attempts were more prevalent in the earlier studies (Batchelor & Napier, 1953; O'Neal et al., 1965). More recent studies however, suggest drug overdose as the most common method (> 90%) (Pierce, 1987; Hawton & Fagg, 1990). Drugs employed include minor tranquillizers, hypnotics, antidepressants and analgesics (Pierce, 1987; Hawton & Fagg, 1990). Barbiturate self-poisoning has declined with a concomitant increase in nonopiate analgesic poisoning, particularly paracetamol and paracetamol containing analgesics (Hawton & Fagg, 1990). Attempts tend to be less impulsive than in younger people (Burston, 1969; Benson & Brody, 1975) and the elderly rarely tell others of their intention (O'Neal et al., 1965).

Gardiner et al. (1964) reported that suicide rates were 18 times greater than general population among those over the age of 55 years, who had attempted suicide previously. Kreitman (1976) reported that 8% of his attempters completed suicide within three years. Pierce (1987), however, reported only 2.8% of his sample completed suicide over a variable follow-up period.

The evidence presented suggests that, in the elderly, there is a considerable overlap between attempted suicides and suicides. The two are not, however, synonymous. Pierce (1987) using validated scales showed high intention scores among his attempters, but with a wide scatter. Lindesay (1991) argued that this wide scatter suggests motives other than death may exist. Clearly, further research is needed to explore the various hypotheses discussed in this section.

Pathways to suicide

In this section, based on the above review of the literature, a broad pathway to suicide is hypothesized, which requires rigorous scientific testing. Shimizu (1990) suggested the concept of preparatory and trigger factors in the genesis of suicide. Preparatory state was defined as the state of preparedness for suicidal intent (Shimizu, 1990), and this usually develops insidiously. We would like to argue that age, cohort and period effects contribute to this preparatory state. Personality and other constitutional factors may also be important here. Depending upon the intensity and frequency of these factors the suicidal intent in this state will be high or low. As not everyone in the preparatory state proceeds to suicide, however, additional factors must be present. These additional factors are the trigger factors (Shimizu, 1990), which are usually acute. In successful suicides, the intensity of these trigger factors may be high or low depending on the intensity of suicidal intent due to the preparatory state (Shimizu, 1990). Independent life events are such trigger factors. Social adversity and cultural factors may operate both as preparatory and trigger factors. The combination of preparatory and trigger factors will both lead to the development of mental illness, particularly depression.

Moreover, the same two factors, in the presence of mental illness, will lead to the formation of suicidal intent and suicide.

We would like to hypothesize how the combination of such diverse preparatory and trigger factors may lead to suicide. The final common pathway may be via the serotonergic system. A number of studies have reported low levels of various markers of serotonin in brains of suicide victims (Asberg et al., 1987). Similar findings have been reported among those who attempt suicide and are consistent across different diagnostic categories (Asberg et al., 1987). It would, therefore, be reasonable to suggest that suicidal behavior is associated with low levels of serotonin activity. As not everyone with low levels of serotinin activity displays suicidal behaviour it has been suggested that this may be a marker of vulnerability (Asberg et al., 1987). We would argue that the preparatory and the trigger factors, in the presence of low serotonin activity, will precipitate mental illness, resulting in a state of mind which develops suicidal intent. This hypothesis has potential implications for treatment, as at present several selective serotonin reuptake inhibitors are available (Montgomery, 1989). The efficacy of these drugs in elderly depression has been and is being studied. However, where is a case for rigorous evaluation of these drugs in elderly suicide prevention, perhaps through large multicenter studies.

Prevention

Ultimately, the aim of all studies of suicide and related topics is to prevent suicides. All psychiatric services also strive towards this ambition. Two questions need to be answered: can this occur and how? Support for the first point comes from suicide trends over recent years where rates in the elderly have declined. Preventative strategies to facilitate such decline are now addressed.

Negative attitudes towards treatment of old people with mental illness are not uncommon among relatives (Wasserman, 1989) and, surprisingly, medical and paramedical staff (Patel, 1974). Attempts to change such attitudes may help reduce suicide rates (Cattell, 1988; Lindesay, 1991). Adequate mental health education, for all professionals working with the elderly, at undergraduate, postgraduate and in-service level is vital. The acceptance of geriatric psychiatry as a subspeciality and the development of academic geriatric psychiatry units in many centres worldwide should facilitate this. Society as a whole needs to be made aware that mental illness and suicidal behavior in the elderly can be recognised and treated. Friends, family and neighbours are very important in the recognition of symptoms of mental illness. Thus, information on recognition of mental illness, availability of services and 'positive propaganda' about its treatability through public education campaigns may assist. In the United Kingdom, the Royal College of Psychiatrists launched such a public education campaign in 1992 – the Defeat

Depression Campaign. It remains to be seen whether this natural experiment will influence the suicide rates. If this British campaign is successful, then there will be a strong case for such campaigns nationally and internationally, perhaps under the auspices of the WHO, with in-built evaluative studies.

Substantial number of elderly suicides have seen a doctor (general practitioner or psychiatrist) shortly before death. Data on the exact nature of these doctor patient contacts are not available. It is unclear whether obvious evidence of mental illness and suicidal behaviour was missed or if such evidence was subtle or absent. Given that the majority of suicides have potentially treatable mental illness, recognition of their illness and intent during the 'final consultation' is an important target for prevention. Diekstra and Van Egmond (1989) argued that it would be difficult for general practitioners to predict such an uncommon event. In the elderly, however, there are a number of risk factors including age, marital status, social isolation, recent life events, physical illness, and first and prolonged episode of depression with a certain symptom profile. Presence of such risk factors should alert the doctor to assess suicide risk. Those general practitioners with superior interview skills, good previous knowledge of their patients, and a favorable attitude towards mental illness are better able to detect mental illness, and this ability can be modified by training (Morriss, 1992; Gask, 1992). In Britain, this may be facilitated by the recent introduction of legislation requiring general practitioners to offer annual physical and mental examination to all their patients over the age of 75 years. The impact of this requirement on suicide rates remains to be evaluated as a natural experiment. Training of general practitioners to improve detection of mental illness (Morriss, 1992; Gask, 1992) could be a useful adjunct to this measure.

Interestingly, the poor sensitivity of psychiatrists in predicting suicides (Pokorny, 1983; Cattell, 1988) has not come under criticism. As a significant number of elderly suicides have had recent contact with a psychiatrist or psychiatric services, the same issues as those for general practitioners need to be addressed.

There are no specific instruments to measure suicidal intent in the elderly. The existing instruments have been reported to have variable sensitivity, specificity and positive predictive values (Pokorny, 1983) and their specific applicability to the elderly has not been evaluated. There is a need to direct research in developing such instruments for use with the elderly with good sensitivity, specificity and positive predictive value.

Once mental illness and suicide risk are identified what should be done next to prevent suicide? Macdonald (1986) reported that general practitioners are good at identifying depression but less good at treating it. There is a clear need to eradicate therapeutic nihilism so that potentially reversible mental illnesses are adequately treated. This can realistically occur through undergraduate and postgraduate education and closer liaison between psychiatry and primary care (Shah, 1991).

Aggressive approaches in treating mental illness and physical illness are vital in preventing suicides. Where possible, the correction of any social adversity will also be helpful. Under utilization of psychiatric services by elderly victims of suicide has been reported (Barraclough, 1971; Cattell, 1988). Should a general practitioner feel out of depth then a referral to a specialist psychogeriatric service should be made. Specialist community psychiatric services can reduce suicide rates (Walk, 1967), but this has not been reported in the elderly. An approach bridging the gap between primary care and psychogeriatric services is to use a community psychiatric nurse (CPN) to treat and coordinate the treatment of mental illness. A trial evaluating the efficacy of CPNs in this endeavor is currently in progress (see Chapter 11). Close collaboration between psychogeriatricians, geriatricians and general practitioners is required for patients with physical illness (Cattell, 1988).

Only a small number of elderly suicides are on antidepressants, usually in inadequate doses, despite a diagnosis of depression. Furthermore, many of these depressive episodes are prolonged episodes. Therefore, aggressive treatment of depression with efficacious antidepressants in adequate doses is vital. Concern has been expressed about providing potential victims with iatrogenic means of suicide with the old-fashioned tricyclic antidepressants. However, mianserin (Cassidy & Henry, 1987; Henry, 1989), lofepramine (Cassidy & Henry, 1987; Henry, 1989), several of the selective serotonin reuptake inhibitors (Montgomery, 1989) and moclobemide, are less toxic in overdose. Furthermore, for noninpatients, weekly supplies of psychotropic drugs, under close psychiatric and primary care supervision, should be prescribed to reduce the risk of toxic overdose of prescribed drugs.

Removal of means of suicide, such as domestic gas, resulted in reduction of suicide rates. Thus, there is reason to believe that removal of other means of suicide may reduce rates (Lindesay, 1991). Although it would be difficult to control prescriptions of drugs such as aspirin and paracetamol, as they can be purchased over the counter, dextropropoxephene can be more closely monitored in general practice (Lindesay, 1991). Suicides due to benzodiazepines can be reduced by simply avoiding their prescription in the first instance and by tailing off the drug. Benzodiazepines have only a limited role in geriatric psychiatry. Similarly, reducing the availability of firearms, through legislation, may be effective in reducing suicide rates. This is supported by the observation that suicide by firearms is uncommon in countries where their access is limited (Shimizu, 1990; Kua & Ko, 1992).

If the patient cannot be managed out of hospital because of the severity of suicidal intent, severity of mental illness and poor social support, admission should be immediate, and involuntary if necessary. The patient should be carefully observed on the ward and a management plan should be agreed by all members of the treating team. Moreover, an important risk period for suicide is just after discharge. Research is needed to identify those individuals at risk of killing themselves in the post discharge period. It may be possible to reduce this by appropriate planning of discharge and close monitoring after discharge, but this requires formal evaluation.

Organizations such as the Samaritans (in the United Kingdom) provide telephone access to people in distress. There is evidence to suggest that they attract a significant number of people at risk of suicide. There is mixed evidence of their efficacy (Bagley, 1968; Jennings, Barraclough & Moss, 1978). Although, they attract suicidal patients (Barraclough & Shea, 1970), it is likely that the elderly do not utilise them adequately (Atkinson, 1971). The efficacy of pilot developments of such organizations however, with targeting of the elderly should be evaluated. Cattell (1988) suggested that organizations, like EXIT, supporting euthanasia attract elderly depressives. Therefore, such organizations should be banned until the effect of legalizing euthanasia on suicide rates is established from countries like the Netherlands.

Once suicide has occurred many preventative issues can be inferred from a detailed case analysis (Alexopoulos, 1991). All members of the treating team need to discuss the details of the case and attempt to identify avenues for improvement. All psychiatric centres should have procedures and policies which automatically invoke an audit of suicides. Barraclough (1971) referred to an important observation made by Krammer: coroners do not always inform their findings to everyone involved with the case and as a result any preventable strategies may not reach the 'shop floor'. There is a clear need to impose such a responsibility upon the coroner so that inquest findings are useful in preventing future suicides.

Another preventative strategy rests with the identification of factors which are protective towards suicide (Appleby, 1992). In the elderly, as discussed in earlier sections, cultural factors, lifelong adversity and improvement of socioeconomic factors are thought to be protective towards suicide. Further research is required to identify the exact nature of these protective factors. Moreover, ways of increasing the presence of such protective factors in the community, with inbuilt evaluative studies, should be a priority for research on the prevention of elderly suicides.

Conclusions

The literature reviewed illustrates that a wide body of data on elderly suicides, from diverse sources, is now available. To date, there has rightly been emphasis on the collection of basic data about elderly suicides. Despite many authors discussing preventative strategies, there is however, a paucity of evaluative data on the effectiveness of preventative measures. There is now an urgent need for such evaluative studies. Ideally, any program designed to prevent suicide should have inbuilt evaluation. This will allow expansion of effective strategies and elimination of ineffective strategies. Due to cross-national variations in elderly suicide rates and correlates, there is a need for cross-national evaluative studies of preventative strategies.

References

Adityanjee, D. R. (1986). Suicide attempts and suicides in India: cross cultural aspects. *International Journal of Social Psychiatry*, **32**, 64–73.

Aldestein, A. & Marden, C. (1975). Suicides 1961–74. In *Population Trends 2*, ed. Office of Population Censuses and Surveys, p. 13, London: Her Majesty's Stationery Office.

Alexopoulous, G. S. (1991). Psychological autopsy of an elderly suicide. *International Journal of Geriatric Psychiatry*, **6**, 45–50.

Appleby, L. (1992). Suicide in psychiatric patients: risk and prevention. *British Journal of Psychiatry*, **161**, 749–58.

Asberg, M., Schalling, D., Traskman-Bendz, L. & Wagner, A. (1987). Psychobiology of suicide, impulsivity, and related phenomena. In *Psychopharmacology the Third Generation of Progress*, ed. H. Y. Meltzer, pp. 655–668. New York: Raven Press.

Atkinson, M. (1971). The Samaritans and the elderly: some problems in communication between a suicide prevention scheme and a group with high suicide risk. *Social Science and Medicine*, **5**, 483–90.

Bagley, C. (1968). The evaluation of suicide prevention scheme by an ecological method. *Social Science and Medicine*, **2**, 1–14.

Baldwin, R. C. & Jolley, D. J. (1986). The prognosis of depression in old age. *British Journal of Psychiatry*, **149**, 574–83.

Barraclough, B. M. (1971). Suicide in the elderly. *British Journal of Psychiatry*, Special supplement **6**, 87–97.

Barraclough, B. M., Bunch, J., Nelson, J. & Sainsbury, P. (1974). 100 cases of suicides – clinical aspects. *British Journal of Psychiatry*, **125**, 355–73.

Barraclough, B. M. & Shea, M. (1970). Suicide and samaritan client. *Lancet*, **ii**, 868–70.

Batchelor, I. R. C. & Napier, M. B. (1953). Attempted suicide in old age. *British Medical Journal*, **ii**, 1186–90.

Benson, R. A. & Brody, D. C. (1975). Suicides by overdosage of medicines in the elderly. *Journal of the American Geriatric Society*, **23**, 304–8.

Bhatia, S. C., Khan, M. H. & Mediratta, R. P. (1987). High risk suicide factors across cultures. *International Journal of Social Psychiatry*, **33**, 226–36.

Blazer, D. G., Bachar, J. R. & Manton, K. G. (1986). Suicide in late life: review and commentary. *Journal of the American Geriatric Society*, **34**, 519–25.

Brain, W. R. (1963). The neurological complications of neoplasms. *Lancet*, **i**, 179–84.

Brent, D. A., Perper, J. A., Kolko, D. J. & Zelenak, J. P. (1988). The psychological autopsy: methodological considerations for the study of adolescent suicide. *Journal of the American Academy of Child and Adolescent Psychiatry*, **27**, 362–6.

Burston, G. R. (1969). Self poisoning in elderly patients. *Gerontologica Clinica*, **11**, 279.

Capstick, A. (1960). Recognition of emotional distubance and the prevention of suicide. *British Medical Journal*, **i**, 1179–82.

Carraci, G. & Miller, N. S. (1991). Epidemiology and diagnosis of alcoholism in the elderly. *International Journal of Geriatric Psychiatry*, **6**, 511–15.

Cassidy, S. & Henry, J. (1987). Fatal toxicity of antidepressant drugs in overdose. *British Medical Journal*, **295**, 102–4.

Cattell, H. R. (1988). Elderly suicide in London: an analysis of coroners' inquests. *International Journal of Geriatric Psychiatry*, **3**, 251–61.

Chynoweth, R., Tonge, J. I. & Armstrong, J. (1980). Suicide in Brisbane – a retrospective psychosocial study. *Australian and New Zealand Journal of Psychiatry*, **14**, 37–45.

Conwell, Y., Olsen, K., Caine, E. D., Flannery, C. (1991). Suicide in later life: psychological autopsy findings, *International Psychogeriatrics*, **3**, 59–66.

Conwell, Y., Rotenberg, M. & Caine, E. D. (1990). Completed suicides at age 50 and over. *Journal of the American Geriatrics Society*, **38**, 640–4.

Copas, J. B. & Robin, A. (1982). Suicide in psychiatric inpatients *British Journal of Psychiatry*, **141**, 503–11

Copeland, J. R. M., Dewey, M. E., Wood, N., Searle, R., Davidson, I. & McWilliam, C. (1987). Range of mental illness among the elderly in the community. Prevalence in Liverpool using the GMS AGECAT package. *British Journal of Psychiatry*, **150**, 815–23.

Crombie, I. K. (1990). Suicide in England and Wales and Scotland. An examination of divergent trends. *British Journal of Psychiatry*, **157**, 529–32.

Daradkeh, T. K. (1989). Suicide in Jordan 1980–1985. *Acta Psychiatrica Scandinavica*, **79**, 241–4.

Diekstra, R. F. W. (1989). Suicide and attempted suicide: an international perspective. *Acta Psychiatrica Scandinavica*, **80** (suppl 354), 1–24.

Diekstra, R. F. W. & Van Egmond, M. (1989). Suicide and attempted suicide in general practice, 1979–1986. *Acta Psychiatrica Scandinavica*, 79, 268–75.

Dorpat, T. L. & Ripley, H. S. (1960). A study of suicide in the Seattle area. *Comprehensive Psychiatry*, **1**, 349–59.

Durkheim, E. (1951). *Suicide*. New York: Free Press of Glencoe.

Ebert, B. W. (1987). Guide to conducting a psychological autopsy. *Professional Psychology: Research and Practice*, **18**, 52–6.

Freud, S. (1949). Mourning and melancholia. In *Collected Papers Volume VI*, ed. Ernest Jones, pp. 152–170. London: Hogarth Press.

Ganesvaran, T. & Rajarajeswaran, R. (1988). Fatal deliberate self-harm seen in a Sri Lankan hospital. *British Journal of Psychiatry*, **152**, 420–3.

Ganesvaran, T., Subramaniam, S. & Mahadevan, K. (1984). Suicide in a northern town of Sri Lanka. *Acta Psychiatrica Scandinavica*, **69**, 420–5.

Gardiner, E. A., Bahn, A. K. & Mack, M. (1964). Suicide and psychiatric care in the elderly. *Archives of General Psychiatry*, **10**, 547–53.

Gask, L. (1992). Training general practitioners to detect and manage emotional disorders. *International Review of Psychiatry*, **4**, 293–300.

Harkey, B. & Hyer, L. (1986). Suicide among psychiatric patients of older ages. *Psychological Reports*, **58**, 775–82.

Hawton, K. & Fagg, J. (1990). Deliberate self poisoning and self injury in older people. *International Journal of Geriatric Psychiatry*, **5**, 367–73.

Hendon, H. (1982). *Suicide in America*. New York: Norton.

Henry, J. (1989). A fatal toxicity index for antidepressant poisoning. *Acta Psychiatrica Scandinavica*, suppl 354, 37–46.

Holding, T. A. & Barraclough, B. M. (1975). Psychiatric morbidity in a sample of a London coroner's open verdicts. *British Journal of Psychiatry*, **127**, 133–43.

Jennings, C., Barraclough, B. M. & Moss, J. R. (1978). Have the Samaritans lowered the suicide rate? A controlled study. *Psychological Medicine*, **8**, 413–22.

Kreitman, N. (1976). Age and parasuicide ('attempted suicide'). *Psychological Medicine*, **6**, 113–21.

Kua, E. H. & Ko, S. M. (1992). A cross-cultural study of suicide among the elderly in Singapore. *British Journal of Psychiatry*, **160**, 558–9.

Lindesay, J. (1991). Suicide in the elderly. *International Journal of Geriatric Psychiatry*, **6**, 355–61.

Lindesay, J., Briggs, K. & Murphy, E. (1989). The Guy's/Age Concern survey. Prevalence rates of cognitive impairment, depression and anxiety in an urban community. *British Journal of Psychiatry*, **155**, 317–29.

Lindesay, J. & Murphy, E. (1987). Suicide in old age. *International Journal of Geriatric Psychiatry*, **2**, 71–2.

Livingston, G., Hawkins, A., Graham, N., Blizzard, R. & Mann, A. (1990). The Gospel Oak study: prevalence rates of dementia, depression and activity limitation among elderly residents in inner London. *Psychological Medicine*, **20**, 137–46.

Loebel, J. P., Loebel, J. S., Dager, S. R., Centerwall, B. S. & Reay, D. T. (1991). Anticipation of nursing home placement may be a precipitant of suicide among the elderly. *Journal of the American Geriatrics Society*, **39**, 407–8.

Macdonald, A. J. D. (1986). Do general practitioners miss depression in elderly patients? *British Medical Journal*, **292**, 1365–7.

MacMohan, B. & Pugh, T. (1965). Suicide in the widowed. *American Journal of Epidemiology*, **81**, 23–31.

Manton, K. G., Blazer, D. G. & Woodbury, M. A. (1987). Suicide in middle age and later life: sex and race specific life table and cohort analysis. *Journal of Gerontology*, **42**, 219–27.

Marshall, J. R. (1978). Changes in aged white male suicide: 1948–1972. *Journal of Gerontology*, **5**, 763–8.

McClure, G. M. G. (1987). Suicides in England and Wales, 1975–1984. *British Journal of Psychiatry*, **150**, 309–14.

McIntosh, J. L. (1984). Components of the decline in elderly suicides: suicide in the young old and the old old by race and sex. *Death Education*, **8**, 113–24.

McIntosh, J. L. & Santos, J. F. (1985–1986). Methods of suicide by age: sex and race differences among the young and the old. *International Journal of Ageing and Human Development*, **22**, 123–39.

Modestin, J. (1989). Completed suicide in psychogeriatric inpatients. *International Journal of Geriatric Psychiatry*, **4**, 209–14.

Montgomery, S. (1989). New antidepressants and 5-HT uptake inhibitors. *Acta Psychiatrica Scandinavica*, **80** (suppl 350), 107–16.

Morgan, H. G., Burns-Cox, C. J., Pocock, H. & Pottle, H. (1975). Deliberate self-harm: clinical and socioeconomic characteristics of 368 patients. *British Journal of Psychiatry*, **127**, 564–74.

Morriss, R. K. (1992). Interviewing skills and the detection of psychiatric problems. *International Review of Psychiatry*, **4**, 287–92.

Murphy, E. (1982). Social origins of depression in old age. *British Journal of Psychiatry*, **141**, 135–42.

Murphy, E. (1983). The prognosis of depression in old age. *British Journal of Psychiatry*, **142**, 111–19.

Murphy, E., Lindesay, J. & Grundy, E. (1986). 60 years of suicide in England and Wales: a cohort study. *Archives of General Psychiatry*, **43**, 969–76.

Murphy, E., Smith, R., Lindesay, J. & Slattery, J. (1988). Increased mortality rates in late life depression. *British Journal of Psychiatry*, **152**, 347–53.

Murphy, G. E. & Wetzel, R. D. (1980). Suicide risk by birth cohorts in the United States, 1949 to 1974. *Archives of General Psychiatry*, **37**, 519–23.

Nelson, F. L. & Farberow, N. L. (1980). Indirect self destructive behaviour in the elderly nursing home patient. *Journal of Gerontology*, **35**, 949–57.

Nowers, M. & Irish, M. (1988). Trends in the reported rates of suicide by self poisoning in the elderly. *Journal of the Royal College of General Practitioners*, **38**, 67–9.

O'Neal, P., Robins, E. & Schmidt, E. H. (1965). A psychiatric study of attempted suicide in persons sixty years of age. *Archives of Neurological Psychiatry*, **75**, 275–84.

Overstone, I. & Kreitman, N. (1974). Two syndromes of suicide, *British Journal of Psychiatry*, **124**, 336–45.

Patel, N. S. (1974). A study on suicide. *Medicine, Science and the Law*, **14**, 129–32.

Pierce, D. (1987). Deliberate self-harm in the elderly. *International Journal of Geriatric Psychiatry*, **2**, 105–10.

Pokorny, A. D. (1983). Prediction of suicides in psychiatric patients. *Archives of General Psychiatry*, **40**, 249–57.

Raleigh, V. S., Bulusu, L. & Balarajan, R. (1990). Suicides among immigrants from the Indian subcontinent. *British Journal of Psychiatry*, **156**, 46–50.

Rich, C. I., Young, D. & Fowler, R. C. (1986). San Diego suicide study I. Young versus old subjects. *Archives of General Psychiatry*, **43**, 577–82.

Robins, E., Murphy, G. E., Wilkinson, R. H., Gassner, S. & Kayes, J. (1959). Some clinical considerations on the prevention of suicide based on a study of 134 successful suicides. *American Journal of Public Health*, **49**, 888–99.

Sainsbury, P. (1955). *Suicide in London*. Maudsley Monograph No 1. London: Chapman & Hall.

Seagar, C. P. & Flood, R. A. (1965). Suicide in Bristol. *British Journal of Psychiatry*, **111**, 919–32.

Seiden, R. H. (1981). Mellowing with age; factors influencing the non-white suicide rate. *International Journal of Ageing and Human Development*, **13**, 265–84.

Sendbuehler, J. M. (1977). Suicide and attempted suicide among the aged. *Canadian Medical Association Journal*, **117**, 418–19.

Sendbuehler, J. M. & Goldstein, S. (1977). Attempted suicide among the aged. *Journal of the American Geriatrics Society*, **25**, 245–8.

Shafii, M., Carrigan, S., Whittinghill, J. R. & Derrick, A. (1985). Psychological autopsy of completed suicide in children and adolescents. *American Journal of Psychiatry*, **142**, 1061–64.

Shah, A. K. (1991). An aspect of community psychiatry training: a senior registrar's experience, *Psychiatric Bulletin*, **14**, 424–5.

Shah, A. K. (1992*a*). Experience of death in psychiatry: a registrar's experience. *British Journal of Clinical and Social Psychiatry*, **8**, 80–2.

Shah, A. K. (1992*b*). Aggressive and violent behaviour among psychogeriatric inpatients: an overview. *Care of the Elderly*, **4**, 396–400.

Shah, A. K., Fineberg, N. A. & James, D. V. (1991). Violence among psychiatric inpatients. *Acta Psychiatrica Scandinavica*, **84**, 304–9.

Shimizu, M. (1990). Depression and suicide in late life. In *Psychogeriatrics: Biomedical and Social Advances*, Eds. K. Hasegawa & A. Homma, pp. 330–334. Amsterdam: Excerpta Medica.

Shulman, K. (1978). Suicide and parasuicide in old age: a review. *Age and Ageing*, **7**, 201–9.

Solomon, M. I. & Hellon, C. P. (1977). Suicide and age in Alberta, Canada 1951 to 1977: a cohort analysis. *Archives of General Psychiatry*, **37**, 511–13.

Stengel, E. (1977). *Suicide and Attempted Suicide*. Ringwood: Penguin.

Stewart, I. (1960). Suicide: the influence of organic disease. *Lancet*, **ii**, 919–20.

Surtees, P. G. & Duffy, J. C. (1989). Suicide in England and Wales 1946–1985: an age-period-cohort analysis. *Acta Psychiatrica Scandinavica*, **79**, 216–23.

Walk, D. (1967). Suicide and community care. *British Journal of Psychiatry*, **105**, 1381–91.

Wasserman, D. (1989). Passive euthanasia in response to attempted suicide: one form of aggressiveness by relatives. *Acta Psychiatrica Scandinavica*, **79**, 460–7.

Wetzel, R. D., Reich, T., Murphy, G. E., Province, M. & Miller, J. P. (1987). The changing relationship between age and suicide rates: cohort effect, period effect or both? *Psychiatric Development*, **3**, 179–218.

Whitlock, F. A. (1978). Suicide, cancer and depression. *British Journal of Psychiatry*, **132**, 269–74.

Woodbury, M. A., Manton, K. G. & Blazer, D. (1988). Trends in US suicide mortality rates 1968 to 1982: race and sex differences in age, period and cohort components. *International Journal of Epidemiology*, **17**, 356–62.

Wolff, K. (1969). Depression and suicide in the geriatric patient. *Journal of the American Geriatrics Society*, **17**, 668–73.

World Health Organization. (1992). *World Health Statistics Annual*. Geneva: World Health Organization.

Zarit, S. W. (1980). *Ageing and Mental Disorders: Psychological Approaches to Assessment and Treatment*. New York: Free Press.

Part 5

Psychosexual disorders

15

Psychosexual disorders

JOHN KELLETT

Introduction

A Darwinian might question the role of sexual behavior in the elderly, pointing out that the purpose of any species was to increase its kind, and coitus beyond the menopause had little to contribute to this aim. If so, he would be mistaken, because the sexual act is not only penetration and fertilization, but is preceded by grooming, whose purpose in primates is to reinforce social bonds. As the human child takes at least 15 years to reach physical maturity, the survival of the last born will depend on this bond lasting until the mother is 65, and the male 70 (due to the need of the female to chose her mate on his status he is usually older by five years (OPCS, 1992)). The earlier death of the male (his expectation of life in the UK in 1988 was 72.4 compared to 78 for the female (OPCS, 1992)) might suggest that he plays a lesser role in child-rearing, or is not really adapted to monogamy (Reynolds & Kellett, 1991). The advantage to the species of prolonging life beyond this point is more controversial, though the elderly may stabilize society as carriers of the culture and provide support for their progeny in rearing their children. Either way, the preservation of the marriage bond can improve the quality of the couple's lives as they compensate for their declining abilities. Male carers of demented wives do better when the sexual contact is retained (Morris, Morris & Britton, 1988).

The emphasis on the bonding role of this behavior can help us to understand the changes of ageing, so that a loss of genital function is not perceived as a personal catastrophe but as an invitation to increase manual and oral contact, thus extending and even increasing the pleasures of intimacy.

Classification of the dysfunctions

Though Table 15.1 lists most sexual dysfunctions, they are far from discrete. Thus a low libido can lead to erectile failure, and repeated anorgasmia can cause a woman to lose her libido, though this may be specific to the partner. Each condition

Table 15.1. *Sexual disorders*

	Male		Female
Phobias	Heterophobia		Vaginismus
Arousal	Erectile failure		Vaginal dryness Dyspareunia
Ejaculation	Retrograde		
Libido		Increase Decrease Incompatibility of levels	
Orgasm		Anorgasmia Reduction of sensation	
Gender		Transsexualism	
Paraphilias	Pedophilia Exhibitionism Frotteurism Voyeurism		
Perversions	Rape Sadomasochism Fetishism Sexual asphyxia Obscene telephone callers Cross-dressing		

has organic and psychological causes, and can be made worse by performance anxiety. Often the attempt to separate the organic and psychological factors leads to a false dichotomy (Kellett, 1990; Gregoire 1990), especially in the elderly where organic causes almost always play a part. In any condition, however, one must establish whether it is primary or secondary, and whether it is general or situational. Thus venous leak syndrome will prevent full erection from infancy, whilst at the other extreme a row about a new color scheme will cause erectile failure limited to that partner at that time.

Changes of aging

To identify these changes one would need to collect a group of young people, and question them yearly about their sexual function for the next 50 years, hoping that their behavior would not be affected by this intrusion into privacy and that the investigator would live to tell the tale. Not surprisingly, this has not happened, and we are largely dependent on cross-sectional surveys where generational effects

Table 15.2. *Sexual activity in the male by age and marital status (Kinsey et al., 1948)*

	Age	N	a		b		c		d		e		f		g		h	
			%	freq	%	freq	%	freq	%	freq	%	freq	%	freq	%	freq	%	freq
Single	21–25	1535	99	2.7	81	1.4	61	1.2			29	0.4	59	1.3	15	1.1	81	0.4
Married	21–25	751	100	3.9	48	0.5	100	3.5	100	3.2	13	0.2	24	1.3	8	0.4	59	0.2
Single	41–45	56	96	1.9	61	1.0	66	1.1			39	0.5	52	0.8	38	1.2	48	0.2
Married	41–45	272	100	2.0	33	0.3	99	1.9	99	1.6	9	0.2	24	0.5	2	0.8	54	0.2
Married	56–60	67	99	1.1	19	0.2	97	1.1	94	0.9	8	0.3	22	0.7			28	0.1

Key: N, sample size; %, reporting activity in that sector; freq, Mean number per week of those active; a, total outlets to orgasm; b, masturbation; c, total intercourse; d, marital intercourse; e, intercourse with prostitutes; f, nonmarital intercourse excluding e; g, homosexual orgasm; h, nocturnal emissions.

such as exposure to the 'Victorian' or 'Carnaby Street' ethic may swamp the effects of aging.

The first such survey was by Kinsey and colleagues (1948,1953) shortly after the Second World War. Although they had large samples of the young (2886 males and 1211 females aged 21–25) the sample over 60 consisted of only 87 white and 39 black males, and 56 females. The impression that three-quarters of males at 80 were impotent was based on a sample of four.

From Table 15.2 one can see a decline in activity of the male in all outlets except intercourse with prostitutes and other nonmarital partners. Table 15.3 documents a similar decline in females, but an increase in masturbation which is responsible for 14% of orgasms in the 20s and 26% aged 51–55. Unlike single males, single females were markedly less active than their married sisters.

Total outlets give a clearer picture and, in case the reader is puzzled by the disparity between males and females, this is largely accounted for by more masturbation and homosexuality in males (see Table 15.4).

Often more information can be obtained by sampling a smaller range of age. Thus Hallstrom (1977) sampled 800 women from Gothenburg in four age strata: 38, 46, 50 and 54. He noted a decline in interest and activity with age but, separating the effects of age and menopause, found the latter to be responsible. As, however, the decline was much greater in the lower social classes he agrees with Masters and Johnson (1966) 'that the psyche plays a part at least equal to, if not greater than that of an unbalanced endocrine system in determining the sex drive of women during the postmenopausal period of their lives'.

Cutler, Garcia & McCoy (1987) also found a decline in sexual activity in perimenopausal women with the lowest levels of estrogen. Riley, however, (1991), in a comprehensive review of the subject, states 'reduced levels of vaginal lubrication and hence dyspareunia are the only features... that have been confirmed to be associated with decreased estrogen levels'.

Hallstrom & Samuelsson (1990) followed up his sample for six years. Two-thirds reported no change in desire. Loss of desire was associated with a poorer relationship whilst an increase was associated with resolution of the problem. Social class had no effect.

Persson (1980) studied a random sample of 166 men and 226 women aged 70, resident in Gothenburg and compared the characteristics of married subjects (66 men (52%) and 33 women (32%)) who had had intercourse in the preceding three months with those who had not. Not surprisingly the active of both sexes were more likely to approve of sexual activity in old age, whereas the active older women were more likely to have had premarital sex and to have enjoyed intercourse. Physical health did not relate to activity except worsening of symptoms in women, though poorer mental health was found in the inactive. Confirming the view of Pfeiffer and Davis (1972) that activity is usually governed by the male, women

Table 15.3. *Sexual activity in the female by age and marital status (Kinsey et al., 1953)*

			a		b		c		d		e	
	Age	N	%	freq	%	freq	%	freq	%	freq	%	freq
Single	21–25	2810	60	1.1	—	—	11	0.18	35	0.9	5	1.0
Married	21–25	1654	88	2.8	99	3.0	15	0.22	27	0.6	1	0.9
Ex*	21–25	238	76	2.3	—	—	21	0.32	41	1.0	6	1.1
Single	41–45	179	68	1.6	—	—	18	0.14	50	1.0	—	—
Married	41–45	497	93	2.0	94	1.8	31	0.13	36	0.6	—	—
Ex	41–45	195	84	1.8	—	—	36	0.24	58	0.7	—	—
Single	56–60	27	44	0.9	—	—	—	—	—	—	—	—
Married	56–60	49	82	0.8	80	1.3	29	0.19	35	0.2	—	—
Ex	56–60	53	55	0.6	—	—	30	0.16	42	0.4	—	—

Key: Ex* means previously married; a, total orgasm; b, marital coitus with or without orgasm; c, dreams to orgasm; d, masturbation to orgasm; e, homosexual orgasm; %, percentage reporting activity in that sector; freq, mean number per week.

Table 15.4. *Outlets per week by age and sex (figures for females in parentheses)*

Age	Number	Percentage active	Mean of those active
16–20	3750 (5649)	99.3 (50)	2.89 (1.1)
41–45	440 (810)	99.1 (87)	2.00 (1.9)
61–65	58 (53)	81 (47)	1.04 (0.5)
71–75	12 (10)	42 (30)	0.3 (0.03)

with younger husbands were more active. Pfeiffer, Verwoerdt & Wang (1968) had earlier sought factors related to continued activity in their nonrandom longitudinal study from Duke University. In men, age was by far the most important factor, though enjoyment and interest were increased in those with higher incomes and social class, with better health the third factor. For women, the findings were similar though higher education took the place of social class.

The frequency of intercourse is not the only measure of sexuality and Weizman and Hart (1987) found that healthy married men in Israel aged 66–71 had intercourse less often but masturbated more often than those aged 60–65.

Obviously cross-sectional studies do not have the strength of longitudinal ones on the effect of aging. The first of these, over six years (Pfeiffer et al., 1968), showed that, despite strong correlations of decline with age, 14% showed an increase in sexual interest and intercourse. The median age for stopping

Table 15.5 *Sexual activity by age and year of follow-up*

Age at start	N	Male 1969	1971	1973	1975	N	Female 1969	1971	1973	1975
46–55	63	2.03	1.98	19.5	1.94 (1.69)	57	1.70	1.71	1.69	1.66 (1.42)
56–65	74	1.47	1.54	1.45	1.32 (1.27)	36	1.23	1.24	1.20	1.16 (0.92)
66–71	33	1.18	1.21	1.19	1.17	15	0.79	0.77	0.76	0.67

Key: 0, never; 1 < 1/week; 2, 1–2 × /week; 3, 3 × /week, 4, > 3/week.
Figures in parentheses indicate level of activity predicted by cross-sectional data.

Table 15.6. *Frequency of sexual activity by age and sex in subjects aged over 80 expressed as percentage*

		Never	Once to several times per year	Several times per month to several times per week	Once per day to several times per day
Masturbation	M	28	31	41	0
	F	60	27	11	2
Foreplay	M	18	17	38	28
	F	36	25	22	17
Coitus	M	30	34	26	3
	F	70	20	10	0

intercourse was 68 for men and 60 for women, usually due to the male. Though every study shows the decline in activity with age, the second study from Duke University by George and Weiler (1981), which was largely random except for only including those who were with their partner throughout, indicated that the effect of aging was only a quarter of that expected from the cross-sectional data of the males, and one-seventh that expected from the females. This implies that cross-sectional studies have been exaggerating the effects of aging, by attributing the different activity of different generations to age rather than upbringing (see Table 15.5).

This conclusion is reinforced by the study of Bretschneider and McCoy (1988) who surveyed the sexual activity of residents in retirement facilities in California. Here subjects were selected for health but were aged 80 to 102. The sample of 100 men and 102 women reported frequent sexual activity as shown in Table 15.6.

The rates for males were twice those for females which probably reflects the sex ratio in the homes of one man to six women. Of men 88% and of women 71% admitted to sexual fantasies.

All these studies are based on interviews or questionnaires and depend on the honesty of the informant. One might predict that men would exaggerate and women minimize their ratings.

Pfeiffer's survey, however, included 54 paired ratings from 31 couples where the data had been obtained from separate interviews. The reported frequency of sexual intercourse (five categories) correlated 0.87 between husband and wife. Where there were differences, in eight cases it was the husband and three the wife who reported higher activity. Bearing in mind that some discrepancy might be caused by extramarital liaisons, the level of agreement is most reassuring. Similarly, Kinsey found high rates of inter-rater and reinterview reliability.

Bald statistics of the frequency of sexual acts may tell us little of the quality and intensity of sexual union in the elderly. For this the reader is referred to the consumer union report by Brecher (1988), a 'Hite report' for the elderly.

The decline in erectile potency with age ultimately affects the majority of the population but this is not necessarily 'sexual dysfunction'. Dysfunction, like disease is defined by the patient whose expectations are not fulfilled. A loss of interest by both partners, which coincides with a loss of erections will lead to cessation of coitus without distress. Sexual dysfunction in the elderly can thus be caused as much by unrealistic expectations as by a decline in function. Osborn, Hawton & Gath (1988) surveyed 600 women stratified into age bands from 35 to 59. Half of those aged 50 to 59 had operationally defined sexual problems (compared to only 14% aged 35–39) but only 21% complained of them. However the discrepancy between having and recognizing a problem was not related to age, only just under a fifth of the 33% with objective problems making a complaint.

Physical changes

These have been detailed by Masters and Johnson (1966), who studied the sexual response of 34 female volunteers aged 51 to 80, and 39 males aged 51 to 90. A summary of their findings is laid out in Tables 15.7 and 15.8. In both sexes there were a few exceptions to the general rule, who maintained regular and frequent sexual contact, and whose physiological reactions were closer to younger age groups. The cause of this decline is unknown.

Though there is a gradual reduction in levels of free testosterone in males, Davidson et al. (1983) found that it only accounted for 4% of the variance in sexual activity to orgasm, whilst age accounted for 12%. It has been suggested that, despite normal levels of testosterone, aging causes a loss of receptor sensitivity, from which one would predict that increasing levels above normal would restore function (Riley, 1991). Weizman et al. (1983) have proposed a rise in prolactin as the cause of decreased desire in men. In their sample of 28 men aged 60–64 and 44 aged 65–70 they found a significant negative correlation between

Table 15.7. *Aging changes in the male*

Retained	
Nil	
Retained but reduced	
Excitement phase	
	Penile erection often only complete at orgasm
Plateau phase	
	Nipple erection
	Testicular elevation
Orgasmic phase	
	Ejaculatory power, especially if prolonged plateau phase
	Rectal and ejaculatory contractions
Lost	
Plateau phase	
	Sexual flush
	Re-erection
	Scrotal vasocongestion
Orgasmic phase	
	Ejaculatory inevitability
	Prostatic contractions
NB Though resolution is quicker, the refractory period may extent to 24 hours	

prolactin level and frequency of sexual intercourse, but the effect on libido was only apparent in the older cohort. Though 27 were impotent, there was only a trend for prolactin to be higher in this group. As prolactin levels are increased by stress it could be argued that nonspecific factors were more important than prolactin itself.

Genital engorgement requires a quadrupling of blood supply making this function dependent on a lack of atheromatous narrowing of the pudendal arteries. The initiation of this increased flow is by the parasympathetic nervous system whose activity is known to decline with age (O'Brien, O'Hare & Corrall, 1986). Finally the rigidity of the collagenous sacks may be lost leading to the loss of rigidity in th engorged penis. Though erectile failure may well represent true malfunction, it is of interest that the variation in frequency of intercourse in men fits a curve of normal distribution (Vallery Masson, Valleron & Potrenaud, 1981), something which occurs with most healthy activities, and implies that the causes are multifactorial.

Most of the above account refers to male function. Though there are changes in the female, these would seem to be more the result, than the cause of abstinence. The dramatic fall in levels of estrogen at the menopause does not stop activity, and hormone replacement therapy keeps the genitalia healthy without having much effect on libido. Sherwin & Gelfand (1987) have shown that testosterone restores

Table 15.8. *Aging changes in the female*

Retained
- Excitement phase
  - Nipple erection
  - Clitoral tumescence, though delayed if no direct stimulation
- Plateau phase
  - Clitoral retraction

Retained but reduced
- Excitement phase
  - Vasocongestion of labia minora
  - Vaginal lubrication
  - Expansion of inner two-thirds of vagina (moves from excitement to plateau phase)
  - Uterine elevation
- Plateau phase
  - Engorgement of areolae
  - Secretion from Bartholin's glands
  - Orgasmic platform
- Orgasmic phase
  - Rectal and orgasmic contractions

Lost
- Excitement phase
  - Breast engorgement, especially if pendulous
  - Sexual flush
  - Swelling of labia majora

NB Resolution is much quicker, apart from nipple erection

sexual drive to normal levels after oophorectomy, but its role in the natural menopause is open to doubt (Dow, Hart & Forrest, 1983).

Medical factors

Chronic disease, malaise, and pain are likely to suppress libido, except to the extent that they promote dependency and intimacy. Most of the epidemiological studies showed little effect of illness. Nevertheless if a disease does not affect sexuality, the treatment probably will. Some drugs like the opiates so saturate the endorphin receptors that orgasmic endorphins have little effect. Others such as the benzodiazepines reduce arousal in a dose-related manner (Riley & Riley, 1986). Recently, Taylor Segraves (1989) has reviewed the mechanisms by which neuroleptics and antidepressants affect function. Dopamine is probably the essential intermediary neurotransmitter between testosterone and libido (Hyppa, Rinne & Sonnine, 1970) and drugs which block it, e.g. neuroleptics, suppress libido. Serotonin, though important in reducing depression also reduces libido which is therefore a little mentioned effect of the newer selective serotonin reuptake inhibitors. Other drugs act peripherally, e.g. thiazides and beta blockers to inhibit engorgement, whilst others e.g. clonidine, clomipramine, phenelzine inhibit orgasm. Drugs which counter testosterone reduce libido in men, e.g. progestogens, cyproterone acetate. Though this may be seen as a relatively short list, these drugs are widely used, often in combination with other remedies. Thus opiates are found in many analgesics, thiazides are the most widely used diuretics for hypertension, neuroleptics are used to control vomiting and vertigo as well as psychosis and agitation, benzodiazepines are still the most widely used hypnotics, and antidepressants are used in general medicine for pain control and to replace the old-fashioned tonic. Morgan et al. (1988) found that 16% of those over 65 were taking benzodiazepine hypnotics, whilst Cartwright and Smith (1988) found that 40% of those over 80 were on diuretics.

Diabetes mellitus is common in the elderly and can present with almost any dysfunction though erectile failure is the commonest (Fairburn, McCulloch & Wu, 1982). As it causes atheroma, autonomic neuropathy, vaginal thrush, malaise and sympathetic overactivity during hypoglycemia, explanations for dysfunction are not difficult to find. Sexual dysfunction precedes as well as follows myocardial infarction though the cause for the former is unknown (Kellett, 1987). Some of the latter is due to misinterpretation of the breathlessness of orgasm as a strain on the heart, rather than physiological overbreathing (as a means of erotic imprinting). In practice, once the patient can climb a flight of stairs he can resume coitus.

Neurological disease can effect sexuality in four ways. First paralysis from, for example, a stroke, makes it physically difficult to make love. Second, spinal and neuropathic disorders affect direct control over the physical processes of arousal and orgasm. The parasympathetic outflow is at S2 at which level orgasm is sensed. Ejaculation is caused by the sympathetic outflow at L2. A lesion above L2 will allow reflex responses without sensation, whilst lower lesions affect erections. Third, dementia usually causes a loss of libido associated with a reduction in LHRH (Oram, Edwardson & Millard, 1981; Zeiss et al., 1990). Subcortical dementias, e.g. Huntington's, retain libido but coarsen behavior often causing sexual deviance, e.g. child abuse. Poorly controlled temporal lobe epilepsy also leads to a lower libido (Spark, Wills & Royal, 1984), though is not inevitable with epilepsy (Jensen et al., 1990). Fourth, is depression which commonly follows nondominant hemisphere lesions, though it is more often the result of stress, bereavement or illness.

Other diseases associated with sexual dysfunction include myxedema, sickle cell disease, hypertension and neurofibromatosis.

Surgical factors

Many diseases which lead to surgery are likely to cause sexual dysfunction if not so treated. Examples include spinal cord compression, rectal carcinoma and ulcerative colitis. Sometimes, however, trauma from the surgery itself can be the final straw. The parasympathetic plexus supplying the penis is closely related to the rectum and prostate so that operations on either can damage these nerves. Major surgery inevitably has effects on body image but in the past these effects may have been exaggerated. The high incidence of dysfunction after total mastectomy was blamed on this, but when this operation was compared to lumpectomy loss of sexual interest was complained of by 28 % of the mastectomy group and 32 % of the lumpectomy patients. The authors (Fallowfield et al., 1990) conclude that fear of cancer is the predominant emotion causing loss of desire.

Surgery shares with medicine the effects of admission to hospital which may separate a couple for the first time. The return home, often with stitches in place and a scar, leaves the couple in doubt if, and when, to resume coitus. These doubts will be reinforced if the issue is not addressed, or if dressings, a catheter, or an ileostomy bag directly interfere with intercourse. Silence from the surgeon and nurses about sexual contact will leave a message that further sexual contact is unmentionable and beyond the pale.

The loss of estrogen secretion at the menopause leads to a reduction and delay of vaginal lubrication and thinning of the mucosa, leading to cystitis. As a result, older women can find intercourse painful. This may be eased by artificial lubricants, prolonged petting, and hormone replacement. The estrogen-lacking vagina is also more prone to infection.

Overweight and weakness of the muscles of the pelvic floor can lead to prolapse of the bladder into the anterior wall of the vagina, leading to discomfort on coitus and stress incontinence. Though surgical repair is made via the vagina, sexual function is usually not affected, provided the couple are advised when to resume coitus. Rectal prolapse repair is more likely to lead to narrowing of the vagina (Francis & Jeffcoate, 1966) though problems are rare.

More serious conditions like cancer may present with sexual dysfunction and Anderson et al. (1986) found that 75% of patients had developed sexual problems before the diagnosis was made, even when they were no different from the normal population before the onset of symptoms. Major surgery and, to an even greater extent, radiotherapy damage the sexual function of the vagina leading to stenosis and dyspareunia. As with any disfiguring operation, much will depend on the attitude and support of the sexual partner. The emphasis on feminine beauty makes the female more vulnerable to these physical insults than her partner. Clearly the imperative with cancer is to save life, but awareness of the sexual function of her genitalia by her therapists can soften the blow.

Cultural pressures

Though the anxiety aroused by adolescent sexuality is absent in the elderly, the biological drive to consummate a relationship is weaker, leaving the individual more subject to social pressure. Apart from medical influence, pension arrangements may discourage the widow from formalizing her new relationship, yet extramarital sex may incur the wrath of her virtuous children. Increasing disability requiring institutional care further denies a couple the privacy needed for intimacy. The growth of sexual imagery in the media is confined to the young, especially for women. Older models are dressed in sensible tweeds rather than diaphanous ball dresses, whilst naked elderly people are only portrayed as objects of deformity. Though the cessation of coitus is determined by the male, the proceptive sexuality of youth merges into the receptive profile of the female, so that any reluctance of either partner is less likely to be overridden.

The relative lack of attention given to sex and the elderly is not typical of the world as a whole. Winn and Newton (1982) looked at such attitudes in 106 traditional societies. They conclude: 'though some decline in the sexual activity of aged males is recorded in a significant proportion of the societies studied, many cultural groups have expectations for continued sexual activity for older men that imply little, if any, loss of their sexual powers until very late in life'. Regarding females they state: 'older women frequently express strong sexual desires and interests, ... engage in sexual activity in many instances until extreme old age ... and may form liaisons with much younger men.'

Institutions

Though only 2.5% of British people of pensionable age are in residential homes (Age Concern, 1990) this rises to a much higher proportion of those aged over 80. Nevertheless, the vast majority of the elderly live in their own homes. Those who enter institutions are too frail to care for themselves because of dementia, weakness or arthritis. Not surprisingly, therefore, these homes are not designed to facilitate sexual contact, and sexual behavior by residents can arouse considerable anxiety. Most surveys show that staff are quite liberal in their attitudes. Damrosh (1984) gave qualified nurses enrolled in a graduate nursing course case vignettes of a 68 year-old woman which differed in one respect. Half mentioned that she was sexually active, and this client was preferred in all ten ratings except popularity with staff. Earlier Kaas (1978), in another American study had tested the attitudes of 85 nursing home residents and 207 nursing staff to sexuality. The staff were more liberal than the residents except in their agreement with the statement 'most people over 55 masturbate some of the time.' The statement 'sexually active elderly are dirty old men and women' provoked definite disagreement from the staff but residents were nearer neutrality. Statements about sex in the young also elicited more liberal views from the staff which suggests that differences may be generational.

Szasz (1983) gave all grades of nursing staff working in a long-stay unit for elderly men the task of citing two sorts of behavior which would cause a problem and one sort which should be encouraged. Most staff were not concerned with sexual behavior of a patient in private, but found it difficult to cope with overt sexual approaches.

Human coitus, like childbirth, must have exposed primitive man to attack from predators. Presumably the latter tends to occur at night for this reason, and couples equally seek a place of safety and privacy to enjoy their intimacy. Most institutions do not provide this, either through a lack of individual rooms, or by staff walking into rooms without knocking and waiting for a response. There is a narrow line between respecting personal choice, and allowing sexual exploitation of a confused woman. By allowing a relationship to develop, staff can incur the anger of relatives who fear the loss of their inheritance and resent the implied insult to the other parent. As a result, the success of such a contact lies more often in the lap of others than the couple themselves. Residents may feel that their ability to remain in the home depends on staff approval.

Homes need to provide double rooms but allow an estranged couple to occupy single ones. Many homes do have such facilities, in marked contrast to the long-stay hospital which may still segregate the sexes. The married visitor's flat can expose the patient to ridicule, and a policy of liberal leave may be the best way of allowing a couple to continue coital contact.

Treatment

For a fuller coverage of this area, the reader is referred to treatment manuals such as those by Fairburn, Dickerson & Greenwood (1983) and Hawton (1985). The first essential is to establish the nature of the complaint, which is often complicated by both the embarrassment of the patient and their unfamiliarity with sexual jargon. The author spent some time designing a treatment program for anorgasmia for an elderly Asian man who complained of 'no emission' only to discover that he meant he could not obtain an erection. A full history is essential and should include details about the onset of the condition, its variability and relation to circumstances. Organic dysfunctions are improved by higher eroticism unlike most psychogenic ones, for which reason most organic cases attribute their problem to the psyche. The sexual history should include the length of petting, the effect and fantasies of masturbation, the ages of physical maturation, first date, and first coitus, and list of partners including current ones which may be unknown to the accompanying spouse (an important reason for interviewing each partner on their own, which also gives them the opportunity to describe their true feelings for each other and intentions). One must obtain a detailed medical history, and if one is likely to be using psychotherapy a family and career history. A thorough history may take over an hour to compile but also aids rapport. Examination includes the style of verbal and nonverbal communication of the couple, e.g. one can offer them a choice of chairs to see if they choose to sit close. The extent of the physical examination will depend on the nature of the complaint. Thus a vaginal examination might be insensitive in a woman who had developed secondary vaginismus after a rape, but might be offered in case she thought she had incurred physical damage. A male with erectile failure should have the checks itemized in Table 15.9.

Though there is little place for hormone assays in patients whose libido is well maintained, those with such a complaint should have an assay of testosterone, sex hormone binding globulin or luteinizing hormone and prolactin. Physical remedies are described in Table 15.10.

The squeeze technique is a method of delaying ejaculation by placing firm pressure across the shaft of the penis behind the glans. The 'stop-start technique' is the use of intermittent stimulation to prolong the erection usually during masturbation. Vacuum systems are rigid tubes into which the penis is sucked by a pump and when engorged a band is slipped onto the base of the penis to maintain the erection. Another method is the use of a thickened condom into which the penis is sucked, the condom remaining in place during coitus. 1.0 mg of phentolamine can be mixed with the papaverine to reduce its acidity and stinging after injection. (see Table 15.11)

For most couples, coital failure has led to a discomfort with all sexual contact. Sensate focus exercises are designed to reverse this. Initially, a ban is placed on coitus and heavy petting, and the couple are taught to use caressing as a means of relaxation rather than for arousal. The timing, place, and order of type of massage are specified. The couple are instructed to avoid distraction, and each to seek pleasure primarily for themselves. As relaxation is achieved, in further sessions the massage can become more intimate until finally coitus is allowed. The process throws up problems in communication that can be interpreted with the emphasis on each partner taking responsibility for their feelings. Sexual release by masturbation is allowed until coitus returns. The process works best where the couple are given the task of learning about each other and a therapist who is seduced into interpretive psychotherapy can retard the process. The arousal circuit is based on a diagram of the brain and genitals to show how the two interact. The guided tour can be based on a real examination of the sex organs of each, or a fantasy trip into the bodies of each.

Briefly, the ladder concept (Stanley, 1981) is used to demonstrate how a couple can satisfy each other on different rungs of sexual arousal, without always having

Table 15.9. *Physical examination of the male*

1. Pulse and blood pressure including testing from sinus arrythmia and pulse on valsalva manoeuvre
2. Check for signs of general disease, e.g. clubbing, pallor, dyspnea, lymphadenopathy, hepatosplenomegaly, etc.
3. Peripheral pulses in the legs
4. Limitation of straight leg raising and tendon reflexes of legs
5. Appearance of external genitalia, consistency and size of testicles, and other scrotal masses
6. Ability to detect light touch and pinprick over feet and genitalia
7. Fundoscopy
8. Test urine for glucose or check blood glucose
9. Intracavernosal injection of 30 mg of papaverine (after checking that patient can obtain injection of metaraminol 6 hours later if priapism occurs)

Table 15.10. *Physical remedies*

Low libido
    Testosterone, antidepressants (trazodone or viloxazine), selegiline, or an L dopa preparation
Premature ejaculation
    Clomipramine, clonidine. Squeeze and 'stop–start' technique
Erectile failure
    Yohimbine, self-intracavernosal injection (with papaverine, phentolamine, or prostaglandin E), vacuum system, surgical implant
Anorgasmia
    Midodrine
Dyspareunia
    KY jelly, estrogen creams or tablets

Table 15.11. *Psychological remedies*

1. Education including anatomy, age norms, guided tour and arousal circuit
2. Sensate focus program
3. Ladder concept
4. Communication pattern
5. Token system
6. Vaginal trainers to desensitize for vaginismus
7. Shaping by masturbation
8. Masturbation prior to penetration for anorgasmia

to have intercourse. A token system can be used to establish means by which a couple can learn to satisfy each other's needs in their social life together. Thus, by bringing his wife tea in bed, a husband may earn sufficient tokens for his wife to give him a cuddle before getting up. Vaginal trainers are phallic objects of different sizes which the woman learns to insert into her vagina starting from the smallest. Masturbatory shaping can be used to reinforce bonding. Thus, if the husband is no longer attracted by his wife, he can use his most erotic fantasies to initiate masturbation provided that ejaculation is associated with thoughts or pictures of his wife. Similarly, a woman with low self-esteem can masturbate or arouse herself to reflections of herself in a mirror, and regain confidence in her body as an erotic stimulus. The man who ejaculates normally on masturbation but not inside his partner uses masturbation until, at the point of ejaculation, he inserts his penis.

These tools of therapy need to be used flexibly so that a couple who enjoy intercourse, but suffer anorgasmia, do not necessarily have to go through the whole sensate focus program.

After the death of a partner, the survivor may wish to remarry but find the process of finding a new partner more difficult than in youth. They should be encouraged to exploit their interests in order to meet people, from evening classes to evensong, from a conservation society to the Conservative party, from a Saga singles holiday to the resident's association. Active encouragement is necessary to thwart the greater reticence of the elderly.

The simplicity and effectiveness of many of these techniques has led to a trial comparing treatment with a manual to treatment with a live therapist where both were effective (Carney, Bancroft & Mathews, 1978). An excellent self-help manual for the elderly is published by Age Concern (Greengross & Greengross 1989).

Deviance

The boundaries of normal sexual behavior are defined by society, so that the treatment for deviance is often at the request of society rather than the patient. Those whose inclinations break the law find relief in the lower libido of aging. Others who may have been distressed by their inclinations when young are reconciled to them when older. A few struggle through a form of marriage and welcome the chance to be themselves thereafter by being homosexual or transsexual. Counselling may be necessary to help the person overcome their guilt. Those that do present in old age are usually suffering from some brain damage which is removing their natural inhibitions. The alcoholic starts to make obscene phone calls, the subcortical dement attempts to touch up his grandchild. Sometimes confused behavior can be wrongly interpreted as sexual as when a demented old lady attempts to undress in public. Patients with Parkinson's disease are prone to a Lewy body dementia, whilst dopaminergic treatment will stimulate the libido

(Barbeau, 1969; Harvey, 1988) of at least a quarter of those receiving it. The combination invites sexual display, and such patients have to be protected from the consequences of their actions.

Conclusion

As Oscar Wilde has said 'the tragedy of old age is not that one is old, but that one is young'. If so it is the job of the doctor to make sure that the young person within has the opportunity to enjoy the pleasures of sexuality without inducing guilt in those who feel there can be life without it. These pleasures are not dependent on vaginal penetration but require a trust in, and affection for human kind. The absence of a confidant (Murphy 1982) remains a major risk factor for mental illness in old age, and there is no better confidant than the one with whom one shares a bed.

References

Age Concern (1990). *Older People in the United Kingdom, some Basic Facts*. London, Age Concern.

Anderson, B., Lachenbruch, P., Andersen, B. & Deprosse, C. (1986). Sexual dysfunction and signs of gynaecologic cancer. *Cancer* **57**, 1880–6.

Barbeau, L. (1969). L-Dopa therapy in Parkinson's Disease: a critical review of nine years' experience. *Canadian Medical Association Journal*, **101**, 59–68.

Brecher, E. M. (1988). *Love, Sex and Ageing*. Boston, Little Brown.

Bretschneider, J. G. & McCoy, N. L. (1988). Sexual interest and behavior in healthy 80 to 102 year olds. *Archives of Sexual Behavior*, **17**, 109–29.

Carney, A., Bancroft, J. & Mathews, A. (1978). Combination of hormones and psychological treatment for female sexual unresponsiveness: a comparative study. *British Journal of Psychiatry*, **133**, 339–46.

Cartwright, A. & Smith, C. (1988). *Elderly People: Their Medicines, and Their Doctors*. London, Routledge.

Cutler, W. B., Garcia, C. R., McCoy, N. (1987). Perimenopausal sexuality. *Archives of Sexual Behavior*, **16**, 225–34.

Damrosch, S. R. (1984). Graduate nursing students' attitudes toward sexually active older persons. *Gerontologist*, **24**, 299–302.

Davidson, J. M., Chen, J. J., Crapo, L., Gray, G. D., Greenleaf, W. J. & Catania, J. A. (1983). Hormonal changes and sexual function in ageing men. *Journal of Clinical Endocrinology*, **57**, 71–7.

Dow, M. G. T., Hart, D. M. & Forrest, C. A. (1983). Hormonal treatment of sexual unresponsiveness in postmenopausal women: a comparative study. *British Journal of Obstetrics and Gynaecology*, **90**, 361–6.

Fairburn, C. G., Dickerson, M. G. & Greenwood, J. (1983). *Sexual Problems and Their Management*. London, Churchill-Livingstone.

Fairburn, C. G., McCulloch, D. K. & Wu, F. C. W. (1982). The effects of diabetes on male sexual function. *Clinics of Endocrinology and Metabolism*, **11**, 749–68.

Fallowfield, L., Hall, A., Maguire, G. & Baum, M. (1990). Psychological outcomes of different treatment policies in women with early breast cancer outside a clinical trial. *British Medical Journal*, **301**, 575–80.

Francis, W. & Jeffcoate, T. (1966). Dyspareunia following vaginal operations. *Journal of Obstetrics and Gynaecology of the British Commonwealth*, **68**, 1–10.

George, L. K. & Weiler, S. J. (1981). Sexuality in middle and late life. *Archives of General Psychiatry*, **38**, 919–23.

Gregoire, A. (1990). Physical or psychological, an unhealthy splitting, in theory and practice. *Sexual and Marital Therapy*, **5**, 103–4.

Greengross, W. & Greengross, S. (1989). *Living, Loving, and Ageing: Sexual and Personal Relationships in Later Life*. Mitcham, Age Concern.

Hallstrom, T. (1977). Sexuality in the climacteric. *Clinics in Obstetrics and Gynaecology*, **4**, 227–39.

Hallstrom, T. & Samuelsson, S. (1990). Changes in womens' sexual desire in middle life: the longitudinal study of women in Gothenburg. *Archives of Sexual Behavior*, **19**, 259–68.

Harvey, N. S. (1988). Serial cognitive profiles in levodopa induced hypersexuality. *British Journal of Psychiatry*, **153**, 833–6.

Hawton, K. (1985). *Sex Therapy: A Practical Guide*. Oxford: Oxford University Press.

Hyppa, M., Rinne, O. K. & Sonnine, V. (1970). The activating effect of L-Dopa treatment on sexual functioning and its experimental background. *Acta Neurologica Scandinavica*, **43** (suppl. 46), 232–4.

Jensen, P., Jensen, S. B., Sorensen, P. S. et al. (1990). Sexual dysfunction in male and female patients with epilepsy: A study of 86 outpatients. *Archives of Sexual Behavior*, **19**, 1–14.

Kaas, M. J. (1978). Sexual expression of the elderly in nursing homes. *Gerontologist*, **18**, 372–8.

Kellett, J. M. (1990). Physical or psychological, time we bridge the divide. *Sexual and Marital Therapy*, **5**, 103–4.

Kellett, J. (1987). Treatment of sexual disorders; a prophylaxis for major pathology? *Journal of the Royal College of Physicians*, **21**, 58–60.

Kinsey, A. C., Pomeroy, W. B. & Martin, C. E. (1948). *Sexual Behavior in the Human Male*. Philadelphia: Saunders.

Kinsey, A. C., Pomeroy, W. B., Martin, C. E. & Gebhard, P. H. (1953). *Sexual Behavior in the Human Female*. Philadelphia: Saunders.

Masters, W. G. & Johnson, V. E. (1966). *Human Sexual Response*. London: Churchill.

Morgan, K., Dalloso, H., Ebrahim, S., Arie, T. & Fentem, P. (1988). Prevalence, frequency, and duration of hypnotic drug use among the elderly living at home. *British Medical Journal*, **296**, 601–2.

Morris, L. W., Morris, R. G. & Britton, P. G. (1988). The relationship between marital intimacy, personal strain, and depression in spouse care-giver of dementia sufferer. *British Journal of Psychiatry*, **61**, 231–6.

Murphy, E. (1982). Social origins of depression in old age. *British Journal of Psychiatry*, **141**, 135–42.

O'Brien, I., O'Hare, P. & Corrall, R. (1986). Heart rate variability in healthy subjects: effect of age and the derivation of normal ranges for tests of autonomic function. *British Heart Journal*, **53**, 348–53.

Office of Population, Census and Surveys (1992). *Population Trends*, London: OPCS.

Oram, J. J., Edwardson, J. & Millard, P. H. (1981). Investigation of cerebrospinal fluid neuropeptides in idiopathic senile dementia. *Gerontology*, **27**, 216–23.

Osborn, M., Hawton, K. & Gath, D. (1988). Sexual dysfunction among middle aged women in the community. *British Medical Journal*, **296**, 959–62.

Persson, G. (1980). Sexuality in a 70 year old urban population. *Journal of Psychosomatic Research*, **19**, 335–42.

Pfeiffer, E. & Davis, G. C. (1972). Determinants of sexual behavior in middle and old age. *Journal of the American Geriatrics Society*, **20**, 151–8.

Pfeiffer, E., Verwoerdt, A. & Wang, H. (1968). Sexual behavior in aged men and women. *Archives of General Psychiatry*, **38**, 919–23.

Reynolds, V. & Kellett, J. (1991). *Mating and Marriage*. Oxford: Oxford University Press.

Riley, A. J. (1991). Sexuality and the menopause. *Sexual and Marital Therapy*, **6**, 135–46.

Riley, A. & Riley E. (1986). The effect of single dose diazepam on female sexual response induced by masturbation. *Sexual and Marital Therapy*, **1**, 49–53.

Sherwin, B. B. & Gelfand, M. M. (1987). The role of androgen in the maintenance of sexual functioning in oopherectomized women. *Psychosomatic Medicine*, **49**, 397–409.

Spark, R. F., Wills, C. A. & Royal, H. (1984). Hypogonadism, hyperprolactinaemia and temporal lobe epilepsy in hyposexual men. *Lancet*, **i**, 413–17.

Stanley, E. (1981). Dealing with fear of failure. *British Medical Journal*, **282**, 1281–4.

Szasz, G. (1983). Sexual incidents in an extended care unit for aged men. *Journal of the American Geriatrics Society*, **31**, 407–11.

Taylor Segraves, R. (1989). Effects of psychotropic drugs on human erections and ejaculation. *Archives of General Psychiatry*, **46**, 275–84.

Vallery Masson, J., Valleron, A. & Potrenaud, J. (1981). Factors related to sexual intercourse frequency in a group of French pre-retirement managers. *Age and Ageing*, **10**, 53–9.

Weizman, R. & Hart, J. (1987). Sexual behavior in healthy married elderly men. *Archives of Sexual Behavior*, **16**, 39–44.

Weizman, A., Weizman, R., Hart, J., Maoz, B., Wijsenbeek, H. & Ben David, M. (1983). The correlation of increased serum prolactin levels with decreased sexual desire and activity in elderly men. *Journal of the American Geriatrics Society*, **31**, 485–8.

Winn, R. L. & Newton, N. (1982). Sexuality and ageing: a study of 106 cultures. *Archives of Sexual Behavior*, **11**, 283–98.

Zeiss, A. M., Davies, H. D., Wood, M. & Tinklenberg, J. R. (1990). The incidence and correlates of erectile problems in patients with Alzheimer's Disease. *Archives of Sexual Behavior*, **19**, 325–33.

Part 6

Substance use and abuse

16

Substance use and abuse

STEPHEN TICEHURST

Introduction

In recent times the abuse of substances by the elderly has received an increasing amount of interest. The impetus for this lies no doubt in the increasing numbers of elderly persons and their contacts with medical and psychiatric services. Despite this, clinicians still have a limited amount of information on which to base assessment and management plans.

The bulk of alcohol research is concerned with younger and middle aged persons. Alcohol abuse and dependence, however, in the elderly has a prevalence sufficient to warrant greater attention. It presents more often in unusual ways and to services not used to dealing with such problems. As a result, such abuse is often unrecognized and the patient falls between services when treatment is required.

Illicit substance abuse is a rarity in the elderly. This may change with the ageing of different generations over the next few decades. The 'abuse' of over the counter and prescribed medications is an emerging concern.

This chapter will summarize available information to aid physicians in their contacts with elderly substance abusers.

Alcohol

Defining the problem

There is a lack of consensus as to when a person's drinking habits become unusual, a problem, or a disease. Clarity of operational criteria may enable us to communicate better. One such attempt is in the Diagnostic and Statistical Manual (DSM-III-R) of the American Psychiatric Association (1987) which has moved away from strict physiological criteria to an acceptance that dependence causes variable levels of disability and is affected by social and psychological variables.

Dependence has behavioral components. Behaviors surrounding drug taking become more important than others previously preferred.

The following criteria (paraphrased) are offered in DSM-III-R.

Abuse

A. A maladaptive pattern of psychoactive substance use with one of:
1. continued use despite knowledge of having a persistent or recurrent social, occupational, psychological, or physical problem that is caused or exacerbated by use
2. recurrent use in hazardous situations

B. Symptoms persist for longer than a month or have occurred repeatedly over a longer period of time.

C. Never met criteria for dependence.

Dependence

At least three of the following criteria over a period of at least one month.

1. use in larger amounts or over longer time than is intended
2. persistent desire or unsuccessful attempts to cut down
3. a great deal of time spent procuring the substance or recovering from its effects
4. intoxication at times when major roles are expected to be met or when it is hazardous
5. reduced social, occupational or recreational activities
6. continued use despite persistent or recurrent related social, psychological or physical problems
7. marked tolerance
8. withdrawal
9. frequent ingestion to relieve or avoid withdrawal symptoms

Alcoholism and *addiction* are usually, but not always, used to describe dependence. Consensus has not been reached that such definitions are valid. Terminology is constantly evolving.

One effect of the lack of consensus regarding definition is the difficulty in interpreting prevalence data from studies using different concepts and rating systems. Studies of community prevalence of alcohol problems among the elderly show a range from 0.7% to 27% (Saunders et al., 1989; Bridgewater et al., 1987; Cahalan & Cisin, 1968; Edwards et al., 1973). Much of this range can be accounted for by different selection criteria concerning 'problem drinking', 'heavy drinking' and 'abuse/dependence'.

The problem of definition is compounded in the elderly because the physiological, pathological and social changes accompanying aging affect the criteria that have been adopted in younger patients. For example, work absenteeism, marital discord and driving under the influence may be less common simply because the elderly are less likely to work and drive and more likely to have lost their partners. Physiological changes in metabolism mean that a frail elderly woman drinking three sherries a day may be at more risk than a fit young man drinking six beers. Many factors have been suggested as the cause of increased physical vulnerability to alcohol in the elderly. These include: decreased body water and volume of distribution; increased neurochemical and neuronal sensitivity; changed absorption, metabolism and excretion; target organ cell loss; decreased excitatory phase with quicker entry to the sedative phase; higher peak levels; increased impairment with same blood levels; decrease in euphoric effects; decreased capacity to develop tolerance; aggravation of other illness; cognitive decline and interaction with other drugs. (Atkinson, 1987; Nordstrom & Berglund, 1987; Chiu, 1986; Ritzmann & Melchior, 1984; Drew, 1968; Jolley & Hodgson, 1985; Zimberg, 1984). Therefore, the effects of aging may mean that criteria for abuse and dependence derived from younger populations are no longer valid in the elderly. The comorbidity of age related diseases makes it more difficult to decide whether it is the alcohol abuse that is causing harm.

Difficulties in measuring the problem

Apart from the problem of definition, numerous other difficulties arise when estimating the number of elderly people with alcohol problems. Rates of recognition are lowered because older patients present in unusual ways. One clinical survey found that alcohol was recognized as a problem on admission in only half the elderly patients later found to have major alcohol difficulties (Rosin & Glatt, 1971). A general hospital study found only 37% of those over 60 with an alcohol problem were recognized by house staff. The recognition rate was 60% in those under 60 (Curtis et al., 1989). A London survey revealed under-reporting by a factor of between 4 and 9 (Edwards et al., 1973).

Elderly problem drinkers may admit to their predicament in only a half of cases (Saunders et al., 1989). For older people, particularly women, the stigma may be an important factor. Relatives can collude with attempts to hide the problem. In these cases, the relative may also abuse alcohol or simply be embarrassed.

Prevalence of alcohol abuse/dependence

Despite the difficulty of determining the extent of problem drinking in the elderly, there is agreement that increased age is associated with decreased alcohol intake. This has been found for both sexes in community, outpatient and inpatient settings (Mishara & Kastenbaum, 1980; Reifler, Raskind & Kethley, 1982; Cahalan & Cisin, 1968; Hagnall & Tunving, 1972; Myers et al., 1984).

The American Environmental Catchment Area (ECA) study found alcohol related diagnoses were less prevalent in the elderly than in younger adults. The six-month prevalence of alcohol abuse/dependence was 3–4% in men over the age of

Table 16.1. *Elderly patients with alcohol-related problems in various treatment agencies*

Type of service dealing with alcohol problems	Proportion of patients of the service who were aged over 65
Outpatient nonmedical service (open referral drug and alcohol service)	Less than 1%
Outpatient general hospital service (Medical referral needed)	12% (15/135 over 3 months)
Inpatient psychiatric hospital addiction service (open referral for admission)	5% (7/153 over 3 months)
Inpatient general hospital alcohol service (open referral of inpatients, usually by nurses)	40% (60/150 over 3 months)

Source: Ticehurst S., unpublished survey result, Newcastle, Australia.

65 and 1% in women. For men, this was the third most common psychiatric diagnosis (Myers et al., 1984). Alcohol abuse/dependence rates in the 25–44 year age group were at least three times higher than in the over 65s for both men and women.

There are differences between and within countries, but the rate remains consistently higher for men. Community studies in Great Britain have found that 3–4% of elderly persons consume alcohol at rates above those considered safe (Iliffe et al., 1991; Saunders et al., 1989).

Elderly alcohol abusers constitute a significant minority of patients in a broad range of treatment facilities. They congregate in general medical rather than psychiatric or generic alcohol treatment settings (Table 16.1). This difference may reflect the predominance of physical, rather than behavioral, complications in the elderly. Alcohol abuse has been found to be the third most common mental disorder in geriatric mental health outreach programs (Reifler et al., 1982; Wattis, 1981). In one study the local doctor was aware of the situation in only 50% of cases (Malcolm, 1984). As distinct from catchment area studies, clinical studies have often found a preponderance of females amongst elderly drinkers (Rosin & Glatt, 1971). This could represent referral bias combined with the increase in female to male ratio with age.

What causes alcohol problems in the elderly?

The problem of drug use has been seen throughout history and across cultures. Why some people *abuse* rather than *use* psychoactive substances remains a mystery. Very little light has been shed on etiology in late life. It is probable that

Table 16.2. *The indirect presentation of alcohol related problems in the elderly*

Medical	Psychological	Forensic	Social
Falls	Wernicke's delirium	Driving under the influence	Family disharmony
Incontinence	Amnesic syndrome	Offensive behavior	Presentation of a family member with depression, etc.
Seizures	Dementia	Assault	Poverty
Liver disease	Aggression	Theft	Self-neglect
Neuropathy	Disinhibition		
Exposure	Depression		
Hypertension	Attempted suicide		
Diabetes	Paranoia		
Burns	Hallucinosis		
Myopathy			
Diarrhea			
Gait abnormality			
Blackouts			
Trauma			
Leg ulcers			
Peptic disease			
Malnutrition			

alcohol abuse and dependence among the aged are related to overall use in the community. Despite this, there is strong evidence of a genetically transmitted predisposition for some individuals to becoming dependent on alcohol. This is perhaps less important in late onset cases who have lower rates of alcoholism in their families (Goodwin, 1985).

Psychosocial stressors have been posed as etiological factors in late onset cases. Retirement is probably not an epidemiological risk factor, but bereavement may be. Clinical studies suggesting a late onset type of alcoholism secondary to psychosocial stressors have not received a great deal of epidemiological support (Caracci & Miller, 1991).

Being male remains a risk factor in advanced age. Depression is a possible risk factor. About one in ten patients admitted for alcoholism will also be depressed, but which comes first is often unclear (Finlayson et al., 1988). Agoraphobia is another psychiatric illness which may predispose to abuse of alcohol.

How do alcohol problems present in the elderly?

The elderly alcohol abuser is unlikely to present directly to an alcohol unit asking for help. They come to the attention of a variety of agencies under the guise of numerous symptoms. Some of the indirect ways in which alcohol problems may present in the elderly are presented in Table 16.2. (Wattis, 1981; Glatt, 1985, Harris et al., 1987; Schuckit & Pastor, 1978).

In the general hospital, elderly alcohol abusers may present with physical signs and symptoms that do not directly point to alcohol. They can suffer a range of cognitive impairments (Wattis, 1983). Finlayson et al. (1988) found 25% of admitted elderly alcoholics to havc dementia. A review concluded that approximately 6% of elderly patients with dementia were diagnosed as suffering from alcohol related dementia (McLean, 1987). There is some evidence that alcohol is a risk factor for Alzheimer type dementia, but this remains controversial (Saunders et al., 1991). King (1986) found that in a clinic sample patients with dementia of the Alzheimer type aged over 80 were more likely to be abusing alcohol than younger patients in the same setting.

As benzodiazepine and other drug abuse also occur in the alcohol abuser (Finlayson, 1984), patients may present with problems due to mixed intoxication, drug interactions, or unrecognized combined withdrawal states. Fourteen percent of the elderly inpatients of one alcohol treatment unit were also abusing prescription medications (Finlayson et al., 1988).

Other atypical presentations include delirium occurring several days postoperatively and the 'senile recluse' or 'Diogenes' syndrome (Post, 1984).

In the psychiatric setting, elderly alcohol abusers very often present with depression (Schuckit & Pastor, 1978). Clinically significant depression in alcohol abusers may be due to a number of factors. These include reaction to the social consequences of alcohol abuse, awareness of losses, insight into one's chronic relapsing behavior and loss of control, lowered self esteem, failing physical health, or the possible toxic effects of alcohol. One longitudinal study found that previous drinking was related to the later development of depression in subjects who were no longer abusing alcohol (Saunders et al., 1991). Cook et al. (1991) found that the depression in such ex-drinkers was more likely to be of the 'neurotic – reactive' type and tended to be more chronic and of a less severe form. The elderly widower living alone is at high risk of both alcoholism and suicide (Maletta, 1982). Alcohol hallucinosis, morbid jealousy, and withdrawal states are not uncommon psychiatric manifestations of alcohol abuse and may mimic functional disorders.

Depression, confusion, and suspiciousness were the most common presenting symptoms in problem drinkers who were not recognized as such in an outreach setting (Reifler et al., 1982).

In a forensic setting, up to a third of elderly offenders may suffer from alcoholism. In one study, 20% of older offenders had been drinking at the time of the offence. This was a larger percentage than for the younger population (Taylor & Parrott, 1988). The majority of arrests of the elderly in the US were either for drunkenness or driving under the influence (Glynn et al., 1984). While other crimes decline with age, arrests for drunkenness increase.

These findings suggest that elderly alcohol abusers are likely to present their problems indirectly. Clinical suspicion must remain high when dealing with elderly patients with any of the medical, psychiatric or forensic presentations listed above and in Table 16.2. The possibility that they will be overlooked or misdiagnosed is heightened by indirect referral patterns. When they are recognized, they are often seen as somebody else's problem and may fall between services.

What is the clinical course of alcohol abuse in the elderly?

Drinking behavior is strongly influenced by cultural, ethnic, socioeconomic and geographical factors. Despite such variations, community surveys show that alcohol consumption in general moderates with age (Ticehurst, 1990). Cost and social pressures as well as the physiological changes discussed previously work towards reduced consumption. Cohorts of the future, however, may not behave in the same way as attitudes, availability and affluence change.

Little systematic study of the natural course of alcohol abuse or dependence in the elderly has been undertaken. There have been several patterns documented in younger people (Vaillant, 1983). Chronic unremitting drinkers are perhaps the least likely to survive into old age (Drew, 1968). Many younger alcohol abusers reduce their consumption as a result of the pathological effects of prolonged consumption. Some elderly people take up drinking after a break of years or months and some start de novo. Rarely, others will gradually escalate consumption in their old age.

Many patients presenting to a psychogeriatric unit do so after years of clinically 'silent drinking' when brain damage or social breakdown intervenes. This can lead to abandonment by the family or a pattern of intense ambivalence about ongoing care.

Case history

Mr P's wife cried at the family interview. 'We didn't have much of a life together.' She revealed a long pattern of heavy drinking by her husband, pathological jealousy and domestic violence. Mrs P had placed and then removed her husband from care on several occasions since he became moderately demented. She was torn between her feelings of guilt in not caring for him and her unresolved anger over his treatment of her throughout their marriage.

Assessment of elderly alcohol abusers

Assessment rests on history, mental state examination, physical examination and an evaluation of the patient's social resources. Gaining a corroborative history may be necessary to overcome memory deficits and denial. The home visit can provide information concerning alcohol consumption as well as evidence for the impact of such consumption on the patient's ability to care for themselves. The history should involve quantification of the amount and patterns of consumption. Evidence for physical and psychological dysfunction should be gathered.

A careful evaluation of the mental state can reveal underlying depression, cognitive impairment and an appreciation of the use of defence mechanisms such as denial and projection. The insight of the patient can affect approaches to therapy. Personality disturbances and paranoid disorders should be assessed.

The physical complications of the disorder may be revealed by examination.

Urine and other assays uncover denied consumption but their use is problematic because of the need for trust in the therapeutic alliance.

Inpatient admission is of use in confused patients to aid in assessment and in those patients with medical or psychiatric problems that require closer scrutiny.

Management of elderly patients who abuse substances

Although the following comments concern the treatment of alcohol abuse, the general principles are relevant for other psychoactive substances.

One focus of intervention is at the community level. The social factors which affect substance abuse include advertising, attitudes, availability, affordability and drinking patterns. Health promoting campaigns are adjuncts to financial disincentives in reducing abusive patterns.

The deleterious effects of alcohol on cognitive functioning may be ameliorated by advocating the addition of thiamine to beer and bread. Encouragement to maintain an adequate diet can also help. Social activities which do not rely on alcohol should be encouraged. It is possible that a reduction in alcohol advertising will be of benefit.

The approach to the individual patient revolves around setting achievable goals. In some patients this may be to alleviate psychiatric, social and medical factors precipitating, perpetuating or resulting from the drinking. The importance of establishing a treatment alliance cannot be overstated. This may be tenuous and cover only aspects of what the treating professional would like. It will suffer setbacks. With some patients, there will be agreement only to pursue specific goals rather than accepting that the substance abuse is the root problem. For example, a patient may be convinced that decreased consumption is worthwhile in order to reduce depressive symptoms, reduce elevated blood pressure or increase social attractiveness. The family physician may be invaluable in implementing suggested treatment strategies because of the need to develop trust over time and the probability of relapse and remission.

Some techniques useful for the individual patient include simple advice, social interventions, day centres, bereavement counselling, replacing the addiction with a nonpharmacological activity and participation in Alcoholics Anonymous and religious groups. Behavioral techniques include positive reinforcement of any step forward, problem solving techniques and cognitive therapy. Groups, preferably elder specific, provide valuable extra peer pressure. Nonconfrontational techniques are probably more acceptable to the old people.

Relatives, meals on wheels, home help and volunteer groups can all help to support the patient and encourage adherence to treatment goals.

Inpatient treatment may be an effective circuit breaker. Treatment resistant patients and those likely to suffer from severe withdrawal or major medical and psychiatric problems may also need admission. Detoxification becomes increasingly risky with age and accompanying disease. Nevertheless, nonmedical detoxification remains a valid option for selected elderly patients. Intramuscular thiamine (50–100 mg) for three days is necessary in patients with poor oral intake or confusion. Oral supplements may suffice in other patients, but glucose loads should not be given before adequate thiamine stores are ensured. Given that the half-life of benzodiazepines may be prolonged in the elderly, care should be taken that they do not accumulate. Benzodiazepine dosage should be empirically determined with the aim of reduction in distressing symptoms over a period of no more than a week. Dosage should begin as much as two-thirds lower than for a fit younger patient. One approach is to give 5 mg of diazepam and then monitor the response, particularly signs of autonomic hyperactivity. Approximately one patient in ten may develop delirium tremens two to three days after cessation of drinking. Such patients must be managed in an inpatient medical setting owing to the high mortality rate of this condition.

In general, disulfiram has not been recommended for use in the elderly. The risks involved with ingesting alcohol whilst taking the drug rise with age. Given the questions as to the efficacy of its use, these risks would weigh against its general use in late life. Disulfiram may also interact with medication commonly prescribed to the elderly such as phenytoin, anticoagulants and benzodiazepines.

Whether total abstinence or controlled drinking is the most appropriate goal is a controversial question. Longitudinal studies show that elderly patients can, and do, moderate their drinking even when their previous levels constitute abuse. However, many patients find it easier to see their abuse as a disease in which abstinence must be permanent. Those patients who present with a picture of dependence, particularly if it is longstanding, should be encouraged to accept abstinence as their goal. Patients whose drinking falls more at the abuse end of the spectrum may find controlled drinking both more acceptable and obtainable.

Involuntary treatment in institutions is sometimes available through guardianship or inebriate orders. In general, this is not found acceptable in most societies except in extreme cases. Ethical issues are often crucial in decision-making. For example, when brain damage occurs, guardianship may be invoked on the grounds that the person can no longer make an informed decision to continue drinking when it is already causing damage. The point at which it is valid to override individual rights, however, is difficult to define.

Case history

Mr E is a chronically institutionalized elderly man with minor amnestic deficits. He presented to a psychogeriatric ward after a fire had destroyed his boarding house for similarly brain-damaged drinkers. He had then been placed in a less tolerant environment where his 'wandering' was treated with three different psychotropics. He became confused. Inpatient assessment revealed minor deficits in his cognitive functioning when his delirium cleared. His family resisted his discharge, but it was felt that there were no longer any grounds to keep the patient against his will. He was discharged to another boarding house where he resumed drinking.

Institutionalization in a hostel or nursing home often provides limits to consumption that help the isolated drinker moderate or cease drinking. However, caution must be exercised that one addiction is not replaced by another to benzodiazepines. Hostels and boarding houses play an increasing role in the provision of long-term accommodation for brain-damaged alcohol abusers. The congregation of such patients is not without risk. A recent fire in such a boarding house in Australia cost the lives of 12 residents.

Even with the most diligent treatment, relapses are common. This is especially so when drinking habits are lifelong and social manipulation is not successful.

Does intervention improve the prognosis?

Evaluation of elder specific intervention is rare. The limited information which exists suggest that elderly patients do no worse with treatment than younger ones and may do better (Janik & Dunham, 1983). There have been suggestions that age specific treatment groups offer good results (Kofoed et al., 1984). Much of the research has been hampered by highly selected groups, high drop-out rates and difficulty in maintaining appropriate controls. Comorbidity with other psychiatric, personality and medical disorders also complicates the picture.

In one study of behavioral intervention, elderly patients who completed treatment did well at 12 month follow-up. However, the vast majority of referred patients either refused treatment or failed to complete the protocol (Dupree, Broskowski & Schonfeld, 1984). Those who continued in treatment were quite socially isolated, late onset drinkers, often widowed and highly motivated. Dropouts had a lower expectation of success at commencement, were more depressed, drank more and had a more external locus of control than those who stayed in treatment. One factor associated with improvement was an expansion in the social network of those who completed therapy.

Other substances

Over the counter medications

The modern pharmacy has a vast array of potentially abusable items for sale. Many elderly patients have a lifetime's experience with various purgative agents that seem to have the effect of putting their bowels to sleep. Likewise cough mixtures could theoretically be abused by the elderly. Drugs with anticholinergic effects are also potential targets of abuse. In the elderly they may cause delirium and psychotic symptoms. Two-thirds of American elders take over the counter substances and this proportion increases with age, particularly among women (Miller, 1991). Such patients do not usually present themselves to psychiatric services for treatment. The management of problems arising from over the counter medications could best be addressed by family physicians routinely inquiring about their use and providing information on the possible dangers of such substances.

Tobacco

Tobacco is probably the most commonly abused substance and a major cause of physical ill health. There are, however, few psychiatric ramifications. Elderly patients may be able to give up smoking at least as easily as younger persons, but the techniques are beyond the scope of this chapter.

Benzodiazepines

There is little doubt that these drugs have been used too commonly in old patients for insomnia and also for behavioral control in institutional settings. Their long-term use for either indication has little to recommend it.

Case history

A general practitioner's mother presented to a psychiatric hospital with delusions, hallucinations and psychomotor agitation. She was diagnosed as having a delirium. History revealed that her son had been prescribing benzodiazepines for insomnia. A circle of tolerance and increasing doses had followed. Confusion became marked and the son felt his mother was dementing. As she became more confused, she became less able to keep her benzodiazepine intake up and developed a withdrawal characterized by delirium with hallucinations and delusions. After a month in hospital she was a cognitively intact alert lady who could give little history about the preceding months.

One-quarter of elderly Americans use psychoactive medication (Beardsley et al., 1988). Salzman et al. (1992) have shown that memory impairment can improve when benzodiazepines are discontinued over two weeks in nursing home patients and that more than half of such patients remained free of the medication at 12 months.

Benzodiazepines are probably prescribed more frequently for women than men in contrast to the situation with alcohol. Rebound anxiety and insomnia can occur after very brief periods of use. Prolonged use leads to tolerance and lack of clinical efficacy. Side-effects of overuse include ataxia, drowsiness, memory impairment, depressed mood and loss of spontaneity. Home visits provide an opportunity to detect tell tale signs of multiple packets of different types of benzodiazepines from multiple doctors. Tablets left can be checked against prescription date and dosage to monitor for overuse.

Elderly patients in nursing homes are often prescribed benzodiazepines, especially if they are not demented. Dementing patients tend instead to receive antipsychotics. The reason for this is not clear.

Withdrawal of long-term benzodiazepines is problematic in the elderly. If there is dependence, inpatient treatment is preferable due to the risk of convulsions, confusional states and the length of the withdrawal. Outpatient withdrawal is best reserved for patients with short histories of use in the absence of dependence. Gradual tapering of the dose over many weeks or months may be necessary.

Doctor shopping is another problem in patients dependent on benzodiazepines. Education for doctors, nurses and patients is a vital part of a strategy for a reduction in inappropriate benzodiazepine prescription.

Other prescribed substances

Analgesics, anti-inflammatory and anti-giddiness agents can be used by patients in a manner dissimilar to that which the doctor has instructed. Sometimes this is the result of beliefs in peer groups concerning the supposed beneficial effects of particular drugs. Ongoing education is the best approach to this problem. Barbiturates have almost disappeared as substances of abuse in most countries. This provides evidence that prescription habits can change and one wonders whether the benzodiazepines are headed the same way.

Illicit drugs

The abuse of illicit drugs is a rare phenomenon amongst the elderly. The reasons for this are unclear. The trend for antisocial personality disorder to become less prevalent with advancing age may be one factor. Others include lack of availability in their social settings, expense, and the possibility that elderly persons do not seek the mind altering effects of psychoactive substances. The harmfulness of many of the drugs works against a long lifespan for chronic abusers. When it does occur it often coexists with alcohol abuse.

Conclusion

The escalating number of elderly people means that substance abuse will become more widespread. As the generation of the prohibition era are replaced by those of the 1960s and 1970s, quite different patterns of substance abuse may emerge. Recent evidence suggesting that young women are drinking larger amounts of alcohol relative to men could presage the end of male dominance amongst elderly alcohol abusers (Oppenheimer, 1991).

Even now, the extent of substance abuse in the elderly is sufficient to warrant more attention and research. The atypical presentation and high degree of missed diagnosis point to the need for heightened awareness by health professionals.

Case histories

Mrs M was drinking moderately at the club in a social setting with her husband from the age of 40 to 60. When he died suddenly she began to consume half a flagon of sherry each day. Despite this she continued to hold down a job as a manageress of a coffee lounge. Gradually it became clear to her employers that her mental abilities were declining. She was sacked for not being able to balance the books and order appropriately. As she became progressively demented in her sixties her alcohol consumption gradually declined and ceased altogether. Despite this, she continued to dement.

Mrs D was a barmaid for most of her life. She drank and swore with the men. Late in her career her memory began to fade. She developed a bizarre system of delusions concerning her past life that had a confabulatory air. She became related to the Queen, said she had been kidnapped from her harbourside hotel by the Japanese navy and parachuted with a team of commandoes, defending her suburb with a mounted machine gun. These beliefs did not respond to antipsychotics. Her abusive nature meant that she lived out her life in a psychiatric hospital.

A man in his sixties was referred by the geriatric team after their efforts to modify his drinking were unsuccessful. He had gross advanced myopathy. He violently abused anyone who attempted to counsel him and his drinking was constant. When no one could be found to obtain his alcohol, he arranged home delivery from various bottle shops. He abused the home help to the point where no volunteers could be found to clean his incontinence. Despite the destructive nature of his drinking he could not be called mentally ill under the local mental health act and he was not cognitively impaired. No intervention was found to be effective.

A 76 year old lady presented to a hospital intoxicated, needing gastric lavage. There was no past history of alcohol abuse. Investigation revealed she was dementing and that a local delinquent was using her house to store implements for housebreaking. On several occasions he had induced her to drink alcohol and try illicit drugs. Appropriate legal intervention ensured her safety and drinking was no longer a problem.

A 77 year old widow presented to a doctor with back pain. She was living in squalor, had not changed her clothes for eight weeks and all the food in the house was rotten. She was assessed by the psychiatric team who could find no evidence of mental illness, but did confirm a short term memory deficit. She was admitted to a psychogeriatric ward for investigation. Her old notes revealed an admission in her sixties for 'alcoholism'. Further inquiry revealed that she had begun drinking heavily at that time after a family dispute. This was reduced following her previous admission but she had continued to have two beers a day until this presentation. In hospital she gained weight but her memory deficit persisted.

References

American Psychiatric Association. (1987). *Diagnostic and Statistical Manual of Mental Disorders*, 3rd ed, rev. Washington DC: APA.

Atkinson, R. M. (1987). Alcohol problems of the elderly. *Alcohol and Alcoholism*, **22**, 415–17.

Beardsley, R. S., Gardocki, G. L., Larson, D. B. & Hidalgo, J. (1988). Prescribing of psychotropic medication by primary care physicians and psychiatrists. *Archives of General Psychiatry*, **45**, 1117–19.

Bridgewater, R., Leigh, S., James, O. F. W. & Potter, J. F. (1987). Alcohol consumption and dependence in elderly patients in an urban community. *British Medical Journal*, **295**, 884–5.

Cahalan, D. & Cisin, I. H. (1968). American drinking practices: Summary of findings from a national probability sample. I. Extent of drinking by population subgroups. *Quarterly Journal of Studies on Alcohol*, **29**, 130–51.

Caracci, G. & Miller, S. (1991). Epidemiology and diagnosis of alcoholism in the elderly (a review). *International Journal of Geriatric Psychiatry*, **6**, 511–15.

Chiu, E. (1986). Alcohol, drugs and the elderly. In *Proceedings of Seminars and of Scientific Sessions. Autumn School of Studies on Alcohol*, ed. J. Santamaria, Melbourne. Dept. of Community Medicine, St Vincent's Hospital.

Cook, B. L., Winokur, G., Garvey, M. & Beach, V. (1991). Depression and previous alcoholism in the elderly. *British Journal of Psychiatry*, **158**, 72–5.

Curtis, J. R., Geller, G., Stokes, E. J., Levine, D. M. & Moore, R. D. (1989). Characteristics, diagnosis, and treatment of alcoholism in elderly patients. *Journal of the American Geriatrics Society*, **37**, 310–16.

Drew, L. R. H. (1968). Alcoholism as a self-limiting disease. *Quarterly Journal Studies on Alcohol*, **29**, 956–67.

Dupree, L. W, Broskowski, H. & Schonfeld, L. (1984). The Gerontology alcohol project: A behavioral treatment program for elderly alcohol abusers. *The Gerontologist*, **24**, 510–16.

Edwards, G., Hawker, A., Hensman, C., Peto, J. & Williamson, V. (1973). Alcoholics known or unknown to agencies: epidemiological studies in a London suburb. *British Journal of Psychiatry*, **123**, 169–83.

Finlayson, R. E. (1984). Prescription drug abuse in older persons. In *Alcohol and Drug Abuse in Old Age*. ed. R. M. Atkinson, p. 61. Washington DC:American Psychiatric Press, Inc.

Finlayson, R. E., Hurt, R. D., Davis, L. J. & Morse, R. M. (1988). Alcoholism in elderly persons: a study of the psychiatric and psychological features of 216 inpatients. *Mayo Clinic Proceedings*, **63**, 761–8.

Glatt, M. M. (1985). Experiences with elderly alcoholics in England. *Alcoholism: Clinical and Experimental Research*, **2**, 23–6.

Glynn, R. J., Bouchard, G. R., LoCastro, J. S. & Hermos, J. A. (1984). Changes in alcohol consumption behaviors among men in the normative ageing study. In *Nature and Extent of Alcohol Problems Among the Elderly*, ed. G. Maddox, L. N. Robins & N. Rosenberg N., New York: Springer.

Goodwin, D. W. (1985). Alcoholism and geriatrics: the sins of the father. *Archives of General Psychiatry*, **42**, 171–4.

Hagnall, O. & Tunving, K. (1972). Prevalence and nature of alcoholism in a total population. *Social Psychiatry*, **7**, 190–201.

Harris, M., Sutherland, D., Cutter, G. & Ballangarry, L. (1987). Alcohol related hospital admissions in a country town. *Australian Drug and Alcohol Review*, **6**, 195–8.

Iliffe S., Haines A., Booroff A., Goldenberg E., Morgan P. & Gallivan S. (1991). Alcohol consumption by elderly people: A general practice survey. *Age and Ageing*, **20**, 120–3.

Janik, S. W. & Dunham, R. G. (1983). A nationwide examination of the need for specific alcoholism treatment programs for the elderly. *Journal of Studies on Alcohol*, **44**, 307–17.

Jolley, D. & Hodgson, S. (1985). Alcoholism in the elderly: a tale of women and our times. In *Recent Advances in Geriatric Medicine* (3rd ed). B. Isaacs, pp. 113–122. Edinburgh: Churchill Livingstone.

King, M. B. (1986). Alcohol abuse and dementia. *International Journal of Geriatric Psychiatry*, **1**, 31–6.

Kofoed, L. L., Tolson, R. L., Atkinson, R. M., Turner, J. A. & Toth, R. F. (1984). Elderly groups in an alcoholism clinic. In *Alcohol and Drug Abuse in Old Age*, ed. R. M. Atkinson, pp. 35–60. Washington DC: American Psychiatric Press, Inc.

Malcolm, M. T. (1984). Alcohol and drug use in the elderly visited at home. *The International Journal of the Addictions*, **19**, 411–18.

Maletta, G. J. (1982). Alcoholism in the aged. In *Encyclopedic Handbook of Alcoholism*, ed. E. M. Pattison & E. Kaufman, pp. 779–791. New York: Gardner Press.

McLean, S. (1987). Assessing dementia. Part I. Difficulties, definitions and differential diagnosis. *Australian and New Zealand Journal of Psychiatry*, **21**, 142–74.

Miller, N. S. (1991). Alcohol and drug dependence. In *Comprehensive Review of Geriatric Psychiatry*, ed. J. Sadavoy, L. W. Lazarus & L. Jarvik, pp. 387–401. Washington: American Psychiatric Press, Inc.

Mishara, B. L. & Kastenbaum, R. (1980). *Alcohol and Old Age*. New York: Grune and Stratton.

Myers, J. K., Weissman, M. M., Tischler, G. L. et al. (1984). Six-month prevalence of psychiatric disorders in three communities. *Archives of General Psychiatry*, **41**, 959–70.

Nordstrom, G. & Berglund, M. (1987). Ageing and recovery from alcoholism. *British Journal of Psychiatry*, **151**, 382–8.

Oppenheimer, E. (1991). Alcohol and drug misuse among women – An overview. *British Journal of Psychiatry*, **158** (suppl. 10), 36–44.

Post, F. (1984). Schizophrenic and paranoid psychoses. In *Handbook of Studies on Psychiatry of Old Age*, ed. D. W. Kay & G. D. Burrows. Amsterdam: Elsevier.

Reifler, B., Raskind, M. & Kethley, A. (1982). Psychiatric diagnoses among geriatric patients seen in an outreach program. *Journal of the American Geriatrics Society*, **30**, 530–33.

Ritzmann, R. F. & Melchior, C. L. (1984). Age and development of tolerance to and physical dependence on alcohol. In *Alcoholism in the Elderly*, eds. J. T. Hartford and T. Samorajski, pp.117–138. New York: Raven Press.

Rosin, A. J. & Glatt, M. M. (1971). Alcohol excess in the elderly. *Quarterly Journal of Studies on Alcohol*, **32**, 53–9.

Salzman, C., Fisher, J., Nobel, K., Glassman, R., Wolfson, A. & Kelley, M. (1992). Cognitive impairment following benzodiazepine discontinuation in elderly nursing home residents. *International Journal of Geriatric Psychiatry*, **7**, 89–93.

Saunders, P. A, Copeland, J. R. M., Dewey, M. E. et al. (1991). Heavy drinking as a risk factor for depression and dementia in elderly men. Findings from the Liverpool longitudinal community study. *British Journal of Psychiatry*, **159**, 213–16.

Saunders, P. A., Copeland, J. R. M., Dewey, M. E. et al. (1989). Alcohol use and abuse on the elderly: findings from the Liverpool longitudinal study of continuing health in the community. *International Journal of Geriatric Psychiatry*, **4**, 103–8.

Schuckit, M. A. & Pastor, P. A. (1978). The elderly as a unique population: alcoholism. *Alcoholism: Clinical and Experimental Research*, **2**, 31–8.

Taylor, P. J. & Parrott, J. M. (1988). Elderly offenders. *British Journal of Psychiatry*, **152**, 340–6.

Ticehurst, S. (1990). Alcohol and the elderly. *Australian and New Zealand Journal of Psychiatry*, **24**, 252–60.

Vaillant, G. E. (1983). *The Natural History of Alcoholism*. Cambridge: Harvard University Press.

Wattis, J. P. (1981). Alcohol problems in the elderly. *Journal of the American Geriatrics Society*, **24**, 131–4.

Wattis, J. P. (1983). Alcohol and old people. *British Journal of Psychiatry*, **143**, 306–7.

Zimberg, S. (1984). Diagnosis and management of the elderly alcoholic. In *Alcohol and Drug Abuse in Old Age*, ed. R. M. Atkinson, pp. 23–34. Washington D. C.: American Psychiatric Press, Inc.

Part 7

Schizophrenia and related psychoses

17

The elderly with schizophrenia

HEINZ HÄFNER MARTIN HAMBRECHT

Historical developments

Several factors have contributed to a growing interest and concern for elderly individuals with a history of schizophrenia. Demographic changes in an aging society as well as the reduced hospital mortality of schizophrenic patients, once at a very high risk especially for tuberculosis, have enabled an increasing number of these persons to become of age. Due to more active strategies in treatment and rehabilitation, such as effective control of productive symptomatology by antipsychotic medication as well as the provision of outpatient and complementary facilities, the duration of inpatient stay has dramatically decreased. Thus, individuals with a history of schizophrenia have become more visible in the community. Extensive long-term follow-up research has revitalized therapeutic activity and optimism even for the chronically hospitalized, because the outcome of schizophrenia was found to be more favorable than expected. '*It is worth trying to help schizophrenics*' (Bleuler, 1974) once thought to suffer from a disease process inevitably leading to dementia.

Epidemiology of the elderly with schizophrenia

The incidence of schizophrenia in the elderly (i.e. onset of the disorder after age 65) is considered to approximate zero if the frequent paranoid states in the elderly, organic psychoses and similar delusional disorders without first-rank symptoms of schizophrenia are carefully ruled out (Bleuler, 1972; Huber, Gross & Schüttler, 1979).

Community studies on the prevalence of schizophrenia among the elderly (Krauss, 1989) have found rates ranging from 0.1% to 1.7%. For an overall estimate of the prevalence, some of these figures are possibly too low, because many chronic patients live quite adapted in homes and most prevalence studies did not include individuals in residential care.

A review of true prevalence studies assessing individuals with schizophrenia aged 60 and over, living in the community or in institutions (Neugebauer, 1980) yielded rates between 0.00% and 2.22% with a median of 0.32%, but most studies only included acute cases and no residual states. These estimates, therefore, are conservative, too.

The hospital prevalence of schizophrenia in elderly psychiatric patients depends highly on mental health policy and the utilization pattern of psychiatric institutions and services. The rate is still high in many countries although decreasing in recent years. In the 1960s, the hospital prevalence was 60% in the USA (Reddick, Kramer & Taube, 1973) decreasing to 44% in the 1980s (Goodman & Siegel, 1986). In the Rhineland county of West Germany about 35% of psychiatric inpatients over 60 years have a diagnosis of schizophrenia (Landschaftsverband Rheinland, 1989).

Long-term course of schizophrenia

Five extensive follow-up studies have investigated the long-term course of schizophrenia. The three European studies were conduced at Lausanne (Ciompi & Müller, 1976), Zurich (M. Bleuler, 1972) and Bonn (Huber et al., 1979). The two American studies were carried out in Iowa (Tsuang, Woolson & Fleming, 1979) and in Vermont (Harding et al., 1987). The mean length of the follow-up in these studies varied between 22.4 years (Bonn) and almost 37 years (Lausanne).

In spite of several methodological shortcomings, in particular, regarding representativeness and diagnostic inclusion criteria, the principal results of these studies have very much in common and contradict the Kraepelinian assumption that schizophrenia is usually a progressive disease leading to an increasingly severe dementia. The rates of full remission or mild residual states at follow-up were very similar in the three European studies and ranged from 53% (Zurich) to 59% (Lausanne). One half to two-thirds of the Vermont patients (Harding et al., 1987) that formerly had been selected from the long-stay wards of the state hospital for chronicity, had achieved considerable improvement or recovered, depending on the areas of outcome considered, such as work performance, social relationships, symptoms, and hospitalizations.

The European studies also indicate that several years after onset, two-thirds of schizophrenics reach a certain stability and nearly one-third recover. In 73% of the Bonn cases, psychopathology remained stable from 5 years after first hospitalization onwards. A stabilising effect of age on symptomatology was discerned only after age 50. In most cases, acute psychosis transformed to residual syndromes by mid-life or even in earlier years.

Huber et al. (1979) concluded from their follow-up data that schizophrenia tends to develop into a certain stage and to remain relatively stable or to show a remission from a characteristic schizophrenic disorder to more or less uncharacteristic syndromes. Even very chronic patients exhibit fluctuations in their condition, sometimes manifesting sudden improvements in psychopathology. The cause of improvement, however, is an enigma in many cases (Janzarik, 1959; Bleuler, 1974).

In Zurich, Bleuler (1972) also observed that, within the last 5 years of the 23-year follow-up about one-third of the patients clearly improved, while in only 5% the condition became worse. Bleuler speculates that aging as well as moving to other institutions and new active treatment methods might have brought about the change.

The social outcome, however, is unsatisfying in a number of cases. In the Bonn study, 25% of the patients were unable and 20% only partly able to support themselves at follow-up and 13% were chronically hospitalized. In the Zurich study, 22.5% of the patients were hospitalized (10% chronically in mental hospitals), while 50% were living independently in the community supporting themselves (Bleuler, 1972). The Iowa study (Tsuang et al., 1979) like many others discerned a considerably worse outcome of schizophrenia on several psychosocial criteria compared to affective psychoses.

Age at onset of schizophrenia and outcome in old age

Symptomatology and course of schizophrenia differ in several aspects between patients with an onset before and after the age of 40. The ABC-Schizophrenia-Study (Häfner et al., 1993), investigating a large representative sample of first admissions with a diagnosis of schizophrenia or related disorders found a higher prevalence of paranoid delusions in (predominantly female) schizophrenics with late onset. Female patients with late onset had an unexpectedly long period of negative symptomatology prior to first hospitalization – probably a predictor for chronicity. From their comprehensive literature review on late-onset schizophrenia, Harris and Jeste (1988) draw conclusions that corroborate the findings of the ABC-Study: schizophrenia with an onset after age 40 is characterized by paranoid symptomatology, high female-male ratio, schizoid or paranoid premorbid personality traits, and a higher risk for a chronic course.

The predictive quality of the age at onset on later outcome is, however, controversial. While Harris & Jeste (1988) concluded a tendency towards chronicity in late-onset schizophrenia from their review, Ciompi & Müller (1976) and Huber et al. (1979) found no correlation between age at onset and late-life outcome. In the Lausanne Study, a 'personality factor' (i.e. premorbid personality traits, adjustment, professional and marital status, accomplishment of vocational training) as well as type of onset and course, length of first hospitalization and productive symptomatology were predictive for the outcome up to old age. The Zurich study, in contrast, only found a loose connection between premorbid personality disorders and outcome of schizophrenia (Bleuler, 1972).

While the long-term outcomes in psychopathology of early and late onset schizophrenia appear to converge (Ciompi & Müller, 1976; Huber et al., 1979), the social outcome might be different in old age because late-onset patients usually have achieved a certain stability of social status and living conditions when they are affected by the disorder for the first time. In contrast, early-onset patients suffer earlier in life the breaks in their social biography that frequently happen during the early course of the disorder. The ABC-Schizophrenia-Study (Häfner et al., 1993) showed that more than three-quarters of first admitted schizophrenics had already suffered such breaks in their social career prior to first hospitalization.

Symptomatology of the elderly with schizophrenia

The Lausanne study (Ciompi & Müller, 1976) was the only follow-up study that solely included patients aged 65 and older (289 cases). This study, therefore, provides the most solid data base on schizophrenia in the elderly. Possible geriatric conclusions from the Bonn, Zurich, Iowa and Vermont studies (Huber et al., 1979; Bleuler, 1972; Tsuang et al., 1979; Harding et al., 1987) are limited, because these studies were more interested in the long-term course and neither investigated nor reported the specific condition of the elderly in their samples (only one-tenth of the Bonn sample, about one-third of the Zurich sample and less than half of the Iowa and Vermont cases were 65 years or older). The studies, however, yielded similar results. Symptomatology and social functioning are very heterogeneous in old people with a history of schizophrenia. Besides remissions, the most common symptomatology is a nonspecific residual state with predominantly nonproductive/negative symptomatology, i.e. indifference, abulia, withdrawal, negativism, mutism, mannerisms, and stereotypies, but rarely delusions or hallucinations. Persisting or reappearing paranoid symptomatology and cognitive decline are associated with emerging sensory deficits (Cooper & Curry, 1976).

In the Zurich study, the residual states were rated as very severe in 24%, moderately severe in 24%, and mild in 33%, while 20% of the cases were considered as fully remitted. Bleuler (1972) describes a shift from severe to milder residual states from the 1940s to the 1960s.

Negative symptoms accounted for most of the psychopathology in the Vermont study (Harding et al., 1987) which included 82 patients diagnosed as schizophrenic in the mid 1950s and rediagnosed according to DSM-III criteria. The study found negative symptoms in 18% and positive symptoms of schizophrenia in 10% of the cases upon follow-up. No psychiatric symptoms were seen in 45% and symptoms of alcoholism, affective, or organic disorders dominated in the rest of the sample.

Subtypes that once could be differentiated in schizophrenic conditions become quite equalized. Aging results in general calming-down and improvement or, if schizophrenic symptoms persist, in unspecific and flattened states (Ciompi & Müller, 1976). Nevertheless, these negative symptoms are quite specific to patients with schizophrenia, can be distinguished from senile dementia (see below), and are not a result of the normal aging process (Meeks & Walker, 1990).

In summary, aging is characterized by a reduction of positive symptoms and a trend towards undifferentiation of negative symptoms. If positive symptoms persist, they become less influential on daily functioning. Patients get subjectively more relaxed and socially better adapted. Impulsive acts and hallucinations will be rarer, and some patients use 'amnesia' for psychotic episodes as a coping strategy. The frequency of acute episodes also diminishes.

The Lausanne Study (Ciompi & Müller, 1976) describes this general trend as a pacification in elderly schizophrenics. The initial symptoms of schizophrenia had vanished in 62% of the sample, were milder in 11% and unchanged or stronger in 20% of the cases. An initial presence of stupor, anxiety, or excitement was related to a better long-term prognosis, whereas social withdrawal, emotional indifference, delusions, and hallucinations predicted poorer outcome.

While positive symptoms are reduced or better integrated into daily living, negative symptoms, in contrast, show a tendency towards chronicity, although unexpected improvements in later years are observed (Janzarik; 1959, 1968).

While new positive symptoms rarely develop in elderly patients with a long history of schizophrenia, negative symptoms such as indifference, abulia, thought disturbance, stereotypical behaviors, mutism, or negativism may occasionally emerge as new symptoms in late-life. These symptoms, however, almost always remain within the frame of the preexisting more or less nonspecific residual state. The rarity of new events is demonstrated by Ciompi & Müller's (1976) showing not one single case where a truly new symptom did appear in late life.

Symptomatology affects the social course of schizophrenia in the elderly, in particular, the negative syndrome, when accompanied by social withdrawal, loneliness, isolation, and dependency on others. The reduction of and better coping with positive symptoms, on the other hand, foster social adjustment in elderly schizophrenics who experience less conflicts in the social field. The chronicity and social consequences of negative symptomatology, however, reduce the quality of life in the majority of elderly schizophrenics. In the Lausanne Study (Ciompi & Müller, 1976), their overall wellbeing (as a combined measure of psychopathology and social outcome) was rated as good or satisfying in only one-third, while two-thirds of the patients were found to experience a moderate or bad quality of life.

Diagnostic problems in the elderly with schizophrenic disorders

Although Chapter 18 is devoted to the discussion of late-onset paranoid disorders, the diagnostic and nosological differentiation of delusional disorders in the elderly cannot be omitted in this description of schizophrenia in the elderly, since paranoid states, paranoid reactions and paraphrenias are quite frequent in old age and differentiation from schizophrenia may sometimes be a problem.

The diagnosis of schizophrenia is feasible when marked positive symptoms (in particular, the Schneiderian first-rank symptoms) and the characteristic negative syndrome pattern are present, fulfilling the criteria of an ICD-10 or DSM-III-R diagnosis of schizophrenia in a person with clear consciousness when organic causes are ruled out. In residual states, a careful psychiatric history and, in particular, the evaluation of negative symptoms, supported, for instance, by the Scale for the Assessment of Negative Symptoms (SANS) of Andreasen (1982), are helpful (Meeks & Walker, 1990; Meeks, 1990).

Among the schizophrenic spectrum disorders, 'late paraphrenia' is the most relevant differential diagnosis in the elderly. Paraphrenia (Kraepelin, 1919) is characterized by systematized, mostly paranoid delusions that far exceed other clinical features while clearcut negative symptoms are absent. Kraepelin coined this term in contrast to the typical schizophrenic 'dementia praecox' because patients with paraphrenia did not show progressive deterioration of mental functioning.

Roth (1955) readopted the term to describe a syndrome pattern frequently found in patients with a late onset of a delusional/schizophrenic disorder. Although in late paraphrenia delusions and hallucinations are common, most patients show a far better preseveration of social and emotional functioning than younger schizophrenics with a characteristic positive and negative symptomatology.

A descriptive study of 47 nonrepresentative cases of paranoid psychosis with an onset after age 60 by Holden (1987) found paraphrenia to be a heterogeneous syndrome giving the appearance of a spectrum of overlapping conditions with paranoid delusions. As a consequence, 'confusion over terms such as late-onset schizophrenia, paraphrenia, late paraphrenia, and paranoid states has persisted to this date' (Harris & Jeste, 1988, p.40). A lack of population-based and systematically analysed data is obvious, and long-term epidemiological studies are also necessary in order to differentiate paraphrenia and paranoid schizophrenia reliably or to prove the existence of a continuum of delusional psychoses.

Uncertainty about valid diagnostic criteria for late paraphrenia limits the value of investigations such as a recent admission study by Pitt (1990), who found paraphrenia to be the most frequent 'schizophrenic' condition with an onset after age 65. The question whether paraphrenia is a subtype of schizophrenia or a distinct disease entity remains to be answered (Harris & Jeste, 1988). An even selection-biased neuropsychiatric study by Miller et al. (1986) advocates the view that paraphrenia might rather be an organic syndrome because it was accompanied by neurological deficits in all of the few presented cases. These patients apparently belong to a subgroup. Two probable subtypes were identified in a sample of 48 patients with late paraphrenia (Förstl et al., 1991), where patients without first-rank symptoms showed significantly more cortical atrophy in cranial computed tomography than patients with first-rank symptoms.

Biological influences on schizophrenia in the elderly

Aging is a biological process that influences the course of a preexisting schizophrenic disorder in various ways: Decreasing drive and generally calmed-down temperament might mitigate affective involvement in the schizophrenic process as described in the Lausanne study (Ciompi & Müller, 1976). Sensory impairments, especially hearing losses, lead to a higher susceptibility to delusional disorders in old people with no psychiatric history. Impaired hearing or vision might also result in an exacerbation of preexisting schizophrenia.

Severe medical illnesses sometimes mitigate the course of schizophrenia or even bring about improvement of psychopathology (Bleuler, 1972; Ciompi & Müller, 1976).

The relationship between schizophrenia and dementia was a major focus of schizophrenia research in the elderly. Kraepelin postulated 'dementia' to be mandatory in the schizophrenic disease process and did not differentiate between dementia caused by organic brain dysfunctions and the 'defect syndrome of dementia praecox' (the cognitive and social deficits due to schizophrenia) in his early writings (1896). Riemer (1950), in contrast, was convinced that schizophrenics cannot become demented in the same way as patients suffering from Alzheimer's disease or other types of brain atrophy.

Because frequent symptoms of schizophrenia (mostly negative symptoms, formal thought disturbances, etc.) are cognitive, the diagnosis of a dementia in chronically ill schizophrenic patients is difficult. The usual test batteries for assessing dementia in the general population might not differentiate sufficiently. Case examples illustrate that pseudodementia might be present not only in depression but also in schizophrenia (Wright & Silove, 1988).

In the large Lausanne sample, clinicians rated the presence and severity of dementia in elderly schizophrenic patients (Ciompi & Müller, 1976). Severe degrees of dementia were observed in 8% of the cases, moderate or mild forms in 17% and 35%, while 23% of the patients were without any signs of dementia, but frequent association of dementia with an unfavorable outcome of schizophrenia reported in this study easily could be a selection artefact.

Not only clinical ratings but also structured dementia assessment scales demonstrate that cognitive impairments are more frequent in elderly schizophrenic outpatients than in the general elderly population (Cohen et al., 1988), but the power of discrimination between signs of a defect syndrome and a beginning of dementia is still weak with all the dementia scales presently in use. It has therefore not been determined whether the higher susceptibility for cognitive decline among groups of aging schizophrenic patients is part of the psychosis itself, a byproduct of psychosocial factors (like social isolation and lack of intellectual stimulation), or an ongoing dementia, independent from schizophrenia. Benos (1984) reported marked psychopathometric differences between elderly schizophrenics, younger schizophrenics, and organic syndromes. Ciompi & Müller (1976) found all combinations of severity between the cognitive deficits and schizophrenia but concluded an independence of the two syndromes. In theoretical terms this assumption is likely but not yet proven.

Cognitive deficits in most elderly schizophrenics indeed seem to exhibit a certain pattern differing from organic syndromes of dementia. According to Cohen et al. (1988), cognitive impairments in elderly patients with schizophrenia particularly concern initiation, flexibility and memory, while attention, construction and conceptualization appear relatively unaffected.

Causes of death in patients with schizophrenia

Few specific factors have been identified determining the risk of fatalities in schizophrenic patients: suicide, infectious diseases, complications of acute states like fatal catatonia, and accidents. Sudden deaths of unknown cause are also more prevalent in schizophrenic patients than in the general population.

In the Bonn study, 25% of the patients who had died during the follow-up period (mean: 22.3 years) committed suicide (Huber et al., 1976). Suicide is more frequent in younger and middle-aged schizophrenics (Allebeck, Varla & Wistedt, 1986), but the long-term follow-ups have shown that chronic and elderly patients with schizophrenia still are at a higher risk for suicide than the general population (Ciompi & Müller, 1976; Bleuler, 1972).

Tuberculosis was a major cause of death in schizophrenic patients until the 1970s. While earlier speculations about the reasons for this excess mortality concerned the lean, often asthenic constitution ('leptosomal type' according to E. Kretschmer) of schizophrenic patients, it is now accepted that bad hygiene and very close physical contact in mental hospitals and in many families with a schizophrenic member led to an elevated risk of infection.

The incidence of tuberculosis and other severe infectious diseases decreased during the last decades. In the Lausanne sample, first hospitalized in the first half of the century, the risk for lethal tuberculosis was fourfold in male patients and twofold in female patients compared to the general population (Ciompi & Müller,

1976). The Zurich sample, first admitted in 1942/43, already included less cases with tuberculosis, although the rate was still higher than in the general population (Bleuler, 1972). The Bonn study, a follow-up of first admissions between 1945 and 1959, does not report a higher relative risk for tuberculosis in schizophrenic patients (Huber et al., 1979).

In fatal catatonia, death is caused by complications including infections, dehydration and other metabolic disturbances. Fatal catatonia, however, is extremely rare in the elderly and therefore considered irrelevant as a cause of death in this group of patients.

Accidents and hidden suicides certainly represent some of the relatively frequent undetermined deaths in schizophrenic patients. Elderly patients with schizophrenia undergo more lethal accidents than younger schizophrenics and the general elderly population (Allebeck et al., 1986). Motor vehicle and home accidents are significantly more frequent in elderly schizophrenics (Edlund, Conrad & Morris, 1989).

Pharmacotherapy

In patients of any age, neuroleptics have been shown to control schizophrenic symptomatology effectively, especially positive symptoms (agitation, delusions and hallucinations) while pharmacotherapy is usually less successful in treating negative symptoms, residual states and chronic paranoid states. Elderly patients often receive higher doses of neuroleptics than needed for maintenance therapy, although this medication is more difficult to use in the elderly (Raskind & Risse, 1986; Rosen, Bohon & Gershon, 1990). A clear positive response is less likely to occur, especially in underlying dementia, and there is a higher incidence of adverse effects of neuroleptic medication in the elderly even at lower dosage levels. Excessive sedation, syncope and falls secondary to orthostatic hypotension, urinary retention, constipation and ileus, impaired visual accommodation and dry mouth, disorientation and occasional delirium, as well as movement disorders, especially tardive dyskinesia are more frequent in elderly patients. The risk for tardive dyskinesia (TD) (involuntary movements appearing late in neuroleptic treatment) increases dramatically with age. Under age 40, about 5% of patients treated with neuroleptics develop TD; beyond age 60, the prevalence of TD is 35% (Kane et al., 1986) but the rate of 1–5% of spontaneous TD in old people never exposed to neuroleptic treatment has to be deducted from this figure. Tan & Tay (1991), Woerner et al. (1991), and Baldessarini (1988) report the same age effect and similar high rates of TD in elderly with schizophrenia. The risk for TD in the elderly seems to be associated with length of treatment, female sex, Eurasian race (vs. Chinese or Indian), and with cognitive impairment and negative symptoms (Kane & Smith, 1982; Tan & Tay, 1991; Karson et al., 1990).

Akathisia is another probably age-related adverse effect of neuroleptics with a high prevalence in schizophrenic patients and was present in 32.5% of schizophrenic inpatients according to Sandyk & Kay (1990).

Because of the higher risk for adverse effects in the elderly, 'dosage of an antipsychotic should start low and the dose should be titrated gradually upwards until either therapeutic effect is reached or adverse effects become significant' (Raskind & Risse, 1986).

Electroconvulsive therapy

Age itself is no contraindication for electroconvulsive therapy (ECT). Due to relatively poor results of ECT in schizophrenia and because of a higher incidence of medical and neurological problems in the elderly, ECT is used in the treatment of elderly patients with schizophrenia only in very exceptional cases (Huang et al., 1989; Benbow, 1991).

Social situation and social management

The ABC-Schizophrenia-Study (Häfner et al., 1993), a large-scale epidemiological investigation of a representative sample of 267 schizophrenic patients, found a high prevalence of social withdrawal, loneliness, single marital status, unemployment and lack of a stable income in schizophrenics prior to first admission in the early course of the disease. These conditions are also characteristic for the social situation of many elderly nonschizophrenics. Schizophrenia and old age therefore both are conditions with an increased risk for social isolation and declining social status, and in elderly schizophrenics the two risk factors are combined. The consequences of these social stresses largely depend on the social structure and the availability of social and economic support in a society, on cultural norms, and on the individual living conditions of the elderly.

Social relations and social behaviors often demonstrate the schizophrenic patient's deficits more sensitively than pure psychopathology, although symptomatology and social biography are interdependent. Meeks (1990), for example, observed that negative symptoms were strongly related to daily functioning while positive symptoms were not. The Lausanne study (Ciompi & Müller, 1976) found 57% of the elderly patients living in peaceful social relations with few conflicts, but in spite of this 72% were socially withdrawn and 65% depending on others. The Vermont study (Harding et al., 1987) yielded more positive results, but the sample was younger and the patients (once included because of severe signs of chronicity) all had completed a comprehensive program of rehabilitation: About two-thirds of the patients met with friends at least every two weeks, led moderate to very full lives, or had one or more moderately to very close friends. Eighty percent were able to meet basic needs.

Elderly patients with schizophrenia require a variety of services – in many cases more than young schizophrenics. These services have to be adapted to the individual needs of the patients and may include housing, custodial care, assistance in everyday needs and activities, occupational therapy or simply control of medication. The living conditions of elderly patients with a history of schizophrenia are quite variable and have considerably changed in recent years. In the Lausanne study, 26% of elderly schizophrenics lived with their families, 17% in homes for elderly citizens, 13% individually, but about 40% were hospitalized (Ciompi & Müller, 1976).

Deinstitutionalization of the chronic mentally ill was the principal social policy issue in psychiatry all over the world during the last 20 years. Much effort was put into discharging these (mostly schizophrenic) patients to families, rest homes, or individual housing projects and this was possible due to effective medication, improved funding, and the 'natural course' of the disorder, i.e. the reduction of symptoms with increasing age leading to remission in some cases and permitting community placement in many others.

The assumption that paranoid schizophrenics remain longer in the hospital than nonparanoid schizophrenics could not be supported (Goodman & Siegel, 1986). Careful reevaluation of diagnoses revealed that patients with chronic undifferentiated schizophrenia have poorer outcomes and are hospitalized for longer.

The possibility to discharge long-term hospitalized patients is not unlimited. Chances for discharge from inpatient treatment are determined by behavioral conduct (particularly assaultiveness and wandering) and cognitive functioning and not by presence or absence of delusions (Moak, 1990), although a diagnosis of schizophrenia is less common among elderly offenders with psychiatric disorders (Taylor & Parrott, 1988). Discharge from long-term custodial care units is easier for those patients who have a guardian and good financial assets.

Intermediate care facilities, like nursing homes, special care units or other long-term care institutions, have been established for those patients who do not need permanent custodial care but are unable to live by themselves in the community. A well-developed network of community based complementary facilities permits service of the individual needs and abilities of patients according to their level of mental and social functioning. Prior to these efforts, within the dichotomy of hospital-care versus self-care in the community, the options in the rehabilitation of chronic elderly inpatients were limited and individuals were too often misplaced in sometimes remote settings that either demanded too much or not enough from them. Nevertheless, a hardcore of extremely challenging geriatric patients is likely to remain in the mental hospitals and some locked facilities will still be needed in the future.

Stress on carers

Long-term follow-up research (presented above) has shown that symptomatology tends to calm down and social adjustment may even increase as schizophrenics grow old. In many cases, episodes of acute psychosis become less frequent and prodromal symptoms of exacerbation are detected earlier. During the previous course of the disorder, patients as well as family and mental health professionals have learnt to cope better with an upcoming crisis. Worsening can often be inhibited by an early intervention with anti-psychotic medication, by individual, family or social support, and by relief of current stress. The majority of elderly patients with schizophrenia, therefore, are easier to manage and care for than other elderly psychiatric groups, especially those with dementia.

Some residual syndromes, however, have a high prevalence of negative symptoms such as self-neglect, withdrawal, or lack of drive which tend to resist active treatment, even with high personal involvement as in psychotherapeutic interventions. Therapeutic efforts in these conditions have to be well adjusted to the individual needs of the patient and require good knowledge of the patient's psychiatric history, social biography and the present social background in order to avoid relapse because of stress, destabilization or loss of support. As one example, the unprepared intrahospital relocation of chronic elderly patients from larger to less spacious, smaller wards significantly increased behavior problems such as aggressiveness or medication refusal (Lichtenberg & McGrogan, 1989).

Research perspectives

Future research on schizophrenia in the elderly has to address a spectrum of questions most of which have been covered in this chapter. Mental health policy in a society with a growing portion of elderly citizens has a need for knowledge of true prevalence and incidence rates of mental disorders in this group. Valid diagnostic criteria are necessary prerequisites not only for this purpose, in particular in the schizophrenia – paranoia – late paraphrenia spectrum. The assessment of signs of dementia in elderly schizophrenics is another relevant issue. More effective therapies, especially pharmacotherapy with less side-effects, are urgently needed in the treatment of the frequent delusional disorders in the elderly.

To answer these and other important questions, will require several methods of psychiatric research. The identification of common and differing symptoms in schizophrenia and paranoid syndromes in the elderly plays a central role. The epidemiological distribution of common and specific signs and symptoms should be investigated together with the related risk factors. Neuroimaging may help to differentiate schizophrenic syndromes from organic brain disorders.

Epidemiology should provide sufficiently large and representative samples for establishing systematic long-term follow-up studies to assess course and outcome of these disorders and the stability or change of the syndromes in old age. The influence of ageing on symptomatology and its course over time should be followed prospectively, as well as the consequences of the disorder on social competence and the quality of life in schizophrenic patients as they become older.

Postmortem studies will be another promising approach if a standardized clinical assessment before death is related to neuropathology after death in order to investigate the specific brain morphology in carefully characterized functional psychoses. Förstl et al. (1992) have successfully applied the strategy in a prospective study with Alzheimer's disease. Other examples for research with autopsy material are the measurement of central catecholamine concentrations and their relation to symptomatology, cognitive functioning, and other variables assessed before death (Bridge et al., 1987) and receptor binding studies in schizophrenia (Hashimoto et al., 1991).

References

Allebeck, P., Varla, A. & Wistedt, B. (1986). Suicide and violent death among patients with schizophrenia. *Acta Psychiatrica Scandinavica*, **74**, 43–9.

Andreasen, N. C. (1982). Negative symptoms in schizophrenia. Definition and reliability. *Archives of General Psychiatry*, **39**, 784–8.

Baldessarini, R. J. (1988). A summary of current knowledge of tardive dyskinesia. *Encephale*, 14 (Spec. No.), 263–8.

Benbow, S. M. (1991). ECT in late life. Special issue: Affective disorders in old age. *International Journal of Geriatric Psychiatry*, **6**, 401–6.

Benos, J. (1984). Psychopathometrische Querschnittsuntersuchung bei chronischen Schizophrenen im Alter. *Fortschritte der Neurologie und Psychiatrie*, **52**, 223–36.

Bleuler, M. (1972). *Die schizophrenen Geistesstörungen im Lichte langjähriger Kranken- und Familiengeschichten*. Stuttgart: Thieme.

Bleuler, M. (1974). The long-term course of the schizophrenic psychoses. *Psychological Medicine*, **4**, 244–54.

Bridge, T. P., Kleinman, J. E., Soldo, B. J. & Karoum, F. (1987) Central catecholamines, cognitive impairment, and affective state in elderly schizophrenics and controls. *Biological Psychiatry*, **22**, 139–47.

Ciompi, L. & Müller, C. (1976). *Lebensweg und Alter der Schizophrenen. Eine katamnestische Langzeitstudie bis ins Senium. Monographien aus dem Gesamtgebiete der Psychiatrie*; *Bd.* 12. Berlin: Springer.

Cohen, C. I., Statsny, P., Perlick, D., Samuelly, I. & Horn, L. (1988). Cognitive deficits among ageing schizophrenic patients residing in the community. *Hospital and Community Psychiatry*, **39**, 557–9.

Cooper, A. F. & Curry, A. R. (1976). The pathology of deafness in the paranoid and affective psychoses of later life. *Journal of Psychosomatic Research*, **20**, 97–105.

Edlund, M. J., Conrad, C. & Morris, P. (1989). Accidents among schizophrenic outpatients. *Comprehensive Psychiatry*, **30**, 522–6.

Förstl, H., Howard, R., Almeida, O. et al. (1991). Cranial computed tomography findings in late paraphrenia with and without first rank symptoms. *Nervenarzt*, **62**, 274–6.

Förstl, H., Burns, A., Luthert, P., Cairns, N., Lantos, P. & Levy, R. (1992). Clinical and neuropathological correlates of depression in Alzheimer's disease. *Psychological Medicine*, **22**, 877–84.

Goodman, A. B. & Siegel, C. (1986). Elderly schizophrenic inpatients in the wake of deinstitutionalization. *American Journal of Psychiatry*, **143**, 204–7.

Häfner, H., Maurer, K., Löffler, W. & Riecher-Rössler, A. (1993). The influence of age and sex on the onset and early course of schizophrenia. *British Journal of Psychiatry*, **162**, 80–6.

Harding, C. M., Brooks, G. W., Ashikaga, T., Strauss, J. S. & Breier, A. (1987). The Vermont Longitudinal Study: II. Long-term outcome of subjects who once met the criteria for DSM-III schizophrenia. *American Journal of Psychiatry*, **144**, 718–27.

Harding, C. M. & Strauss, J. S. (1985). The course of schizophrenia: An evolving concept. In *Controversies in Schizophrenia – Changes and Constancies*, ed. M. Alpert, pp. 339–350. New York: The Guilford Press.

Harris, M. J. & Jeste, D. V. (1988). Late-onset schizophrenia: an overview. *Schizophrenia Bulletin*, **14**, 39–55.

Hashimoto, T., Nishino, N., Nakai, H. & Tanaka, C. (1991). Increase in serotonin 5-HT-sub(1A). receptors in prefrontal and temporal cortices of brains from patients with chronic schizophrenia. *Life Sciences*, **48**, 355–63.

Holden, N. L. (1987). Late paraphrenia or the paraphrenias? A descriptive study with a 10-year follow-up. *British Journal of Psychiatry*, **150**, 635–9.

Huang, K. C., Lucas, L. F., Tsueda, K. et al. (1989). Electroconvulsive therapy. Special issue: ECT in the high-risk patient. *Convulsive Therapy*, **5**, 17–25.

Huber, G., Gross, G. & Schüttler, R. (1979). *Schizophrenie. Verlaufs- und sozialpsychiatrische Langzeituntersuchungen an den* 1945–1959 *in Bonn hospitalisierten schizophrenen Kranken*. Berlin, Heidelberg, New York: Springer.

Janzarik, W. (1959). *Dynamische Grundkonstellationen in endogenen Psychosen. Ein Beitrag zur Differentialtypologie der Wahnphänomene*. Berlin: Springer.

Janzarik, W. (1968). *Schizophrene Verläufe. Eine strukturdynamische Interpretation. Monographien aus dem Gesamtgebiete der Psychiatrie*; *H*. 126. Berlin: Springer.

Kane, J. M. & Smith, J. M. (1982). Tardive dyskinesia. Prevalence and risk factors 1959–1979. *Archives of General Psychiatry*, **39**, 473–81.

Kane, J. M., Woerner, M., Borenstein, M., Wegner, J. T. & Lieberman, J. A. (1986). Integrating incidence and prevalence of tardive dyskinesia. *Psychopharmacological Bulletin*, **22**, 254–8.

Karson, C. N., Bracha, H. S., Powell, A. & Adams, L. (1990). Dyskinetic movements, cognitive impairment and negative symptoms in elderly neuropsychiatric patients. *American Journal of Psychiatry*, **147**, 1646–9.

Kraepelin, E. (1896). *Lehrbuch der Psychiatrie. 5. Auflage*. Leipzig: Abel.

Kraepelin, E. (1919). *Dementia Praecox and Paraphrenia*. Edinburgh: Livingstone.

Krauss, B. (1989). Epidemiologie. In *Psychiatrie der Gegenwart 8: Alterspsychiatrie*, ed. K. P. Kisker, H. Lauter, J.-E. Meyer et al., pp. 59–84. Berlin, Heidelberg, New York: Springer.

Landschaftsverband Rheinland (1989). *Zahlen, Fakten und Tendenzen. Materialen zur Rheinischen Psychiatrie*. Düsseldorf: Landschaftsverband Rheinland.

Lichtenberg, P. A. & McGrogan, A. (1989). Relocating elderly patients (Letter). *Hospital and Community Psychiatry*, **40**, 755.

Meeks, S. (1990). Positive and negative symptoms in elderly schizophrenics: a case discussion. *Clinical Gerontologist*, **10**, 38–42.

Meeks, S. & Walker, J. S. (1990). Blunted affect, blunted lives? Negative symptoms, ADL functioning, and mental health among older adults. *International Journal of Geriatric Psychiatry*, **5**, 233–8.

Miller, B. L., Benson, D. F., Cummings, J. L. & Neshkes (1986). Late-life paraphrenia: An organic delusional syndrome. *Journal of Clinical Psychiatry*, **47**, 204–7.

Moak, G. S. (1990). Discharge and retention of psychogeriatric long-stay patients in a state mental hospital. *Hospital and Community Psychiatry*, **41**, 445–7.

Neugebauer, R. (1980). Formulation of hypotheses about the true prevalence of functional and organic psychiatric disorders among the elderly in the United States. In *Mental Illness in the United States*, ed. B. P. Dohrenwend, B. S. Dohrenwend, M. S. Gould, et al. pp. 95–113. New York: Praeger.

Pitt, B. (1990). Schizoaffective disorders in the elderly. In *Affective and Schizoaffective Disorders – Similarities and Differences*, ed. A. Marneros & M. T. Tsuang, pp. 102–106. Berlin, Heidelberg, New York: Springer.

Raskind, M. A. & Risse, S. C. (1986). Antipsychotic drugs and the elderly. *Journal of Clinical Psychiatry*, **47**, (5), 17–22.

Reddick, R. W., Kramer, M. & Taube, C. A. (1973). Epidemiology of mental illness and utilization of psychiatric facilities among older persons. In *Mental Illness in Later Life*, ed. E. W. Busse & E. Pfeiffer, Washington, DC: American Psychiatric Association.

Riemer, M. D. (1950). A study of the mental status of schizophrenics hospitalized for over 25 years into their senium. *Psychiatric Quarterly*, **24**, 309–13.

Rosen, J., Bohon, S. & Gershon, S. (1990). Antipsychotics in the elderly. *Acta Psychiatrica Scandinavica*, **82** (Suppl. 358), 170–5.

Roth, M. (1955). The natural history of mental disorder in old age. *Journal of Mental Sciences*, **129**, 281–301.

Sandyk, R. & Kay, S. R. (1990). Relationship of neuroleptic-induced akathisia to drug-induced parkinsonism. *Italian Journal of Neurological Sciences*, **11**, 439–42.

Tan, C. H. & Tay, L. K. (1991). Tardive dyskinesia in elderly psychiatric patients in Singapore. *Australian and New Zealand Journal of Psychiatry*, **25**, 119–22.

Taylor, P. J. & Parrott, J. M. (1988). Elderly offenders. A study of age-related factors among custodially remanded prisoners. *British Journal of Psychiatry*, **152**, 340–6.

Tsuang, M. T., Woolson, R. F. & Fleming, J. A. (1979). Long-term outcome of major psychoses. I. Schizophrenia and affective disorders compared with psychiatrically symptom-free surgical conditions. *Archives of General Psychiatry*, **36**, 1295–1301.

Woerner, M. G., Kane, J. M., Lieberman, J. A. et al. (1991). The prevalence of tardive dyskinesia. *Journal of Clinical Psychopharmacology*, **11**, 34–42.

Wright, J. M. & Silove, D. (1988). Pseudodementia in schizophrenia and mania. *Australian and New Zealand Journal of Psychiatry*, **22**, 109–14.

18

Late onset paranoid disorders:
Part I: Coming to terms with late paraphrenia

OSVALDO P. ALMEIDA ROBERT HOWARD HANS FÖRSTL
RAYMOND LEVY

To some extent, all diagnoses in psychiatry are surrounded by uncertainty, but late paraphrenia is certainly among the most controversial. A number of factors have contributed to late paraphrenia's appararently uncertain position as a diagnostic category. Delusions and hallucinations, the basic clinical features of late paraphrenia, have their onset most frequently in early or middle life, and are then usually associated with the diagnoses of schizophrenia or delusional disorder. Conversely, psychotic symptoms appearing for the first time in late life are frequently associated with organic mental disorders (Burns, Jacoby & Levy, 1990). To complicate this further, the use of the Kraepelinian term 'paraphrenia' is itself surrounded by uncertainties, particularly since Mayer (1921) demonstrated that most paraphrenics became indistinguishable from schizophrenics at follow-up. It is hardly surprising that the diagnostic category of late paraphrenia has been all but abandoned from the current psychiatric nosology (Quintal, Day-Cody & Levy, 1991). Recent evidence, however, suggests that its death sentence may have been premature.

How late paraphrenia came into existence

The term 'paraphrenia' was introduced by Emil Kraepelin (1919) to describe a group of paranoid patients with marked delusions and hallucinations in whom affect, will and personality were largely preserved. Kraepelin (1919) admitted that it was often difficult to separate paraphrenia from dementia praecox and estimated that approximately 40% of his patients would progress to exhibit the features of dementia praecox with time.

Mayer (1921) carried out a follow-up of Kraepelin's original paraphrenic patients and found that only a tiny minority of them had failed to develop the features of dementia praecox. Mayer suggested that a later age at onset for paraphrenia could perhaps account for many of the early differences observed between these patients and those with dementia praecox.

In 1952 Roth and Morrisey described a group of subjects with a well-organized system of paranoid delusions in which signs of organic dementia, sustained confusion or affective disorder were absent. Most of these patients experienced hallucinations, usually of auditory type. Since the onset of the symptoms was predominantly after the age of 60 and the clinical features presented by these patients were very similar to those described by Kraepelin under the heading of 'paraphrenia', the diagnostic term 'late paraphrenia' was introduced for this particular group of elderly patients. Subsequently, Roth (1955) demonstrated that late paraphrenia followed a course that was different from that of the dementias and the affective disorders in terms of mortality and symptomatological remission at 6 month and 2 year follow-up. Late paraphrenia, however, was never firmly established as a diagnostic category in its own right and an interchangeable diagnosis of schizophrenia was frequently used for the same group of patients (e.g. Kay & Roth, 1961). Fish (1960) pointed out that the use of the term 'late paraphrenia' was misleading, as there was no obvious evidence that these patients were at all different from schizophrenics.

Uncertainty about how best to classify the paranoid disorders of late onset persists. Some authors believe that late paraphrenia and allied late onset non-affective psychoses are the form of expression of schizophrenia in old age (Grahame, 1984). Internationally, the current trend seems to be for the abandonment of the diagnosis of late paraphrenia. In the two main diagnostic guidelines manuals, the DSM-IV (American Psychiatric Association, draft 1993) and the ICD-10 (World Health Organization, draft 1992), most cases are now accomodated under the headings of paranoid schizophrenia with late onset or persistent delusional disorder (Quintal et al., 1991).

In the following sections we will present a review of the main features and characteristics of late paraphrenia, late onset schizophrenia and other paranoid disorders with onset in late life.

Epidemiology

The few studies assessing the prevalence of late paraphrenia among the elderly have been mostly hospital based and estimated that such patients contribute to 10% of all elderly patients admitted to a mental hospital (Kay & Roth, 1961; Blessed & Wilson, 1982). Holden's (1987) survey of the Camberwell Case Register suggested that the annual incidence of late paraphrenia was 17–26/100000, depending upon whether or not patients with possible organic aetiology were included.

The few community studies available in the UK have calculated that the prevalence of paraphrenic symptoms in the elderly is between 1% and 2.6% (Kay, Beamish & Roth, 1964; Parsons, 1964; Williamson et al., 1964; Goldberg, 1970).

In the United States, paranoid symptoms were found in 2% (Lowenthal, 1964) to 4% (Christenson & Blazer, 1984) of the population over the age of 65. Post (1966) warned that these figures may underestimate the real prevalence of the disorder in the elderly living in the community, particularly because these patients are often socially isolated and may have symptoms that are not disruptive enough to be noticed.

The clinical features

'Neighbours, landlords, or relatives are implicated in plots to be rid of the patients, or to annoy or interfere with them through jealousy or simply for amusement... Patients feel drugged, hypnotized, have their thoughts read, their minds or bodies worked upon by rays, machines or electricity, complain that they are spied upon, can get no privacy in thought or act...(auditory hallucinations) consist of threatening, accusing, commanding of cajoling voices, jeering commentaries, screams, shouts for help, obscene words and songs, music, loud bangs, rappings, shots or explosions... The thoughts are repeated aloud...God, spirits, distant or deceased relatives, or most often, jealous, hostile neighbours are held responsible (for these phenomena)' (Kay & Roth, 1961).

Delusions of persecution are characteristic and are reported in approximately 85% of patients. Nonetheless, a wide range of delusional activity is observed in late paraphrenics, including delusions of reference, misidentification, delusions of control, hypocondriasis, grandiosity, sexual and religious delusions (for review see Howard, Almeida & Levy, in press).

Auditory hallucinations were originally reported in around 75% of the patients (Kay & Roth, 1961). Visual, olfactory, tactile and somatic hallucinations are less common, but not infrequent. Visual hallucinations, for instance, have been reported in up to 61% of these patients (Pearlson et al., 1989).

First rank symptoms of Schneider, considered one of the cardinal features of schizophrenia, are very frequent in late paraphrenics. Prevalences of 35% (Pearlson et al., 1989) to 64% (Marneros & Deister, 1984) of such symptoms have been reported in late onset cases, although a systematic psychopathological assessment in a large number of patients has only recently been described (Howard et al., in press).

Concomitant affective symptoms have been reported by some workers in up to 60% of cases (Post, 1966; Holden, 1987), although their presence in late paraphrenia has not as yet been systematically evaluated. Post (1966) found 'depressive admixtures' in approximately 60% of his subjects, whereas Holden (1987) considered that 10 of his 24 nonorganic late paraphrenics displayed prominent affective symptoms. The possible overlap of late paraphrenia with mood disorders is still unclear, although strictly speaking doubtful cases should not be included under the diagnosis of late paraphrenia as defined by Kay & Roth (1961).

Diagnosis

Following its introduction, late paraphrenia became a widely used diagnostic category in Great Britain and other European Countries, although its somewhat loose definition and its questionable relationship with schizophrenia hampered universal acceptance of the concept (see above). In the USA only recently psychiatrists became fully aware that schizophreniform symptoms may arise very late in life. This is illustrated by the removal of the upper age limit for the onset of schizophrenia by the DSM-III-R in 1987 (APA, 1987).

Schizophrenia with late-onset and persistent delusional disorder are the diagnostic options offered by DSM-III-R (APA, 1987) and the ICD-10 (WHO, draft 1990).

But are these the most suitable diagnoses for these patients? Persistent delusional disorder, for example, demands the exclusion of those patients with prominent hallucinations. This is, therefore, a very unsatisfactory option as most patients will display such symptoms. The proposed alternative diagnosis of late onset schizophrenia also seems unsuitable for a number of reasons:

1. The psychopathology of early onset schizophrenia and late paraphrenia (and late onset schizophrenia) seem to be distinct. Delusions, the hallmark of late paraphrenia, are present in only a fraction of early onset schizophrenics (Pearlson et al., 1989). Hallucinations tend to affect multiple sensory modalities in late paraphrenics and are also far more frequent in old age than in early onset schizophrenics (Pearlson et al., 1989). Thought disorder is extremely uncommon in late paraphrenics (5.6%), but affects a great proportion of young schizophrenics (51.9%) (Pearlson et al., 1989). Negative symptoms such as constricted affect, withdrawal and impoverishment of thought are rarely seen in late paraphrenics, although they have been reported as present in up to 84.5% of non-elderly schizophrenics (Andreasen et al., 1990);
2. The prevalence of schizophrenia has been falling steadily over the past decades in the population under the age of 55 (Der, Gupta & Murray, 1990; Eagles, Hunter & McCrance, 1988), but has remained surprisingly stable for those aged 55 or over, where indeed a progressive increase in its prevalence is observed (Der et al., 1990). This may indicate that early- and late-onset cases have different etiologies. In fact, it is unlikely that the neurodevelopmental mechanisms proposed for the pathogenesis of early onset schizophrenia (Weinberger, 1987; McNeil, 1991) would play an important role in late paraphrenia, when the involvement of neurodegenerative mechanisms seem more plausible.
3. Neuroimaging findings (reviewed below) indicate that late onset cases present structural brain changes that seem to be qualitatively and quantitatively different from those described in younger schizophrenics.

The question of heterogeneity in late paraphrenia

Several attemps to deal with the apparent heterogeneity of this condition have been made. Kay & Roth (1961) suggested that three subgroups of late paraphrenics could be identified by their symptomatological or etiological patterns, although the points of similarity between the patients seemed more relevant to them than the differences.

1. Paranoid psychoses without hallucinations. These patients exhibited a delusional system that could be considered a 'caricature' of their premorbid deviant personality. They were more likely to be older, present with more associated sensory deficits and with a delusional system confined to situations of daily living;
2. Reactive late paraphrenia, with psychotic symptoms arising after unusual circumstances or prolonged isolation;
3. 'Endogenous' late paraphrenia. This group of patients presented with more systematised and fantastic delusions, persistent auditory hallucinations and social isolation. Hearing impairment was reported in half of these patients.

Post (1966) also proposed the allocation of these patients into three subgroups, not completely different from those previously described by Kay & Roth (1961). The first group of patients was characterized by a paucity of delusional beliefs and other abnormal experiences such as auditory hallucinations. These symptoms were unlikely to interfere with the patients' normal activities. The second and third groups presented a more disabling and widespread psychotic symptomatology, almost always with auditory hallucinations and bizarre delusions. The third group was separated from the second by the presence of first rank symptoms. As a consequence, Post (1966; 1980) described them as more 'schizophrenic' or 'endogenous'. Again, there were no clear long-term differences between the subgroups.

More recently Holden (1987) has retrospectively assessed all subjects with a diagnosis of persistent delusional psychosis using the Camberwell Case Register. He suggested that these patients were best allocated into six subgroups. An '*affective*' subgroup was formed by patients whose symptoms were later considered to be secondary to a depressive illness. In the '*symptomatic*' subgroup there was a strong association between paranoid symptoms and chronic physical illness. A clear cognitive deterioration at 3 year follow-up typified the '*organic*' subgroup. The remaining 'functional' patients were distributed into three different subgroups: '*schizoaffective*' (at least one subsequent episode being diagnosed as affective disorder), '*schizophreniform*' (patients with Schneiderian first rank sympotms) and '*paranoid*' (paranoid symptoms not associated with prominent hallucinations). Holden (1987) found that his 'organic' subgroup had a poorer outcome, and that the presence of affective or first rank symptoms were associated with less instituitionalization and better treatment response.

Further attempts to subdivide late paraphrenia have been recently reported with the use of neuroimaging techniques (reviewed below), although the question of heterogeneity still awaits clarification.

The role of risk factors

Female sex, deviant premorbid personality and sensory impairment have been the most consistent factors associated with the diagnosis of late paraphrenia. Hereditary factors have also been suggested, although their role remains subject to dispute.

Sex

There is a well-established preponderance of women with late paraphrenia. The reported proportion of this imbalance varies widely with rates from 3:1 to 45:2 (Herbert & Jacobson, 1967; Kay et al., 1964). Schizophrenia with paranoid symptoms has been reported to be more prevalent in middle and late life (Larson & Nyman, 1970), when more women are at risk for the development of the disorder (Bland, 1977; Lewine, 1988; Seeman, 1982). However, this late preponderance of women is unlikely to be merely due to some protective factor delaying the onset of illness in this population. Indeed, Castle & Murray (1991) showed that the incidence of schizophrenic symptoms in women after the age of 55 clearly exceeds the expected frequency if the incidence curve had been simply shifted to the right.

Premorbid Personality

Late paraphrenics have been frequently described as quarrelsome, religious, suspicious, sensitive, unsociable and cold-hearted (Kay & Roth, 1961; Post, 1966; Kay, 1972). In some patients, particularly those without hallucinations, the psychotic symptoms may be seen as an exaggeration or caricature of their premorbid personality. Herbert & Jacobson (1967) emphasized that the onset of the illness in their patients ocurred 'against a background of disturbance sufficiently strong to disrupt the personality', which often contained paranoid or schizoid traits. These 'premorbid defects' have been regarded as the source rather than the result of the reported low marriage rate and social isolation of these patients (Kay & Roth, 1961; Post, 1966, 1980).

Sensory Impairment

An association with both visual and auditory impairment has been reported in late paraphrenia (Herbert & Jacobson, 1967; Kay & Roth, 1961). Major ocular pathology (predominantly cataracts) was found in 55% of 54 patients, significantly more than in elderly depressive controls (Cooper & Porter, 1976). Hearing impairment is also more frequent in late paraphrenics than in elderly depressives or age matched controls (Naguib & Levy, 1987; Post, 1966); the etiology being more likely to be conductive than degenerative (Cooper et al., 1974). Cooper (1976) suggested that the characteristics of the hearing impairment more strongly associated with the diagnosis of late paraphrenia were early age of onset, long duration and profound auditory loss. The relevance of hearing impairment in the production of the psychotic symptoms is still uncertain, although significant symptomatological improvement has been described in some patients after the fitting of a hearing aid (Almeida et al., 1993; Eastwood, Corbin & Reed, 1981).

Genetics

Kay (1972) suggested that the risk for developing schizophrenia among the first degree relatives of late paraphrenics was 3.4%, a rate intermediate between that described for the general population (less than 1%) and for the families of young schizophrenics (5.8%). A possible genetic relationship between late paraphrenia and schizophrenia had already been explored by others (Herbert & Jacobson, 1967; Kay & Roth, 1961), although a clear interpretation of their results is hampered by a series of methodological difficulties:

1. No clear diagnostic criteria for late paraphrenia or schizophrenia were used;
2. The source of the information about the family pedigree was unreliable;
3. The retrospective use of delusions and hallucinations as the key-symptoms to detect the illness in the families has possibly produced many 'false positives', particularly when we consider that these symptoms are fairly frequent in many of the organic (Berrios & Brook, 1985; Burns et al., 1990) and affective disorders of the elderly (Charney & Nelson, 1981; Glassman & Roose, 1981);
4. Individuals with the postulated genotype may die of unrelated causes before they reach the age for the expression of the disorder.

Naguib et al. (1987) used the human leucocytic antigen (HLA) technique to explore the possible association of late paraphrenia with genetic factors. There was no obvious relationship between the disorder and the antigens investigated, although the authors suggested that the HLA-B37 could be a possible candidate.

This contrasts with the reported association between HLA-A9 and paranoid schizophrenia (McGuffin, Farmer & Yonace, 1981).

In summary, women particularly those known to have been sensitive, quarrelsome, unmarried and socially isolated, run a greater risk of developing late paraphrenic symptoms. Sensory impairment is also likely to contribute to the formation of the hallucinatory phenomena and its correction may be an important part of the treatment strategy of these patients. The proposed genetic association between late paraphrenia and schizophrenia seems to be highly speculative and it is still uncertain whether there is any inherited predisposition for the development of the disorder.

Neuropsychological findings

To date, only Naguib & Levy (1987) have systematically investigated the cognitive features associated with late paraphrenia. They used the Mental Test Score (MTS), Digit Copying Test (DCT) and Digit Symbol Substitution Test to evaluate 43 subjects. Patients performed worse than normal age-matched controls on both MTS and DCT and showed some deterioration on the MTS at a 3.7 year follow-up (Hymas, Naguib & Levy, 1989), although they remained above the cut-off score for dementia.

More recently, Miller et al. (1991) used a comprehensive neuropsychological assessment battery to evaluate a group of 24 psychotic patients with onset of the symptoms after the age of 45, mean age of 60.1. Patients performed worse than age-matched controls in all tasks (Mini Mental State Examination, Wechsler Adult Intelligence Scale-revised, Wisconsin Card Sorting Test, Logical Memory and Visual Reproduction from the Wechsler Memory Scale, Verbal Fluency, the Stroop Test and Warrington Recognition Memory Test).

In short, late paraphrenics (and late life psychotic patients) do not show an obvious cognitive deterioration, at least not as marked as that observed in demented subjects. Nonetheless, their performance is worse than would be expected for their age in a variety of cognitive tasks, even in those as basic as the Mini Mental State Examination and the Mental Test Score.

Neuroimaging findings

An extensive review of the available neuroimaging studies in late life psychosis is presented elsewhere (Förstl et al., 1992). In this section, we will only consider their most important positive findings.

Miller et al. (1986) observed 'occult organic disorder' in the scans of four of their five patients (mostly white-matter lesions). Naguib & Levy (1987) described normally distributed ventricular enlargement in a group of 43 late paraphrenics which was uncoupled from the usual association with age and cortical atrophy occurring in an age-matched control population (Burns et al., 1989). Rabins et al. (1987) reported similar findings in a sample of 29 late onset schizophrenics (mean age of onset = 62.4), although these abnormalities were not as marked as those observed in an age-matched control group of psychotic patients with Alzheimer's disease. Other CT studies confirmed that psychosis in late life seems to be associated with increased VBR (Pearlson et al., 1987) and white matter lesions (Flint, Rifat & Eastwood, 1991; Kohlmeyer, 1988).

Attempts to discriminate patients with and without manifest CT scan abnormalities have been recently reported. Flint et al. (1991) suggested that late paraphrenics without hallucinations were more likely to show evidence of brain infarction in their scans, whereas Howard et al. (1992) found that those without first rank symptoms of Schneider exhibited more cortical atrophy.

A series of MRI studies of late life psychosis have been recently published and indicate that a great proportion of these patients show evidence of white matter disease (Breitner et al., 1990; Harris, Cullum & Jeste, 1988; Krull et al., 1991; Miller et al., 1991).

In summary, neuroimaging suggests that subtle organic factors may be critical for the development of psychotic symptoms in late life in at least a subgroup of patients. Moreover, these results indicate that the structural brain abnormalities reported in this group of patients seem to be qualitatively and quantitatively different from those observed in young schizophrenics (for review see Lewis, 1990; Waddington et al., 1990).

Management and treatment

Late paraphrenics do not seek treatment spontaneously, but may request action from their relatives, police or other authorities against their persecutors. Many are probably maintained in the community by rehousing or support given by families, friends and social workers, but the effectiveness of this form of management has not as yet been evaluated. Doctors tend to see these patients only when all these measures have failed and distress and disturbance have become intolerable (Post, 1984).

Late paraphrenics only rarely agree to attend a psychiatric appointment in an outpatient clinic and a domiciliary visit is often necessary. The first medical contact with the patient may later prove to be essential for the success of treatment. The psychiatrist should try to establish a good rapport with the patient and be sympathetic to her complaints. He must also ensure that late paraphrenia is the correct diagnosis (investigate cognitive decline, neurological signs or symptoms, associated affective symptoms, etc.) and further interviews should be organized to establish the patient's good compliance with the therapeutic strategy. Medication should be offered as a way to diminish the patient's distress. Unfortunately, compulsory admission may be necessary with noncompliant subjects. In these cases the medical team should try to regain the patient's confidence in order to guarantee an effective future management.

The use of neuroleptics for the treatment of late paraphrenics is widely accepted, although no controlled trials have ever been reported. The risk of side-effects (mainly extrapyramidal) favors the use of oral medication, although Howard &

Levy (1992) have recently suggested that depot intramuscular medication may improve compliance and reduce the required antipsychotic drug dose. Post (1966) found that, of 71 patients who received 10–30 mg of trifluoperazine or 40–500 mg of thioradazine per day, 8.5% showed no response, 31% showed some signs of improvement and 60.5% presented a complete response to treatment. Less optimistic results have been reported by Rabins, Pauker & Thomas (1984) and Pearlson et al. (1989) who found that 14.5% and 24.1%, respectively, of their late onset schizophrenics did not show any signs of improvement after neuroleptic treatment. Howard & Levy (1992) found that, after a minimum of 3 months of antipsychotic treatment, 42.2% of patients showed no response, 31.3% improved partially and 26.6% presented symptomatological remission.

Neuroleptics seem to promote some symptomatological improvement in at least 60% of late paraphrenics. Numerous factors may be involved with failure to respond to the medication and these include non-compliance, the use of ineffective drug-doses, intolerance to the medication (extrapyramidal and anticholinergic side-effects) and the presence of concomitant organic factors.

Post (1966) suggested that immediate response to treatment, the development of insight, younger age and being married were all good prognostic features. Neuroleptics are an essential part of late paraphrenics' treatment. However, it would seem that psychological, occupational, social support and correction of sensory impairment may play a vital role in the patients' future outcome. Untreated late paraphrenics generally pursue an unremitting-chronic course, and once the symptoms have fully developed they are unlikely to change until the patient's death.

Conclusion

Psychotic symptoms in late life result from a complex interaction of factors such as ageing, sex, poor social adjustment and isolation, sensory and cognitive decline and subtle brain lesions. The diagnostic category of late paraphrenia is the only one to take these factors into consideration and seems, therefore, the most suitable to describe such state(s). Moreover, it seems inappropriate to assume that late onset cases are simply a variant of early onset schizophrenia when there is increasing evidence pointing in the opposite direction.

Late paraphrenia remains a surprisingly unexplored category in psychiatry. We are still unsure about its real prevalence and incidence, its natural history, response to treatment, etiological factors, neuropathology, neurochemistry and the significance of the neuroimaging and the neuropsychological abnormalities so far reported. During the past five years we have witnessed a renewed interest in this area, not only from old age psychiatrists but also increasingly from psychiatrists working with schizophrenia. Exciting years lie ahead and we trust that the study of late paraphrenia will provide us with some futher hints on the relationship between the brain and mental disorders.

References

Almeida, O. P., Förstl, H., Howard, R. & David, A. S. (1993). Unilateral auditory hallucinations: a case report and a brief review of the literature. *British Journal of Psychiatry*, **162**, 262–4.

Almeida, O. P.. Howard, R., Förstl, H. & Levy, R. (1992). Should the diagnosis of late paraphrenia be abandoned? *Psychological Medicine*, **22**, 11–14.

American Psychiatric Association (1987). *Diagnostic and Statistical Manual of Mental Disorders. 3rd edition, revised.* Washington, DC.

American Psychiatric Association (draft 1993). *Diagnostic and Statistical Manual of Mental Disorders. 4th edition.* Washington, DC.

Andreasen, N. C., Flaum, M., Swayze, V. W., Tyrrel , M. S. & Arndt, S. (1990). Positive and negative symptoms in schizophrenia: a critical appraisal. *Archives of General Psychiatry*, **47**, 615–21.

Berrios, G. & Brook, P. (1985). Delusions and the psychopathology of the elderly with dementia. *Acta Psychiatrica Scandinavica*, **72**, 296–301.

Bland, R. C. (1977). Demographic aspects of functional psychoses in Canada. *Acta Psychiatrica Scandinavica*, **55**, 369–80.

Blessed, G. & Wilson, D. (1982). The contemporary natural history of mental disorder in old age. *British Journal of Psychiatry*, **141**, 59–67.

Breitner, J. C. S., Husain, M. M., Figiel, G. S., Krishnan, K. R. R. & Boyko, O. B. (1990). Cerebral white matter disease in late-onset paranoid psychosis. *Biological Psychiatry*, **28**, 266–74.

Burns, A., Carrick, J., Ames, D., Naguib, M. & Levy, R. (1989). The cerebral cortical appearance in late paraphrenia. *International Journal of Geriatric Psychiatry*, **4**, 31–4.

Burns, A., Jacoby, R. & Levy, R. (1990). Psychiatric phenomena in Alzheimer's disease. *British Journal of Psychiatry*, **157**, 72–94.

Castle, D. J. & Murray, R. M. (1991). The neurodevelopmental basis of sex differences in schizophrenia. *Psychological Medicine*, **21**, 565–75.

Charney, D. S. & Nelson, J. C. (1981). Delusional and nondelusional unipolar depression: Further evidence for distinct subtypes. *American Journal of Psychiatry*, **136**, 328–33.

Christenson, R. & Blazer, D. (1984). Epidemiology of persecutory ideation in an elderly population in the community. *American Journal of Psychiatry*, **141**, 1088–91.

Cooper, A. F., Curry, A. R., Kay, D. W. K., Garside, R. F. & Roth, M. (1974). Hearing loss in paranoid and affective psychoses of the elderly. *Lancet*, **ii**, 851–4.

Cooper, A. F. (1976). Deafness and psychiatric illness. *British Journal of Psychiatry*, **129**, 216–26.

Cooper, A. F. & Porter, R. (1976). Visual acuity and ocular pathology in the paranoid and affective psychoses of later life. *Journal of Psychosomatic Research*, **20**, 107–14.

Der, G., Gupta, S. & Murray, R. (1990). Is schizophrenia disappearing? *Lancet*, **335**, 513–16.

Eagles, J. M., Hunter, D. & McCrance, C. (1988). Decline in the diagnosis of schizophrenia among first contacts with psychiatric services in North-East Scotland, 1969–1984. *British Journal of Psychiatry*, **152**, 793–8.

Eastwood, M. R., Corbin, S. & Reed, M. (1981). Hearing impairment and paraphrenia. *Journal of Otolaryngology*, **10**, 306–8.

Fish, F. (1960). Senile schizophrenia. *Journal of Mental Science*, **106**, 938–46.

Flint, A. J., Rifat, S. L. & Eastwood, M. R. (1991). Late-onset paranoia: distinct from paraphrenia? *International Journal of Geriatric Psychiatry*, **6**, 103–9.

Förstl, H., Howard, R., Almeida, O. P. & Stadmüller, G. (1992). Psychotic symptoms and the paraphrenic brain. In *Delusions and Hallucinations in Old Age*, ed. C. Katona & R. Levy. London: Gaskell Publications.

Glassman, A. H. & Roose, S. P. (1981). Delusional depression: a distinct clinical entity? *Archives of General Psychiatry*, **38**, 424–7.

Goldberg, E. M. (1970). *Helping the Aged: A Field of Experiment in Social Work*. London: George Allen & Unwin.

Grahame, P. S. (1984). Schizophrenia in old age (late paraphrenia). *British Journal of Psychiatry*, **145**, 493–5.

Harris, M. J., Cullum, C. M. & Jeste, D. V. (1988). Clinical presentation of late-onset schizophrenia. *Journal of Clinical Psychiatry*, **49**, 356–60.

Herbert, M. E. & Jacobson, S. (1967). Late paraphrenia. *British Journal of Psychiatry*, **113**, 461–9.

Holden, N. L. (1987). Late paraphrenia or the paraphrenias? A descriptive study with a 10-year follow-up. *British Journal of Psychiatry*, **150**, 635–9.

Howard, R., Almeida, O. & Levy, R. (in press). Schizophrenic symptoms in late paraphrenia. *Psychopathology*.

Howard, R. J., Förstl, H., Naguib, M., Burns, A. & Levy, R. (1992). First-rank symptoms of Schneider in late paraphrenia: cortical structural correlates. *British Journal of Psychiatry*, **160**, 108–9.

Howard, R. & Levy, R. (1992). Which factors affect treatment response in late paraphrenia? *International Journal of Geriatric Psychiatry*, **7**, 667–72.

Hymas, N., Naguib, M. & Levy, R. (1989). Late-paraphrenia: a follow-up study. *International Journal of Geriatric Psychiatry*, **4**, 23–9.

Kay, D. W. K. & Roth, M. (1961). Environmental and hereditary factors in the schizophrenias of old age and their bearing on the general problem of schizophrenia. *Journal of Mental Science*, **107**, 649–86.

Kay, D. W. K., Beamish, P. & Roth, M. (1964). Old age mental disorders in Newcastle-upon-Tyne. *Journal of Mental Science*, **110**, 668–82.

Kay, D. W. K. (1972). Schizophrenia and schizophrenia-like states in the elderly. *British Journal of Hospital Medicine*, **8**, 369–76.

Kohlmeyer, K. (1988). Periventrikuläre Dichteminderungen des Grosshirnhemisphärenmarks in Computertomogrammen von neuropsychiatrischen Patienten in der zweiten Lebenshälfte: diagnostische Bedeutung und Pathoenese. *Fortschritte der Neurologie und Psychiatrie*, **56**, 279–87.

Kraepelin, E. (1919). *Dementia Praecox and Paraphrenia* (translated by R. M. Barclay from the eighth German edition of the '*Text-Book of Psychiatry*', vol iii, part ii, section on the Endogenous Dementias, 1919). E & S Livingstone: Edinburgh.

Krull, A. J., Press, G., Dupont, R., Harris, J. & Jeste, D. V. (1991). Brain imaging in late-onset schizophrenia and related psychoses. *International Journal of Geriatric Psychiatry*, **6**, 651–8.

Larson, C. A. & Nyman, G. E. (1970). Age of onset in schizophrenia. *Human Heredity*, **20**, 241–7.

Lewine, R. J. (1988). Gender and schizophrenia. In *Handbook of Schizophrenia*, Vol 3, ed. H. A. Nasrallah. Amsterdam: Elsevier Science Publishers.

Lewis, S. W. (1990). Computerised tomography in schizophrenia 15 years on. *British Journal of Psychiatry*, **157** (suppl. 9), 16–24.

Lowenthal, M. F. (1964). *Lives in distress*. New York: Basic Books.

Marneros, A. & Deister, A. (1984). The psychopathology of 'late schizophrenia'. *Psychopathology*, **17**, 264–74.

Mayer, W. (1921). On paraphrenic psychoses. *Zeitschrift für die Gesamte Neurologie und Psychiatrie*, **71**, 187–206.

McGuffin, P., Farmer, A. E. & Yonace, A. H. (1981). HLA antigens and subtypes of schizophrenia. *Psychiatry Research*, **5**, 115–22.

McNeil, T. F. (1991). Obstetric complication in schizophrenic patients. *Schizophrenia Research*, **5**, 89–101.

Miller, B. L., Benson, D. F., Cummings, J. L. & Neshkes, R. (1986). Late-life paraphrenia: an organic delusional syndrome. *Journal of Clinical Psychiatry*, **47**, 204–7.

Miller, B. L., Lesser, I. M., Boone, K. B., Hill, E., Mehringer, C. M. & Wong, K. (1991). Brain lesions and cognitive function in late-life psychosis. *British Journal of Psychiatry*, **158**, 76–82.

Naguib, M. & Levy, R. (1987). Late paraphrenia: neuropsychological impairment and structural brain abnormalities on computed tomography. *International Journal of Geriatric Psychiatry*, **2**, 83–90.

Naguib, M., McGuffin, P., Levy, R., Festenstein, H. & Alonso, A. (1987). Genetic markers in late paraphrenia: a study of HLA antigens. *British Journal of Psychiatry*, **150**, 124–7.

Parsons, P. L. (1964). Mental health of Swansea's old folk. *British Journal of Preventive and Social Medicine*, **19**, 43–7.

Pearlson, G. D., Kreger, L., Rabins, P. V., Chase, G. A., Cohen, B., Wirth, J. B., Schlaepfer, T. B. & Tune, L. E. (1989). A chart review study of late-onset and early-onset schizophrenia. *American Journal of Psychiatry*, **146**, 1568–74.

Post, F. (1966). *Persistent Persecutory States of the Elderly*. Oxford: Pergamon Press.

Post, F. (1980). Paranoid, schizophrenia-like, and schizophrenic states in the aged. In *Handbook of Mental Health and Aging*, ed. J. E. Birren and R. B. Sloane, pp. 591–615. Englewood Cliffs: Prentice Hall.

Post, F. (1984). Schizophrenic and paranoid psychoses. In *Handbook of Studies on Psychiatry and Old Age*, ed D. W. K. Kay & G. D. Burrows, pp. 291–302. Amsterdam: Elsevier Science Publishers.

Quintal, M., Day-Cody, D. & Levy, R. (1991). Late paraphrenia and ICD-10. *International Journal of Geriatric Psychiatry*, **6**, 111–16.
Rabins, P., Pauker, S. & Thomas, J. (1984). Can schizophrenia begin after age 44? *Comprehensive Psychiatry*, **25**, 290–5.
Rabins, P., Pearlson, G., Jayaram, G., Steele, C. & Tune, L. (1987). Increased ventricular-to-brain ratio in late-onset schizophrenia. *American Journal of Psychiatry*, **144**, 1216–18.
Roth, M. (1955). The natural history of mental disorder in old age. *Journal of Mental Science*, **101**, 281–301.
Roth, M. & Morrisey, J. (1952). Problems in the diagnosis and classification of mental disorders in old age. *Journal of Mental Science*, **98**, 66–80.
Seeman, M. V. (1982). Gender differences in schizophrenia. *Canadian Journal of Psychiatry*, **27**, 107–12.
Waddington, J. L., O'Callaghan, E., Larkin, C., Redmond, O., Stack, J. & Ennis, J. T. (1990). Magnetic resonance imaging and spectroscopy in schizophrenia. *British Journal of Psychiatry*, **157** (suppl. 9), 56–65.
Weinberger, D. R. (1987). Implications of normal brain development for the pathogenesis of schizophrenia. *Archives of General Psychiatry*, **44**, 660–9.
Williamson, J., Stokoe, I. H., Gray, S., Fisher, M. & Smith, A. (1964). Old people at home: their unreported needs. *Lancet*, **i**, 1117–20.
World Health Organization (draft 1990). *Tenth Revison of the International Classification of Diseases, ch. V. Mental and behavioral disorders*. Geneva: World Health Organization.

Part II: Paraphrenia, schizophrenia or ?

PETER RABINS GODFREY PEARLSON

Chapter 18 Part I by Almeida et al. thoroughly and comprehensively reviews the classification of mid- and late-life psychiatric disorders that are characterized by the presence of delusions, hallucinations and an absence of depression and progressive cognitive impairment. Their conclusion, that we do not yet have enough knowledge to abandon the concept of late-life paraphrenia, is well supported. Here, the current status of this debate is reviewed and a strategy that might move the debate along is proposed. Most discussions of this topic have framed the question as a choice between limited alternatives: schizophrenia versus paraphrenia; paraphrenia versus late-onset affective disorder; organic versus functional. An alternative approach is offered here. It is suggested that two broad collections of data can be reviewed. First, genetic, treatment response and structural brain change (via neuropathology and neuroimaging) data can be added to the extensive literature on psychopathology (Robins & Guze, 1970). Second, comparisons

Table 18.1. *Early onset schizophrenia (EOS) versus late onset schizophrenia (LOS)*

	Like	Unlike
Genetics	Greater family history of schizophrenia than in general population	EOS: more familial risk than LOS
Epidemiology		EOS: F:M 1:1 LOS: F:M approx. 6:1 LOS: infertility in females in some studies
Risk factors		LOS: associated with sensory deficits and social isolation
Phenomenology	First rank symptoms common	EOS: more thought disorder, affective blunting and negative symptoms LOS: more vivid and multimodal hallucinations
Course		EOS: prognosis variable; better pre-morbid personality have better outcome; positive symptoms become less prevalent LOS: positive symptoms remain prominent
Treatment	Respond to neuroleptics	
Neuropathology		EOS: temporal lobe abnormalities in some cases LOS: no studies
Biological markers		
CT/MRI	Nonspecific white matter changes and ventricular enlargement; superior temporal gyrus atrophy	
SPECT		EOS: no studies LOS: excess of vascular lesions, esp. frontal and temporal lobe
PET	Excess D2 receptors in some studies of drug-native subjects	
EEG/ERP		EOS: P300 changes LOS: not studied
Neuropsychology	Impairments may be similar	

among the disorders that begin in later life and characteristically manifest hallucinations and delusions may help clarify whether this set of symptoms is unique or is a subset of another diagnostic entity.

Tables 18.1 through 18.8 apply this approach to the common functional and

Table 18.2. *Late-onset affective disorder (LOA) versus late onset schizophrenia (LOS)*

	Like	Unlike
Genetics	Fewer similarly affected relatives compared to early onset cases	Each runs true-to-type in families
Epidemiology	Prevalence declines after age 65	F:M 2:1 in LOA F:M 5–7: 1 in LOS LOA: high suicide rates LOS: no reported increase in suicide rates LOA: unassociated with marital status or fertility LOS: some studies show marriage and fertility rates low in LOS
Risk factors		LOA: premorbid personality – no reported associated LOS: premorbid personality – schizoid LOA: social isolation not reported premorbidly LOS: social isolation common LOA: sensory impairment not associated LOS: sensory impairment common
Phenomenology	Somatic delusion common Thought disorder rare	LOA: first rank symptoms uncommon LOS: first rank symptoms common LOA: hallucinations uncommon LOS: hallucinations common LOA: hallucinations unimodal LOS: hallucinations multimodal, vivid LOA: mood change present LOS: mood change absent LOA: vegetative symptoms common LOS: no vegetative symptoms
Course		LOA: increase mortality LOS: mortality rates unknown LOA: acute episodes with relapse LOS: tends to be chronic LOA: associated cognitive impairment which resolves or progresses LOS: stable cognitive defects
Response to treatment	Majority show some response to biological treatment	Respond to appropriate treatment of early onset form of the illness LOA: antidepressants, ECT LOS: neuroleptics
Neuropathology	Neither have excess number of plaques and tangles Both have association with nonspecific changes	
Biological markers CT		Left anterior stroke predisposes to LOA Right posterior stroke predisposes to LOS

Table 18.3. *Alzheimer's disease (AD) versus late onset schizophrenia (LOS)*

	Like	Unlike
Genetics		AD: familial AD dominantly inherited and linked to chromosome 21 LOS: family history of schizophrenia
Epidemiology		AD: equal sex incidence LOS: female predominance
Risk factors		AD: prior head injury for AD in general
Phenomenology	Delusions often paranoid	AD: 'simple' hallucinations and delusions, transient LOS: complex, persistent
Course		AD: hallucinations and delusions late in course
Response to treatment	Hallucinations and delusions respond to low dose neuroleptics	AD: hallucinations and delusions respond to treatment – cognitive disorder does not
Neurobiology		
CT/MRI	Nonspecific white matter changes Ventricular and sulcal enlargement	AD: changes more marked, show obvious progression
EEG/ERP		AD: left temporal slowing LOS: no specific pattern on EEG
SPECT		AD: decreased temporal and parietal relative rCBF LOS: symptomatic cases have frontal and temporal vascular lesions
PET		AD: decreased temporal and parietal glucose metabolism LOS: no glucose studies
Neuropathology		AD: plaques, tangles, granulovacolar degeneration LOS: none of the above

organic syndromes of later life. Based on the data summarized in these Tables (which were compiled from all the references), Chapter 18 Part I, a review published by ourselves (Pearlson & Rabins, 1988), review articles by others (Kay & Roth, 1961; Jeste et al., 1988; Castle & Howard, 1992; Hassett et al., 1992) and long-term follow-up studies of early-onset schizophrenia (Harding et al., 1987; Chiompi, 1987) the following conclusions are drawn:

1. Patients with the late-life syndrome characterized by hallucinations and delusions and absence of cognitive and mood disorder form a heterogeneous group.

Table 18.4. *Multiinfarct disease (MID) versus late onset schizophrenia (LOS)*

Like	Unlike
Genetics	Each runs true to type but weak association
Epidemiology	MID: male predominance LOS: female predominance
Risk factors	MID: vascular risk factors LOS: no symptoms of vascular disease
Phenomenology	MID: more depression, emotional disability, stepwise cognitive impairment LOS: hallucinations and delusions with mild and stable cognitive deficits
Course	MID: stepwise CVAs LOS: resolution or chronic relapsing
Response to treatment	MID: low dose TCAs LOS: low dose neuroleptics
Neuropathology	MID: lucencies, widespread infarcts LOS: no studies
Biological markers	
MRI	MID: infarcts present LOS: infarcts uncommon

2. Schizophrenic patients with illness beginning in early life also form a heterogeneous group in both phenomenology and course.
3. Individuals with late-life onset hallucinations and delusions and no mood or cognitive disorder have a higher prevalence of identifiable brain abnormalities than young individuals with similar symptoms (Miller et al., 1991). However, in the majority of late-onset cases no specific lesion or etiology can be identified.
4. The more careful one is to exclude individuals with identifiable structural brain lesions and progressive cognitive disorder and to require the presence of both hallucinations and delusions, the more comparable the late-onset group is to early-onset schizophrenia. None the less, the low prevalence of thought disorder and affective flattening in late-onset cases (Pearlson et al., 1989) suggests that the early- and late-onset conditions are not fully equivalent. These differences and similarities provide fertile ground for research.

Summary

It is premature to decide whether late-onset paraphrenia is a late life form of schizophrenia or a distinct syndrome. None the less, the data reviewed in Tables 18.1–8 and by others support the conclusion that early-life onset schizophrenia

Table 18.5. *Delusional disorder (DD) versus late onset schizophrenia (LOS)*

	Like	Unlike
Genetics	Slightly increased family history of schizophrenia	
Epidemiology	Rare in population studies	DD: more common in males LOS: more common in females
Risk factors		DD: paranoid premorbid personality LOS: paranoid or schizoid premorbid personality
Phenomenology	Persecutory delusions common	DD: hallucinations rare and insipid LOS: hallucinations prevalent, multimodal and vivid
Course	Chronic course common Personality deterioration uncommon	
Response to treatment		DD: ? poor response to neuroleptics LOS: variable response to neuroleptics; some full resolution
Neuropathology	None	
Biological markers	None	

Table 18.6. *Focal brain disease (FBD) versus late onset schizophrenia (LOS)*

	Like	Unlike
Genetics		FBD: genetics varies by disease LOS: tends to run in families
Epidemiology		
Risk factors		For stroke: hypertension, diabetes and hypercholeslemia
Phenomenology		FBD: onset sudden or subacute LOS: onset rarely sudden or subacute
Course		FBD: focal neurologic signs and symptoms
Response to treatment		
Neuropathology		FBD: pathology of specific disease LOS: no specific neuropathology
Biological markers		

Table 18.7. *Delirium versus late onset schizophrenia (LOS)*

	Like	Unlike
Genetics		Delirium: no reported genetic contribution
Epidemiology		Delirium ● common in medically ill ● increased death rate
Risk factors		Delirium: identifiable metabolic, toxic, infectious or withdrawal states LOS: no associated metabolic, toxic, infectious or withdrawal abnormalities
Phenomenology	Nonauditory hallucinations relatively common	Delirium: fluctuating level of consciousness LOS: fully alert
		Delirium: first rank symptoms rare LOS: first rank symptoms common
Course		Delirium: variable throughout day LOS: rarely variable throughout day
		Delirium: usually reversible with correction of underlying abnormality LOS: often chronic
Response to treatment	Neuroleptics useful in both	Delirium: reassurance and reorientation help briefly LOS: reassurance and reorientation rarely helpful
Biological markers		Delirium: elevated temperature, tachycardia common LOS: no elevated temperature, tachycardia rare
		Delirium: slow EEG LOS: no EEG changes
		Delirium: markers of metabolic, toxic, infectious or focal lesion

and the late-onset condition have many similarities and several important differences. Therefore, we agree with Almeida et al. that closure on this question is premature and that more data is needed before firm opinions are developed.

A comparison with diabetes mellitus reveals some parallels: elevated fasting blood glucose can first manifest at any age. Early-onset cases are more likely to be insulin dependent while later onset cases are less likely to require insulin. These differences reflect different pathophysiologies which are not intrinsically age-dependent but whose age of onset reflect characteristics of the different etiologies.

Table 18.8. *Hallucinosis (HAL) versus late onset schizophrenia (LOS)*

	Like	Unlike
Genetics		HAL: no known genetic predisposition
Epidemiology	Rare in population studies	
Risk factors	Associated with sensory organ impairment	
Phenomenology	Hallucinations vivid	HAL: delusions rare or absent LOS: delusions are necessary for diagnosis
	Insight lacking	HAL: insight sometimes present HAL: usually single modality LOS: multiple modality common
Course	Often chronic	
Response to treatment		HAL: neuroleptic response poor LOS: neuroleptic response better HAL: reassurance sometimes helpful LOS: reassurance rarely helpful HAL: environmental change can elicit (e.g. darkness, isolation) or relieve (e.g. brighter light, interactions with others) LOS: effects of environmental change uncommon
Neuropathology	None	
Biological markers		

That is, age is not the primary determinant of the different etiologies of diabetes but the likelihood of any specific etiology being the initiating event in an individual does vary across the lifespan. Studying symptom patterns, treatment characteristics and molecular biologic correlates across the age span has resulted in a beginning identification of genetic, autoimmune and infectious etiologies. A similar process is now being applied to the syndrome characterized by hallucinations and delusions, chronic course and absence of affective symptoms and progressive dementia. The specific biologic markers that are needed to advance molecular understanding of these diseases are lacking, but an intensive search is ongoing (e.g. Kilidireas et al., 1992). The recognition that syndromic classification is an early step in the search for specific causes of disease should temper arguments about this intriguing condition.

Acknowledgements

Supported by NIMH grants MH40843 to PVR and MH43775 and RR-00722 to GDP. We thank Jessie Roth for discussions over the parallels with diabetes mellitus.

References

Castle, D. J. & Howard, R. (1992). What do we know about the aetiology of late-onset schizophrenia? *European Psychiatry*, **7**, 99–108.

Chiompi, L. (1987). Review of follow-up studies on long-term evolution and ageing in schizophrenia. In *Schizophrenia and Ageing*, pp. 37–51, eds. N. E. Miller & G. D. Cohen. New York: Guilford Press.

Cooper, A. F., Curry, A. R., Kay, D. W. K., Garside, R. F. & Roth, M. (1974). Hearing loss in paranoid and affective psychoses of the elderly. *Lancet*, **ii**, 851–4.

Gold, K. & Rabins, P. V. (1989). Isolated visual hallucinations and the Charles Bonnet syndrome: a review of the literature and presentation of six cases. *Comprehensive Psychiatry* **30**, 90–8.

Harding, C. M., Brooks, G. W., Ashikaga, T., Strauss, J. S. & Breier, A. (1987). The Vermont longitudinal study of persons with severe mental illness. II. Long-term outcome of subjects who retrospectively met DSM-III criteria for schizophrenia. *American Journal of Psychiatry*, **144**, 727–35.

Hassett, A. M., Keks, N. A., Jackson, H. J. & Copolov, D. L. (1992). The diagnostic valdiity of paraphrenia. *Australian and New Zealand of Journal of Psychiatry*, **26**, 18–29.

Hymas, N., Naguib, M. & Levy, R. (1989). Late paraphrenia – a follow-up study. *International Journal of Geriatric Psychiatry*, **4**, 23–9.

Jeste, D. V., Harris, M. J., Pearlson, G. D., Rabins, P., Lesser, I. M., Miller, B., Coles, C. & Yassa, R. (1988). Late-onset schizophrenia: Studying clinical validity. *Psychiatric Clinics of North America*, **11**, 1–13.

Kay, D. W. K. & Roth, M. (1961). Environmental and hereditary factors in the schizophrenias of old age ('late paraphrenia') and their bearing on the general problem of causation in schizophrenia. *Journal of Mental Science*, **107**, 649–85.

Kay, D. W. K., Cooper, A. F., Garside, R. F. & Roth, M. (1976). The differentiation of paranoid from affective psychoses by patients' premorbid characteristics. *British Journal of Psychiatry*, **129**, 207–15.

Kilidireas, K., Latov, N., Strauss, D. H., Gorig, A. D., Hashim, G. A., Gorman, J. M. & Sadiq, S. A. (1992). Antibodies to the human 60 kDa heat-shock protein in patients with schizophrenia. *Lancet*, **340**, 569–72.

McHugh, P. R. & Slavney, P. R. (1983). *The Perspectives of Psychiatry*. Baltimore: Johns Hopkins University Press.

Miller, B. L., Lesser, I. M., Boone, K. B., Hill, E., Mehringer, C. M. & Wong, K. (1991). Brain lesions and cognitive function in late-life psychosis. *British Journal of Psychiatry*, **158**, 76–82.

Naguib, M. & Levy, R. (1987). Late paraphrenia: neuropsychological impairment and structural brain abnormalities on computed tomography. *International Journal of Geriatric Psychiatry*, **2**, 83–90.

Pearlson, G. D. & Rabins, P. (1988). The late-onset psychoses: possible risk factors. *Psychiatric Clinics of North America Journal*, **11**, 15–32.

Pearlson, G. D., Kreger, L. Rabins, P. V., Chase, G. A., Cohen, B., Wirth, J. B., Schlaepfer, T. B. & Tune, L. E. (1989). A chart review of late-onset and early-onset schizophrenia. *American Journal of Psychiatry*, **146**, 1568–74.

Rabins, P. V., Pauker, S. & Thomas, J. (1987). Can schizophrenia begin after age 44? *Comprehensive Psychiatry*, **25**, 290–3.

Robins, E. & Guze, S. B. (1970). Establishment of diagnostic validity in psychiatric illness: its application to schizophrenia. *American Journal of Psychiatry*, **126**, 983–7.

Siegel, C. E. & Goodman, A. B. (1987). Mental illness among the elderly in a large state psychiatric facility: a comparison with other age groups. In *Schizophrenia & Aging*, eds. N. E. Miller & G. D. Cohen. New York: The Guilford Press.

Winokur, G. (1977). Delusional disorder (paranoia). *Comprehensive Psychiatry*, **18**, 511–21.

19

Community or asylum? Finding a place to care for the elderly psychiatric patient

CHRIS GILLEARD

Introduction

The average age of those patients still living in the large mental hospitals of the nineteenth and early twentieth centuries has steadily risen. These 'old long-stay patients' are often left behind in the hospital's remaining wards as younger more active patients are found places in community housing projects, group homes and psychiatric 'hospital' hostels (cf. Jones, 1989). Staff remaining behind with their patients are likely to be older and reluctant to contemplate finding a place for either themselves or their patients 'in the community'. Should the mental health services continue to offer an asylum to these ageing schizophrenic patients whose adult life may well have been shaped by past institutional regimes? Are sheltered work opportunities or group living attractive options for these retirement-age patients? Does living in the community offer any real improvement in the quality of life for an elderly ex-asylum inmate? Or is a hostel or nursing home nothing more than a miniature asylum in the community, a parish madhouse replacing the county asylum? The aim of this chapter is to examine the empirical evidence and consider the policy options surrounding the move out of the asylum for the elderly person with chronic schizophrenia.

The decline of the psychiatric hospital

The number of mental hospital beds in both the United States and Europe has been reducing steadily in recent years and this downward trend seems to be accelerating. What happens to these disappearing patients is a question of concern to clinicians and policy makers alike. How many are successfully placed in the community, and how many are left neglected and even further impoverished in bed and board rooming houses, shelters for the homeless or out on the streets?

Table 19.1 drawn from Scull (1989) illustrates the extent to which the number of long-stay patients in British and North American hospitals fell over the period 1950–1980.

The decline of these last decades has continued. In the UK the process of mental hospital closure has now been reaffirmed as part of the British Government's targets for 'the Nation's Health' (Secretary of State for Health, 1991). In other Western countries similar trends are evident (Balestrieri, Micciolo & Tansella, 1987; Haveman, 1986; Licht, Gouiliaer & Lund, 1991). At the same time voices have been raised critical of this process of 'deinstitutionalization' (Weller, 1985; Gralnick, 1985; Wasow, 1986). Closures continue but now they are proceeding hand in hand with research and evaluation that is helping pave the way for a more informed debate.

As mentioned earlier, surveys of patients left behind in the mental hospitals indicate an increasingly aged and handicapped population. The quinquennial survey conducted since 1960 at Glenside Hospital in Bristol, UK, has shown that while the number of male patients aged under 65 years has dropped from over 350 to under 100 in the space of 25 years, the corresponding number of male patients over 65 has remained almost static at just under 100. The latter group of older patients are described by the authors of the latest survey in the following terms:

> These severely handicapped people continue to live in impoverished ward environments with only minimal staff. They ... suffer personal poverty no longer able to supplement their income from industrial therapy; they survive on a basic allowance which scarcely provides a packet of cigarettes a day (Ford, Goddard & Lansdall-Welfare, 1987)

Where complete closure of psychiatric hospitals has taken place, as in the Worcester Development Project in the British Midlands, the fate of older patients has reflected a policy of 'hospital replacement' rather than 'hospital closure' (Khoosal & Jones, 1990). After one hospital closed, the patients were transferred to another and when that hospital too closed the patients were moved into rehabilitation hostels and nursing homes/community hospitals or transferred to yet another hospital. The reality appears to be that this older population (composed largely of schizophrenic patients) remains within the walls of one type of institution or another. Their disabilities are severe:

> More than a third ... were incapable of walking without assistance and over two thirds suffered from poor mobility and frequent incontinence (Milner & Hassall, 1990)

While these authors are clear about the benefits to younger patients arising from the hospital replacement program they concluded that:

> the benefit for the older patients ... is not yet so apparent ... half do not appear to know that they are in a different environment and only two ... (9%) ... seem to appreciate the change. (Milner & Hassall, 1990)

It is not inevitable that the older long-stay patients remain behind. Recent experience in Massachusetts suggests that often it may be easier to discharge these

Table 19.1. *Resident population of mental hospitals in the United States and United Kingdom 1950–1980*

Year	USA	UK
1951	520 300	143 200
1955	558 000	146 900
1960	535 000	136 200
1965	475 200	123 600
1970	339 000	103 300
1975	191 400	87 000
1980	132 200	75 200

After Scull, 1989, pp. 312–313

older patients from large psychiatric hospitals than it is for younger more disturbed patients (Geller et al., 1990). As a result of legal actions mandating a drastic reduction in the number of patients in Northampton State Hospital, it proved possible to:

> virtually eliminate its geriatric population through the placement of patients in nursing homes (and) ... specialized geriatric residential programs

These authors note, however that, a 'crucial but as yet unanswered question' remains, namely, whether such achievements in reducing this population significantly improved the quality of life they were experiencing. In a telling indictment of the process of transferring chronic patients from state mental hospitals to nursing homes, rest homes and single room occupancy hotels, Brown (1985) points out that these 'community options' can become:

> merely ... mini-institutions which replicate many of the custodial and dehumanising elements of asylum life (Brown, 1985)

The Veterans Administration study report by Linn and her colleagues (Linn et al., 1985) suggests that transfer to nursing home care in the USA can do more clinical harm than transferring patients from ward to ward within the same hospital. It provides one of the few pieces of evidence in support of the long-stay mental institution – though the 'community nursing homes' described are a long way from the idealized forms of specialist residential care settings often envisioned in hospital 'resettlement' plans.

Extent of disabilities among old long-stay patients

A significant factor restricting the benefits of hospital closure or replacement for older patients is their frailty and limited ability to participate in and enjoy the experience of a less monotonous and impoverished environment. Evidence of 'creaming off' (Carson, Shaw & Wills, 1989) amongst patients moved out of the long-stay wards of the psychiatric hospital suggests that age-compounded disability can make transfer harder reducing the quality of hospital care to that of a welfare/warehousing function. Stewart (1991) in a survey of the health status of the old long-stay patients in one Scottish psychiatric hospital found only 20% free of significant physical illness, with a quarter unable to walk without assistance and a similar number doubly incontinent. It is difficult to envisage how such a group of patients could manage outside of an institution and such patients who are moved tend to be transferred either to nursing homes or other hospitals rather than to a noninstitutional environment.

The problem is accentuated by the combined effects of disease progression, institutionally determined deprivations of normal developmental opportunities and the cumulative effects of treatment regimes that themselves induce iatrogenic disabilities. Research on tardive dyskinesia – a syndrome of abnormal involuntary movements particularly affecting the muscles of the mouth, tongue and jaws – has shown the importance of both age and the cumulative effects of neuroleptic medication on the incidence of this socially disabling neurological disorder (McClelland et al., 1991). There is evidence that progressive cognitive impairment may accompany such neurological deficits. The implications of such disability are profound, affecting the patient's ability to communicate effectively, to eat hygienically, and to present him or herself in a socially normal manner.

How much cognitive impairment in aging schizophrenic patients reflects the natural history of the disease is almost impossible to determine. Studies suggest that dementia is common, in some cases affecting up to as many as 60% of elderly hospitalized schizophrenic patients but this intellectual deterioration seems unrelated to indices of structural abnormality of the brain as indexed by cortical volume and ventricular widening, (Pakkenberg, 1987; see also Chapter 17). The possibility cannot be dismissed that such 'end states' in schizophrenia are in part an artefact of both care and treatment. That dementia develops in the later stage of some patients' illness, and that it appears to be associated with increasing length of illness (and hence treatment) raises the question of whether the asylum has produced this 'end state' or whether the prevalence of end-state schizophrenia is simply greater in those most in need of asylum.

Whatever the relationship between the treatment and care offered to patients suffering from schizophrenia and the nature of their disabilities in old age, it is apparent that a large number of elderly hospital patients are neurologically, intellectually and socially disabled and that these disabilities can be progressive. Community living for such patients may inevitably mean living in a sheltered care environment which has to support both their disability and their dependency.

Of course, there are many elderly patients in hospital who are not so severely disabled and who are able to move to more autonomous residential settings. Of the

463 patients aged 60 and over moved out of Northampton State Hospital, 198 went into 'independent' accommodation and only 68 to Nursing Homes (Sommers et al., 1988). The costs and benefits that may accrue from such moves have not always been well documented but one can gain some understanding from studies examining the impact of relocation on an aging psychiatric patient population.

Relocation of the elderly patient: Opportunity or threat?

As noted above, the reality of many hospital closure programs has been that patients are moved from one institutional setting to another, though more often than not a smaller one. Such interinstitutional transfer of older patients has been associated with heightened morbidity and mortality, especially for the more disabled (Schulz & Brenner, 1977; Rowland, 1977). However the transfer of older patients may have beneficial as well as harmful effects and much may depend upon the nature of the place people are moved to, where they are moved from and how much preparation there has been for the move. Some studies have examined the effect of transferring older psychiatric patients from 'out of the way' hospital annexes or small mental hospitals into a larger psychiatric hospital (Morris, Bowie & Spencer, 1988). Others have examined transfer from one psychiatric hospital to another (Chanfreau et al., 1990), or from psychiatric hospital to nursing homes and residential homes (Jasnau, 1967; Perkins, King & Hollyman 1989*b*) while others have looked at transfers within the same hospital (Linn et al., 1985). The results provide little support for the view that either intra- or interinstitutional transfer causes enhanced mortality. When contrasted with the mortality of control groups or with premove mortality rates there seems no evidence of high mortality following relocation (Morris et al., 1988; Chanfreau et al., 1990).

Evidence of 'deterioration' in health or level of functioning is less straightforward. In one study Chanfreau et al. (1990) found some deterioration in behavior following interhospital transfer in the immediate aftermath of the move which one year later had not completely reversed itself. In contrast, in a study of elderly patients transferred from hospital to private residential homes, Perkins et al. (1989*b*) noted an improvement in behavioral functioning. Since the ages of the patients in these last two studies were similar (mean *c*. 70 years), and the same measure of functioning was used (the CAPE Behavior Rating Scale) with both groups of patients obtaining similar rating scale totals (between 7 and 10 points) one is led to conclude that the posttransfer environment is of particular significance in determining whether improvement or deterioration results.

What is also of importance in this latter report is that the process of identifying the alternative (nonhospital) accommodation, preparing both patients and care staff in advance of the move and retaining key-worker links with familiar staff from the parent hospital served to enhance the continuity of care while ensuring an improved home environment in private and voluntary nursing, residential and hostel settings (Perkins et al., 1989*a*). In another study of 18 old long-stay patients moved from a large mental hospital to smaller hospital hostels, Kingdon et al. (1991) also reported clinical improvements and a reduction in 'deviant' behavior. This contrasts with an equally recent study (Chong & Abbott, 1992) examining the impact of interhospital moves on patient symptomatology. The authors reported that while negative symptoms declined after the move, positive symptoms (hallucinations and to a lesser degree delusions) actually worsened. Most of these studies, however, suggest that measured purely in terms of clinical status, transfer, relocation or resettlement can achieve some observable benefit in so far as the transfer is to a 'nonhospital' residential setting. This does not seem to be so true for moves between hospitals. On the other hand intrahospital moves can also prove of temporary benefit (Linn et al., 1985).

As noted earlier, those elderly patients who move to smaller homes or hostels may not be representative of the total elderly hospitalized population, and it may be that part of the positive effects of transfer can be ascribed to the relative fitness of those moved. In a report on the reprovision of Cane Hill Hospital, Holloway (1991) noted that elderly patients found places in supported housing or private residential or nursing homes were less disabled than those not found places. He was led to conclude:

> Given the difficulties encountered in discharging the 'elderly graduate' patients and an apparent reluctance to fund specialist purpose built local services, the outlook for the more disabled patients remaining within the declining psychiatric hospital is very uncertain (Holloway, 1991).

The fact that more than half of the elderly patients left behind had died within a three-year period is one indication of the gloomy future that such patients may face. One must conclude that despite some early evidence of negative effects, relocation from psychiatric hospitals does provide an opportunity for positive change, at least for those older patients fortunate enough to be considered 'suitable' for alternative accommodation. For those merely shifted from one hospital to another there seems little evidence of any beneficial changes. Improvements that do occur may have more to do with an improved quality of life rather than any improvement in the underlying severity of the illness.

Relocation: What do the patients really want?

One must ask whether these attempts to find alternative accommodation are really what patients wish for. Perkins et al. (1989*b*) found a very positive response from their relocated patients to a move from hospital to homes and hotels. More studies of user satisfaction with services are needed to fully appreciate the impact of community-oriented policies on these older patients. The new consumerism in health care is percolating into the mental hospitals and asylums of yesteryear. Already, it is possible to identify studies that have asked elderly residents of long-stay wards what they want and where they would like to be living (Abrahamson, Swatton & Wills, 1989; Hughes et al., 1991; MacDonald, Sibbald & Hoare, 1988). Although as many as half of the patients have been found unable or unwilling to take part in such interviews, the views of the vocally coherent patients suggest that many do find their living environment unsatisfactory and would like to live elsewhere even if they are not always able to identify a 'realistic' alternative place to live. Abrahamson et al. (1989) have shown that those with more knowledge of outside resources are more likely to express a wish to move out than those without such knowledge. While disability may make it difficult for many older long-stay psychiatric patients to express clear views about their preferred living environment, and although the years in hospital may deprive patients of the knowledge and experience that home, work and family confer on most other adults, many still express a wish to not be there; and to be in a better place.

MacDonald et al. (1988) found that nearly two-thirds of the residents on long-stay wards in one South London hospital expressed a wish to live somewhere else. While age itself was not a factor in influencing the desire to live elsewhere, they found that increasing length of stay tended to dampen the wish to move. Clearly, some older patients have lived long enough in hospital to believe that these places are their home, and hence treat community placement as a kind of 'eviction'. There is evidence that such 'predischarge' attitudes predict the subsequent breakdown of community care (Drake & Wallach, 1988) but evidence collected after a move into the community suggests that the experience of life outside the mental hospital more often than not strengthens the desire not to return.

After community placement, very few patients wish to return to their old 'home' (Kingdon et al., 1991; Perkins et al., 1989*a*; MacGilp, 1991). Indeed, most studies indicate that patients continue to move further into the community, and away from the shelter of hostels and group homes. There are some patients who will need to be readmitted, but the numbers concerned may be less than the rate of readmissions amongst acutely admitted patients. Of course, it would be foolish to argue that every elderly patient is willing to consider a move out of an environment that may have served as their home for decades, but the fact that some are reluctant to move should not lead us to minimize the opportunities that do exist for even frail elderly patients to experience an improved quality of life outside the mental hospital.

Psychiatric hospitals, quality of care and quality of life

Examination of the quality of life of elderly patients in large psychiatric institutions has become a topical issue along with all the other issues arising out of the deinstitutionalization movement. Nevertheless, attempts to measure quality of life and quality of care have lagged behind other measurement concerns such as those concerned with symptomatology or behavioral functioning. One of the first attempts to assess the quality of care and quality of life of chronic seriously ill psychiatric patients was the study of three mental hospitals conducted in the early 1960s by Wing & Brown (1970). Guided by the hypothesis that the 'poverty' of social care influenced the extent of schizophrenics' impairment and fostered deterioration in their mental health, they used a number of measures to assess the 'social poverty' of the three hospitals. Table 19.2 illustrates the five measures of 'social poverty' that these authors developed.

While their study concentrated upon a young (age 60 and below) hospital population, the substantive findings and general methodological approach have continuing relevance to an older population who some 30 years earlier, were the middle-aged subjects of these very studies. Subsequent developments in the fields of quality of care and quality of life in long-term psychiatric care have reflected similar concerns (Lavender, 1985). The openness or restrictiveness of the environment, the degree of patients' engagement in their environment and the degree of concern and support shown for the patient as an individual seem enduringly important dimensions by which to judge what constitutes 'quality' of care, and 'quality' of life. While these areas have been selected by researchers largely on the basis of their own clinical experiences, similar themes have emerged in more recent consumer-oriented studies. Thus privacy, choice and independence are chief among patients' own accounts of what they value in their return to the community as is the escape from the restrictive routines of large institutions (MacGilp, 1991; MacDonald et al., 1988). Having a room of one's own, for example, figures high on the list of patients' expressed needs of community placement (Abrahamson et al., 1989; MacGilp, 1991).

Most of the 'quality of life' studies contrasting life in a mental hospital and life outside suggest that the material bases of life – food, shelter, hygiene facilities – rarely serve as the arbiter of choice for a place of residence. Goffman's original critique of the total institution (Goffman, 1961) seems to be echoed in measures of consumer choice and quality of life. However, the patients involved in these studies while often in their late fifties, sixties and seventies, are not representative of all the older psychiatric patients living in psychiatric hospitals. How far disability and dependency shift the salient features that constitute 'quality' in life is an important but largely unaddressed issue in the psychiatry and sociology of later life. Perhaps choice, privacy and independence eventually give way to safety, security and

Table 19.2. *Measuring quality of care: Wing and Brown's indicators of environmental poverty*

Variable	Illustrative content
Personal possessions	Inventory of 70 items, e.g. toothbrush, handbag, underwear etc.
Time budget	What time patients rise, how long they wait for breakfast, etc.
Ward restrictiveness	Inventory of 35 items, e.g. time outside door locked, times when bathroom available, etc.
Nurses' attitudes	13 item questionnaire examining nursing view of what the patient could manage to do
Patients' occupation	Nature of patient's daytime activities; ward work, OT, gardens, etc.

From Wing & Brown, 1970, pp. 33–43.

sympathy when age and illness combine to weaken the spirit. One of the few studies that has addressed this question involved elderly nursing home residents. It may have relevance for older psychiatric patients too. Cohn and Sugar (1991) surveyed staff, residents and family from five different nursing home settings. They found basic needs more important to residents than staff anticipated, and issues of choice and autonomy less so. Their findings led them to suggest that:

> each group tended to define quality of life in terms of domains over which they had responsibility and which therefore validated their roles (Cohn & Sugar, 1991)

It seems as if people are reluctant to place central value on aspects of their life which they cannot control. The implication would seem to be that those domains where autonomy cannot be exercised atrophy as sources of esteem and value. An impoverished and restrictive environment may lead to a decline in the value attached to freedom and choice; poor health and disability may have similar effects. Increased freedom may in turn restore 'choice' and 'privacy' to more centrally valued concerns for patients, and so may improvements in health and reductions in disability. Perhaps one should acknowledge that the opportunity to value choice and independence depends equally on the degree to which a care setting provides such opportunity and illness restricts it. A total lack of care combined with a total lack of control may come to encapsulate the fears of many professionals about the deteriorating quality of life that may await patients following 'deinstitutionalization'. The issues around life on the street for older ex-patients are therefore examined next.

Hospital closure and homelessness

While the evidence might suggest that the quality of life for elderly psychiatric patients after hospital discharge is not obviously worse and may be rather better than it was in hospital, some authors have claimed that patients may 'drop through the net' of community care and end up homeless on the streets. What price then they ask are choice and freedom if a person has nowhere to live and no effective means of taking care of him or herself? Studies of homelessness and mental health now are appearing in response to these concerns. The findings suggest that few older people with serious mental illness are actually sleeping rough on the streets (Reed et al., 1992). While it is true that a proportion of the urban homeless are of pensionable age (George, Shanks & Westlake, 1991; Kelling, 1991) elderly people in hostels and shelters for the homeless seem less likely to be seriously mentally ill than do younger adults. According to one recent report:

> mental health problems and psychiatric disorders (are) proportionately less of a problem among the older homeless people ... compared to other homeless age groups (Kelling, 1991).

It is difficult to know the reasons for this; recent studies indicate that the typical 'psychiatric patient' found among the homeless is a middle-aged man (Marshall (1989). It may be that local authorities are better able to provide older men and women with permanent accommodation, while the effort of remaining homeless and rootless may become too wearisome in later life. Risks of physical disease may result in greater rates of admission to general hospitals and subsequent rehousing. Whatever the precise reasons, there seems little justification to believe that the closures of psychiatric wards and hospitals have particularly raised the numbers of homeless mentally ill amongst those relatively few old people who remain part of the homeless population.

The ethos of asylum

So far this chapter has examined the empirical literature on the consequences of a policy that has been implemented slowly, spasmodically but inexorably, closing down the large mental hospitals of the late nineteenth and early twentieth centuries and replacing them with smaller, less custodial care settings. Numbers of psychiatric in-patients have fallen, the average age of the asylum population has risen and disability has increased within the asylum walls. For many older patients, there is little evidence that this process has been more than a transfer of care from large hospital asylums to smaller residential and nursing home settings and hostels typically managed by nonstatutory private or charitable bodies. Nevertheless, the process has rarely been harmful to health or destructive to the quality of life available to these patients and in an important number of cases it has been positively beneficial. There appears to be no serious reason to fear that these older patients (most of whom suffer from schizophrenic illnesses) are in danger of finding themselves without food or shelter as a result of these hospital closures. One must ask what all the fuss has been about.

The dismantling of the psychiatric hospital/lunatic asylum is on the agenda of almost every Western government's health department. The recent shocking relevations about the 'mental health care' institutions of Eastern Europe surely confirm the view that the provision of asylum can never be separate from the need to protect the social order and maintain the facade of social hygiene. If we worry now that the mentally ill litter our streets and raise concerns over our personal safety how much more reason do we have to worry about the ease with which hundreds of thousands of citizens have been excluded from any form of social or cultural national life by the policies of asylum?

Elderly psychiatric patients are an economic cost to every state. Their adult years may seem to have produced little more than concern and worry to others and private misery to themselves; their very appearance seems to testify to our failure to treat them properly. The more intolerant a society is to its own failings, the more it seeks to lock away its long-term mentally ill and disabled citizens. The totalitarian nature of welfare institutions was expressed early on by Goffman (1961) but the link between the nature of mental institutions and the ethos of a society is brought out most clearly in the writings of Franco Basaglia:

> Opening the institution is not opening the door, it is opening one's mind when faced with a sick person (Basaglia, 1979).

The need for asylum is not, and can never be a clinical need. It is a societal decision, perhaps a societal need, in the sense that society needs to offer asylum to those whom it cannot treat or care for through other formal and informal institutions and when it cannot or dare not leave them alone. The size of an institution, its hidden place and its closed door policies reflect this lack of tolerance for both our failure to treat and our failure to care. If we can develop a greater tolerance for our own limitations as a society, then perhaps we can offer less solid institutions more accessible to the community that will encourage an openness of mind to the problems of mental sickness that Basaglia worked so hard to achieve for his own society.

The introduction of case management approaches, together with the new consumerism in health care, and a health service operating within socially agreed limits of human and material resources seems to provide a sensible basis for moving forwards. Recognition that managing care involves a financial as well as a clinical and social responsibility is embodied in the principle of case management. The discipline of financially accounting for care provides one of the most visible ways by which the state can demonstrate its agreement to care. Viewing the patient and his or her family as key 'stakeholders' in this process along with the providers and purchasers of welfare, enhances the principle of accountability.

If we can be guided by the belief that the institutions of society should offer all of us the opportunity to develop throughout our adult lives, and that even those presenting the most serious disabilities or the most serious dangers to society retain this potential for lifelong development, then we cannot accept a return to the closed doors of the mental asylums. The challenge is to understand what social and health care systems can do and what society is prepared to spend to make such systems a reality for all those who approach their old age having lived with the shadow of mental illness across most of their adult lives.

References

Abrahamson, D., Swatton, J. & Wills, W. (1989). Do long stay psychiatric patients want to leave hospital? *Health Trends*, **21**, 17–19.

Balestrieri, M., Micciolo, R. & Tansella, M. (1987). Long stay and long-term psychiatric patients in an area with a community-based system of care: a register follow-up. *International Journal of Social Psychiatry*, **33**, 251–63.

Basaglia, F. (1979). Liberta e Terapeutica? Milan: Feltrinellii. cited by Giannichedda, M.G. (1988). A future of social invisibility, In *Psychiatry in Transition. The British and Italian Experiences*, ed. S. Ramon. London: Pluto Press.

Brown, P. (1985). *The Transfer of Care: Psychiatric Deinstitutionization and its Aftermath.* London: Routledge and Kegan Paul.

Carson, J., Shaw, L. & Wills, W. (1989). Which patients first: a study from the closure of a large psychiatric hospital. *Health Trends*, **21**, 117–20.

Chanfreau, D., Deadman, J. M., George, H. & Taylor, K. E. (1990) Transfer of long-stay psychiatric patients: a preliminary report of inter-institutional relocation. *British Journal of Clinical Psychology*, **29**, 59–70.

Chong, L. S. & Abbott, P. M. (1992). Relocation of long stay general psychiatric in-patients. *Psychiatric Bulletin*, **16**, 22.

Cohn, J. & Sugar, J. A. (1991). Determinants of quality of life in institutions: Perceptions of frail older residents, staff and families. In *The Concept and Measurement of Quality of Life in the Frail Elderly*, (eds.). J. E. Birren, J. E. Lubben, J. C. Rowe and D. E. Detuchman, pp. 28–48. New York: Academic Press.

Drake, R. E. & Wallach, M. A. (1988). Mental patients' attitude toward hospitalization: a neglected aspect of hospital tenure. *American Journal of Psychiatry*, **145**, 29–34.

Ford, M., Goddard, C. & Lansdall-Welfare, R. (1987). The dismantling of the mental hospital? Glenside Hospital surveys 1960–1985. *British Journal of Psychiatry*, **151**, 479–85.

Geller, J. L., Fisher, W. H., Wirth-Cauchon, J. L. & Simon, L. J. (1990). Second-generation deinstitutionalization: the impact of Brewster versus Dukakis on State Hospital Case Mix. *American Journal of Psychiatry*, **147**, 982–7.

George, S. L., Shanks, N. J. & Westlake, I. (1991). Census of single homeless people in Sheffield. *British Medical Journal*, **302**, 1387–9.

Goffman, E. (1961). *Asylums: Essays on the Social Situation of Mental Patients and Other Inmates.* New York: Doubleday.

Gralnick, A. (1985). Build a better state hospital, deinstitutionalization has failed. *Hospital and Community Psychiatry*, **36**, 738–45.

Haveman, M. J. (1986). Dehospitalization of psychiatric care in the Netherlands. *Acta Psychiatrica Scandinavica*, **73**, 456–63.

Holloway, F. (1991). 'Elderly graduates' and a hospital closure program: the experience of the Camberwell resettlement team. *Psychiatric Bulletin*, **15**, 321–3.

Hughes, I. C. T., McLackland, B. M., Oles, G. S., Pryce, I. G. & Griffiths, R. D. P. (1991). The long-stay psychiatric patient as consumer. *Psychiatric Bulletin*, **15**, 662–3.

Jasnau, K. F. (1967). Individualized versus mass transfer of nonpsychotic geriatric patients from mental hospitals to nursing homes with special reference to the death rate. *Journal of the American Geriatric Society*, **15**, 280–4.

Jones, D. (1989). The selection of patients for reprovision. In *TAPS, Moving Long Stay Patients into the Community: First Results*. London: NETRHA.

Kelling, K. (1991). *Older homeless people in London*. London: Age Concern Greater London.

Kelly, G. R. (1983). Minimising the adverse effects of mass relocation among chronic psychiatric inpatients. *Hospital and Community Psychiatry*, **34**, 150–4.

Khoosal, D. & Jones, P. (1990). Worcester Development Project: where do patients go when hospitals close? *Health Trends*, **22**, 137–41.

Kingdon, D., Turkington, D., Malcolm, K., Szulecka, K. & Larkin, E. (1991). Replacing the mental hospital: Community provision for a district's chronically psychiatrically disabled in domestic environment? *British Journal of Psychiatry*, **158**, 113–17.

Lavender, A. (1985). Quality of care and staff practices in long-stay settings. In New Developments in Clinical Psychology, ed. F. N. Watts. London: Wiley and Sons.

Licht, R. W., Gouiliaev, G. & Lund, J. (1991). Trends in long stay hospitalization in Denmark: a descriptive register study, 1972–1987. *Acta Psychiatrica Scandinavica*, **83**, 314–18.

Linn, M. W., Gurel, L., Williford, W. O., Overall, J., Gurland, B., Laughlin, P. & Barchiese, A. (1985). Nursing home care as an alternative to psychiatric hospitalization. *Archives of General Psychiatry*, **42**, 544–51.

McClelland, H. A., Metcalfe, A. V., Kerr, T. A., Dutta, D. & Watson, P. (1991). Facial dyskinesia: a 16 year follow-up. *British Journal of Psychiatry* **158**, 691–6.

MacDonald, L., Sibbald, B. & Hoare, C. (1988). Measuring patient satisfaction with life in a long stay hospital. *International Journal of Social Psychiatry*, **34**, 292–304.

MacGilp, D. (1991). A quality of life study of discharged long-term psychiatric patients. *Journal of Advanced Nursing*, **16**, 1206–15.

Marshall, M. (1989). Collected and neglected: Are Oxford hostels for the homeless filling up with disabled psychiatric patients? *British Medical Journal*, **299**, 706–9.

Milner, G. & Hassall, C. (1990). Worcester Development Project: the closure and replacement of a mental hospital. *Health Trends*, **22**, 141–5.

Morris, R. K., Bowie, P. C. W. & Spencer, P. V. (1988). The mortality of longstay patients following inter-hospital relocation. *British Journal of Psychiatry*, **152**, 705–6.

Pakkenberg, B. (1987). Post-mortem study of chronic schizophrenic brains. *British Journal of Psychiatry*, **151**, 744–52.

Perkins, R., Fahey, K., Shinner, M. & Hollyman, J. (1989*a*). Barriers broken down. *The Health Services Journal*, **99**, 1432–3.

Perkins, R., King, S. & Hollyman, J. (1989*b*). Resettlement of old long-stay psychiatric patients: the use of the private sector. *British Journal of Psychiatry*, **155**, 233–8.

Reed, A., Ramsden, S., Marshall, J. et al. (1992). Psychiatric morbidity and substance abuse among residents of a cold weather shelter. *British Medical Journal*, **304**, 1028–9.

Rowland, K. F. (1977). Environmental effects predicting death for the elderly. *Psychological Bulletin*, **84**, 349–72.

Schulz, R. & Brenner, G. (1977). Relocation of the aged: a review and theoretical analysis. *Journal of Gerontology*, **32**, 323–33.

Scull, A. (1989). *Social Order/Mental Disorder: Anglo-American Psychiatry in Historical Perspective*. London: Routledge.

Secretary of State for Health (1991). *The Health of the Nation*. London: HMSO.

Sommers, I., Baskin, D., Specht, D. & Shively, M. (1988). Deinstitutionalization of the elderly mentally ill: factors affecting discharge to alternative living arrangement. *The Gerontologist*, **28**, 653–8.

Stewart, M. (1991). The physical health of old long stay in-patients in one psychiatric hospital. *Psychiatric Bulletin*, **15**, 404–6.

Wasow, M. (1986). The need for asylum for the chronically mentally ill. *Schizophrenia Bulletin*, **12**, 162–7.

Weller, M. P. I. (1985). Friern hospital: where have all the patients gone? *Lancet*, **i**, 869–71.

Wing, J. K. & Brown, G. W. (1970). *Institutionalism and Schizophrenia*. Cambridge: Cambridge University Press.

Part 8

Psychological, biological and medical issues

20

A developmental psychology of old age

SID WILLIAMS

Introduction

Many writers use the term 'developmental' mainly to refer to psychological events occurring in childhood (Bowlby, 1988; Rutter, 1988). There is, of course, a logical nexus between psychological and physical development so that it could be argued that they are active concurrently and therefore cease at the same time. The corollary to such a view, taken in the extreme, would have it that psychological change in adulthood represents a passive response to current inputs, the form of that response having been already determined by childhood experiences. This is a linear model of behavior, which would see the individual adult person's role in behavioral and psychological change as essentially passive. A developmental model, in contrast, seeks to view the behavioral and psychological response of the person themselves as a significant factor in influencing both their own state and their environment through homeostatic and adaptive mechanisms.

In a model which equates physical with psychological development, old age is likely to be viewed as a period of involution and decay, rather than one of continued development. Superficially there is no innate reason that old age should be seen as more than a period of deterioration.

Comfort (1965) suggested that an old person was like 'a space probe that has been "designed" by selection to pass Mars, but that has no further built-in instructions once it has done so, and no components specifically produced to last longer than that. It will travel on, but the failure rate in its guidance and control mechanisms will steadily increase – and this failure of homeostasis, of self-righting, is exactly what we see in the aging organism.'

Human beings, however, appear to be the longest-lived species of mammal (Comfort,1979) and survive long after they have ceased to be maximally fertile, physically mature and vigorous. In general, in nature, the average age of a species at death is related to evolutionary forces. Usually, individual animals who no longer serve any function in continuing the species then die or become particularly vulnerable to predators. Indeed, the male of some spiders is usually ingested by the female after mating – apparently then having maximal value as food.

It appears that humankind evolved in its present form while living as hunter–gatherers, and that any human physical and behavioral features, such as longevity, had some survival value in a hunter–gatherer setting. Even in this setting there probably were some 'old' people, forming a much smaller proportion of the group than they do in the twentieth century, but present none the less. Indeed, it has been suggested that the transition from hunter–gatherer society to early farming cultures resulted in a shortening of the lifespan (Ross, 1992). Comfort (1979) quoting anthropological studies emphasizes that though there may be relatively few aged in 'primitive' societies, these few are very likely to be active, productive and essential to the society.

Comfort also says that 'it is clear throughout phylogeny that there is a relation between survival into the senile period and the existence of a social mode of life. In some cases, longevity has evolved as a prerequisite of social organization, in others, social organization itself increases the possibility of survival into old age, while the social group very probably draws adaptive benefits from the existence of old individuals.' Human longevity may thus be a result of the increased protection given by human groups to their older and infirm members, related to the human ability to adapt the environment rather than adapting to the environment. In other words, it may be a result of the particular human form of evolutionary success. Or this longevity may be a significant cause of the relative evolutionary success of human beings. Even if the first explanation is true, this does not exclude the second explanation – since there is still likely to be some evolutionary advantage in human longevity, whatever mechanisms may contribute to it. Biological characteristics shaped by evolutionary forces are, in general, parsimonious and usually fulfil some function.

Old people in a hunter–gatherer society probably had, among other roles, the care of young children at the potentially difficult ages when they can no longer be carried by their parents but still cannot safely take part in hunting and gathering activities. Old people may then have had a valuable educational role while child-minding and may have helped to provide a protective and productive environment for the group through the transmission of essential knowledge, attitudes and behaviors.

With the availability of language but without substantial permanent (especially written) records, the older persons in the hunter–gatherer group would presumably have been a valuable source of information particularly to young children, but also to people of all ages. This information probably encompassed the obvious factual matters helpful for survival (such as the location of food in particular seasons), as well as more subtle questions relevant to the social mode of human life. These questions may have included ethical, moral and legal issues;

matters of individual and group identity, and philosophical or spiritual issues. All these matters overlap in practice and may have been conveyed (as they are today) in song, work, story, ritual, or religious observance, in all of which the act of communication may hold significance equal to or greater than its content. The act of communication for instance may involve the modelling of useful attachment behaviors, which Bowlby (1988) has particularly emphasized.

These communications, as the process of 'symbolic interactionism' (Victor, 1987) become the glue which holds a society together, help it to function effectively and to adapt appropriately.

It is the philosophical or spiritual issues which will be the focus of this chapter. They include the 'meaning of life' issues – the nature of humankind, of the world, of god(s), of life and of death. They interweave and are inextricable from the ethical, moral, legal and identity issues but it is the significance of these 'meaning of life' issues to the developmental psychology of old age which will be addressed particularly here. The hypothesis to be developed is that old people have an important, even essential role in providing both a source of information about the 'meaning of life' issues and a testbench for a philosophy of life or worldview particularly where it relates to these 'great issues'.

This hypothesis is offered in part to challenge the reader to address the issue of the psychology of old age beyond considerations of cognitive change and apart from any preconception of involution and decay.

Some theories and ideas

The following is a brief and selective review of some of the ideas which contribute to the hypothesis proposed later in this chapter.

Successful aging

Inherent to the discussion of patterns of psychological aging are judgements of what constitutes 'successful aging'. An important distinction between 'usual and successful aging' has been made by Rowe and Kahn (1987). They emphasize that, in studying the biology of aging it is worth discriminating between what is common or statistically 'usual' and what can be judged as 'successful'. Thus while it may be usual at the age of 90 years to be suffering from several significant illnesses or disorders, it may not be considered successful. On the other hand the performance on parameters of cardiovascular fitness of a group of very fit old persons may demonstrate successful but not usual aging.

Disengagement, activity and continuity theories

Disengagement theory was based on the observation in a USA study by Cumming and Henry (1979) that old people who had disengaged seemed more content than those who had not so disengaged. Their hypothesis was that 'aging is an inevitable mutual withdrawal or disengagement, resulting in decreased interaction between the aging person and others in the social systems he belongs to'. It has since been suggested that those disengaged old people in the study were fulfilling the role expectations of their particular society and that although disengagement may be the modal tendency in the developmental process beyond age 50 in the US society studied ('usual aging'), there was nothing inherently beneficial to the individual ('successful aging') in adopting disengagement as a pattern of behavior in old age. It has been argued that disengagement theory has been successful in justifying social policies which marginalize old people.

A contrary activity theory (Maddox,1964) suggests that old people who remain as active, productive and socially integrated as possible are most likely to have a sense of life satisfaction. Although sounding more attractive at face value than disengagement theory, there is a dangerous corollary to activity theory: that those who don't manage or wish to remain 'active' have, in some sense, failed the test of aging and are not entitled to the help of the rest of society. There are inherent value judgments in this as in disengagement theory, both are hard to test with empirical research and both are at the least, simplistic.

Continuity theory probably best fits the available data (Atchley, 1972) – that people attempt to continue on a trajectory of disengagement, or activity, or other behavior pattern depending on the lifestyles and personalities they have established in younger life. Certainly, many observations suggest that successful and indeed usual responses of old people to aging may be quite diverse.

Symbolic interactionism

This is a theory fundamental to sociology which suggests that the process of social interaction, and in particular the exchange of language, results in human beings living in a symbolic as well as a physical environment (Victor,1987). According to this theory, the human social world and subjective reality is constructed by a process of interaction with others. There are echos in this concept of a number of psychological theories such as Kelly's personal construct theory (Kelly, 1955). The interpersonal process described by symbolic interactionism seems similar also to the 'syntaxic mode of experience' involving 'consensual validation', as described by Sullivan (Weiner,1989). Russell (1981) used the concept of symbolic interactionism to describe the social processes occurring in 'Senior Citizens'

Centres' in an Australian city in a way which illustrates the utility of this approach.

Aging and the family

Clearly, the old person exists in a social matrix, usually a family, and families can be seen as functional entities with their own developmental history and process (Brody, 1974). As an individual reaches 'old age', their children are often entering middle or late adulthood. Their own parent or parents may be of very advanced years. The individual's psychological changes associated with aging need to be seen in such contexts.

Stresses of old age

The stresses of old age are many. The old person may have to adapt to a changed role or roles, loss, approaching death, self acceptance, dependency, and loss of autonomy, mastery or agency. Losses are perhaps more likely to be 'irretrievably hopeless, in a way which was rare for younger people' (Murphy, 1982). The elderly may in fact, however, experience less adverse events (both in number and severity) than younger persons and report less subjective distress when so exposed (Henderson, 1990). There may be a possibly related fall in the prevalence of depression in very old age (Myers et al., 1984), although this finding has been questioned (see Chapter 7).

Ethology and attachment behaviors

Bowlby (1988) has used ethological concepts, particularly those related to attachment behaviors to provide models of aspects of human psychology. The old person's ability to form and maintain secure and mutually beneficial attachments is likely to be of great significance both to the person themselves and as a role model for younger persons. There appears to be an association between good social ties and reduced mortality at all ages (Henderson, 1988).

Developmental epigenetic model

Using a developmental epigenetic model based loosely on embryological principles, Freud wrote of development occurring up to the end of adolescence. Erik Erikson took developmental theory much further, producing a theory for the whole of life in eight stages (Lofgren,1989). In the eighth stage of 'later adulthood' he emphasized the importance of approaching death which he said drove the old person to review and attempt to integrate their life experience with their world view and expectations, leading to either 'ego-integrity' or 'despair'. This model has intuitive appeal and has influenced many writers since, although Erikson may have given too much weight to death as a significant concern of the old person. It is also probably significant that Erikson saw this phase as beginning usually around 51 years, which is quite young in gerontological terms. The concern with the issue of death is more likely to be associated with these 'young old' years, as will be discussed further below.

The life review

Butler (1963) emphasized the importance in old age of 'the life review as a naturally occurring, universal mental process characterized by the progressive return to consciousness of past experiences, and, particularly, the resurgence of unresolved conflicts; simultaneously, and normally, these revived experiences and conflicts can be surveyed and reintegrated'. Butler also presumed that 'this process is prompted by the realization of approaching dissolution and death, and the inability to maintain one's sense of personal invulnerability' which has obvious similarities to the Eriksonian concept and is subject to the same criticisms (see below). It is also not established that the tendency to reminisce and review is as characteristic of old age as Butler suggests. It may be a lifelong phenomenon and it may not be as common an occurrence in old age as proposed.

Death and the mid-life crisis/transition

Other writers have emphasized the importance of the issue of death and vulnerability, not to the old person, but to the person in their middle adulthood – which can be said to begin about the age of 35 (Turner & Helms, 1987). Many will face the challenges associated with this stage at an earlier or later time in life. About this time the individual is often particularly confronted with the facts of aging in their own body and those of their parents or elders and often also of the facts of death in their parents/elders. Although an individual may be confronted by these facts earlier in life, there seems to be an ability to deny these issues through early adulthood as is apparent in many risk-taking behaviors at an earlier age. During the mid-life transition (Turner and Helms, among others, have objected to the term 'crisis'), the person in their middle years either confims or develops a philosophy of life or world-view – so that by the time old age is reached, there is little concern about or fear of death. The old appear to fear dependency and pain, loss of dignity and autonomy, and are saddened that they will be separated from family and friends, but the issue of death itself does not seem to exercise them greatly. Thus in Cumming and Henry's study: 'One question – whether the respondent often thought of dying – was a failure because only a tiny fraction admits ever thinking of death or dying.' The theme of the relationship between the mid-life transition and old age will be further discussed later.

Some aspects of human brain function and their significance

The search for meaning

The neurosciences present one of the most rapidly enlarging and most exciting areas of the human sciences. As has been put forward by Changeux (1985) in his book 'Neuronal Man', if we take care not to give way to 'simplistic reductionism', there may be utility in seeking a model of human behavior in the nature of the human brain.

The relative success of humans as a species depends, at least in part, on two related characteristics. First, the power of problem-solving in the abstract and second, the tendency to search for closure, explanations and models for observed phenomena.

Like a satiated rat which spontaneously explores a maze, humans have a propensity to engage in exploratory behavior when there is no immediate reason so to do. Humans, however, explore their world in an abstract as well as a concrete sense.

The tendency to explore and manipulate objects is exaggerated and disinhibited by some frontal lesions to produce 'Utilization Behavior' as part of the 'Environmental Dependency Syndrome' described by Lhermitte, Pillon & Serdaru (1986), where among other behaviors, 'the sight of an object implies the order to use it'. This behavior can be viewed as the result of a combination of the disinhibited drive to explore and understand, and a failure of the capacity for abstraction, so that the usual abstract exploration is made concrete and physical, and therefore visible to an observer. Like other behaviors and reflexes associated with impaired brain function, the behaviors of the environmental dependency syndrome are apparent in, indeed are characteristic of, young children. They probably also contribute substantially to some problem behaviors of patients with dementia.

The same tendency to explore and engage the abstract and semantic environment is a feature of the human experience. It too may become exaggerated and disinhibited in some persons with temporal lobe epilepsy and then be expressed as religiosity, philosophical interests and hypermoralism (McLelland, 1991).

The general human tendency to explore abstract issues with the expectation of closure is described by Hawking (1990) as follows:

> We want to make sense of what we see around us and to ask: What is the nature of the universe? What is our place in it and where did we come from? Why is it the way it is?

These questions imply the presence of an answer, an assumption engendered by these characteristics of the human brain rather than necessarily by the presence of an answer. For after all, mankind seems to have always searched for answers to these 'great issues' and to have been variably satisfied with a wide variety of 'answers'.

The sense of self

The abstract concept of the 'self' is probably a direct consequence of the human ability to develop complex abstract concepts. Thus, as well as having abstract concepts of items and occurrences in the external environment, humans possess the capacity to develop sophisticated concepts of themselves.

The limits of self; the awareness of death; The Limits of Control

With the experience of abstract awareness, several potentially disturbing and interrelated issues confront the human species as follows: that the self is apparently finite and limited; that all humans die; that many humans will experience illness and impairment during their lives; that human beings have only limited control over the time and nature of their death and many other aspects of their life and circumstances.

The resultant dilemma was bluntly and graphically described by Gould (1970):

> That far from being a creature created by an omnipotent God who has made him but a little lower than the angels, (man) is in fact, an accident of nature, clinging to an ephemeral perch on an all too mortal speck of fragile cosmic grit. To an animal with an instinct for survival this is a pretty frightening idea.

The limits of understanding; the illusion of control

There is an added difficulty, in that the limitations of the human brain make it difficult, if not impossible, to fully comprehend issues of the infinite – words such as 'transcendental' are available to allow description of such phenomena. Such words and concepts provide a sense of closure and perhaps satisfy the drive or search for meaning: '*Wo die Begriffe fehlen stellt des Wort sich ein*' (Where comprehension is lacking, words readily appear: Goethe).

Indeed, it could be argued that most human beings maintain an illusion of control over their lives and circumstances. When this illusion is breached by some personal or natural disaster most become temporarily or partially incapacitated by a crisis response or grief reaction (Sifneos, 1985).

Existential threats

It could be argued that the fear of death, and philosophic preoccupation with these related issues of meaning and the nature of things are confined to self-indulgent middle-class intellectuals. Becker (1975) however puts arguments for the universality of what he dramatically calls 'the terror of death'.

It is also noticeable that the families of patients with dementia or other malignant condition often show a propensity to explore issues of 'meaning', and this process of exploration becomes an important part of clinical management of these conditions. Also, a significant part of the assessment process in a geriatric service, as elsewhere in medicine, involves the provision of diagnostic labels and explanations of observed phenomena in a process of negotiation described by Balint (1968). This provides a sense of closure, and an illusion of control which, the relatives and the patient appear to seek. This process of negotiated 'meaning' probably long preceded scientific medicine and is the province of the Shaman in many cultures to this day.

Thus, the brain characteristics which have led to the evolutionary success of the human species can, and do, pose a threat to the individual and to the human group. In the individual this threat can find expression in alienation and suicide as well as in other dysfunctional behaviors such as substance abuse and hedonism. At a group level, the threat may be apparent in the form of cult movements, civil unrest and/or the blind devotion to leaders and social movements which claim to provide simple 'answers'.

Old age as the source of the solution to transcendental dilemmas

If the phenomenon of longevity as a human characteristic developed about the same time as the changes or developments which led to the evolutionary success of the species, it is likely, as previously argued, that the two may be related in some way. It is quite conceivable that the development of language and the associated ability to use and manipulate knowledge and ideas led to an exponential increase in survival and adaptation skills. This may have been associated with relatively rapid cultural evolution (Dawkins,1989), or in other words the evolution of ideas and behaviors. If this were so, there would be considerable advantage in having old individuals in the group who could act as sources of knowledge and experience – particularly in the long period (largely as hunter–gatherers) of human history before the development of written language.

If, however (as previously argued) the same neuropsychological characteristics which led to evolutionary success also led to threats to the individual and the group, perhaps the experience and knowledge of elders could hold the additional potential to counteract these threats. Perhaps old age provided some solutions to these potential threats.

These solutions may have been in two forms. The old person may have been a source of information about the 'great issues' and the old person may also have provided a testbench for a philosophy of life.

Perhaps when humans faced an awareness of death and relative lack of control over their fate at various times during their lives, they could avail themselves of the views of their elders and they could also observe the success or otherwise of their elders in dealing with the facts of infirmity and death. The elders may have had many ways of coping with the joys and vicissitudes of old age – some by disengagement, some by activity, by accommodation and detachment, by angry protest, or despair, by a belief in a particular political system or supernatural force. The younger person could choose or affirm whatever belief system seemed most successful, coherent or attractive, or indeed reject the belief system of their elders on the basis of its apparent failure.

This process is still apparent in twentieth century society, during life crises, both accidental and developmental. For instance, during adolescence when first the human brain allows a fully developed abstract attitude, when issues of identity seem to be of particular importance and when many find contact with grandparents or other elders particularly constructive. And again, during the mid-life transition, when the young person's denial of mortality and morbidity falls away and many people seem to develop or consolidate a philosophy of life, an attitude to, and a belief about, the transcendental issues confronting them.

A developmental psychology of old age

To summarize the proposed model of psychological development in old age: the main task of old age is similar in most senses to that proposed by Erikson, that is, to review one's life, and to come to terms with the results of that review while coping with the stresses particularly associated with old age. However, approaching death is not seen in this model as a major preoccupation of the old person, the issues of mortality and morbidity having been dealt with at an earlier time of life, particularly during the mid-life transition. Rather, the philosophy or world view developed earlier in life is being tested in old age, the relative success of that philosophy being observed by younger members of the family and group who are themselves developing or affirming their own philosophy.

All this is made necessary because of the nature of the human brain, which by developing to a high degree an abstract consciousness and spirit of enquiry at the same time advantages and threatens the human individual and the group. The advantages are augmented by the availability of the old person as a source of information. The threats are counteracted by the old person who acts again as an information source as well as a role model.

References

Atchley, R. C. (1972). *The Social Forces in Later Life: An Introduction to Social Gerontology.* Belmont, California: Wadsworth.

Balint, M. (1968). *The Doctor, his Patient and the Illness.* 2nd ed. London: Pitman Medical.
Becker E. (1975). *The Denial of Death.* New York: The Free Press, Macmillan.
Bowlby, J. (1988). Developmental psychiatry comes of age. *American Journal of Psychiatry*, **145**, 1–10.
Brody, E. M. (1974). Ageing and family personality: a developmental view. *Family Process*, **13**, 1, 23–7.
Butler, R. N. (1963). The life review: an interpretation of reminiscence in the aged. *Psychiatry*, **26**, 65–76.
Changeux, J. (1985). *Neuronal Man. The Biology of Mind.* New York: Oxford University Press.
Comfort, A. (1965). *The Process of Ageing.* London: Weidenfeld & Nicholson.
Comfort, A. (1979). *Ageing:The Biology of Senescence.* Edinburgh & London: Churchill Livingstone.
Cumming, E. & Henry, E. W. (1979). *Growing Old.* Reprint Edition. New York: Arno Press.
Dawkins, R. (1989). *The Selfish Gene.* Oxford: Oxford University Press.
Gould, D. (1970). A Groundling's Notebook, *New Scientist*, **48**, 729, 457.
Hawking, S. W. (1990). *A Brief History of Time.* Sydney: Bantam Press – Transworld Publishers.
Henderson, A. S. (1988). *An Introduction to Social Psychiatry*, Oxford: Oxford University Press.
Henderson, A. S. (1990). The social psychiatry of later life. *British Journal of Psychiatry*, **156**, 645–53.
Kelly, G. (1955). *The Psychology of Personal Constructs.* New York: Norton.
Lhermitte, F., Pillon B., & Serdaru, M. (1986). Human autonomy and the frontal lobes. Part I: imitation and utilization behavior: a neuropsychological study of 75 patients. *Annals of Neurology*, **19**, 326–34.
Lofgren, L. B. (1989), Erik H. Erikson. in *Comprehensive Textbook of Psychiatry/V*, 5th edn, ed. H. I. Kaplan & B. J. Sadock pp. 403–10. Baltimore: Williams & Wilkins.
McLelland, R. J. (1991), Psychiatric aspects of epilepsy. *Current Opinion in Psychiatry*, **4**, 127–30.
Maddox, G. L. (1964). Disengagement theory: A critical evaluation. *The Gerontologist*, **4**, 80–2.
Murphy, E. (1982). Social origins of depression in old age. *British Journal of Psychiatry*, **141**, 135–42.
Myers, J. K., Weissman, M. M., Tischler, G. L. et al. (1984). Six-month prevalence of psychiatric disorders in three communities: 1980–1982. *Archives of General Psychiatry*, **41**, 959–67.
Ross, E. P. (1992) Trends in molecular archeology. Eloquent remains. *Scientific American*, **266**, 72–81.
Rowe, J. W. & Kahn, R. L., (1987). Human ageing: usual and successful. *Science*, **237**, 143–9.
Russell, C. (1981) *The Ageing Experience.* Sydney: George Allen & Unwin.

Rutter, M. (1988). Epidemiological approaches to developmental psychopathology. *Archives of General Psychiatry*, **45**, 486–95.

Sifneos, P. E. (1985). Brief dynamic and crisis theory.in *Comprehensive Textbook of Psychiatry/V*, 5th edn, ed. H. I. Kaplan & B. J. Sadock pp. 1562–7. Baltimore: Williams & Wilkins.

Turner, J. S. & Helms, D. B. (1987). *Lifespan Development*, 3rd edn. New York: Holt, Rinehart and Winston.

Victor, C. R. (1987). *Old Age in Modern Society: A Textbook of Social Gerontology*. London: Croom Helm.

Weiner, M. F. (1989). Harry Stack Sullivan. In *Comprehensive Textbook of Psychiatry*, 5th edn, ed. H. I. Kaplan, & B. J. Sadock, pp. 424–6. Baltimore: Williams & Wilkins.

21

The biology of functional psychiatric disorders

MICHAEL PHILPOT

Introduction

Why study the biological aspects of psychiatric illness in elderly people? The question leads to three others.

(i) Are there features specific to psychiatric illness in elderly patients?
(ii) Are the biological features in young patients also present in elderly patients?
(iii) Can evidence obtained from such study help determine whether aging itself is a factor in the late onset of psychiatric illness?

Answers to the first two questions might help show whether late onset disorders are materially different from early onset disorders. Some still believe this to be the case with depression (Teicher et al., 1988) and it remains an issue in relation to the para-/schizo-phrenias (Almeida et al., 1992). The last question is perhaps the most interesting but difficult to examine.

In the case of affective disorders, the notion that the process of physical aging acts as a risk factor has long been held (Burton, 1652; Maudsley, 1879; Charcot, 1881). In modern times, Post (1968) eloquently laid out the argument. Given that the genetic contribution was thought to diminish with increasing age of first onset and that there was little evidence to suggest personality weakness was of any importance, he wrote:

> Why, then, is it that some people respond with depressive reactions ... A deceptively simple answer might be that in some individuals there occur changes due to aging which make them particularly liable to succumb to stresses in a depressive fashion.

Post dismissed the possibility of endocrinological disorder and favored structural changes of the brain, which was reasonable given the state of knowledge at the time. Although he was referring to affective disorder the argument also has been cited in the context of paraphrenia (Post, 1992).

Several methodological problems present themselves to the study of the aging-vulnerability hypothesis. The most serious concerns the widespread use of cross-sectional research designs. Cohort factors are usually ignored or mentioned in passing and yet, in other areas of scientific endeavour, have long been acknowledged to have powerful effects. In some fields, longitudinal studies are precluded on practical or ethical grounds such as in postmortem brain or lumbar puncture research but would otherwise be perfectly possible.

As with any study in psychiatry, it is worth repeating that diagnostic issues are of importance. Careful attention needs to be paid to inclusion and exclusion criteria, including the concurrent use of psychotropic drugs, and yet this is often not the case.

The development of the psychiatry of old age as a speciality in its own right has had a confounding effect such that patient samples might only include those over 65 years of age who are accessible to the researcher–clinician. General psychiatrists, on the other hand, tend to exclude 'adults' over 65 years specifically in an attempt to avoid the distortion of results by the greater variability of biological data in older persons. Such practices make the adoption of a developmental perspective difficult. Similarly, little attention is paid to the representativeness of patients volunteering for research studies. Are those agreeing to have lumbar punctures while severely depressed typical of sufferers or is their apparent submissiveness an important factor in determining the experimental results?

It is beyond the scope of this chapter to review the entire field of psychobiology so mention has been confined to those studies involving elderly subjects. The reader will notice that little space is devoted to anything but depression: this reflects the dearth of studies involving other conditions.

Neurochemistry

Neurochemical research in humans involves the analysis of postmortem brain tissue, cerebrospinal fluid (CSF), blood cells (leucocytes and platelets) and urine. Subjects, dying of natural causes, used in postmortem studies are often considerably older than those investigated in other studies, a factor which may account for some of the discrepancies in results.

The monoamine hypothesis of depression (Schildkraut, 1965) appears to have stood the test of time albeit in a modified form which not only places greater emphasis on the role of serotonin but incorporates the interaction with noradrenergic and glucocorticoid systems and changes in receptor sensitivity (Pryor & Sulser, 1991).

Serotonin (5-hydroxytryptamine, 5-HT)

Postmortem studies

Serotonin cell bodies are situated in the raphe nuclei of the brainstem. Robinson, Davies & Nies, (1972) showed that the concentration of the 5-HT metabolite, 5-hydroxyindole acetic acid (5-HIAA), as measured in the brainstem of normal subjects, increased after the age of 65. Monoamine oxidase (MAO) activity also correlated positively with age suggesting an increased turnover of monoamines. Serotonin itself did not change but the results seemed to suggest that the abnormalities might make the elderly susceptible to depression. However, later studies have failed to confirm this and no consistent age effect has been demonstrated (Cheetham, Katona & Horton, 1991).

A number of studies have measured 5-HT and 5-HIAA in the brains of elderly depressed patients dying from natural causes compared to controls (Crow et al., 1984; Ferrier et al., 1986). No differences were found except that frontal 5-HIAA was lower in patients who had been drug-free for at least one year before death (Ferrier et al., 1986). Reductions of 5-HT and 5-HIAA in the brain stem and other brain areas such as frontal cortex or basal ganglia are more obvious in suicide victims (Cheetham et al., 1991).

5-HT_1 and 5-HT_2 receptor binding sites decrease in number with age (Sparks, 1989), a finding which has also been demonstrated in vivo using positron emission tomography (Wong et al., 1984). 5-HT_2 receptors in the frontal cortex, however, were raised in number in elderly depressed patients (McKeith et al., 1987; Yates et al., 1990) while 5-HT_1 receptors were normal in number and distribution (McKeith et al., 1987; Yates & Ferrier, 1990). Raised receptor numbers had previously only been reported in patients committing or attempting suicide (Stanley & Mann, 1983). Further evidence of reduced 5-HT uptake in the frontal cortex of elderly depressed patients has suggested that either a downregulation of presynaptic sites or a reduction in the number of 5-HT neurons occurs (Leake et al., 1991).

CSF and peripheral markers

CSF 5-HIAA has consistently been shown to increase with age (Meek et al., 1977) but results from depressed patients have been more variable. Reduced levels may be restricted to those with coexisting anxiety or suicidal behavior (Mann et al., 1989). Molchan et al. (1991*a*) found no difference in CSF 5-HIAA in elderly depressed patients but CSF 5-HIAA was reduced in elderly patients who had attempted suicide (Jones et al., 1991).

Blood platelets are derived from tissue which has the same embryonic origins as CNS neurons. Neurochemically, they function like brain tissue but do not synthesise their own 5-HT, which is absorbed from the blood (Elliott, 1991).

Platelet 5-HT receptors resemble the 5-HT_2 type and are reduced in number in unipolar or endogenous depression (Healy, Carney & Leonard, 1985). A number of research groups have found reductions in the numbers of 5-HT uptake sites using [^{3}H]-imipramine in elderly depressed patients (Schneider, Severson & Sloane, 1985; Suranyi-Codotte et al., 1985; Nemeroff et al., 1988*c*). The precise significance of these findings is unclear but Husain et al. (1991) reported a positive correlation between platelet [^{3}H]-imipramine binding and the number of areas of subcortical hyperintensity demonstrated by magnetic resonance imaging.

Platelets also contain MAO-B which converts 5-HT to 5-HIAA. In general, studies have shown reduced levels in bipolar affective disorders but increased levels in endogenous-type depression (Sandler, Reveley & Glover, 1981). Alexopoulos et al. (1987) compared platelet MAO-B activity in elderly patients with depression, dementia and combinations of the two with healthy controls. Patients with depression alone had reduced MAO activity and those with dementia had increased activity compared to control subjects. MAO activity was also raised in demented patients with depressive symptoms and those with depressive pseudodementia so that the marker had little diagnostic value.

Norepinephrine (NE)

Post-mortem studies

Robinson et al. (1972) demonstrated an age-related reduction in NE concentration in the brain-stem of normal subjects at postmortem together with the previously described increase in MAO activity. Riederer et al. (1980) found reduced concentration of NE in the red nucleus of the brain-stem and reduced concentration of 3-methoxy-4-hydroxyphenylethylene glycol (MHPG), the chief metabolite of NE, in six of 14 brain regions, particularly the globus pallidus. Brain receptor and uptake studies have not revealed any consistent changes in this system (Ferrier et al., 1986; Gross-Isseroff, Israeli & Biegon, 1989).

CSF and peripheral markers

MHPG may be measured in CSF and plasma. Gerner et al. (1984) found increased CSF MHPG in depressed patients aged over 40 years but in another study levels were similar to those found in patients with Alzheimer's disease and healthy controls (Molchan et al., 1991*a*). Halbreich et al. (1987) found that plasma MHPG increased significantly with age in healthy subjects and in endogenously depressed patients but was not related to symptom severity or clinical subtype. However, Azorin et al. (1990) found *reduced* plasma MHPG in elderly patients whose cortisol hypersecretion was not suppressed by dexamethasone.

The number of beta-adrenoreceptor binding sites on leucocytes increases with age, although binding affinity does not change (Gietzen et al., 1991). Binding is consistently reduced in depressed patients and in some studies correlates with the severity of the illness (Elliott, 1991).

Platelets carry $alpha_{2A}$ receptors which are very similar to central $alpha_2$ receptors found on pre- and postsynaptic neurones. Two studies carried out in groups of elderly patients report contradictory results. Doyle et al. (1985) found binding capacity to high affinity sites almost doubled in depressed patients but Georgotas et al. (1987) found no abnormality.

Dopamine (DA)

Although age-related reductions in function in the dopaminergic system have been demonstrated in postmortem brains (Rogers & Bloom, 1985) and in vivo using positron emission tomography (Wong et al., 1984) this system has been neglected with regard to depression and while homo-vanillic acid (HVA), the metabolite of DA, was increased in depressed patients over the age of 40 years in one study (Gerner et al., 1984) others have failed to confirm this finding (Molchan et al., 1991*a*).

In schizophrenia research, the DA hypothesis has just about survived despite many inconsistencies and disappointments. (For a critical review the reader is referred to Healy, 1991.) There is no consistent evidence from postmortem schizophrenia studies that DA or its metabolites differ in concentration from normal (Deakin, 1988) although the number of D_2 receptors may be increased in brain areas such as the striatum (Pilowsky, 1992).

Owen et al. (1987) found a reduction in MAO-B activity in the brains of elderly schizophrenic patients. The reductions were found in frontal and temporal regions and the amygdala and were associated with negative symptomatology. However, the authors concluded that the changes were probably not related to an alteration in monoamine metabolism but to a disruption of glial function.

Other neurotransmitters

There is circumstantial evidence to suggest a role for the cholinergic system in the etiology of depression (Dilsaver, 1986) but few controlled research studies have been carried out.

Other systems researched in older depressed subjects include the gamma-amino-butyric acid (GABA) system but no clear pattern has emerged (Crow et al., 1984). Sunderland et al. (1987) demonstrated a reduction in somatostatin-like immuno-reactivity (SLI) in elderly depressed patients which was similar to that found in demented patients. Although somatostatin interacts with other neurotransmitter systems important in depression and dementia its precise significance is not yet known.

Lastly, abnormalities of histamine H_1 (Nakai et al., 1991), glutamate (Harrison, McLaughlin & Kerwin, 1991; Simpson et al., 1992) and GABA (Simpson et al., 1992) receptors have all been described in schizophrenia.

Neuroendocrinology

In contrast to the more direct methods described above, this section deals with dynamic tests of neurotransmitter function, determining the output of each system in response to a neuroendocrine challenge under controlled conditions. The methods have the advantage of being easy to perform and repeat in the living subject.

Hypothalamic–pituitary–adrenal axis (HPA)

More detailed reviews of this field are provided elsewhere (Braddock, 1986; Philpot, 1986). Carroll (1982) developed the dexamethasone suppression test (DST) in which the administration of dexamethasone at 23.00 hours to normal subjects results in suppression of the diurnal variation of cortisol secretion over the next 18–24 hours. It was noted that patients with melancholia or endogenous depression were less likely to show this suppression, that is, they were 'nonsuppressors'. Unfortunately, after 20 years of experimentation, it is clear that an abnormal DST response is far from specific to melancholia and is also influenced by factors such as age, cognitive state and the ability to absorb dexamethasone (Georgotas et al., 1986; Hunt, Johnson & Caterson, 1989).

McKeith (1984) found that the DST differentiated well between elderly patients with endogenous and nonendogenous depression but that a significant percentage of patients with dementia also had abnormal responses reducing the clinical efficacy of the test in psychogeriatric practice. Two studies have demonstrated that demented patients with significant depression are more likely to be nonsuppressors (Katona & Aldridge, 1985; Abou-Saleh et al., 1987). Conversely, Shrimankar, Soni & McMurray (1989) found that nonsuppression was equally prevalent in demented patients with and without depression. Leake et al. (1990) measured *N*-pro-opiomelanocortin (*N*-POMC), adrenocorticotrophic hormone (ACTH) and cortisol before and after the DST in dementia and depression. Different patterns of response were found: elderly depressed patients had raised cortisol concentrations before and after dexamethasone, demented patients had raised cortisol only after DST, ACTH was raised after DST in both groups, but *N*-POMC was raised after DST only in depressed patients. The authors suggested that the mechanism of cortisol hypersecretion in dementia differed from that in depression and further evidence of this comes from a study in which the alpha adrenergic agonist, clonidine, was used as the challenge. Postclonidine cortisol secretion was reduced in elderly depressed patients and demented patients with hypercortisolemia but demented patients with normal cortisols at baseline had raised cortisols after clonidine (Vollhardt et al., 1989).

The HPA axis can also be stimulated by corticotrophin releasing factor (CRF) which acts directly on the anterior pituitary. The ACTH response is blunted in depression but the cortisol release is exaggerated and similar to that of controls (Holsboer, 1989). As a result it has been suggested that raised CRF is the basis for hypersecretion of cortisol. This is borne out by the increased CRF levels in the CSF of depressed patients (Nemeroff, 1988*a*). In a complex study, von Bardeleben & Holsboer (1991) administered the CRF test to a group of depressed patients with a wide age range after pretreatment on the previous day with dexamethasone. In normal subjects, cortisol response to CRF was inhibited, but in depressed subjects cortisol rose sharply as expected. The magnitude of the rise correlated positively with age and severity of depression. The age association was absent in the normal group. This seemed to indicate that impairment of glucocorticoid receptors in depression could be accelerated or accentuated by the aging process.

Hypothalamic–pituitary–thyroid axis

Thyroxine is thought to be an important cofactor in the action of monoamines (Whybrow & Prange, 1981) and is clinically useful in the management of rapid cycling affective disorder (Bauer & Whybrow, 1990). The thyroid-stimulating hormone (TSH) response to thyrotrophin-releasing hormone (TRH) is usually blunted in depression (Szabadi, 1991) and in normal elderly subjects (Snyder & Utiger, 1972). However, recent studies in elderly depressed subjects have reported conflicting results. Molchan et al. (1991*b*) found that mean stimulated TSH was lower in elderly depressed patients than in those with Alzheimer's disease and healthy controls but Targum, Marshall & Fishman (1992) found no such difference between elderly depressed patients and controls although the response was significantly reduced in men.

Electrophysiology

The electroencephalogram (EEG)

Changes in the EEG with age may be determined by visual or computerized quantitative analysis. In summary, they are as follows: a reduction in alpha wave frequency and amplitude, an increase in beta frequency and a less consistent increase in theta and delta wave activity (Muller, 1984; Williamson et al., 1990). The changes may be related to subclinical abnormalities of white matter associated with arteriosclerosis (Visser, 1985).

On visual inspection the EEG in depression appears 'normal' but quantitative analysis has revealed subtle changes. O'Connor, Shaw & Ongley (1979) compared EEG spectra from elderly depressed patients, demented patients and healthy controls. EEG coherence (the degree to the EEG is synchronized within a given brain region) was significantly greater in the parietal and temporal areas in depressed patients compared to healthy controls. Others have found a relative increase in alpha power and a decrease in theta power in similar areas of cortex (Brenner et al., 1986; Guidi, Scarpino & Angleri, 1989). Brenner et al. (1986) used a combination measure of delta and theta power in an attempt to discriminate between depressed and mildly demented patients. Although achieving 100% specificity the method was only 27% sensitive which is no improvement on the results obtained by traditional methods (Wright, Harding & Orwin, 1986). Have, Kolbeinsson & Petursson (1991) found no quantitative EEG variable which discriminated between depressed patients and controls.

Sleep EEG

Increasing interest has been accorded to the significance of sleep abnormalities in psychiatric disorders (Benca et al., 1992) and the clinical use of sleep EEG recordings is becoming more practical with the development of compact recording devices which can be used in the patient's home and decoded later. Sleep changes with age are reviewed elsewhere (Spiegel, 1991) but can be summarised as follows: a reduction in total night-time sleep with frequent awakenings, reduced slow-wave sleep and some reduction in rapid eye movement (REM) sleep. These features contribute to the increased tendency of older persons to complain of insomnia.

Clinical changes in sleep during depressive illness are well known and include delayed sleep onset and early morning waking. Sleep EEG studies have shown that REM sleep onset occurs much sooner in depressed patients, there is reduced REM latency (Reynolds et al., 1985), and this feature becomes more pronounced with ageing (Lauer et al., 1991). REM% (the proportion of total sleep spent in REM) increases (Reynolds et al., 1985, 1988). Reynolds et al. (1988) used four sleep measures in a discriminant function analysis between demented and elderly depressed patients. Of cases, 78% were successfully allocated to their diagnostic group. When comparing patients with depressive pseudodementia and those with Alzheimer's dementia and depressive features the method still classified 64% of cases correctly. The validity of the diagnosis was checked over a two year follow-up period suggesting that the technique is the most powerful yet in differentiating between the two groups. More recently, Lauer et al. (1991) have shown that REM latency and REM% change with age, not only in depressed adults but also in healthy individuals whereas REM density (essentially a measure of the frequency of eye movements with REM sleep) remains stable across age groups suggesting that it is a more appropriate marker of depression per se. Lastly, Reynolds et al. (1992) have determined that elderly patients experiencing bereavement uncomplicated by major depression could not be differentiated from healthy controls on the basis of sleep EEG parameters.

Evoked potentials

The EEG response to the passive perception of discrete repeated sensory stimuli may be recorded and averaged by computer to construct a waveform known as the evoked potential (EP). EPs are made up of peaks and troughs reflecting electrical activity at successive levels of the central nervous system. Shape and duration of responses varies with the sensory modality used (Halliday, 1982). The latencies of visual EPs to flash and pattern reversal stimuli become gradually more delayed with age and responses to increasing intensity of flash correspondingly increase in amplitude possibly reflecting a reduction in cortical inhibition (Dustman, Snyder & Schlehuber, 1981). VEPs have been reported as normal in elderly depressed patients (Friedman & Meares, 1979; Wright et al., 1986) but studies of melancholic patients have revealed consistent abnormalities in the latency and amplitude of the flash VEP (Duffy, Burchfiel & Lombroso, 1979; Vasile et al., 1989, 1992).

Hendrickson, Levy & Post (1979) reported delayed auditory EPs in elderly depressed patients which failed to return to normal after treatment. Abnormalities of somatosensory EPs were not found.

Early reports of abnormalities in the somatosensory EPs of schizophrenics implying faulty callosal transmission (Jones & Miller, 1981) have not been replicated (Fenwick, Brennan & Philpot, 1983; Furlong et al., 1990).

Event related potentials (ERPs)

Whereas EPs require no active participation from the subject other than attention to the stimulus, ERPs require active problem-solving and are thus thought to be a closer marker of cognitive function. The most basic auditory paradigm simply requires the subject to differentiate between low tones (occurring frequently) and high tones (occurring rarely). The resulting ERP consists of a large positive wave peaking at around 300 ms after the stimulus, and known by convention as the P300 or P3. Tasks may be made more complex and can be presented in other modalities although auditory ERPs have been used in the majority of studies. P300 latency increases with age (Brown, Marsh & LaRue, 1982; Pfefferbaum et al., 1984) and elderly patients with depression have a greater variability of response, presumably as some may be in the early stages of dementia (Have et al., 1991). Brown et al. (1982) found that P300 discriminated well between demented patients and controls and similar findings have been replicated more recently by others (Have et al., 1991). Unfortunately, the P300 latency correlates with cognitive performance so that patients with mild dementia show few significant abnormalities (Kraiuhin et al., 1990) and the clinical value of the technique has been challenged (Patterson, Michalewski & Starr, 1988; Pfefferbaum, Ford & Kraemer, 1990). The method used to generate the P300 is probably crucial in this respect (Gottlieb, Wertman & Bentin, 1991).

Blackwood et al. (1987) have demonstrated significant abnormalities in the P300 in younger schizophrenics (compared to depressed and healthy controls) which do not normalize during treatment with antipsychotic drugs. These investigations have yet to be extended to late-onset schizophrenics.

Immunology

This area is of interest to psychobiologists for three reasons: firstly, the interaction between mood and resistance to infection (Fox, 1985); secondly the increased death rate following bereavement and depression (Clayton, 1979; Murphy et al., 1988) and thirdly the theoretical similarities between the central nervous system and the immune system (Fudenberg et al., 1984).

Schleifer et al. (1983) demonstrated significant impairment of lymphocyte function in vitro in a prospective study of bereaved men. Reduced lymphocyte activities were also described in patients suffering from major depressive disorder (Schleifer et al., 1984) but these changes were found to be limited to patients with unipolar depression aged over 60 years (Schleifer et al., 1989). Similarly, Aldwin et al. (1991) demonstrated that older depressed men who had experienced recent life events were more likely to have abnormalities of thymosin-alpha-1 (TA-1; which is required for the differentiation and development of T cells).

Maes et al. (1989) found that abnormal lymphocyte responses in major depression were correlated negatively with age, severity of depression and post-DST cortisol. There is evidence to suggest that these changes occur as a result of hypercortisolemia (Lowy et al., 1984), a factor which may be more evident in older patients (Maes et al., 1989). In apparent contrast, the same group have identified selective increases in white cell populations which may differentiate between subtypes of depression and which suggest a state-related immune activation (Maes et al., 1992*a*, *b*).

Circadian rhythms

Research in biological rhythms has been stimulated by the development of techniques measuring periodic fluctuations in bodily functions and markers and the identification of the suprachiasmatic nucleus (SCN) as the principal internal pacemaker (Anderson & Wirz-Justice, 1991). Work on affective disorders has suggested a number of hypotheses concerning the etiological significance of abnormalities in circadian rhythms such as phase advance, phase delay and changes in the amplitude of rhythms or their periodicity (Anderson & Wirz-Justice, 1991). The daily sleep–wake cycle is, perhaps, the most obvious circadian rhythm. There is evidence that REM sleep shows a phase advance (particularly in elderly depressed patients, Lauer et al., 1991) and that some stages of sleep may be 'depressogenic' accounting for the antidepressant effect of sleep deprivation (Wu & Bunney, 1990).

In a pilot study of eight elderly depressed patients, Teicher et al. (1988) found that total 24-hour motor activity was greater than in an age-matched control group and that peak activity, known as the acrophase, occurred about two hours later than expected. The duration of phase delay correlated with post-DST cortisol level. This contrasted with previous findings in younger depressed patients where the acrophase, as indicated by motor activity, body temperature and MHPG excretion, was *advanced* by approximately 1.5 hours (Wehr & Wirz-Justice, 1982). The authors believed that this difference between young and old could reflect the different pattern of depressive symptoms seen in older patients, although the evidence that there is a clinical difference is not compelling.

Melatonin secretion from the pineal gland is regulated by the SCN and has a marked diurnal variation which peaks shortly after midnight. The amount secreted decreases with age (Nair et al., 1986; Rubin et al., 1992) and the timing of the peak concentration may show a phase advance in elderly subjects (Thomas & Miles, 1989). Reduced melatonin secretion has been hailed as a marker for depression (Arendt, 1989) but this role has not always been borne out (Rubin et al., 1992) and studies have yet to be extended to elderly depressed subjects.

Genetics

Affective disorders

It is a feature of many conditions that the genetic contribution to etiology tends to decrease the later the onset. Hopkinson (1964) found that the prevalence of depression among the first-degree relatives of depressed probands whose illness began after the age of 50 was less than half of that of probands with early onset depression. This finding has been duplicated a number of times (Mendelwicz, 1976; Weissman et al., 1984; Maier et al., 1991). Interestingly, Rice et al. (1984) found that mothers with depression had a greater influence on the liability of children to depression than fathers but the differential risk also decreased with age of onset of the proband.

First-degree relatives of patients with Alzheimer's disease and major depression have a significantly higher lifetime risk of depression than Alzheimer disease patients without depression suggesting that the dementia may increase the likelihood of the genetic susceptibility to depression (Pearlson et al., 1990). However, these findings could be the result of cohort effects and there is now evidence that lifetime risk has risen and age of onset has fallen throughout the twentieth century so far (Burke et al., 1991; Warshaw, Klerman & Lavori, 1991).

Similar age-related trends apply to results from family studies of mania (Weissman et al., 1984). Studies have reported that 25–50% of first degree relatives of elderly manic patients have affective illness (Stone, 1989; Broadhead & Jacoby, 1990; Shulman, Tohen & Satlin, 1992). Stone (1989) found that elderly manic patients with a positive family history had an earlier age of onset than those without.

Schizophrenia and Paranoid Psychoses

Kay (1972) calculated the risks of schizophrenia to first-degree relatives of paraphrenics versus young schizophrenics to be 3.4 and 5.8%, respectively. This figure was not age adjusted, so that the observed difference may have resulted from the paraphrenics relatives not living through the risk period. Careful age-corrected studies show that early illness onset is associated with greater risk to siblings but not children and that age of onset within families is closely correlated (Kendler & Maclean, 1990).

HLA studies demonstrated that HLA-A9 was more common in paranoid schizophrenia (McGuffin, Farmer & Yonace, 1981) and in older schizophrenics with onset after 50 years of age (Eberhard, Franzen & Low, 1975). Naguib et al. (1987) did not confirm this association in a group of paraphrenics but found other antigens, B37, Bw55 and Cw6 to be more common. This was not a particularly robust finding and has not been replicated to date. Given the variability of HLA studies it is too early to use this information to justify the assertion that paraphrenia is genetically distinct from paranoid schizophrenia. Chromosomal markers linking schizophrenia to chromosome 5 have not been confirmed and interest is now also focusing on chromosomes 11, 18 and 19 (Bassett, 1992).

The excess of women presenting with late-onset paranoid psychoses is marked (Lewis, 1992). Speculation has concerned the reduction in D_2 receptors with age which may be less marked in women and thus leave them with a relative excess (Pearlson & Rabins, 1988). Estrogens have an antidopaminergic function in the central nervous system and their loss may account for the increase in incidence after menopause (Seeman & Lang, 1990). In addition, it has been observed that the incidence is increasing in younger cohorts but remaining stable in older groups (Eagles, 1991). This may be related to a companion hypothesis suggesting a genetically determined type of schizophrenia associated with late onset and being female and an environmentally determined/neurodevelopmental type associated with early onset and being male (Castle & Murray, 1991).

Conclusions

In view of the paucity of psychobiological research carried out in elderly patients with schizophrenia, mania, primary anxiety states and other neuroses, the conclusions presented here can really only apply to depression. Sadly, it is not yet possible to give firm answers to the questions posed at the outset. It is unlikely that there are specific markers of depressive illness in old age although immunological changes come closest in this respect and most postmortem studies of patients dying from natural causes are, of necessity, restricted to the elderly. It appears that other biological features of depression found in younger patients are also present in the elderly, albeit, on occasion, in an exaggerated form. The evidence that aging is a risk factor for depression is the weakest and as mentioned in the introduction, there are many methodological pitfalls. Perhaps the ideal protocol would involve the use of a trait marker for depression in a community study, identifying its prevalence among healthy elderly individuals and following the group carrying the marker to determine the incidence of depression. Unfortunately, no trait markers of depression yet exist.

On a practical clinical level the use of biological markers to aid differential diagnosis also reveals inconsistencies. Many researchers seem content to compare groups of dementia sufferers with groups of depressed patients or healthy controls. The acid test is surely to compare demented patients with cognitively impaired depressed patients: after all, this is where the diagnostic problems lie. But even if a method is 60–70% successful in classifying cases, as with the sleep EEG (Reynolds et al., 1988), this represents only a modest improvement on chance. In any event it is doubtful whether many clinicians would abandon a trial of an antidepressive treatment in difficult cases merely because of a negative result in such a test.

Lastly, Post (1968) may have been right to single out structural brain changes as the important etiological factor as others, more recently, have done (e.g. Alexopoulos, 1990; see also Chapter 22). It may be boring but inevitable to conclude as Nemeroff has (1988*b*):

> The relationship between the biology of aging and the biology of affective disorders remains obscure.

References

Abou-Saleh, M. T., Spalding, E. M., Kellett, J. M., Coppen, A. (1987). Dexamethasone suppression test in dementia. *International Journal of Geriatric Psychiatry*, **2**, 59–65.

Aldwin, C. M., Spiro, A., Clark, G. & Hall, N. (1991). Thymic peptides, stress and depressive symptoms in older men: a comparison of different statistical techniques for small samples. *Brain, Behavior and Immunology*, **5**, 206–18.

Alexopoulos, G. S., Young, R. C., Lieberman, K.W & Shamoian, C. A. (1987). Platelet

MAO activity in geriatric patients with depression and dementia. *American Journal of Psychiatry*, **144**, 1480–83.

Alexopoulos, G. S. (1990). Late-life depression: a neurological brain disease. *International Journal of Geriatric Psychiatry*, **4**, 187–90.

Almeida, O. P., Howard, R., Förstl, H. & Levy, R. (1992). Should the diagnosis of late paraphrenia be abandoned? *Psychological Medicine*, **22**, 11–14.

Anderson, J. L. & Wirz-Justice, A. (1991). Biological rhythms in the pathophysiology and treatment of affective disorders. In *Biological Aspects of Affective Disorders*, ed. R. Horton & C. Katona, pp. 223–270. London: Academic Press.

Arendt, J. (1989) Melatonin: a new probe in psychiatric investigation? *British Journal of Psychiatry*, **155**, 585–90.

Azorin, J. M., Michel, B., Chave, B., Raucoules, D., Valli, M & Lancon, C.(1990). Total plasma 3-methoxy-4-hydroxyphenylglycol (MHPG) in Alzheimer's disease. Comparison with depressives and normal controls. *International Journal of Geriatric Psychiatry*, **5**, 389–94.

Bassett, A. S. (1992). Chromosomal aberrations and schizophrenia. Autosomes. *British Journal of Psychiatry*, **161**, 323–34.

Bauer, M. S. & Whybrow, P. C. (1990). Rapid cycling bipolar affective disorder. II. Treatment of refractory rapid cycling with high dose liothyronine: a preliminary study. *Archives of General Psychiatry*, **47**, 435–40.

Benca, R. M., Obermeyer, W. H., Thisted, R.A & Gillin, J. C. (1992). Sleep and psychiatric disorders. A meta-analysis. *Archives of General Psychiatry*, **49**, 651–68.

Blackwood, D. H. R., Whalley, L. J., Christie, J. E., Blackburn, I. M., St. Clair, D. M. & McInnes, A. (1987). Changes in auditory P3 event-related potential in schizophrenia and depression. *British Journal of Psychiatry*, **150**, 154–60.

Braddock, L. (1986). The dexamethasone suppression test: fact and artifact. *British Journal of Psychiatry*, **148**, 363–74.

Brenner, R. P., Ulrich, R. F., Spiker, D. G. et al. (1986). Computerised EEG spectral analysis in elderly normal, demented and depressed subjects. *Electroencephalography and Clinical Neurophysiology*, **64**, 483–92.

Broadhead, J. & Jacoby, R. (1990). Mania in old age: a first prospective study. *International Journal of Geriatric Psychiatry*, **5**, 215–22.

Brown, W. S., Marsh, J. T. & LaRue, A. (1982). Event-related potentials in psychiatry: differentiating depression and dementia in the elderly. *Bulletin of the Los Angeles Neurological Society*, **47**, 91–107.

Burke, K. C., Burke, J. D., Rae, D. S. & Regier, D. A. (1991). Comparing age at onset of major depression and other psychiatric disorders by birth cohorts in five US community populations. *Archives of General Psychiatry*, **48**, 789–95.

Burton, R. (1652). *The Anatomy of Melancholy*, 13th edn. 1827. London: Longman, Rees, Orme & Co.

Carroll, B. J. (1982). The dexamethasone suppression test for melancholia. *British Journal of Psychiatry*, **140**, 292–304.

Castle, D. J. & Murray, R. M. (1991). The neurodevelopmental basis of sex differences in schizophrenia. *Psychological Medicine*, **21**, 565–75.

Charcot, J. M. (1881). *Clinical Lectures on Senile and Chronic Diseases*. London: The New Sydenham Society.

Cheetham, S. C., Katona, C. L. E. & Horton, R. W. (1991). Post-mortem studies of neurotransmitter biochemistry in depression and suicide. In *Biological Aspects of Affective Disorders*, ed. R. Horton & C. Katona, pp. 191–222. London: Academic Press.

Clayton, P. J. (1979). The sequelae and nonsequelae of conjugal bereavement. *American Journal of Psychiatry*, **136**, 1530–4.

Crow, T. J., Cross, A. J., Cooper, S. J., Deakin, J. F., Ferrier, I. N., Johnson. J. A., Joseph, M. H., Owen, F., Poulter, M. & Lofthouse, R. (1984). Neurotransmitter receptors and monoamine metabolism in the brains of patients with Alzheimer-type dementia, depression and suicide. *Neuropharmacology*, **23**, 1561–9.

Deakin, J. F. W. (1988). The neurochemistry of schizophrenia. In *Schizophrenia: The Major Issues*, ed. P. Bebbington & P. McGuffin, pp. 56–72. Oxford: Heinemann.

Dilsaver, S. C. (1986). Pathophysiology of 'cholinoceptor supersensitivity' in affective disorders. *Biological Psychiatry*, **21**, 813–29.

Doyle, M. C., George, A. J., Ravindran, A. V. & Philpott, R. (1985). Platelet $alpha_2$ adrenoreceptor binding in elderly depressed patients. *American Journal of Psychiatry*, **142**, 1489–90.

Duffy, F. H., Burchfiel, J. L. & Lombroso, C. T. (1979). Brain electrical activity mapping (BEAM): a method for extending the clinical utility of EEG and evoked potential data. *Annals of Neurology*, **5**, 309–21.

Dustman, R. E., Snyder, E. W. & Schlehuber, C. J. (1981). Life-span alterations in visually evoked potentials and inhibitory function. *Neurobiology of Aging*, **2**, 187–92.

Eagles, J. M. (1991). Is schizophrenia disappearing? *British Journal of Psychiatry*, **158**, 834–35.

Eberhard, G., Franzen, G. & Low, B. (1975). Schizophrenia susceptibility and HLA antigens. *Neuropsychobiology*, **1**, 211–17.

Elliott, J. M. (1991). Peripheral markers in affective disorders. In *Biological Aspects of Affective Disorders*, ed. R. Horton & C. Katona, pp. 78–94. London: Academic Press.

Fenwick, P., Brennan, D. & Philpot, M. (1983). Function of the corpus callosum in schizophrenia. *British Journal of Psychiatry*, **143**, 524.

Ferrier, I. N., McKeith, I. G., Cross, A. J., Perry, E. K., Candy, J. M. & Perry, R. H. (1986). Postmortem neurochemical studies in depression. *Annals of the New York Academy of Sciences*, **487**, 128–42.

Fox, R. A. (1985). Immunology of aging. In *Textbook of Geriatrics and Gerontology*, 3rd. edition, ed. J. C. Brocklehurst, pp. 82–104. Edinburgh: Churchill Livingstone.

Friedman, J & Meares, R. (1979). Cortical evoked potentials and severity of depression. *American Journal of Psychiatry*, **136**, 1218–20.

Fudenberg, H. H., Whitten, H. D., Arnaud, P. & Khansari, N. (1984). Is Alzheimer's disease immunological disorder? Observations and speculations. *Clinical Immunology and Immunopathology*, **32**, 127–31.

Furlong, P., Barczak, P., Hayes, G. & Harding, G. (1990). Somatosensory evoked potentials in schizophrenia. A lateralization study. *British Journal of Psychiatry*, **157**, 881–7.

Georgotas, A., McCue, R. E., Kim, M. et al. (1986). Dexamethasone suppression in dementia, depression and normal aging. *American Journal of Psychiatry*, **143**, 452–6.

Georgotas, A., Schweizer, J., McCue, R. E., Armour, M. & Friedhoff, A. S. (1987). Clinical and treatment effects on ^{3}H-clonidine and ^{3}H-imipramine binding in elderly depressed patients. *Life Sciences*, **40**, 2137–43.

Gerner, R. H., Fairbanks, L., Anderson, G. M. et al. (1984). CSF neurochemistry in depressed, manic and schizophrenic patients compared with that of normal controls. *American Journal of Psychiatry*, **141**, 1533–40.

Gietzen, D. W., Goodman, T. A., Weiler, P. G. et al. (1991). Beta receptor density in human lymphocyte membranes: changing with aging? *Journal of Gerontology*, **46**, B130–4.

Gottlieb, D., Wertman, E. & Bentin, S. (1991). Passive listening and task related P300 measurement for the evaluation of dementia and pseudodementia. *Clinical Electroencephalography*, **22**, 102–7.

Gross-Isseroff, R., Israeli, M. & Biegon, A. (1989). Autoradiographic analysis of tritiated imipramine binding in the human brain post mortem: effects of suicide. *Archives of General Psychiatry*, **46**, 237–41.

Guidi, M., Scarpino, O. & Angleri, F. (1989). Topographic EEG and flash visual evoked potentials in elderly subjects, depressed patients and demented patients. *Psychiatry Research*, **29**, 403–6.

Halbreich, U., Sharpless, N., Asnis, G. M. et al. (1987). Afternoon continuous plasma levels of 3-methoxy-4-hydroxyphenolglycol and age. *Archives of General Psychiatry*, **44**, 804–12.

Halliday, A. M. (1982). *Evoked Potentials in Clinical Testing*. Edinburgh: Churchill Livingstone.

Harrison, P. J., McLaughlin, D. & Kerwin, R. W. (1991). Decreased hippocampal expression of a glutamate receptor gene in schizophrenia. *Lancet*, **i**, 450–2.

Have, G., Kolbeinsson, H. & Petursson, H. (1991). Dementia and depression in old age: psychophysiological aspects. *Acta Psychiatrica Scandinavica*, **83**, 329–33.

Healy, D., Carney, P. A. & Leonard, B. E. (1985). Peripheral adrenoreceptors and serotonin receptors: changes associated with response to treatment with trazodone or amitriptyline. *Journal of Affective Disorders*, **9**, 285–96.

Healy, D. (1991). D_1 and D_2 and D_3. *British Journal of Psychiatry*, **159**, 319–24.

Hendrickson, E., Levy, R. & Post, F. (1979). Averaged evoked responses in relation to cognitive and affective state of elderly psychiatric patients. *British Journal of Psychiatry*, **134**, 494–501.

Holsboer, F. (1989). Psychiatric implications of altered limbic-hypothalamic-pituitary-adrenocortical action. *European Archives of Psychiatry and Neurological Sciences*, **238**, 302–22.

Hopkinson, G. (1964). A genetic study of affective illness in patients over 50. *British Journal of Psychiatry*, **110**, 244–54.

Hunt, G. E., Johnson, G. F. S. & Caterson, I. D. (1989). The effect of age on cortisol and plasma dexamethasone concentrations in depressed patients and controls. *Journal of Affective Disorders*, **17**, 21–32.

Husain, M. M., Knight, D. L., Doraiswamy, P. M. et al. (1991) Platelet [^{3}H]-imipramine binding and leukoencephalopathy in geriatric depression. *Biological Psychiatry*, **29**, 665–70.

Jones, G. H. & Miller, J. J. (1981). Functional tests of the corpus callosum in schizophrenia. *British Journal of Psychiatry*, **139**, 553–7.

Jones, J. S., Stanley, B., Mann. J. J. et al. (1991). CSF 5-HIAA and HVA concentrations in elderly depressed patients who have attempted suicide. *American Journal of Psychiatry*, **148**, 1225–7.

Katona, C. L. E. & Aldridge, C. R. (1985). The dexamethasone suppression test and depressive signs in dementia. *Journal of Affective Disorders*, **8**, 83–9.

Kay, D. W. K. (1972). Schizophrenia and schizophrenia-like states in the elderly. *British Journal of Hospital Medicine*, **8**, 369–76.

Kendler, K. S. & Maclean, C. J. (1990). Estimating familial effects on age at onset and liability to schizophrenia. I. Result of a large sample family study. *Genetics and Epidemiology*, **7**, 409–17.

Kraiuhin, C., Gordon, E., Coyle, S. et al. (1990). Normal latency of the P300 event-related potential in mild-to-moderate Alzheimer's disease and depression. *Biological Psychiatry*, **28**, 372–86.

Lauer, C. J., Riemann, D., Wiegand, M. & Berger, M. (1991). From early to late adulthood. Changes in EEG sleep of depressed patients and healthy volunteers. *Biological Psychiatry*, **29**, 979–93.

Leake, A., Charlton, B. G., Lowry, P. J., Jackson, S., Fairburn, A. & Ferrier, I. N. (1990). Plasma *N*-POMC, ACTH and cortisol concentrations in a psychogeriatric population. *British Journal of Psychiatry*, **156**, 676–9.

Leake, A., Fairburn, A. F., McKeith, I. G. & Ferrier, I. N. (1991). Studies on the serotonin uptake binding site in major depressive disorder and control post-mortem brain: neurochemical and clinical correlates. *Psychiatry Research*, **39**, 155–65.

Lewis, S. (1992). Sex and schizophrenia. *British Journal of Psychiatry*, **161**, 445–50.

Lowy, M. T., Reder, A. T., Antel, J. P. & Meltzer, H. Y. (1984). Glucocorticoid resistance in depression. The DST and lymphocyte sensitivity to dexamethasone. *American Journal of Psychiatry*, **141**, 1365–8.

McGuffin, P., Farmer, A. E. & Yonace, A. H. L. (1981). HLA antigens and subtypes of schizophrenia. *Psychiatry Research*, **5**, 115–22.

McKeith, I. R. (1984). The clinical use of the DST in a psychogeriatric population. *British Journal of Psychiatry*, **145**, 389–94.

McKeith, I. G., Marshall, E. F., Ferrier, I. N. et al. (1987). 5-HT receptor binding in post-mortem brains from patients with affective disorder. *Journal of Affective Disorders*, **13**, 67–74.

Maes, M., Bosmans, E., Suy, E., Minner, B. & Raus, J. (1989). Impaired lymphocyte stimulation by mitogens in severely depressed patients. A complex interface with HPA-axis hyperfunction, noradrenergic activity and the ageing process. *British Journal of Psychiatry*, **155**, 793–8.

Maes, M., Van der Planken, M., Stevens, W. J. et al. (1992*a*). Leukocytosis, monocytosis and neutrophilia: hallmarks of severe depression. *Journal of Psychiatric Research*, **26**, 125–34.

Maes, M., Lambrechts, J., Bosmans, E. et al. (1992*b*). Evidence for a systemic immune activation during depression: results of leukocyte enumeration by flow cytometry in conjunction with monoclonal antibody staining. *Psychological Medicine*, **22**, 45–53.

Maier, W., Lichtermann, D., Minges, J., Heun, R., Hallmayer, J. & Klinger, T. (1991). Unipolar depression in the aged: determinants of familial aggregation. *Journal of Affective Disorders*, **23**, 53–61.

Mann, J. J., Arango, V., Marzuk, P. M., Theccanat, S. & Reis, D. J. (1989). Evidence for the 5-HT hypothesis of suicide. A review of post-mortem studies. *British Journal of Psychiatry*, **155** (suppl. 8), 7–14.

Maudsley, H. (1879) *The Pathology of Mind*. London: Macmillan.

Meek, J. L., Bertilsson, L., Cheney, D. L., Zsilla, G & Costa, E. (1977). Aging-induced changes in acetylcholine and serotonin content of discrete brain nuclei. *Journal of Gerontology*, **32**, 129–31.

Mendelwicz, J. (1976). The age factor in depressive illness: some genetic considerations. *Journal of Gerontology*, **31**, 300–4.

Molchan, S. E., Lawlor, B. A., Hill, J. L. et al. (1991*a*). CSF monoamine metabolites and somatostatin in Alzheimer's disease and major depression. *Biological Psychiatry*, **29**, 1110–18.

Molchan, S. E., Lawlor, B. A., Hill, J. L. et al. (1991*b*). The TRH stimulation test in Alzheimer's disease and major depression: relationship to clinical and CSF measures. *Biological Psychiatry*, **30**, 567–76.

Muller, H. F. (1984). Electrical brain activity in psychogeriatrics. In *Handbook of Studies in Psychiatry and Old Age*, ed. D. W. K. Kay & G. D. Burrows, pp. 120–139. Amsterdam: Elsevier.

Murphy, E., Smith, R., Lindesay, J. & Slattery, J. (1988). Increased mortality rates in late-life depression. *British Journal of Psychiatry*, **152**, 347–53.

Naguib, M., McGuffin, P., Levy, R., Festenstein, H. & Alonso, A. C. (1987). Genetic markers in late paraphrenia: a study of HLA antigens. *British Journal of Psychiatry*, **150**, 124–7.

Nair, N. P. V., Hariharasubramaniam, N., Pilapil, C., Isaac, I. & Thavundayil, J. X. (1986). Plasma melatonin – an index of brain aging in humans? *Biological Psychiatry*, **21**, 141–50.

Nakai, T., Kitamura, N., Hashimoto, T. et al. (1991). Decreased histamine H_1 receptors in the frontal cortex of brains from patients with chronic schizophrenia. *Biological Psychiatry*, **30**, 349–56.

Nemeroff, C. B. (1988*a*). The role of corticotrophin-releasing factor in the pathogenesis of major depression. *Pharmacopsychiatry*, **21**, 76–82.

Nemeroff, C. B. (1988*b*). The neurobiology of aging and the neurobiology of depression: is there a relationship? *Neurobiology of Aging*, **9**, 120–2.

Nemeroff, C. B., Knight, D. L., Krishnan, R. R. et al. (1988*c*). Marked reduction in the number of platelet-tritiated imipramine binding sites in geriatric depression. *Archives of General Psychiatry*, **45**, 919–23.

O'Connor, K. P., Shaw, J. C. & Ongley, C. O. (1979). The EEG and differential diagnosis in psychogeriatrics. *British Journal of Psychiatry*, **135**, 156–62.

Owen, F., Crow, T. J., Frith, C. D. et al. (1987). Selective decreases in MAO-B activity in post-mortem brains from schizophrenic patients. *British Journal of Psychiatry*, **151**, 514–19.

Patterson, J. V., Michalewski, H.J & Starr, A. (1988). Latency variability of the components of auditory event-related potentials to infrequent stimuli in aging, Alzheimer-type dementia and depression. *Electroencephalography and clinical Neurophysiology*, **71**, 450–60.

Pearlson, G. & Rabins, P. (1988). The late onset psychoses – possible risk factors. *Psychiatric Clinics of North America*, **2**, 15–31.

Pearlson, G. D., Ross, C. A., Lohr, W. D., Rovner, B. W., Chase, G. A. & Folstein, M. F. (1990). Association between family history of affective disorder and the depressive syndrome of Alzheimer's disease. *American Journal of Psychiatry*, **147**, 452–6.

Pfefferbaum, A., Ford. J. M., Wenegrat, B. G., Roth, W. T. & Koppell, B. S. (1984). Clinical applications of the P3 component of event-related potentials. I. Normal aging. *Electroencephalography and clinical Neurophysiology*, **59**, 85–103.

Pfefferbaum, A., Ford, J. M. & Kraemer, H. C. (1990). Clinical utility of long-latency 'cognitive' event-related potentials (P3): the cons. *Electroencephalography and Clinical Neurophysiology*, **76**, 6–12.

Philpot, M. (1986). Biological factors in depression in the elderly. In *Affective Disorders in the Elderly*, ed. E. Murphy, pp. 53–78. Edinburgh: Churchill Livingstone.

Pilowsky, L. (1992). Understanding schizophrenia. *British Medical Journal*, **305**, 327–8.

Post, F. (1968). The factor of ageing in affective illness. In *Recent Developments in the Affective Disorders: a Symposium*, ed. A. Coppen and A. Walk. Royal Medico-Psychological Association Special; Publication No. 2. pp. 105–116. Ashford: Headley Brothers.

Post, F. (1992). Changing concepts: persistent delusions. In *Delusions and Hallucinations in Old Age*, ed. C. Katona & R. Levy, pp. 43–49. London: Gaskell.

Pryor, J. C. & Sulser, F. (1991). Evolution of the monoamine hypotheses of depression. In *Biological Aspects of Affective Disorders*, ed. R. Horton & C. Katona, pp. 78–94. London: Academic Press.

Reynolds, C. F., Kupfer, D. J., Taska, L. S. et al. (1985). EEG sleep in elderly depressed, demented and healthy subjects. *Biological Psychiatry*, **20**, 431–42.

Reynolds, C. F., Kupfer, D. J., Houck, P. R. et al. (1988). Reliable discrimination of elderly depressed and demented patients by electroencephalographic sleep data. *Archives of General Psychiatry*, **45**, 258–64.

Reynolds, C. F., Hoch, C. C., Buysse, D. J. et al. (1992). Electroencephalographic sleep in spousal bereavement and bereavement-related depression of late-life. *Biological Psychiatry*, **31**, 69–82.

Rice, J., Reich, T., Andreasen, N. C. et al. (1984). Sex-related differences in depression. Familial evidence. *Journal of Affective Disorders*, **71**, 199–210.

Riederer, P., Birkmayer, W., Seemann, D. & Wuketich, S. (1980). 4-hydroxy-3-

methoxyphenolglycol as an index of brain noradrenaline turnover in endogenous depression. *Acta Psychiatrica Scandinavica*, **61** (suppl. 280), 251–7.

Robinson, D. S., Davies, J. M. & Nies, A. (1972). Ageing, monoamines and monoamine oxidase levels. *Lancet*, **ii**, 368–70.

Rogers, J. & Bloom, F. E. (1985). Neurotransmitter metabolism and function in the aging central nervous system. In *Handbook of the Biology of Aging*, 2nd edition, ed. C. E. Finch & E. L. Schneider, pp. 645–668. New York: Van Nostrand, Reinhold.

Rubin, R. T., Heist, E. K., McGeoy, S. S., Hanada, K. & Lesser, I. M. (1992). Neuroendocrine aspects of primary endogenous depression. XI. Serum melatonin measures in patients and matched control subjects. *Archives of General Psychiatry*, **49**, 558–67.

Sandler, M., Reveley, M. A. & Glover, V. (1981). Human platelet monoamine oxidase activity in health and disease: a review. *Journal of Clinical Pathology*, **34**, 292–302.

Schildkraut, J. J. (1965). The catecholamine hypothesis of affective disorders: a review of the supporting evidence. *American Journal of Psychiatry*, **122**, 509–22.

Schleifer, S. J., Keller, S. E., Camerino, M., Thorton, J. C. & Stein, M. (1983). Suppression of lymphocyte stimulation following bereavement. *Journal of the American Medical Association*, **250**, 374–7.

Schleifer, S. J., Keller, S. E., Meyerson, A. T., Raskin, M. J., Davis, K. L. & Stein, M. (1984). Lymphocyte function in major depressive disorder. *Archives of General Psychiatry*, **41**, 484–6.

Schleifer, S. J., Keller, S. E., Bond, R. N., Cohen, J. & Stein, M. (1989). Major depressive disorder and immunity. Role of age, sex, severity and hospitalisation. *Archives of General Psychiatry*, **46**, 81–7.

Schneider, L. S., Severson, J. A. & Sloane, R. B. (1985). Platelet [^{3}H]-imipramine binding in depressed elderly patients. *Biological Psychiatry*, **20**, 1232–4.

Seeman, M. V. & Lang, M. (1990). The role of oestrogens in schizophrenia gender differences. *Schizophrenia Bulletin*, **16**, 185–95.

Shrimankar, J., Soni, S. D. & McMurray, J. (1989). Dexamethasone suppression test in dementia and depression: clinical and biological correlates. *British Journal of Psychiatry*, **154**, 372–7.

Shulman, K., Tohen, M. & Satlin, A. (1992). Mania revisited. In *Recent Advances in Psychogeriatrics* 2, ed. T. Arie, pp. 71–79. Edinburgh: Churchill Livingstone.

Simpson, M. D. C., Slater, P., Royston, C. & Deakin, J. F. W. (1992). Regionally selective deficits in uptake sites for glutamate and gamma-aminobutyric acid in the basal ganglia in schizophrenia. *Psychiatry Research*, **42**, 273–82.

Snyder, P. J. & Utiger, R. D. (1972). Response to thyrotropin releasing hormone (TRH) in normal man. *Journal of Clinical Endocrinology and Metabolism*, **34**, 380–5.

Sparks, L. D. (1989). Aging and Alzheimer's disease. Altered cortical serotonergic binding. *Archives of Neurology*, **46**, 138–40.

Spiegel, R. (1991). Sleep and its disorders. In *Principles and Practice of Geriatric Medicine*, 2nd. edition, ed. M. S. J. Pathy, pp. 205–227. Chichester: Wiley.

Stanley, M. & Mann, J. J. (1983). Increased serotonin-2 binding in frontal cortex of suicide victims. *Lancet*, **i**, 214–16.

Stone, K. (1989). Mania in the elderly. *British Journal of Psychiatry*, **155**, 220–4.

Sunderland, T., Rubinow, D. R., Tariot, P. N. et al. (1987). CSF somatostatin in patients with Alzheimer's disease, older depressed patients, and age-matched control subjects. *American Journal of Psychiatry*, **144**, 1313–16.

Suranyi-Codotte, B. E., Gauthier, S., Lafaille, F. et al. (1985). Platelet [^{3}H]-imipramine binding distinguishes depression from Alzheimer's dementia. *Life Sciences*, **37**, 2305–11.

Szabadi, E. (1991). Thyroid dysfunction and affective illness. *British Medical Journal*, **302**, 923–4.

Targum, S. D., Marshall, L.E & Fishman, P. (1992). Variability of TRH test response in depressed and normal elderly subjects. *Biological Psychiatry*, **31**, 787–93.

Teicher, M. H., Lawrence, J. M., Barber, N. I., Finkelstein, S. P., Lieberman, H. R. & Baldessarini, R. J. (1988). Increased activity and phase delay in circadian motility rhythms in geriatric depression. *Archives of General Psychiatry*, **45**, 913–17.

Thomas, D. R. & Miles, A. (1989). Melatonin secretion and age. *Biological Psychiatry*, **25**, 365–7.

Vasile, R. G., Duffy, F. H., McAnulty, G. et al. (1989). Abnormal visual evoked response in melancholia. *Biological Psychiatry*, **25**, 785–8.

Vasile, R. G., Duffy, F. H., McAnulty, G., Mooney, J. J., Bloomingdale, K. & Schildkraut, J. J. (1992). Abnormal flash visual evoked response in melancholia: a replication study. *Biological Psychiatry*, **31**, 325–36.

Visser, S. L. (1985). EEG and evoked potentials in the diagnosis of dementias. In *Senile Dementia of the Alzheimer Type*, ed. J. Traber and W. H. Gispen, pp. 102–116, Berlin: Springer-Verlag.

Vollhardt, B. R., Alexopoulos, G. S., Young, R. C., Kream, J. & Shamoian, C. A. (1989). Clonidine challenge of cortisol secretion in dementia and geriatric depression. *International Psychogeriatrics*, **1**, 167–75.

von Bardeleben, U. & Holsboer, F. (1991). Effects of age on the cortisol response to human corticotrophin-releasing hormone in depressed patients pretreated with dexamethasone. *Biological Psychiatry*, **29**, 1042–50.

Warshaw, M. G., Klerman, G. L. & Lavori, P. W. (1991). The use of conditional probabilities to examine age-period-cohort data: further evidence for a period effect in major depressive disorder. *Journal of Affective Disorder*, **23**, 119–29.

Wehr, T. A. & Wirz-Justice, A. (1982). Circadian rhythm mechanisms in affective illness and in antidepressant drug action. *Pharmacopsychiatry*, **15**, 31–9.

Weissman, M. M., Gershon, E. S., Kidd, K. K. et al. (1984). Psychiatric disorders in the relatives of probands with affective disorders. *Archives of General Psychiatry*, **41**, 13–21.

Whybrow, P. C. & Prange, A. J. (1981). A hypothesis of thyroid-catecholamine receptor interaction. *Archives of General Psychiatry*, **38**, 106–13.

Williamson, P. C., Merskey, H., Morrison, S. et al. (1990). Quantitative electroencephalographic correlates of cognitive decline in normal elderly subjects. *Archives of Neurology*, **47**, 1185–8.

Wong, D., Wagner, H. N., Dannals, R. F. et al. (1984). Effects of age on dopamine and serotonin receptors measured by positron tomography in the living human brain. *Science*, **226**, 1393–6.

Wright, C. E., Harding, G. F. A. & Orwin, A. (1986). The flash and pattern VEP as a diagnostic indicator of dementia. *Documenta Ophthalmologica*, **62**, 89–96.

Wu, J. C. & Bunney, W. E. (1990). The biological basis of an antidepressant response to sleep deprivation and relapse: review and hypothesis. *American Journal of Psychiatry*, **147**, 14–21.

Yates, M. & Ferrier, I. N. (1990). 5-HT_1 receptors in major depression. *Journal of Psychopharmacology*, **4**, 69–74.

Yates, M., Leake, A., Candy, J. M., Fairburn, A. F., McKeith, I. G. & Ferrier, I. N. (1990). 5-HT_2 receptor changes in major depression. *Biological Psychiatry*, **27**, 489–96.

22

Brain imaging in functional psychiatric disorders of the elderly

ROBERT HOWARD BARBARA BEATS

The development of noninvasive computerized brain imaging techniques and their application to functional psychiatric disorders such as depression and schizophrenia represents one of the most important research advances in psychiatry over the past two decades. This chapter reviews the results of reported brain imaging studies of depression, schizophrenia and schizophrenia-like illnesses in the elderly.

X-ray computer tomography studies

In cranial Computed Tomography (CT), an X-ray source is moved around the head in the transverse plane, and detectors directly opposite the source record the quantity of radiation that has passed through the head. From a large series of such readings, a two-dimensional image made up of scanned squares, or pixels, is built up and represents a transverse slice of the head 5–10 mm thick. Most CT scanners produce an image of 256 × 256 pixels. CT scanning is cheap, widely available, involves a scanning time of only around 10 minutes and is generally well tolerated by subjects. There have been a large number of studies of CT in depression in both young, elderly and mixed age populations of patients. Despite varying methodology, both in terms of patient and control selection and method of measurement of anatomical structures (hand tracing, mechanical planimetry or computerized quantification), the results are in general agreement.

Depression

In an early CT study of elderly depressed patients, Jacoby & Levy (1980) examined the scans of 41 patients diagnosed with the Geriatric Mental State Schedule (GMS) (Copeland et al. 1976) and 50 healthy age-matched controls. Depressed patients as a whole had a brain radiodensity which was intermediate between that of normal controls and patients with dementia. Furthermore, there was a subgroup of depressed patients with an increased ventricle-to-brain ratio (VBR) who were older, had a late onset of depression, more endogenous features and a high mortality from cerebrovascular and cardiovascular disease (Jacoby & Levy, 1980, Jacoby, Levy & Bird, 1981, Jacoby et al., 1983).

Ames, Dolan & Mann (1990) used the GMS and CT scans to examine 20 depressed and 14 demented patients with a mean age of 83 years and compared them with 18 age-matched controls. The depressed subjects could not be distinguished from the dementia sufferers on VBR or cortical atrophy score, but both patient groups had bigger ventricles than controls. Five of the depressed patients were dead two years later and fewer than one third had recovered from depression.

Pearlson et al. (1989) scanned 26 elderly patients with major depression (DSM-III-R, American Psychiatric Association, 1987), together with a control group of 31 matched healthy individuals. Depressed subjects had increased lateral ventricle size and reduced brain radiodensity. These changes were most marked in those patients who had the lowest mini mental state (MMSE) (Folstein, Folstein & McHugh, 1975) scores. These MMSE scores returned to control levels with recovery from depression.

Abas, Sahakian & Levy, (1990) CT scanned 19 elderly depressed patients and found increased ventricle-to-brain ratio to be positively correlated with cognitive impairment, which did not return to control levels on clinical recovery of mood.

Beats, Förstl & Levy, (1991) in a study of 25 elderly depressed patients, all of whom scored 24 or more on the MMSE reported significantly larger third ventricles compared with controls. Radiodensity was increased in the caudate heads and decreased in the dorso-medial thalamus. Areas of the lateral and third ventricles correlated with age, duration of depressive illness, age at onset and degree of cognitive impairment.

In CT studies of age-mixed depressed populations, similar results to those detailed above have been reported. Schlegel & Kretschmar (1987) examined 60 depressed patients of all ages and 60 matched healthy controls. They found increased lateral and third ventricle sizes in the depressed group. These changes were most marked in a subgroup of elderly male psychotic patients. Dolan, Calloway & Mann (1985) found that increasing age and male sex were associated with larger cerebral ventricular size among 101 patients who met Research Diagnostic Criteria for major depression (Spitzer, Endicott & Robins, 1978) and 52 normal controls. Depressed patients had larger ventricles than normals after controlling for age and sex. Kellner, Rubinow & Post (1986) CT scanned 21 depressed subjects with widely varying ages (25 – 63 years), and confirmed the association between degree of cognitive impairment and VBR.

Schizophrenia and schizophrenia-like illnesses

More than 20 studies using CT scanning in young patients have shown that schizophrenics, in comparison with matched healthy controls, show slight enlargement of the lateral and third ventricles and a mild degree of cortical sulcal widening (for a review see Lewis, 1990). The results of CT studies of patients with late-onset schizophrenia and other schizophrenia-like illnesses fall into two groups. First, mostly early studies which demonstrated dramatic focal brain damage in small series of patients and second, larger populations of patients in whom subtle brain abnormalities, analogous to those in early-onset schizophrenia have been found.

The first CT study to specifically examine patients with schizophrenic symptoms with an onset in late life was by Miller et al. (1986). Five female patients, whose age at onset of symptoms ranged from 58 to 81 years were scanned. Three of the patients had extensive cortical and subcortical infarcts and one had normal pressure hydrocephalus. The scan appearances were so abnormal that the authors titled their paper 'Late life paraphrenia: an organic delusional syndrome'. It has to be said that better selection of patients, with scrupulous exclusion of a history or clinical signs of neurological disease or dementia, has not confirmed this conclusion. Three CT studies of better selected patients were published in 1987 and all had very similar results. Pearlson et al. (1987) compared the scans of eight patients with late-onset schizophrenia, whose MMSE score was greater than 24, with those of 14 normal age-matched controls. Rabins et al. (1987) examined 29 patients who satisfied DSM-III (APA, 1980) criteria for schizophrenia, but had a mean age at onset of symptoms of 66 years, and 23 normal controls. Naguib & Levy (1987) compared 43 late paraphrenics with 40 age-matched controls. All three studies reported that the mean VBR of patients exceeded that of controls. Naguib & Levy (1987) found no correlation between increased VBR and clinical parameters such as illness duration or degree of cognitive impairment: a finding that contrasts with the situation in the late-onset depression CT studies. Late paraphrenics have uniform and normally distributed lateral ventricular dilatation on CT, which is uncoupled from the usual association with cortical sulcal widening seen in an age-matched control group (Burns et al., 1989). Those late paraphrenics who do not have Schneiderian first-rank symptoms have more cortical atrophy on CT scan than patients with these symptoms (Howard et al., 1992).

Exclusion from CT studies of patients with obvious neurological signs or a history of stroke, alcohol abuse or dementia has shown that structural abnormalities on CT in patients with late paraphrenia are probably no more common than in controls. Despite adhering to these exclusions, however, Flint, Rifat & Eastwood, (1991) found unsuspected cerebral infarction on the scans of 5 out of 16 of their late paraphrenic patients. Most of these infarcts were subcortical or frontal and they were more likely to occur in patients with delusions but no hallucinations.

Magnetic resonance imaging

Whilst CT depends on absorption of X-rays, magnetic resonance imaging (MRI) has as its principle the absorption of radio waves by hydrogen nuclei. All the hydrogen nuclei in water and organic molecules spin around their own axes. In MRI, the subject's head is placed in a magnetic field 10 000 times stronger than that of the earth. This causes all the spinning nuclei to line up with their axes pointing in the same direction. Pulses of radio waves are then administered which are absorbed by the spinning hydrogen nuclei, causing their angle of spin to tilt. When this pulse is switched off, the nuclei relax back to their original angles of spin and an energy signal is released. This energy signal decays in a particular pattern which forms the basis of the final image. The relaxation time has two main components, T1 and T2, and these vary according to tissue characteristics such as the density of hydrogen nuclei. This enables MRI to discriminate between grey and white matter in a way that CT cannot and to yield high resolution images in any plane. Compared with CT, MRI is expensive and not widely available. Patients must lie within a claustrophobia-inducing tube for scan times of 30 minutes to one hour. MR examination may be impossible in patients who are agitated or uncooperative.

Late onset depression

The superiority of MRI over CT imaging, both in terms of grey/white matter resolution and visualization of deep white matter regions is undoubted. A large number of MRI studies of the brains of elderly patients with depression have taken advantage of this feature to specifically examine changes in periventricular and deep white matter. The results need to be interpreted with caution, since few of the studies have assessed abnormalities in the white matter in any kind of standardized manner and appropriate control populations, matched for cerebrovascular disease risk factors are rarely used.

Patchy periventricular high signal intensity lesions on MRI were initially reported in 30% of those over the age of 60, and were considered to accompany normal aging (Bradley, Waluch & Wycoff, 1984, Sze, DeArmond & Brant-Zawadski, 1985). Periventricular and deep white matter MRI abnormalities are now known to be associated with both risk factors for, and symptoms of, cerebrovascular disease (Gerard & Weisberg 1986; Awad et al., 1986*a*; Erkinjuntti et al., 1987; Hershey et al., 1987; and Hunt et al., 1989). It may be therefore, that any study purporting to show that elderly depressed patients have more white matter abnormalities than healthy matched controls is doing little more than confirming the established association between late-onset depression and cerebrovascular disease in an expensive high-technology fashion.

The commonly reported 'white matter lesions' are areas of white matter that demonstrate prolonged T2 relaxation times and so appear as areas of hyperintensity on the T2 image (Miller et al., 1991). They almost certainly represent volumes of brain tissue where water content is increased by edema, demyelinating disease, subcortical atherosclerotic encephalopathy or gliosis (Awad et al., 1986*b*).

There has been little agreement between MRI studies of white matter hyperintensities in elderly depressed patients as to exactly what should be considered abnormal or how such changes should be measured. Ratings of MRI scans of elderly depressed patients using modifications of graded assessments developed for examining scans of patients with Alzheimer's disease (Fazekas et al., 1988; CERAD, 1989) have been the most standardized. As an example, Coffey et al. (1988, 1990) have rated white matter lesions on scans as follows:

1. Periventricular hyperintensity (absent, pencil-thin cap, halo, and irregular periventricular hyperintensity extending into the deep white matter).
2. Deep white matter hyperintensity (absent, punctate foci, beginning confluence of foci, and large confluent areas).
3. Changes in subcortical grey matter nuclei.

Unfortunately, most of the reported studies have not used standardized grading assessments in their identification of white matter abnormality and there is dispute as to exactly what should constitute an abnormality.

Many of the studies of MRI in elderly depressed patients have not used age-matched controls, but where controls have been included, it is often not clear that these have been appropriately matched for the presence of cerebrovascular risk factors.

Coffey et al. (1988) examined 67 depressed inpatients whose mean age was 71.6 years with MRI and found subcortical white matter changes in 66% of them. Krishnan et al. (1988) found white matter lesions in 80% of depressed inpatients over the age of 60. White matter lesions were present in 83% of patients of all ages who had hypertension in this study. Coffey et al. (1990) in a later study MRI scanned 51 depressed inpatients with a mean age of 71.7 years. These included 16 patients with Parkinson's disease, dementia or stroke and 27% of patients were hypertensive. Not suprisingly, severe white matter lesions were more common in patients than in age-matched healthy community volunteers.

Churchill et al. (1991) examined 47 depressed patients with a mean age of 71.6 and found white matter lesions in 77% of them. Dupont and colleagues (1990) looked at 19 younger depressed patients using T2-weighted images and found an increase in subcortical hyperintensities even in this group compared to controls. The abnormal findings were associated with certain clinical features (impaired verbal fluency and recall) and with a higher number of admissions for affective disorder.

The best designed study of white matter lesions in elderly depressed patients is that of Rabins et al. (1991). Twenty one depressed inpatients over the age of 60 were examined to exclude stroke and a median blood pressure reading was taken from five measures. Any history of hypertension or cardiovascular disease was recorded. A control group was used, consisting of 14 age-matched healthy individuals. There was significantly more white matter disease in the depressed patients than in the controls and, surprisingly, there was no relationship between the presence of hypertension and white matter lesions in the depressed group. This study was also the first to report MRI changes in cortical brain structure in elderly depressed patients. Compared to control subjects, depressed patients had greater cerebral sulcal and temporal sulcal atrophy, larger sylvian fissures, lateral and third ventricles and temporal horns.

Late-onset schizophrenia and schizophrenia-like illnesses

In late-onset schizophrenia, as well as depression, there have been several reports of increased white matter abnormality in patients demonstrated by MRI scanning. Miller et al. (1989) found extensive white matter lesions on the MRI scans of five out of 27 patients with late life psychosis. They recognized a subset of such patients who performed poorly on psychometric tests of frontal lobe function, had extensive white matter lesions, delusions and a frontal syndrome. In a further report of white matter lesions in late life psychosis, Miller et al. (1991) found white matter lesions in 42% of 24 patients. Severe white matter lesions were present in 28% of patients and only 8% of controls, but cerebrovascular risk factors were inadequately excluded or controlled for inpatients.

Breitner et al. (1990) found more white matter changes in eight female late onset schizophrenics than in eight healthy age-matched controls. Since four of the schizophrenics had cognitive impairment, four of them were hypertensive, one had a history of myocardial infarction and one was a diabetic, again any differences between patients and controls are most likely to reflect increased cerebrovascular disease risks in the patients, rather than a specific cerebral disease substrate for late-onset schizophrenia.

Quantitative anatomical analysis of MRI scans in elderly patients with schizophrenia has begun to be reported only very recently. Jeste et al. (1991) in a population of DSM-III-R (APA, 1987) late-onset schizophrenics, found larger lateral ventricles, more white matter abnormalities and smaller caudate nuclei than in normal controls.

Pearlson et al. (1991) take the view that late- and early-onset schizophrenia are clinically similar and probably represent the same thing. They have therefore hypothesized that structural brain changes in schizophrenics with an early or late onset should be the same. Using both computerized analysis and visual analog rating scales they have estimated medial and lateral temporal lobe volumes and the size of other brain structures in fourteen late onset schizophrenics. Late-onset schizophrenics had smaller superior temporal gyri than a population of normal controls or a group of patients with Alzheimer's disease. The volumes of hippocampus, amygdala and entorrhinal cortex were reduced in patients with Alzheimer's disease and late-onset schizophrenia compared with controls. On a visual rating scale, the late-onset schizophrenia patients had more temporal lobe pathology than depressed patients.

Functional imaging

To date, clinicians have less experience of techniques for imaging brain function rather than structure. This is unfortunate, since alterations in brain function must underly all the symptoms and signs of psychiatric disorders.

Positron emission tomography (PET) depends on the decay of a nucleus of an administered isotope such as oxygen-15 or fluorine-18. These isotopes can be used to label oxygen or glucose molecules which are taken up by the brain, where their regional concentration is directly related to the pattern of metabolic activity. As each nucleus decays, it emits a positron, which collides with an electron. From the point of collision, a pair of gamma rays are emitted in opposite directions. These are detected by opposing pairs of detectors placed around the head, so that the source of emission is pinpointed. Two-dimensional slices are created with a resolution of about 6 mm, showing regional cerebral metabolism in terms of blood flow, glucose or oxygen metabolism. Neurotransmitter systems can be imaged by radiolabeled ligands with specific binding for receptor sites. PET is expensive and requires short-lived isotopes that need a nearby cyclotron for their production.

Single photon emission tomography (SPET) relies on more conventional radioisotopes with longer half-lives, such as xenon-133 and technetium-99. As they decay, a single gamma ray is emitted. Multidetector SPET scanners can achieve resolutions that are comparable to PET. Intravenous injectable radioamines, such as HMPAO, remain trapped in the brain and are stable in distribution for several hours. Specific ligands are becoming available for SPET that will allow investigation of individual neurotransmitter receptors.

Studies of cerebral blood flow using SPET in young depressed patients have been reported to show reduced global blood flow, most marked in frontal and anterior temporo-parietal regions. In addition, this pattern of blood flow has been related to both age and severity of depression (Sackeim et al., 1990). Other studies have reported cerebral blood flow to be unchanged in depressed patients (Reisches, Hedde & Drochner, 1989).

PET studies have shown that a reduction in the brain's metabolic activity during episodes of depression can be localized to the dorsal anterior lateral prefrontal cortex. This reduced metabolism is related to the severity of depressive symptoms in unipolar and bipolar patients as well as those with obsessive–compulsive disorder (Baxter et al. 1989).

There are good reasons to suppose that functional imaging of elderly depressed patients will yield similar results. We have recently examined nine patients with late-onset depression using SPET. Compared to age-matched healthy controls, left anterior frontal and anterior temporal blood flow was reduced in the depressed patients. In a further recent SPET study of elderly depressives, Kumar et al. (1991) found an increase in the ratio of cerebral/cerebellar blood flow in nine patients following treatment and recovery of mood.

There is thus good reason to conclude that functional imaging has demonstrated abnormalities in blood flow and metabolism in the brain of depressed patients of all ages. It is not clear how these patterns relate to particular depressive symptoms such as delusions or psychomotor retardation. Studies of regional cerebral blood flow in schizophrenics, using both PET and SPET, have revealed a characteristic difference from controls when both groups are occupied on a task associated with frontal lobe activity. Schizophrenics have a pattern of reduced metabolism and blood flow, particularly in the left dorso-lateral frontal region (Weinberger, Bergman & Zec, 1986).

PET scanning has been used in attempts to determine the number of dopamine receptors in the brains of schizophrenics. In the simplest terms, a logical component of the dopamine hypothesis of schizophrenia would be that the number of D2 receptors should be increased in the brains of patients who had not received medication. So far, the reports of such PET studies in young schizophrenics have been conflicting.

Studies of regional cerebral blood flow and metabolism in late-onset schizophrenics are still awaited. There has been, however, a preliminary PET study report of increased dopamine D2 receptor numbers in the brains of eight neuroleptic-naive late-onset schizophrenics (Pearlson et al., 1991).

The future

The application of new brain imaging techniques to functional psychiatric disorders in the elderly seems always to have lagged behind investigation of younger patients with the same diagnoses. It is thus simple to identify two areas of imaging research where old age psychiatrists need to 'catch up'. These are the extension of PET and SPET studies and quantitative MRI to populations of elderly patients with late-onset schizophrenia and depression. New imaging techniques are under development and assessment, but the most urgent goals for old age psychiatrists with an interest in neuroimaging must be to determine whether or not the changes in brain structure and function found in younger patients have their analogs amongst older people. A challenge faced uniquely by those investigators who image the brains of elderly patients is the separation of physiological changes associated with normal aging from pathological changes that may represent the cerebral substrate of psychiatric disorder.

References

Abas, M. A., Sahakian, B. J. & Levy, R. (1990). Neuropsychological deficits and CT scan changes in elderly depressives. *Psychological Medicine*, **20**, 507–20.

American Psychiatric Association (1980). *Diagnostic and Statistical Manual of Mental Disorders*, 3rd edition, Washington, DC, American Psychiatric Association.

American Psychiatric Association (1987). *Diagnostic and Statistical Manual of Mental Disorders*, third edition revised. Washington, DC: American Psychiatric Association.

Ames, D., Dolan, R. & Mann, A. (1990). The distinction between depression and dementia in the very old. *International Journal of Geriatric Psychiatry*, **5**, 193–8.

Awad, I. A., Spetzler, R. F., Hodak, J. A., Awad, C. A. & Carey, R. (1986*a*). Incidental subcortical lesions identified on magnetic resonance imaging in the elderly. 1. Correlation with age and cerebrovascular risk factors. *Stroke* **17**, 1084–9.

Awad, I. A., Johnson, P. C., Spetzler, R. S. & Hodak, J. A. (1986*b*) Incidental subcortical lesions identified on magnetic resonance imaging in the elderly. 2. Post mortem pathological correlations. *Stroke*, **17**, 1090–7.

Baxter, L. R., Schwartz, J. M., Phelps, M. E. et al. (1989). Reduction of prefrontal cortex glucose metabolism common to three types of depression. *Archives of General Psychiatry*, **46**, 243–50.

Beats, B., Förstl, H. & Levy, R. (1991). Ventricular enlargement and caudate hyperdensity in elderly depressives. *Biological Psychiatry*, **30**, 452–8.

Bradley, W. G., Waluch, V. & Wycoff, R. R. (1984). Differential diagnosis of periventricular abnormalities in MRI of the brain. *Noninvasive Medical Imaging* **1**, 35–41.

Breitner, J. C. S., Husain, M. M., Figiel, G. S., Krishnan, K. R. R. & Boyko, O. B. (1990). Cerebral white matter disease in late-onset paranoid psychosis. *Biological Psychiatry*, **28**, 266–74.

Burns, A. Carrick, J., Ames, D., Naguib M. & Levy R. (1989). The cerebral cortical appearance in late paraphrenia. *International Journal of Geriatric Psychiatry*, **4**, 31–4.

Consortium for Establishing a Registry for Alzheimer's Disease (CERAD). (1989). *Protocol for Neuroimaging Assessment of Alzheimer's Disease*. Durham, NC: CERAD.

Churchill, C. M., Priolo, C. V., Nemeroff, C. B., Krishnan, R. R. & Breitner, J. C. S. (1991). Occult subcortical magnetic resonance findings in elderly depressives. *International Journal of Geriatric Psychiatry*, **6**, 213–6.

Coffey, C. E., Figiel, G. S., Djang, W. T., Cress, M., Saunders, W. B. & Weiner, R. D. (1988). Leukoencephalopathy in elderly depressed patients referred for ECT. *Biological Psychiatry*, **24**, 143–61.

Coffey, C. E., Figiel, G. S., Djang, W. T. & Weiner, R. D. (1990). Subcortical hyperintensity on magnetic resonance imaging: A comparison of normal and depressed elderly subjects. *American Journal of Psychiatry*, **147**, 187–9.

Copeland, J. R. M., Kelleher, M. J., Kellett, J. M. et al. (1976). A semi-structured interview for the assessment of diagnosis and mental state in the elderly: The Geriatric Mental State Schedule: 1. Development and reliability. *Psychological Medicine*, **6**, 439–49.

Dolan, R. J., Calloway, S. P. & Mann, A. H. (1985). Cerebral ventricular size: depressed subjects. *Psychological Medicine*, **15**, 873–8.

Dupont, R. M., Jernigan, T. L., Butters, N., Hesselink, J. R., Heindel, W. & Gillin, J. C. (1990). Subcortical abnormalities detected in bipolar disorder using magnetic resonance imaging: Clinical and neuropsychological significance. *Archives of General Psychiatry*, **47**, 55–9.

Erkinjuntti, T., Ketonen, L., Sulkava, R., Sipponen, J., Vuorialho, M. & Hvanainen, M. (1987). Do white matter changes on MRI and CT differentiate vascular dementia from Alzheimer's disease? *Journal of Neurology, Neurosurgery and Psychiatry*, **50**, 37–42.

Fazekas, F., Niederkorn, K., Schmidt, R. et al. (1988). White matter signal abnormalities in normal individuals: correlation with carotid ultrasonography, cerebral blood flow measurements and cerebrovascular risk factors. *Stroke*, **19**, 1285–8.

Flint, A. J., Rifat, S. L. & Eastwood, M. R. (1991). Late-onset paranoia: distinct from paraphrenia? *International Journal of Geriatric Psychiatry*, **6**, 103–9.

Folstein, M. F., Folstein, S. E. & McHugh, P. R. (1975). 'Mini-mental state', a practical method for grading the cognitive state of patients for the clinician. *Journal of Psychiatric Research*, **12**, 189–98.

Gerard, G. & Weisberg, L. A. (1986). MRI periventicular lesions in adults. *Neurology*, **36**, 998–1001.

Hershey, L. A., Modic, M. T., Greenough, P. G. & Jaffe, D. F. (1987). Magnetic resonance imaging in vascular dementia. *Neurology*, **37**, 29–36.

Howard, R. J., Förstl, H., Naguib, M., Burns, A. & Levy, R. (1992). First-rank symptoms of Schneider in late paraphrenia. Cortical structural correlates. *British Journal of Psychiatry*, **160**, 108–9.

Hunt, A. L., Orrison, W. W., Yeo, R. A. et al. (1989). Clinical significance of MRI white matter lesions in the elderly. *Neurology*, **39**, 1470–4.

Jacoby, R. J., Dolan, R. J., Baldy, R. & Levy, R. (1983). Quantitative computed tomography in elderly depressed patients. *British Journal of Psychiatry*, **143**, 124–7.

Jacoby, R. J. & Levy, R. (1980). Computed tomography in the elderly: 3. Affective disorder. *British Journal of Psychiatry*, **136**, 270–5.

Jacoby, R. J., Levy, R. & Bird, J. M. (1981). Computed tomography and the outcome of affective disorder: a follow-up study of elderly patients. *British Journal of Psychiatry*, **139**, 288–92.

Jeste, D. V., Dupont, R., Jernigan, T., Sewell, D., Heindel, W. & Harris, M. J. (1991).

Clinical and brain-imaging studies of late-onset schizophrenia. *Proceedings of American College of Neuropsychopharmacologists*, 30th Annual Meeting, San Juan, Puerto Rico.

Kellner, C. H., Rubinow, D. R. & Post, R. M. (1986). Cerebral ventricular size and cognitive impairment in depression. *Journal of Affective Disorders*, **10**, 215–9.

Krishnan, K. R. R., Goli, V., Ellinwood, E. H., France, R. D., Blazer, D. G. & Nemeroff, C. B. (1988). Leukoencephalopathy in patients diagnosed as major depressive. *Biological Psychiatry*, **25**, 519–22.

Kumar, A., Mozley, D., Dunham, C., Velchik, M., Reilley, J., Gottlieb, G. & Alavi, A. (1991). Semiquantitative I-123 IMP SPET studies in late onset depression before and after treatment. *International Journal of Geriatric Psychiatry*, **6**, 775–7.

Lewis, S. W. (1990). Computerized tomography in schizophrenia 15 years on. *British Journal of Psychiatry*, **157** (suppl. 9), 16–24.

Miller, B. L., Benson, F., Cummings, J. L. & Neshkes, R. (1986). Late-life paraphrenia: An organic delusional syndrome. *Journal of Clinical Psychiatry*, **47**, 204–7.

Miller, B. L., Lesser, I. M., Boone, K. et al. (1989). Brain white-matter lesions and psychosis. *British Journal of Psychiatry*, **155**, 73–8.

Miller, B. L., Lesser, I. M., Boone, K., Hill, E., Mehringer, C. M. & Wong, K. (1991). Brain lesions and cognitive function in late-life psychosis. *British Journal of Psychiatry*, **158**, 76–82.

Naguib, M. & Levy, R. (1987). Late paraphrenia: neuropsychological impairment and structural brain abnormalities on computed tomography. *International Journal of Geriatric Psychiatry*, **2**, 83–90.

Pearlson, G. D., Garbacz, D., Tompkins, R. H., Ahn, H. O. & Rabins, P. V. (1987). Lateral cerebral ventricle size in late-onset schizophrenia. In *Schizophrenia and Ageing*, Ed. N. E. Miller & G. D. Cohen, pp. 246–8: New York: Guildford Press.

Pearlson, G. D., Rabins, P. V., Kim, W. S. et al. (1989). Structural brain changes and cognitive deficits in elderly depressives with and without reversible dementia ('pseudodementia'). *Psychological Medicine*, **19**, 573–84.

Pearlson, G. D., Barta, P. E., Tune, L. E. et al. (1991). Quantitative MRI and PET in late life onset schizophrenia. *Proceedings of American College of Neuropsychopharmacology*, 30th Annual Meeting, San Juan, Puerto Rico.

Rabins, P. V., Pearlson, G., Jayaram, G., Steele, C. & Tune, L. (1987). Increased ventricle-to-brain ratio in late-onset schizophrenia. *American Journal of Psychiatry*, **144**, 1216–8.

Rabins, P. V., Pearlson, G. D., Aylward, E., Kumar, A. J. & Dowell, K. (1991). Cortical magnetic resonance imaging changes in elderly inpatients with major depression. *American Journal of Psychiatry*, **148**, 617–20.

Reisches, F. M., Hedde, J. P. & Drochner, R. (1989). Clinical correlates and cerebral blood flow in depression. *Psychiatric Research*, **29**, 323–6.

Sackeim, H. A., Prohovnik, I., Moeller, J. R. et al. (1990). Regional cerebral blood flow in mood disorders. 1. Comparison of major depressives and normal controls at rest. *Archives of General Psychiatry*, **47**, 60–70.

Schlegel, S. & Kretschmer, K. (1987). Computed tomography in affective disorders. Part 1. Ventricular and sulcal measurements. *Biological Psychiatry*, **22**, 4–14.

Spitzer, R. L., Endicott, J. & Robins, E. (1978). Research Diagnostic Criteria: rationale and reliability. *Archives of General Psychiatry*, **35**, 773–82.

Sze, G., DeArmond, S. & Brant-Zawadski, M. (1985). 'Abnormal' MRI foci anterior to the frontal horns: pathologic correlates of a ubiquitous finding. *American Journal of Neuroradiology*, **6**, 467–8.

Weinberger, D. R., Berman, K. F. & Zec, R. F. (1986). Physiological dysfunction of dorsolateral prefrontal cortex in schizophrenia. 1. Regional cerebral blood flow evidence. *Archives of General Psychiatry*, **43**, 114–24.

23

Medical comorbidity: presentation in a general hospital setting

BRICE PITT

Introduction

Improved public health and a lower birthrate (because of contraception and abortion) mean that the world is ageing. Although the nations with the oldest populations are also, at present, the most developed, the rate of ageing is most striking in the less developed countries. The prosperity of Japan, together with a distinctive diet and a free health service for old people, has been reflected in an astonishing increase in the number of those old people and the highest life expectancy in the world; this is both good news and bad (Okamoto, 1992), in that there is a major problem of where and how to place those old people who are in hospital because of infirmity.

In Britain, which shares with North-Western Europe the distinction of having the highest proportion of old people in the world, the process has been more gradual. In 1901 5% were aged 65 or more, in 1991 15%. In response to the kind of difficulties now reported by the Japanese, the last 30 years have seen the appointment of ever-increasing numbers of old age psychiatrists, from about three in 1966 to well over 300 at the time of writing (Royal Colleges of Physicians & Psychiatrists, 1989). The College and the Department of Health finally recognized old age psychiatry as a full specialty in 1990.

Although originally based in large psychiatric hospitals, more and more of these psychiatrists have moved into departments within general hospitals. This usually means that they are much nearer to the people they serve, as mental hospitals have tended to be well out of sight (and often out of mind!). They are also, appropriately, nearer to general hospital wards. On these wards a large proportion of the patients are elderly, with a high morbidity for psychiatric disorder (chiefly delirium, dementia and depression). There is also a high morbidity for physical illness and disability in those who are referred for psychiatric disorder in old age, so 'psychogeriatrics' has a strong claim to be based on a general hospital site.

This chapter considers the frequent comorbidity of physical and psychiatric illness, *contributory factors*, how nonpsychiatric clinicians may *screen* their patients for common psychiatric disorders, general hospital staff *attitudes* to and knowledge of mental illness among old people in their wards, the importance of close *liaison* between medical and psychiatric services for the elderly and how it may be achieved, and general implications for education and resources.

Comorbidity

According to a number of epidemiological surveys (Copeland et al., 1987; Lindesay, Briggs & Murphy, 1989; Livingston et al., 1990), morbidity for dementia in the community population aged 65 and over is at least 5%, rising to 20% in those over 80. Major depression prevails in 2–3% of those over 65, minor in another 10–12%. Anxiety states are present in about 10% of the over-65s. One would hardly expect a lower psychiatric morbidity than this among old people in general hospital wards; indeed, it might well be expected to be higher.

While this is almost certainly true, there are sometimes problems in establishing the prevalence of psychiatric disorder in such wards. Assessments are often hampered by a lack of quiet and privacy, and the inexorable ward routine, bustle and noise offer many distractions. The patients may be enfeebled, exhausted, preoccupied or discouragingly deaf. They may have been abruptly removed by transfer, discharge or sudden death.

Even so, it is likely that dementia prevails in up to 30% of those over 65 in general hospital wards (Feldman et al., 1987; Johnston et al., 1987; Pitt 1991*a*) which is six times the rate among those of the same age in the community. Demented people tend to neglect themselves and to refuse the help they really need. Thus they may fail to shop or feed themselves or fail to take the medicines they have been prescribed. They are at risk of accidents, subnutrition, hypothermia and the worst effects of the common maladies of later life like hypertension, diabetes and heart disease. Unfortunately they may also be suffering from ill-treatment and injury from 'elder abuse' (Homer & Gilleard, 1991; Pitt, 1992*b*). While their admission to hospital is usually for a sufficient 'medical' reason, it may also signify that the limits of community care have been reached. They are then a risk of being labelled 'social' admissions, signifying that whether or not the admission was justified on medical grounds, they have outstayed their welcome. It is often difficult to regain the level of community support previously provided, or the circumstances of the admission may indicate that level of care no longer suffices. To intensify community care or, more often, arrange transfer to a residential or nursing home or a long-stay ward takes time, during which the old person is in danger of being overlooked, marginalized or even resented as a 'bed-blocker'. Delay in effecting a move to more appropriate care increases the prevalence of demented patients on general hospital wards.

Delirium is a disorder seen far more often in than outside hospital. It has a very low prevalence in the community, lasting for no more than days or weeks, but is a common manifestation of serious physical illness (pneumonia, metabolic upsets, major surgery) in old age which often necessitates admission to hospital. Delirium is more frequent in newly admitted patients than in those who have been in hospital for some time, though drug-induced confusion and intercurrent infections may cause subsequent delirium in a quarter of those who were admitted cognitively intact (Hodkinson, 1973). There was far more delirium – two-thirds of those showing an organic brain syndrome (OBS) – among consecutive newly admitted patients aged 70 and over in Oxford (Feldman et al., 1987) than in a prevalence study of elderly patients in the general wards of the Royal Free Hospital (Johnson et al., 1987). Of consecutive elderly acute medical patients admitted to the Beth Israel Medical Center in New York, 13.5% met the American Psychiatric Association's (1980) diagnostic criteria (DSM-III) for delirium, while another 3.5% became delirious during their stay (Cameron et al., 1987). In Edmonton, Alberta, delirium was found in 16% of people aged 65–91 admitted to acute medical care and appeared in a further 9% during their stay (Rockwood, 1989). The figure for delirium of 16% in newly admitted patients was also reported by Bergmann & Eastham (1974) and Seymour, Henschke & Cape (1980). Gustafson et al. (1988) found delirium in no less than 61% of 111 consecutive patients operated on for fractured neck of femur.

One of the main risk factors for delirium, apart from the severity of the precipitating physical illness, is pre-existing dementia. Koponen et al. (1989) found far more cortical atrophy, focal changes and ventricular enlargement among the CT scans of the brains of 69 delirious elderly patients than in those of control patients.

The outcome of delirium is said to be recovery or death (Bedford, 1959), while dementia is an unusual consequence unless it was already present. Understandably, there seems to be more definite information about death than recovery (Pitt, 1991*b*). Some features of delirium are less transitory than others: Rockwood & Fox (1992) found that memory impairment lasted a mean 28 days. Intriguingly (though probably irrelevantly) Lewy body disease, which some now claim to be more prevalent than multi-infarct dementia (McKeith et al., 1992), has features of both delirium and dementia, and in a sense bridges the gap between the two disorders postulated by those who consider them to be on a continuum rather than wholly separate syndromes (Pitt, 1991*b*).

Depressive illness may be the cause or consequence of physical illness. Dangerous dehydration and malnutrition may arise from the refusal by some severely depressed old people to take fluids or food. Gross self-neglect may result from apathy, retardation and morbid preoccupations; medication for such physical disorders as heart failure, arthritis and diabetes may not be taken. Anorexia and weight loss or atypical pain associated with 'masked' depression may also lead to admission to general hospital wards, for investigation. Unlike suicide (Pitt & Nowers, 1986), deliberate self-harm is much less common in old than young people but is still not rare as a cause of admission to a general hospital.

Physical illness is probably the commonest factor associated with late life depression (Post, 1962; Murphy, 1982). Chronic obstructive airways disease, (Borson & McDonald, 1989; Kukull et al., 1986), malignant disease (Evans, Copeland & Dewey, 1991), myocardial infarction (Koenig et al., 1988) and stroke (Robinson et al., 1983; Dam, Pedersen & Ahlgren, 1989) seem to be especially depressing. While the depression usually takes the form of an adjustment disorder (American Psychiatric Association, 1980), or a major depressive disorder precipitated by the stress of physical illness, occasionally it is intrinsic to the physical condition: endocrine disease such as Cushing's syndrome (Cohen, 1980; Haskett, 1985); hypothyroidism (Tappy et al., 1987); hyperparathyroidism (McAllion & Paterson 1989); occult carcinoma (Whitlock & Siskind, 1979); and stroke where the cerebral lesion is in the anterior left hemisphere (Robinson et al., 1989).

Depression may lower the threshold for physical illness and increases mortality, possibly by effects on the immune system (Lancet, 1987).

For all these reasons the prevalence of depression in general hospital wards might be expected to be a good deal higher than in the community. However, not all surveys agree that this is so. Table 23.1 shows a range in different studies of from 5% to more than 40%. Such a variation may be due to the use of different screening instruments, different cut-points on the same instruments, or different diagnostic criteria; to whether or not cognitively impaired patients were excluded; to the kind of areas served by the hospital and what alternative resources (such as nursing homes) there are; and to whether the hospital is acute or long-stay, and takes its patients from a defined catchment area or selectively from further afield.

Estimates of the prevalence of depression in the community also vary. Recent community surveys in the United Kingdom are pretty consistent: Gurland et al. (1983) found 12% of their elderly London subjects (and 13% of those in New York) to be depressed; Copeland et al. (1987) in Liverpool 11.3%; Lindesay et al. (1989) in South London 13.5%; and Livingston et al. in North London (1990) 16%. However, in the Epidemiological Catchment Area Survey in the USA rates of depression in older people according to the DSM-III based Diagnostic Interview Schedule are low, and consistently less than in those who are younger: Myers, Weissman & Tischler (1984) give six-month prevalence rates for affective disorder in the population aged 65 or more in four communities as ranging from none to 2.6% in women (see Chapter 7).

It is easy to exceed these USA figures in the hospital prevalence studies shown in Table 23.1. On the other hand, the rates given by three of these studies (Bergmann

Table 23.1. *Prevalence of depression among elderly medical in-patients*

Authors	Instrument	Year	Place	Prevalence rates
Bergmann & Eastham	Clinical	1974	Newcastle	5% endogenous
Magni, de Leo & Schifano	Zung, DFS	1985	Padua (geriatric)	42% (> younger)
Cooper	CASE	1987	Mannheim	21%
Feldman et al.	PSE	1987	Oxford	5% (< younger)
Johnston et al.	GHQ	1987	N. London	11.6%
Kay et al.	GMS, ICD-9	1987	Hobart (nursing homes, long-stay patients)	25% M, 30% F
Koenig et al.	DIS	1988	Durham NC	11.5% major
Kafonek et al.	DSM-III	1989	Baltimore (long-stay patients)	21% (all syndromes)
Roohanna & Pitt	BAS	1989	W. London (geriatric)	21% 'caseness'
Pitt	BAS	1991*a*	E. London	6.5% major 5.5% other

& Eastham, 1974; Feldman et al. 1987; Pitt, 1991*a*) – 5% or just over – though well above American levels, appear to be less than those in the UK community studies. Probably this is because they reflect only major depression (which prevails in 2–3% of the elderly in the UK community studies – Lindesay et al., 1989). It is still surprising, that Feldman and colleagues (1987) in Oxford found far less depression in older than in younger medical inpatients: 5%, compared with 12.5% in those 55–69, and 18% in those 17–54. The instrument they used was the Present State Examination (PSE), Wing, Cooper & Sartorius, 1974), and although the nature of depression in old age is not all that different from that in those who are younger, perhaps somatic symptoms of depression might sometimes be ascribed to concurrent physical disorder, and impaired cognition to dementia. An instrument specially designed for the elderly, such as the Geriatric Mental State (GMS, Copeland et al., 1976) might be preferable. It may also be relevant that threshold scores for caseness may need to be modified according to the setting. Goldberg (1985) has pointed out that his General Health Questionnaire (GHQ, Goldberg, 1972) requires a much lower score for likely caseness in general practice than in neurological in-patients. The author's personal experience suggests that the threshold score for 'caseness' of cognitive impairment on the Mini-Mental State Examination (Folstein, Folstein & McHugh, 1975) needs to be set seven points lower among geriatric in-patients than among bright, successful people in their sixties attending a Memory Clinic.

Hospital is a powerful catalyst for the experience of anxiety. Not only is there the disorder requiring admission, but there are unfamiliar routines, mysterious and usually uncomfortable investigations, strange staff in a variety of roles, a communal life with an assortment of fellow-patients and all too much scope for failures in communication. Still greater are the fears of pain, disability, dependency and death.

Anxiety may lead to sleeplessness in hospital, and the ready prescription of a (usually benzodiazepine) hypnotic in the past too often contributed to the already formidable habituation to hypnotics in elderly people. On the other hand, the brusque, sometimes unwitting, withdrawal of a sedative (including alcohol) after admission to hospital may precipitate acute anxiety, or even a fit. Anxiety is one of the commonest consequences of a myocardial infarction, and thus a cause of prolonged invalidism. It also contributes to the 'fear of falling' syndrome (Lindesay, 1991) where, after an attack of giddiness, dizziness or a transient ischaemic attack the patient is afraid of walking without having something or someone to hold on to. Anxiety symptoms may arise directly from thyrotoxicosis, hypoxia in those with cardio-respiratory disease (Schiffer, Klein & Rider, 1988) and cardiac arrhythmias, and the manifold somatic manifestations of anxiety may suggest a host of physical disorders, through overbreathing, tachycardia, frequency of micturition, diarrhoea, palpitations and even faints.

Difficult old people – including those who are personality disordered, paranoid, 'graduate' schizophrenics – are usually left out of morbidity surveys, probably because of difficulty in devising suitable screening instruments and because they are very likely to be among those who refuse to become involved. However, they are likely to be over-represented in general hospital wards because they neglect themselves and have isolated themselves from or fallen out with those who might care for them at home. In a prevalence study of patients over 65 in the general wards of hospitals serving the London borough of Hackney (Pitt, 1991*a*) no less than 30% of the subjects were single, which might reflect such isolation.

Alcohol abuse is often overlooked in the elderly (Schiffer et al., 1988) because it is not expected. Atkinson (1991) points out that many clinicians believe that alcoholics either die prematurely or recover spontaneously and that late addiction is rare. Nevertheless, alcohol abuse contributes to falls, burns, cognitive impairment of various degrees, peripheral neuritis and hepatic cirrhosis, with oesophageal varices and liver failure. Patients are unlikely to mention their drinking unless asked about it, and even then tend to make the least of it. Friends and families may hide heavy drinking because of embarrassment or collusion. The CAGE screening questions (Ewing, 1984) are useful in diagnosis.

Finally, comorbidity may well be iatrogenic. Drugs given for psychiatric disorder may cause physical morbidity, and vice versa. Tricyclic antidepressants, for example, may cause hypotension and drowsiness (both resulting in falls and other accidents)(Blake et al., 1988), cardiac arrhythmias, dental problems, glaucoma, retention of urine and fits. Steroids, propanolol, L-dopa and indomethacin may all cause depression. Anti-Parkinsonian and some hypotensive agents may occasion a variety of psychiatric syndromes, including confusion, depression, visual hallucinations, mania and paranoia.

Screening

Goldberg (1985) explains that the recognition of psychiatric illness in general wards by physicians and surgeons comes about either because a cue suggests such disorder or because the patient's complaints cannot be accounted for by known organic disease. However, in over half such patients, with illnesses diagnosable according to research criteria, the diagnosis is not made. Goldberg suggests five reasons:

1. The patients provide no cue (though they will readily describe their symptoms if asked).
2. The cues are not picked up.
3. Patients lack privacy.
4. Having found an organic disorder, doctors look no further.
5. Even when they suspect psychiatric disorder, the doctors may lack the confidence to pursue the assessment.

Consequently he advocates screening tests, with which general hospital doctors may become familiar and comfortable, thus increasing their alertness.

The use of short cognitive tests for old people in hospital is fairly well established, because they are pretty handy, valid, reliable and sensitive to change, and because cognitive deficits are so common in such patients, with important implications for prognosis and management. The 10-item Abbreviated Mental Test Score (AMTS, Hodkinson, 1972) is widely used by geriatricians in the UK, and for all its obvious limits (it is almost entirely a memory test, with a low 'ceiling', and knowing the name of the ward and recognising two people on it are more or less easy according to how long the patient has been there) has proved useful (Kafetz, 1986); a score of 7 or less is suggestive of cognitive impairment.

Internationally, the most widely used screening instrument for cognitive impairment is the Mini-Mental State Examination (Folstein et al., 1975). The score below which cognitive impairment is likely is 24/30, but this criterion may need to be modified for certain groups of people (see above): as with almost all cognitive tests, more might be expected of those who are intelligent, and well educated, and less of those less advantaged (Brayne & Calloway, 1990). Dysphasic, dysarthric, drugged, psychotic, foreign and uncooperative patients may also score low. Also scores vary a bit according to how hawkish or dove-like is the tester, so in research it is always wise to check inter-rater reliability before and after training, or retraining, in its use.

Other well-established screening tests for cognition are sufficiently similar not to need separate discussion here. The brevity of the AMTS (not only does it not take long to administer but the items are easily remembered by the rater) is likely to keep it a firm favorite with general ward doctors who have got to know it. Cognition, however, is only one aspect of the organic brain syndromes, which also have their important behavioral components. Here the Behavioral Scales of the Clifton Assessment Procedures for the Elderly (CAPE), and the Blessed Dementia Scale (Blessed, Tomlinson & Roth, 1968), which can be completed by the ward nurses, come into their own.

It is also highly desirable to screen for depression, which may retard the patient's progress, increases mortality and is often treatable. Two scales especially designed for the elderly are the Geriatric Depression Scale (GDS, Yesavage et al., 1983) and the Depression Scale of the Brief Assessment Schedule (BAS, Macdonald et al., 1982). The former comprises 30 questions (with a slightly American flavour) which cleverly avoid the 'somatic' features of depression (anorexia, weight loss, insomnia, energy) to which an accompanying physical disorder might contribute. In geriatric inpatients, Adshead, Day-Cody & Pitt (1992) found the sensitivity and specificity of the GDS to be 72% and 88%, the positive and negative predictive values to be 75% and 86% and the mean time taken to administer the test was just under seven minutes. An adaptation of 19 items from the BAS as statements boldly printed on cards to which the patient responds 'true' or 'false' with respect to their current feelings (BASDEC) had very similar sensitivity, specificity, positive and negative predictive values, but took only half as long. It may therefore prove especially popular as a screening instrument for depression in old people in hospital, useable by any member of the ward team.

The author, in an as yet unpublished survey, found that geriatricians were aware of 88% of those of their in-patients who were found independently to have the organic brain syndrome, but only 42% of those who were depressed. Instruments like BASDEC and the GDS have the potential to improve this recognition.

Attitudes

In the general ward the old person with psychiatric disorder is at risk of getting too little attention, or too much of the wrong kind.

Too little results from failure to diagnose the disorder, or labelling and dismissing the patient because of it. Labels such as 'social admission', 'bed-blocker', or the adjectives 'geriatric' or 'psychogeriatric' used as nouns, carry the risk of robbing the person so stigmatized of their humanity, leaving them simply as an obstacle to the proper use of the ward. They are then overlooked or abandoned in a corner while there is a long, fitful, exasperated and frequently inept quest for 'disposal', with mutterings about the deficiencies of families, social workers, psychiatrists and geriatricians as well as the hapless patient! The ever briefer continuation notes comprise such observations as 'i.s.q.' and 'waiting for Godot'! Evidence of discussions with such patients about their future is often lacking, and, in the absence of information and rehabilitation, institutionalization and dependency are insidiously induced. At the time of writing it looks as if changes in the provision of community care in England and Wales (Secretaries of State, 1989), giving the responsibility wholly to social services with limited budgets, may, if anything, continue this dismal scenario.

Too much attention may take the form of oversedation, being placed out of sight (and out of mind) in a side-room and even physical restraint. Binding the elderly, especially those who are confused, even if near to death, is not unknown in the USA (Frengley & Mion, 1986; Robbins et al., 1987) while in the UK the favored form of restraint was the 'geriatric' Buxton chair, which could be tilted backwards to thwart attempts to leave it but also had a table which could be locked across the patient's lap. The culmination of this excess of attention may be precipitate referral to a psychiatrist who arrives to find the patient unrousable after an intramuscular injection of chlorpromazine, and notes which only record the absence of significant physical signs and the mental state as 'confused', 'restless', 'wandering' or 'aggressive'.

Occasionally psychotropic drugs are peremptorily and inappropriately withdrawn when the patient is admitted, there being an assumption that they have been given unnecessarily and for too long, without a proper enquiry into their rationale, which may then become painfully apparent after a week or two.

The attitudes which give rise to such abuses include (Pitt, 1992*a*):

1. Ignorance:
   The lessons learnt during a psychiatric attachment or clerkship seem easily forgotten (partly from lack of reinforcement) in the hurly-burly of life on a busy general ward; or, in the case of old age psychiatry, they may never have been learned in the first place.
2. Prejudice:
   'Mental disorder means madness, trouble, unpredictable, erratic behavior, attention-seeking or even malingering. If the ward is upstairs, then suicidal patients may hurl themselves from the windows. If it is on the ground, restless old people may wander away and get run over or be lost'.
3. Paranoia:
   'We are being used as a dump for problems which belong to the GP, social services, rejecting families, administrators, the geriatricians or the psychiatrists, who don't pull their weight, and pass the buck'. The beleaguered house officer (intern) or registrar (resident) subjects the referring doctor to a hostile interrogation if the patient is old, which may leave all parties bruised and aggrieved.
4. Anxiety:
   'We have not the staff, the training or the facilities to deal with these sorts of problems. The other patients, who are really ill, will be upset by noisiness and interference. There

Table 23.2. *Reasons cited in surveys of why medical patients are not referred to psychiatrists*

(*a*)	The psychiatric service dissatisfies the physician.
(*b*)	Psychiatric language is useless to the physician.
(*c*)	The physician is unaware of the need for psychiatric intervention.
(*d*)	The physician is unaware of the possibility of psychiatric intervention.
(*e*)	The physician believes the psychiatric disorder to be incurable.
(*f*)	The physician fears the patient's emotions.
(*g*)	The physician feels he does not know the patient well enough.
(*h*)	The significance of psychological issues is denied.
(*i*)	There is a poor working relationship between the physician and the psychiatrist.
(*j*)	The physician believes that the patient is disadvantaged by being labelled a psychiatric case.
(*k*)	The patient refuses psychiatric referral.
(*l*)	The physician considers the patient too physically ill.
(*m*)	The physician believes that every doctor should be able to treat psychiatric illness.
(*n*)	The physician cannot or will not spare the time for psychological issues.

From White, 1990.

will be a disaster – a drip will be pulled down, or someone recovering from a myocardial infarction will have a cardiac arrest – and we'll be blamed'.

Such attitudes may not be shown by those who have been properly trained and realise that in most general hospitals in developed countries two-fifths of the patients will be old, and half of these will be confused, depressed or otherwise psychiatrically disordered (Pitt, 1991*a*). A good corrective is a competent consultation–liaison service with old age psychiatry.

White's (1990) analysis of why medical patients with psychiatric disorder may not be referred to psychiatrists is worth citing (see Table 23.2).

Consultation and liaison

The further away the psychiatric base is from the general hospital, the less frequent and effective will be the consultations and liaison. There is a world of difference between what can be provided from a remote psychiatric hospital and from a psychogeriatric unit based in the same general hospital. Also the elderly patients in that general hospital unit will benefit far more from the ease and speed and familiarity of consultations by the general medical and surgical staff than can those perceived as being in a distant 'bin'.

At the most basic level, there is the ward consultation, when the psychiatrist receives a note or phone call explaining the problem more or less adequately and goes to see the patient. He or she may have given notice of the visit, and will therefore hope that the patient will be in the ward, and not at X-ray or an out-patient appointment in another hospital, or discharged! The house officer (intern) or registrar (resident) may be there, but rarely the consultant. There may be a detailed referral in the case-notes, explaining how the patient came to be in hospital, the nature of the current problem and what is hoped for from the consultation. Otherwise the nursing notes may well be more informative than the medical. Perhaps a relative will happen to be visiting at the time of the consultation, or has been actually asked to attend for the occasion. At the end of the consultation an opinion is written in the case-notes, with the probable diagnosis, how it was reached, what further information and investigations are needed and making some recommendations. Often there will be an indication that these are provisional and may be modified in the light of better knowledge. The more such consultations are given, the better the psychiatrist is known and the more frank, friendly and informative the ward staff are likely to be.

This basic model is enriched where the psychiatrist has a regular meeting with the medical firms – not all, because there will usually be too many, but at least with the geriatric team. Such meetings may be at set times, or during ward or day hospital rounds or at out-patient clinics especially where these involve some joint working. If possible, the status of those meeting should be comparable; if it is always the medical registrar who meets the consultant psychiatrist, then the commitment of his consultant may be in doubt, and while day-to-day problems can be tackled, matters of policy may be hard to resolve. It is good, too, if the respective teams can meet, rather than just representative individuals.

However, less comprehensive liaison can still have measurable effects. Scott, Fairbairn & Woodhouse (1988) describe how a senior registrar in the psychiatry of old age started attending the weekly multidisciplinary ward round and case conferences and reviews of a geriatric unit. After two years referrals doubled, from the whole hospital, not just the geriatric unit. The recognition and referral of depression, in particular, increased more than fivefold.

Highly desirable, but sadly elusive, is the joint geriatric/psychogeriatric ward. This was commended in Britain by a Department of Health (GM (70) 11), issued after Kidd's (1962) study suggesting that there was considerable misplacement of old people with psychiatric disorder in geriatric wards, and of those with physical illness in psychiatric wards, which was to the misplaced patients' disadvantage. Although these observations were not confirmed by Hodkinson, Evans & Mezey (1972), the idea of joint units still seemed attractive. It was hoped that avoiding misplacement would reduce the need for long-stay beds and that dual expertise would meet the complex needs of older people with their multiple pathology and co-morbidity for physical and psychiatric disorder.

A detailed account of the operation of such a unit is given by Pitt & Silver (1980). A joint admission ward in the satellite of a London teaching hospital took all acute geriatric admissions and selected patients with psychiatric disorder. These were:

(i) Delirious
(ii) Probably demented
(iii) Those with significant comorbidity, e.g. Parkinson's disease and paranoia, depression and severe dehydration
(iv) Patients with nonspecific disorders such as not eating, falling about, 'failure to thrive'

These were patients for whom the availability of geriatric expertise was especially relevant. Patients with uncomplicated functional psychiatric disorder and dementia were admitted to a small psychiatric hospital close by.

Each consultant did his own, perambulatory ward round and they met for a big multidisciplinary meeting every week. The role of the psychogeriatrician in such a unit is shown in Table 23.3.

The disadvantages are that considerable senior involvement is required, including time, some spent as a spectator; there could be uncertainty about who was in charge; mentally normal patients may be upset by those who clearly are not (though this is so on almost any general ward); and the unit complements other resources, but does not necessarily replace them.

The advantages, though, are that medicine and psychiatry are made simultaneously available to patients who often need both; the threshold for referral from one service to the other is eliminated; psychiatric patients are made more acceptable on the medical wards; mutual teaching and training are enhanced; liaison and reciprocity are intrinsic to the modus operandi; and there is no question of patients falling between stools – 'too ill for a home, too disturbed for a geriatric ward, too feeble for a psychiatric'.

Table 23.3. *The role of the psychogeriatrician in a liaison service*

(*a*)	The identification of psychiatric disorder.
(*b*)	Assessing its relevance to any physical disorder: cause, consequence, coincidental, part of, exacerbating, iatrogenic?
(*c*)	Estimating its effect on prognosis.
(*d*)	Implementing its treatment.
(*e*)	Helping staff understanding of the possible psychodynamics of dependency, 'attention seeking', 'manipulation', 'undue' disability, aggression and failure to cooperate.
(*f*)	Helping with the management of common losses – dying, bereavement, amputation, being rejected.
(*g*)	Arranging transfer to a psychiatric ward when appropriate.
(*h*)	Arranging follow-up.
(*i*)	Teaching nurses and junior doctors about psychiatric illness in old age and when and what to do about it.

From Pitt, 1991*a*).

The ultimate in joint working is the integrated department of health care of the elderly (Arie, 1983) where psychiatrists and physicians work together not so much in the same wards but in the same department and sharing the same professor to provide a 'seamless service'. This provides a coherent, comprehensive service for the consumer and the trainee; constant cross-fertilization, to the advantage of research; and a powerful voice within the health district to assert the needs of the elderly, whose needs for staff, amenities, expertise, technological resources and 'real estate' have constantly to be reaffirmed.

The relationship between geriatric physicians and old age psychiatrists

Despite a strong feeling that, to paraphrase Benjamin Franklin, 'we must hang together, or we shall hang separately', psychiatrists and physicians for the elderly do not always get on! They may not meet often enough, or they may look to the psychiatric or medical 'family' whence they come rather than be prepared to form a partnership with a fantasized alien discipline, or there may have been some bitter, still unresolved dispute about a very difficult but 'immobile' patient, or a fully ambulant demented person without behavioral problems. It was partly to overcome such difficulties that in 1979 a joint committee of the British Geriatrics Society and the Royal College of Psychiatrists approved and published the 'Guidelines for Collaboration between Geriatric Physicians and Psychiatrists in the Care of the Elderly' which had been prepared by Professor Tom Arie (1979).

The main thrust was that services for the elderly should be a unity for 'consumers'. 'Patients should not be bounced back from one part of the service merely because they seem more appropriate for another part: such distribution of referrals should be the internal responsibility of the service'. 'Responsibility should be determined by the assessed needs of the patient and not by the quirks of the referral'. 'Lack of resources does not alter the definition of responsibility. Once a patient's needs are recognized as falling within the province of one service, that service should support that patient within the limits of the feasible – even if this is less than ideal: a 'psychiatric' patient does not become 'geriatric' simply because there are no psychiatric beds or vice versa'. 'No one should be labelled as a "psychiatric patient" by virtue merely of some previous psychiatric episode'.

Kaufman & Bates (1990) looked at how relations were between consultants in the two specialties ten years later. Opinions were obtained from 30 of 33 consultants in geriatric medicine in two health regions, 25 (83%) of whom were aware of the guidelines. Seventeen (57%) felt that relations were unsatisfactory; this was mainly attributed to lack of resources. Twenty-one (70%) reported particular problems with dementia beds. The presence or absence of a psychogeriatrician did not necessarily improve relations; if the psychogeriatrician had been given too few beds, problems remained. However, where there was collaborative activity (joint meetings or rounds, regular visits to each other's units, research, education, staff rotations) there was a marked absence of substantial problems with demented patients.

Conclusions

Old people with psychiatric disorder form a substantial proportion of the patients in a general hospital. In such a hospital with, say, 500 beds (excluding obstetric, paediatric, psychiatric and geriatric) in the UK they could well number 100 (20%). Despite changes in health care (e.g. 'Working for Patients' – Secretaries of State, 1989 – Britain, permitting hospitals to become self-governing trusts) the high proportion of elderly people in the population means that this not only is, but will remain, a fact of hospital life. Psychiatric disorder is associated with a higher mortality, a longer stay in hospital and less likelihood of being at home after discharge than where there is no such disorder (Pitt, 1991*a*), so it needs to be reckoned with.

There is too much psychiatric disorder among old people and it is too closely associated with serious physical illness, to be 'handed over' to the specialist psychogeriatric services (Anderson & Philpott, 1991). So all who deal with older patients in the general hospital – doctors, nurses, social and paramedical workers – need to be trained to recognize, allow for and manage psychiatric disorder in the elderly.

At the same time psychogeriatric expertise needs to be available within the general hospital for speedy consultation, including diagnosis, treatment, management and placement. There should be a psychogeriatric unit in every substantial general hospital, and it should be closely affiliated to the department of geriatric medicine.

References

Adshead, F., Day-Cody, D. & Pitt, B. (1992). BASDEC: a novel screening instrument for depression in elderly medical in-patients. *British Medical Journal*, **305**, 397.

American Psychiatric Association. (1980). *Diagnostic and Statistical Manual of Mental Disorders*, 3rd edition. Washington DC: American Psychiatric Association.

Anderson, D. N. & Philpott, R. M. (1991). The changing pattern of referrals for psychogeriatric consultation in the general hospital: an eight-year study. *International Journal of Geriatric Psychiatry*, **6**, 801–7.

Arie, T. (1979). Guidelines for collaboration between geriatric physicians and psychiatrists in the care of the elderly. *Bulletin of the Royal College of Psychiatrists*, November, 168–9.

Arie, T. (1983). Organization of services for the elderly: implications for education and patient care – experience in Nottingham. In *Gerontopsychiatric Diagnostics and*

Treatment. Multidimensional Approaches. Ed. M. Bergener. New York: Springer Publishing Company.

Atkinson, R. M. (1991). Alcohol and drug abuse in the elderly. In *Psychiatry in the Elderly*, ed. R. Jacoby & C. Oppenheimer. Oxford: Oxford Medical Publications.

Bedford, P. D. (1959). General medical aspects of confusional states in elderly people. *British Medical Journal*, **ii**, 185–8.

Bergmann, K. & Eastham, E. J. (1974). Psychogeriatric assessment and assessment for treatment in an acute medical ward setting. *Age and Ageing*, **3**, 174–88.

Blake, A. J., Morgan, K., Bendall, M. J. et al. (1988). Falls by elderly people at home – prevalence and associated factors. *Age and Ageing*, **17**, 365–72.

Blessed, G., Tomlinson, B. E. & Roth M. (1968). The association between quantitative measures of dementia and senile changes in the grey matter of elderly subjects. *British Journal of Psychiatry*, **114**, 791–811.

Borson, S. & McDonald, G. (1989). Depression and chronic pulmonary disease. In *Depression and Co-existing Disease*, ed. R. Robinson & P. Rabins. New York: Igoaku-Shoin.

Brayne, C. & Calloway, P. (1990). The association of education and socioeconomic status with the Mini Mental State Examination and the clinical diagnosis of dementia in elderly people. *Age and Ageing*, **19**, 91–6.

Cameron, D. J., Thomas, R. I., Mulvihill, M. & Bronheim, H. (1987). Delirium: a test of the Diagnostic and Statistical Manual III on medical in-patients. *Journal of the American Geriatrics Society*, **35**, 1007–10.

Cooper, B. (1987). Psychiatric disorders among elderly patients admitted to general hospital wards. *Journal of the Royal Society of Medicine*, **80**, 13–16.

Cohen, S. I. (1980). Cushing's syndrome: a psychiatric study of 29 patients. *British Journal of Psychiatry*, **136**, 120–4.

Copeland, J. R. M., Kelleher, M. J., Kellett, J. M., Gourlay, A. J., Gurland, B. J., Fleiss, J. L. & Sharpe, L. (1976). A semi-structured clinical interview for the assessment of diagnosis and mental state in the elderly. The Geriatric Mental State Schedule I: development and reliability. *Psychological Medicine*, **6**, 439–49.

Copeland, J. R. M., Dewey, M., Wood, N., Searle, R., Davidson, I. & McWilliam, C. (1987). Range of mental illness among the elderly in the community. Prevalence in Liverpool using the GMS-AGECAT package. *British Journal of Psychiatry*, **150**, 815–23.

Dam, H., Pedersen, H. E. & Ahlgren, P. (1989). Depression among patients with stroke. *Acta Psychiatrica Scandinavica*, **80**, 118–24.

Department of Health & Social Security (1970). *Psycho-geriatric Assessment Units.* Circular HM (70) 11. London: HMSO.

Evans, M. E. Copeland, J. R. M. & Dewey, M. E. (1991). Depression in the elderly in the community: effect of physical illness and selected social factors. *International Journal of Geriatric Psychiatry*, **6**, 787–95.

Ewing, J. A. (1984). Detecting alcoholism: the CAGE questionnaire. *Journal of the American Medical Association*, **252**, 1905–7.

Feldman, E., Mayou, R., Hawton, K., Ardern, M. & Smith, E. B. O. (1987). Psychiatric disorder in medical in-patients. *Quartlerly Journal of Medicine*, **240**, 301–8.

Folstein, M. F., Folstein, S. E. & McHugh, P. R. (1975). 'Mini-mental state'. A practical method for grading the cognitive state of patients for the clinician. *Journal of Psychiatric Research*, **12**, 189–98.

Frengley, J. D. & Mion, L. C. (1986). Incidence of physical restraints on acute general medical wards. *Journal of the American Geriatrics Society*, **34**, 565–8.

Goldberg, D. P. (1972). *The Detection of Psychiatric Illness by Questionnaire*. Oxford: Oxford University Press.

Goldberg, D. (1985). Identifying psychiatric illness among general medical patients. *British Medical Journal*, **291**, 161–2.

Gurland, B., Copeland, J. R. M., Kuriansky, J., Kelleher, M., Sharpe, L. & Dean, L. (1983). *The Mind and Mood of Aging*. New York: Haworth Press.

Gustafson, Y., Berggren, D., Brannstrom, B., Bucht, G., Norberg, A., Hansson, L. I. & Winblad, B. (1988). Acute confusional states in elderly patients treated for femoral neck fracture. *Journal of the American Geriatrics Society*, **36**, 525–30.

Haskett, R. F. (1985). Diagnostic categorization of psychiatric disturbance in Cushing's syndrome. *American Journal of Psychiatry*, **142**, 911–16.

Hodkinson, H. M. (1972). Evaluation of a mental test score for assessment of mental impairment in the elderly. *Age and Ageing*, **1**, 233–8.

Hodkinson, H. M. (1973). Mental impairment in the elderly. *Journal of the Royal College of Physicians*, 305–17.

Hodkinson, H. M., Evans, G. J. & Mezey, A. G. (1972). Factors associated with misplacement of elderly patients in geriatric and psychogeriatric wards. *Gerontologica Clinica*, **14**, 267–73.

Homer, A. C. & Gilleard, C. (1991). Abuse of elderly people by their carers. *British Medical Journal*, **302**, 346.

Johnston, M., Wakeling, A., Graham, N. & Stokes, F. (1987). Cognitive impairment, emotional disorder and length of stay of elderly patients in a district general hospital. *British Journal of Medical Psychology*, **60**, 133–9.

Kafetz, K. M. (1986). *Clinical Tests – Geriatric Medicine*. London: Wolfe.

Kafonek, S., Ettinger, W., Rocca, R. & Kittner, S. (1989). Dementia, depression and functional status in a long-term care facility. *Journal of the American Geriatrics Society*, **37**, 29.

Kaufman, B. M. & Bates, A. B. (1990). Factors affecting provision of psychogeriatric care: a survey of geriatricians' views. *Care of the Elderly*, **2**, **25–7**.

Kay, D. W. K., Holding, T., Jones, B. & Littler, S. (1987). Psychiatric morbidity in Hobart's dependent aged. *Australian and New Zealand Journal of Psychiatry*, **21**, 463–75.

Kidd, C. B. (1962). Misplacement of the elderly in hospital. *British Medical Journal*, **ii**, 1491–5.

Koenig, H., Meador, K., Cohen, H. & Blazer, D. (1988). Self-rated depression scales and screening for major depression in the older hospitalized patient with medical illness. *Journal of the American Geriatrics Society*, **36**, 699–706.

Koponen, H., Stenback, U., Mattila, E., Soininen, H., Reinikinen, K. & Riekkinen, P. J. (1989). Delirium among elderly persons admitted to a psychiatric hospital: clinical course during the acute stage and a one year follow-up. *Acta Psychiatrica Scandinavica*, **6**, 579–85.

Kukull, W., Koepsell, T., Inui, T. S., Borson, S., Okimoto, J., Raskind, M. A. & Gale, J. L. (1986). Depression and physical illness among elderly general medical clinic patients. *Journal of Affective Disorder*, **10**, 153–62.

Lancet (1987). Depression, stress and immunity. *The Lancet*, **i**, 1467–8.

Lindesay, J. (1991). Anxiety disorders in the elderly. In *Psychiatry in the Elderly*, ed. R. Jacoby & C. Oppenheimer. Oxford: Oxford Medical Publications.

Lindesay, J., Briggs, K. & Murphy, E. (1989). The Guy's/Age Concern Survey. Prevalence rates of cognitive impairment, depression and anxiety in an urban community. *British Journal of Psychiatry*, **155**, 317–29.

Livingston, G., Hawkins, A., Graham, N., Blizard, R. & Mann, A. H. (1990). The Gospel Oak study: prevalence rates of dementia, depression and activity limitation among elderly residents in inner London. *Psychological Medicine*, **20**, 137–46.

MacDonald, A. J. D., Mann, A. H., Jenkins, R., Richard, L., Godlove, C. & Rodwell, G. (1982). An attempt to determine the impact of four types of care upon the elderly in London by the study of matched groups. *Psychological Medicine*, **12**, 193–200.

McAllion, S. J. & Paterson, C. R. (1989). Psychiatric morbidity in primary parathyroidism. *Postgraduate Medical Journal*, **65**, 628–31.

McKeith, I., Fairbairn, A., Perry, R., Thompson, P. & Perry, E. (1992). Neuroleptic sensitivity in patients with senile dementia of the Lewy body type. *British Medical Journal*, **305**, 673–8.

Magni, G., De Leo, D. & Schifano, F. (1985). Depression in geriatric and adult medical in-patients. *Journal of Clinical Psychology*, **41**, 337–44.

Murphy, E. (1982). The social origins of depression in old age. *British Journal of Psychiatry*, **141**, 135–42.

Myers, J., Weissman, M. & Tischler, G. (1984). Six-month prevalence of psychiatric disorder in three communities. *Archives of General Psychiatry*, **41**, 959–67.

Okamoto (1992). Health care for the elderly in Japan: medical and welfare in an aging society facing a crisis in long-term care. *British Medical Journal*, **305**, 403–5.

Pattie, A. H. & Gilleard, C. J. (1979). *Manual of the Clifton Assessment Procedures for the Elderly* (*CAPE*). Sevenoaks: Hodder & Stoughton.

Pitt, B. (1991*a*). The mentally disordered old person in the general hospital. In *Studies on General Hospital Psychiatry*, ed. F. K. Judd, G. D. Burrows & D. R. Lipsitt. Amsterdam: Elsevier.

Pitt, B. (1991*b*). Delirium. *Reviews in Clinical Gerontology*, **1**, 147–57.

Pitt, B. (1991*c*). Depression in the general hospital setting. *International Journal of Geriatric Psychiatry*, **6**, 363–70.

Pitt, B. (1992*a*). The liaison psychiatry of old age. In *Recent Advances in Clinical Psychiatry* (8), eds. K. Granville-Grossman. Edinburgh: Churchill Livingstone.

Pitt, B. (1992*b*). Abusing old people. *British Medical Journal*, **305**, 968–9.

Pitt, B. & Nowers, M. (1986). Elderly would-be suicides are more determined, still treatable. *Geriatric Medicine*, **16**, (10), 7–8.

Pitt, B. & Silver, C. P. (1980). The combined approach to geriatrics and psychiatry: evaluation of a joint unit in a teaching hospital district. *Age and Ageing*, **9**, 33–7.

Post, F. (1962). *The Significance of Affective Disorders in Old Age*, Maudsley Monographs 10. Oxford: Oxford University Press.

Robbins, L. J., Boyko, E., Lane, J., Cooper, D. & Jahnigen, D. W. (1987). Binding the elderly: a prospective study of the use of mechanical restraints in an acute care hospital. *Journal of the American Geriatrics Society*, **35**, 290–6.

Robinson, R. G., Starr, L. B., Kubos, K. L. & Price, T. R. (1983). A two-year longitudinal study of post-stroke mood disorders: findings during the initial evaluation. *Stroke*, **14**, 736–41.

Robinson, R. G., Kubos, K. L., Starr, L. B., Rao, K. & Price, T. R. (1984). Mood disorders in stroke patients: importance of lesion location. *Brain*, **107**, 81–93.

Rockwood, K. (1989). Acute confusion in elderly medical patients. *Journal of the American Geriatrics Society*, **37**, 150–4.

Rockwood, K. & Fox, R. A. (1992). The duration of delirium. *Age and Ageing*, **21** (Suppl. 1), 39.

Roohanna, R. & Pitt, B. (1989). Psychiatric morbidity in patients admitted to geriatric wards. In *The 4th Congress of the International Psychogeriatric Association: Programme and Abstracts*. Tokyo: International Psychogeriatric Association.

Royal College of Physicians of London and Royal College of Psychiatrists (1989). *Care of Elderly People with Mental Illness: Specialist Services and Medical Training*. London: Royal College of Psychiatrists.

Schiffer, R. B., Klein, R. F. & Rider, R. C. (1988). *The Medical Evaluation of Psychiatric Patients*. New York: Plenum Medical.

Scott, J., Fairbairn, A. & Woodhouse, K. (1988). Referrals to a psychogeriatric consultation–liaison service. *International Journal of Geriatric Psychiatry*, **3**, 131–5.

Secretaries of State for Health, Social Security, Wales, Scotland (1989). *Working for Patients*. London: Her Majesty's Stationery Office.

Secretaries of State for Health, Social Security, Wales, Scotland (1989). *Caring for People*. London: Her Majesty's Stationery Office.

Seymour, D. G., Henschke, P. J. & Cape, R. D. T. (1980). Acute confusional states and dementia in the elderly: the role of dehydration/volume depletion, physical illness and age. *Age and Ageing*, **9**, 137–46.

Tappy, L., Randin, J. P., Schwed, P., Wertheimer, J. & Lemarchand-Beraud, T. (1987). Prevalence of thyroid disorders in psychogeriatric patients. A possible relationhip of hypothyroidism with neurotic depression but not with dementia. *Journal of the American Geriatrics Society*, **35**, 526–31.

White, A. (1990). Styles of liaison psychiatry: discussion paper. *Journal of the Royal Society of Medicine*, **83**, 506–8.

Whitlock, F. A. & Siskind, M. (1979). Depression and cancer: a follow-up study. *Psychological Medicine*, **9**, 747–52.

Wing, J., Cooper, J. & Sartorius, N. (1974). *The Measurement and Classification of Psychiatric Symptoms*. Cambridge: Cambridge University Press.

Yesavage, J. A., Brink, T. L., Rose, T. L., Lum, O., Huang, V., Adey, M. & Leirer, V. O. (1983). Development and validation of a geriatric depression screening scale: a preliminary report. *Journal of Psychiatric Research*, **17**, 37–49.

24

Psychiatric aspects of cerebro-vascular disease

PETER BURVILL

Historical

Many of the early clinical masters in psychiatry and neurology recognized that depression was frequently associated with cerebro-vascular disease (Kraepelin, 1921; Bleuler, 1951). In spite of this early recognition that cerebro-vascular disease may lead to characteristic mood disturbances, there was by the 1940s a general acceptance of the idea that these mood disturbances represented a psychological response of the organism to severe stress (Starkstein & Robinson, 1989). Many more recent studies of depression after stroke, however, have consistently found that the severity of depression is not closely related to the severity of physical impairment, and it has increasingly been clear that the relationship between stroke and mood change is more complex than once thought. It was not until the late 1960s that systematic evaluation of mood changes in patients with brain injuries was undertaken, when different syndromes between left and right hemisphere lesions were found (Gainotti, 1972). Over the past decade research, mainly from Robinson and his coworkers in Baltimore, has focused on the possible relationship of various mood disorders to specific localization of the lesion in the brain.

Introduction

A number of good reviews of the psychiatric disorders after stroke have been published in the past five years (House, 1987*a*; Dupont, Callum & Jeste, 1988; Primeau, 1988; Starkstein & Robinson, 1989; Robinson & Starkstein, 1990; Johnson, 1991*a*). Apart from the obvious overlap in the two reviews of Robinson and Starkstein, each of these have approached the subject from a different perspective.

The major focus of this chapter is on poststroke depression (PSD) as most research work has been on this topic, although more recent work has paid attention to a wider variety of diagnostic categories (House, 1987*b*; Castillo &

Robinson, 1991). The latter include anxiety disorders, cognitive impairment, disorders such as apathy and neglect, irritability and aggression, and the various forms of organic emotionalism such as emotional lability, catastrophic reactions and pathological laughing and crying. All of these may be specific to the brain damage, but many of these conditions have been poorly described in standard psychiatric nomenclature (House, 1987*b*).

Clinical syndromes

Depression

Depression is the most common psychiatric syndrome following stroke, but there is not a specific PSD syndrome. The range of clinical presentation is the same as for depression from other causes. There may be at least two types of PSD. One is major depression similar to functional major depression. The other is minor depression with a clinical course similar to the chronic characterological depressions termed dysthymic disorder, without necessarily lasting two or more years as is required by DSM-III criteria (Starkstein & Robinson, 1989). Robinson, Lipsey & Pearlson (1984) described a third type of poststroke mood disorder – an indifferent apathetic mental state with inappropriate cheerfulness, said to be more common in right hemisphere lesions. However in the Oxford Community Stroke Study, House (1988) found that the distribution of scores using the Present State Examination and the Beck Depression Inventory one month after stroke were continuously distributed. He described a group of physical symptoms such as tension, insomnia and restlessness, as well as mood changes, such as anxiety, irritability, sadness, and impaired concentration, which he called 'undifferentiated mood disturbance' forming part of an adjustment reaction which is a psychologically understandable response to acute illness. Johnson (1991*a*) pointed to the lack of research in differentiating the various subgroups of PSD.

Coexisting physical conditions, plus general physical debility in the early stages poststroke, can share certain symptoms in common with depressive illness. These include tiredness, lack of energy, poor appetite, weight loss and insomnia, all of which may lead to a false diagnosis of depression (false positives). Alternatively the medical condition may mask symptoms, such as denial or neglect, that may result in a failure to diagnose depression (false negatives) (Robinson & Starkstein, 1990). Fedoroff et al. (1991) claim that the existence of an acute medical illness does not invalidate the use of DSM-III diagnostic criteria for major depression.

Anxiety disorders

The study of anxiety disorders in the elderly, including poststroke, has been relatively neglected. In order of frequency, the commonest disorders are phobic disorders (agoraphobia and/or social phobia), generalized anxiety disorder, and panic disorder. In both the community studies in Oxford (Sharpe et al., 1990) and Perth (Johnson & Burvill, 1990) almost 20% of patients had some degree of phobic anxiety at four months poststroke, although many of these had cleared after 12 months. Patients can become fearful of going out, particularly unaccompanied, thereby greatly restricting their socialization and general quality of life. Generalized anxiety disorder is much less common, and is usually found in association with some degree of depression. Panic disorder, *per se*, is relatively uncommon poststroke.

Cognitive impairment

In the acute-stroke period there is often a stage of confusion, or quiet delirium, which can vary in intensity from very mild to severe and may take many weeks to resolve. Cerebro-vascular disease is widely recognized as a major contributor to the step-wise deterioration of multi-infarct dementia, which is the second most common type of dementia after Alzheimer's disease. Following stroke, there can be a number of specific cognitive impairments, such as difficulty in problem solving, comprehension, topographical orientation and performance of complicated tasks, which may result from focal brain damage, without significantly impairing memory. Global dementia varying in severity from relatively mild to very severe can occur following a single stroke. Patients with concomitant PSD may suffer more severe cognitive impairment than would be explained by the cerebral lesion per se, i.e. one cause of 'pseudodementia', which might improve with treatment of the depression (Robinson, et al., 1986). The latter authors found that all patients with major depression, but only 40% of nondepressed patients, had some degree of intellectual impairment. In the Oxford Community Study, House, Dennis, Warlow et al. (1990*a*), using the Mini-Mental State Examination (MMSE), failed to find evidence of depressive pseudodementia. The difference between these two studies possibly reflects differences in severity of depression between those in the selected in-patient group and those in a community setting. However, tests such as the MMSE often fail to detect those cognitive impairments due to lesions in the right hemisphere which involve language skills. Communication problems and physical impairments can often contribute to the failure to detect the more subtle cognitive impairments. Bolla-Wilson et al. (1989) found that neuropsychological performance was significantly more impaired in patients with major depression following left hemisphere lesions, than in nondepressed patients with comparable left hemisphere lesions, or in both depressed and nondepressed patients with right hemisphere lesions.

Mania

Mania is a relatively rare complication of stroke and the clinical manifestations are almost identical to those in primary mania (Starkstein, Robinson & Price, 1987). These authors found only three cases among 700 stroke patients. The interval between the stroke to the onset of mania can be quite variable, and as long as two years. Although the natural history of poststroke mania has not been systematically examined, it is reported that some patients develop a bipolar disorder and that a proportion of these have a prior history of bipolar disorder (Starkstein & Robinson, 1989).

Paranoid delusions

The association of psychotic conditions following stroke has been briefly reviewed by Dupont et al. (1988). These syndromes include reduplicative paramnesia, Capgras syndrome, various other delusional disorders and paranoia. The onset of psychosis can occur a considerable interval after the stroke. Reported case studies indicate the importance of considering possible right hemisphere infarction as the source of late-onset delusions or reduplicate paramnesia presenting as disorientation. Psychotic symptoms can follow brain-stem strokes.

Personality changes

Personality changes may be a more useful concept than clinical syndromes to describe the complex of emotional, cognitive, perceptual and behavioral disturbance which occur after gross brain lesions, particularly if the changes are permanent (Johnson, 1991*a*). Collection of longitudinal data on prestroke and poststroke functioning from informants should enable this kind of assessment to be made.

Emotional lability

This syndrome has a number of characteristic features: it is usually sudden and unheralded in its appearance, uncontrollable by the patient, socially inappropriate in its expression, usually inappropriate emotionally and occasionally associated with pathological laughter (House, 1987*a*). In the Perth Community Stroke Study emotional lability was observed at interview in 8.5% of patients and a further 8.3% reported that they had experienced it at other times since the stroke. Emotional lability is not the same as depression, but can overlap with it. *Catastrophic reaction* is not easy to distinguish from emotional lability (House, 1987a). It is particularly liable to occur in dysphasic patients. In some patients it is not obvious except in response to being pressed to perform certain tasks, when it appears apparently in direct response to the imminent failure to complete the task.

Indifference reaction

Some patients develop a state of morbid apathy and lack of motivation, which at times can change to euphoria or socially inappropriate jocularity (Kolb & Taylor, 1981).

Prevalence of poststroke depression

Point prevalence of PSD found in various studies has varied widely for a number of reasons (Primeau, 1988), including the use of different assessment instruments and criteria for case identification, and the different settings from which patients have been derived. Almost all studies are of the prevalence of PSD in survivors from the acute stages of stroke as about 25% of stroke patients die within the first two months. Studies based on in-patients have shown that up to 50% of stroke patients may develop depression during the acute poststroke period, and another 30% may develop depression at some time during the first two years following the stroke (Robinson & Starkstein, 1990). The highest prevalence rates have been from studies which have examined only patients admitted to acute hospitals because of the stroke (Robinson & Szetela, 1981; Feibel & Springer, 1982; Robinson et al., 1983; Ebrahim, Barer & Nouri, 1987), or from rehabilitation units (Folstein, Maiberger & McHugh, 1977; Sinyor, et al., 1986*a*; Eastwood, et al., 1989; Morris, Robinson & Raphael, 1990). Among outpatient stroke populations the prevalence of depression is close to 30%. The lowest reported prevalence of major depression has come from the two community-based studies by Wade, Legh-Smith & Hewer (1987) and House (1988), in which all stroke patients in a region, whether hospitalized or not, were assessed. They each reported a prevalence of 32%, which included all cases of depression – mild, minor and probable. Preliminary findings from the Perth Community Stroke Study showed a similar result (27.8%) (Johnson & Burvill, 1990).

Many of the studies have shown a higher prevalence of major depression than of minor depression, which is the reverse of what one would expect. This is possibly a reflection of overestimation of cases of major depression by including many symptoms, which might be due to physical effects of the stroke, among the list of depressive symptoms. If these symptoms were excluded, some cases might have been diagnosed as minor depressions.

The significance of many of the prevalence figures reported is rendered uncertain by the failure to examine control groups in most studies (Johnson, 1991*a*). Exceptions have been both the Oxford and Perth Community Stroke Studies. The former found that rates of PSD were 50–100% above rates in an age-matched control group drawn from the same age/sex register. After reviewing a number of studies, both House (1987*a*) and Primeau (1988) concluded that it is unproven that depression is commoner in an unselected group of patients after strokes than it is among the elderly with other physical illnesses. Factors such as hospitalization, family pressures, bereavement, and socialization make comparison of the two groups especially difficult (Morris & Raphael, 1987).

Most systematic studies of stroke patients have focused on hospitalized cases and patients in rehabilitation programs. Therefore they have been biased towards inclusion of patients with more severe initial strokes and more persistent disabilities; factors likely to have promoted depression (Johnson, 1991*a*). For example, many of the studies of Robinson and his colleagues in Baltimore have been based upon acute in-patients, with severe strokes, who were predominantly male, black and from low socioeconomic areas.

Anxiety

Most studies have not looked at the prevalence of anxiety disorders poststroke. House (1988) reported 8% of anxiety states of some sort in the Oxford Community Stroke Study. The preliminary findings of the Perth Community Stroke Study (Johnson & Burvill, 1990) showed 22.6% have an anxiety state of some type, according to DSM-III-R criteria, the majority (19.3%) being cases of agoraphobia or social phobia, the percentage being much higher in women. About 30% of depressed patients had mixed anxiety and depressive disorders.

Follow-up studies of depression

There has been great variability in reported information by various authors on the duration of PSD. House (1987*a*) claimed that the reported persistence of PSD is sometimes based on follow-up studies with unacceptably high attrition rates. Robinson, Bolduc & Price (1987) reported rising prevalence of depression peaking six months or more after the stroke. Starkstein & Robinson (1989) summarized the Baltimore studies of the longitudinal history of PSD as follows: the natural course of PSD appears to be approximately one year for major depression and more than two years for the majority of minor depressions. Infarcts in the territory of the middle cerebral artery produce longer lasting depressive disorders than brain stem/cerebellar infarcts (posterior circulation). Rapid improvement in depression is much more likely to occur if lesions are located in the subcortex. The authors warned that all studies of PSD to date have excluded a significant group of patients because their comprehension is too severely impaired or because they are unconscious.

Morris et al. (1990) found at 15 month follow-up of their hospitalized patients that the average duration of major depression episodes was 39 weeks and minor depression 12 weeks. The latter was said to be equivalent to that found for adjustment reactions in other medical and nonmedical contexts. They reported a mortality rate of 23% for major depression and 6% for minor depression.

Whereas Robinson et al. (1984) have found that only 5% of cases of PSD detected 2–4 weeks poststroke have recovered by six months, the comparable proportion in the community studies by Wade et al. (1987) and House (1988) were one-third and the majority, respectively. In the community studies, it appears that some people develop their mood disorders early and settle down, whereas others become depressed rather later in the six month poststroke period. A few people have a consistently maintained mood disorder throughout the six month period. Thus it would appear that the severity of the initial PSD can determine the length of that depression, with the community studies detecting a higher proportion of less severe depressions with a shorter duration than those more severely depressed inpatients.

Etiology

The prediction of depression following stroke is a complex undertaking and consideration must be given to a wide range of factors, including the following:

Demographic variables such as age, sex, education level and marital status have not generally appeared important although there have been reports of increased depression in younger patients and women (Johnson, 1991*b*).

Genetic vulnerability

The contribution of past or family history of psychiatric disorder has surprisingly been almost completely neglected in the literature. Starkstein et al. (1989) found stroke patients with major depression following right hemisphere lesions had a higher frequency of family history of a psychiatric illness than patients with either no mood change or major depression following left hemisphere lesions. Eastwood et al. (1989), Dam, Pedersen & Ahlgren (1989) and Morris et al. (1990) found that past history of a psychiatric disorder was associated with increased PSD after both left and right hemisphere lesions.

Life events

House, Dennis, Mogridge et al. (1990) have been the only investigators to systematically study the effects of life events as a cause of stroke. They found a significant excess of severe threatening life events in the 12 months pre-stroke compared with both a control group and the 12 months following the stroke.

These life events were not associated with other known risk factors of stroke. They did not report any relationship between these events and the subsequent onset of depression.

Physical impairment

The relationship between PSD and physical impairment is a complex interactive one. Physical impairment does not appear to cause depression, but once depression occurs the most depressed patients remain the most impaired and vice versa (Robinson et al., 1984; Parikh et al., 1987).

Social functioning

Several studies have found weak positive associations between PSD and impairments of social functioning, but there have also been negative findings (Johnson, 1991*a*). It is difficult to assess whether such impairment is primary or secondary to the depression. Starkstein & Robinson (1989) concluded that impaired social functioning probably did not cause PSD, but that, once the depression occurs, physical or intellectual impairments, as well as depression, can all negatively impact upon the patients' future social functioning.

Psychological factors

The subjective impact of a stroke can be overwhelming, with a wide variety of psychological reactions at different stages after the stroke (Primeau, 1988). Johnson (1991*a*) outlined the case for 'loss' being a cause of PSD. Stroke can be construed as a loss event, involving loss of health, independence and of particular capabilities such as speech and motor skills, together with associated social and occupational activities. The threatening nature of the event is longer standing than the effects of the stroke itself, such that even a mild stroke raises the threat of future strokes, of more permanent loss of function and independence in the future, of further ill health generally and even of death. Morris, Robinson & Raphael (1991) found that PSD patients who perceived their support to be inadequate had a longer duration of depressive illness than those who perceived their support more favorably. They concluded that, following stroke, perception of social support from key relationships may mediate the emotional response to this late life crisis.

Lesion location

Robinson and his coworkers from the Johns Hopkins University in Baltimore have been the strongest advocates for the view that the location of the lesion in the brain is the single most important factor in the etiology of PSD. A contrasting view is that put by House (1987*b*) that the degree of brain damage is only weakly associated with subsequent emotional problems, and that there is no conclusive proof that damage in any specific site is particularly likely to lead to depression. He concluded that the etiology of PSD is probably largely determined by social factors. Robinson & Starkstein (1990) summarized findings of the Baltimore group as follows: the frequency of PSD is higher in patients with left hemisphere than right hemisphere lesions. The highest incidence is in those with damage to the left anterior region of the brain, which may be either cortical (involving the frontal lobe) or sub cortical (involving the basal ganglia). In both cortical and subcortical lesions of the left hemisphere, the closer the left lesion is to the frontal pole, the more severe the depression. When PSD is combined with anxiety disorders, the lesions occur almost exclusively in cortical areas, whereas when PSD occurs without significant anxiety symptoms, it is frequently associated with strokes involving the left basal ganglia. The pathogenesis of PSD in patients with right hemisphere lesions remains more obscure and is more complex. Depression is probably more frequent when the lesion involves the right parietal lobe. Findings in the Oxford Community Study failed to find an association of PSD with left-sided lesions, anterior lesion in the left hemisphere or proximity of the lesion to the left frontal pole (Sharpe et al., 1990). However, there have also been reports of similar rates of PSD with the lesions in either hemisphere (Feibel & Springer, 1982; Sinyor et al., 1986*b*; Ebrahim et al., 1987; House, 1988; House et al., 1989).

Morris, Robinson & Raphael (1992) reported that anterior lesion location in the left hemisphere was associated with both a diagnosis of depression and severity of depressive symptoms, but only after the influence of prestroke vulnerability to depression was removed. They made the point that not all PSD seemed to be related to lesion location, and that some may be related to personal or genetic vulnerabilities, to gender or to social role disruption. *Subcortical atrophy* before the actual stroke (Starkstein & Robinson 1989) may constitute an important risk factor which may explain why some, but not all, patients with lesions in the same locations develop depression.

There have been major reservations about the findings of many of these studies, particularly those of Robinson's group, on the grounds that only highly selected subgroups of stroke patients have been examined and often only very small numbers have been involved. Furthermore, in the particular measures of lesion location which had been used, the topographical approach to lesion location does not conform very closely to anatomical and neurological boundaries and does not satisfactorily separate cortical from subcortical lesions (House, 1988). Initially the identification and localization of lesions relied almost exclusively on computerized tomography (CT), although half of clinically diagnosed strokes do not produce physical changes on CT scans, and those that do require several weeks before swelling and edema subside and a stable image is seen. Magnetic resonance imaging (MRI) is more sensitive than CT in detecting symptomatic cerebral infarctions within 72 hours of onset, as well as infarctions involving the posterior fossa. Another promising technique in the study of post stroke mood disorders is positron emission tomography (PET). PET scanning has the great advantage that it can show metabolic and biochemical changes that may be outside the ischaemic area seen on MRI or CT images. Mood disorders may be mediated through distant effects of lesions, or lesions may play a facilitatory role for another primary mechanism leading to depression. Several PET scan studies have shown hypometabolism in areas distant from the actual lesion location (Feeney & Baron, 1986).

Lesion volume

Some authors have found no association between PSD and lesion volume (Dam et al., 1989; Robinson, Kubos, Starr, et al., 1984), while others have found both positive and negative correlations depending upon which hemisphere was examined (Sinyor et al., 1986*b*; Eastwood et al., 1989).

Severity of depression

Robinson & Starkstein (1990) and Eastwood et al. (1989) reported a significant correlation between severity of the depression and the distance of the lesion in the left hemisphere from the frontal pole, the most frontal being the most severe. Sinyor et al. (1986*b*) reported a similar correlation, irrespective of side involved. Dam et al. (1989) found more severely depressed patients with lesions in the right rather than the left hemisphere.

Type of stroke

Morris et al. (1992) have been the only workers to report an association between diagnosis of depression and type of stroke. They found that none of the PSD patients had a cerebral hemorrhage, in contrast to one-third of nondepressed stroke patients. The phenomenon was not explained by differences in the background demographic or clinical factors, or lesion characteristics, between patients with hemorrhages and those with infarction.

Prior stroke

Prior history of stroke may also constitute an important risk factor for the development of depression (Eastwood et al., 1989; Robinson & Starkstein, 1990). The obvious question of assessing whether some patients were already depressed at the time of the stroke has been poorly studied.

Etiological factors in mania

Studies indicate that mania is more likely to follow right hemisphere lesions (Cummings & Mendez, 1984), especially involving damage to the limbic areas. Starkstein & Robinson (1989) concluded that mania following stroke could be rare because it requires the existence of two factors:

(i) a predisposing factor of either a genetic loading for affective disorder or subcortical atrophy, and
(ii) a specific right hemisphere limbic lesion.

Underlying brain mechanisms in poststroke depression

Robinson & Starkstein (1990) provided a succinct summary of the mechanisms which they hypothesized may underlie the etiology of PSD. They postulated differential disruption of adrenergic and serotonergic pathways in the brain, and greater depletion of biogenic amines in patients with right hemisphere strokes compared with those with left hemisphere damage. Investigations in rats by the Baltimore team (Robinson et al., 1975; Robinson, 1979) demonstrated that the biochemical response to ischemic lesions was lateralized: right hemisphere lesions produced depletions of noradrenaline and spontaneous hyperactivity while comparable lesions of the left hemisphere did not. They have recently found a similar lateralized biochemical response to ischemia in human subjects (Mayberg et al., 1989). Starkstein et al. (1988) speculated that the shorter duration of depression following cerebellar and brain stem lesions may be related to the possibility that biogenic amines are depleted less when lesions are located in the brain stem, perhaps because such lesions are sometimes caudal to the biogenic amine nuclei.

Different studies (Martinot et al., 1990; Baxter et al., 1989; Buchsbaum et al., 1986) on patients with primary (not secondary to brain injury) depression using PET have demonstrated hypometabolism in the left frontal cortex among depressed patients. Lesions that damage similar areas of the frontal cortex, either directly, or indirectly by involvement of basal ganglia structures that project to the cortex, may effectively cause a comparable hypometabolism (Morris, Robinson & Raphael, 1992). In patients with right hemisphere stroke, the relationship of anterior lesion location to mood state is more complex.

Treatment

The same principles and range of available treatments for the treatment of primary depression apply also to PSD. The main barrier towards the treatment of PSD appears to be failure to recognise its existence (Dupont et al., 1988).

Management of PSD needs to be tailored to the individual case, taking into account the severity of the depression, the nature of the symptoms present, the duration of the depression to date, the various etiological factors, the individual's likely compliance with particular treatment approaches, susceptibility to side-effects and, where there is a past history of depression, previous response to treatment (Johnson, 1991*b*). Johnson advocated two therapeutic interventions fundamental to the management of most cases. The first was sympathetic ongoing professional interest and counselling, which was particularly important for those patients who had residual disabilities. The second was alleviation, where possible, of probable etiological factors. Treatment may involve a variety of approaches including physiotherapy, attendance at day centres, provision of home nursing or housekeeping, changed accommodation, and giving advice or support to family members, friends or nursing staff. Adjusting medications such as analgesics or antihypertensives may be helpful. If a patient stays at home or has been discharged after stroke, most of this 'psychotherapeutic' input may be denied as outpatient and domiciliary support is often minimal.

Although tricyclic antidepressants are not without risk in the elderly individual with medical problems, reported studies indicate that the benefits generally outweigh the risks (Dupont et al., 1988). There are only two controlled studies of the treatment of PSD with antidepressants reported in the literature. Lipsey et al. (1984) reported the results of a six-week double blind randomized treatment study of PSD using nortriptyline. The 11 nortriptyline-treated patients who completed the study showed significantly greater improvement in their depressive scores than the 15 placebo treated patients. Reding et al. (1986) conducted a study on 27 patients participating in a stroke rehabilitation program randomly giving either placebo or trazodone hydrochloride. Patients with abnormal dexamethasone suppression test results showed significantly greater improvement with trazadone than with placebo. House (1987*a*) suggested the use of a tricyclic antidepressant, such as dothiepin or amitriptyline, introduced at low dosage (25–50 mg daily) and the dose gradually increased to the maximum tolerated (probably about 100–150 mg daily). He proposed the main indications for the use of antidepressant medication as:

(a) biological or psychotic symptoms of depression;
(b) persistent depressive mood, even without biological symptoms, which does not respond to counselling, or to changes in social setting such as day care; and
(c) atypical depressive presentations such as hypochondriasis or pseudodementia. Reports have suggested that pathological emotionalism might respond to tricyclic medication (Ross & Rush, 1981).

Stroke is not a contraindication to ECT (Karliner, 1978; Murray, Shea & Conn, 1987). Except that it is usually not used within three months of stroke, there are no special contraindications (House, 1987*a*). Murray et al. (1987) treated 14 patients with ECT and reported a marked improvement in all but two cases. Side-effects were rare. It can be used for major depression unresponsive to antidepressants, in patients who have biological or psychotic features, and in those with a high risk of suicide.

Robinson et al. (1986) suggested that treatment of PSD might benefit cognitive function, but House (1987*a*) concluded that there is no clear evidence for this. Morris et al. (personal communication), based on their studies of cortical serotonin receptors using PET, suggested that drugs which improved serotonin neurotransmission, for example fluoxetine, may contribute to the treatment of cognitive impairment associated with cerebrovascular disease.

In the Perth Community Stroke Study the two psychiatrists who interviewed the patients considered that the severity and nature of the depressive illness in the majority of cases did not warrant prescription of antidepressant medication.

Although there are no systematic studies of the treatment of poststroke mania, almost all cases of secondary mania reported in the literature showed good response to treatment with the usual anti-manic drugs (lithium and neuroleptics) (Starkstein, Boston & Robinson, 1988).

Prevention is always better than cure. The best way to prevent the psychiatric sequelae of stroke is to attend to preventative measures for stroke itself. Major risk factors are hypertension, smoking, consumption of alcohol, diabetes and certain dietary practices (Jamrozik, 1991). Attention to all these risk factors is important in preventing stroke.

Rehabilitation

Depression is one of the significant barriers to physical rehabilitation after stroke and treatment of the depression may improve rehabilitation outcome. In a study of stroke patients undergoing physical rehabilitation, Mayo, Korner-Bitensky & Becker (1991) reported depression to be one of four major variables adversely influencing recovery time to independent functioning. The evidence linking depression and functional recovery is conflicting, because it is difficult to untangle whether impaired function leads to depression, or whether depression leads to delayed recovery. However those without evidence of depression progress to independence at a greater rate than those with PSD, suggesting that patients with depression may not have the motivation needed to overcome disability and thus require more time to achieve independence (Mayo et al., 1991). Carnwath & Johnson (1987) found that spouses of stroke patients were more likely to be depressed and had more physical symptoms than an age-sex matched control group. Their depression increased with the severity of the spouse's stroke, and with time, over the three years of the study.

Future directions

The above survey of the field, together with specific suggestions raised in the six review papers, indicate a large number of questions which need to be clarified by future research. Future studies need to be on large samples of patients drawn from all psychosocial classes and different clinical situations – inpatients, outpatient clinics, rehabilitation units and community settings – thereby avoiding small biased samples which have characterized much of the research to date. Appropriate control groups are essential. A wider range of psychiatric and neuropsychiatric conditions should be studied, especially anxiety states, personality changes and cognitive impairment. It is important to determine whether depressive and other disorders are more common poststroke than after a variety of noncerebral physical illnesses. A concerted effort is needed to revise and refine diagnostic systems so that specific aspects of poststroke disability, such as physical and cognitive impairments, are taken into account and their impact on diagnosis re-examined. Standard international interview schedules and diagnostic criteria are essential.

The etiology of depression and other psychiatric conditions poststroke has yet to be satisfactorily determined, including the relevance of the much researched anatomical site of lesion hypothesis. With regard to the latter, the newer localising techniques such as MRI are probably much more effective than CT scanning. In determining lesion localization areas more akin to standard neuro-anatomical boundaries of the brain should be adopted. More attention needs to be paid to the interactions between the site of lesions, prestroke cerebral atrophy, and the complex of nonanatomical factors, such as past personal and family history of psychiatric disorder, psychiatric illness at the time of the stroke, personality, social circumstances and stressful life events pre- and poststroke, physical illness pre- and poststroke, time of onset after the stroke, treatment facilities available poststroke and social and family supports poststroke. More extensive use of PET scanning should help elicit the mechanisms of poststroke psychiatric disorders.

More psychopharmacological agents should be studied in randomized double-blind clinical trials, as should other interactional treatments aimed at family or caregivers, since education and social functioning are important variables in the rehabilitation of stroke patients. Other similar studies include the effect of early treatment of PSD with antidepressants on recovery from cognitive deficits, functional disability and general rehabilitation.

There remain a number of unanswered questions on the long-term history of poststroke psychiatric disorders, for example, the duration of various disorders, whether PSD impairs social or intellectual function in the long term, and whether poststroke mood disorder influences survival as has been claimed for general medical patients and for hemodialysis patients.

Finally, the complexities of the differences in the interaction of poststroke psychiatric disorders, neuropsychological deficits, communication difficulties and anatomical site between right and left hemisphere lesions remain to be unravelled. Psychiatric disorders in poststroke aphasic patients are virtually unexplored, as is any systematic psychiatric study of patients following transient ischemic attacks.

References

Baxter, L. R., Schwartz, J. M., Phelps, M. E. et al. (1989). Reduction of prefrontal cortex glucose metabolism common to three types of depression. *Archives of General Psychiatry*, **46**, 243–50.

Bleuler, E. P. (1951). *Textbook of Psychiatry*, New York: Dover Publications.

Bolla-Wilson, K., Robinson, R. G., Starkstein, S. E. et al. (1989). Lateralization of dementia and depression in stroke patients. *American Journal of Psychiatry*, **146**, 627–34.

Buchsbaum, M. S., Wu, J., De Lisa, L. E. et al. (1986). Frontal cortex and basal ganglia metabolic rates assessed by positron tomography with [18-F] 2-deoxyglucose in affective illness. *Journal of Affective Disorders*, **10**, 137–52.

Carnwath, T. C. & Johnson, D. A. (1987). Psychiatric morbidity among spouses of patients with stroke. *British Medical Journal*, **294**, 409–11.

Castillo, C. S. & Robinson, R. G. (1991). Neuropsychiatric disorders and cerebrovascular disease. *Current Opinion in Psychiatry*, **4**, 101–5.

Cummings, J. L. & Mendez, M. F. (1984). Secondary mania with focal cerebrovascular lesions. *American Journal of Psychiatry*, **142**, 1084–7.

Dam, H., Pedersen, H. E. & Ahlgren, P. (1989). Depression among patients with stroke. *Acta Psychiatrica Scandinavica*, **80**, 118–24.

Dupont, R. M., Cullum, C. M. & Jeste, D. V. (1988). Poststroke depression and psychosis. *Psychiatric Clinics of North America*, **11**, 133–49.

Eastwood, M. R., Rifat, S. L., Nobbs, H. & Ruderman, J.(1989). Mood disorder following cerebrovascular accident. *British Journal of Psychiatry*, **154**, 195–200.

Ebrahim, S., Barer, D. & Nouri, F. (1987). Affective illness after stroke. *British Journal of Psychiatry*, **151**, 52–6.

Federoff, J. P., Starkstein, S. E., Parikh, R. M. et al. (1991). Are depressive symptoms nonspecific in patients with acute stroke? *American Journal of Psychiatry*, **148**, 1172–6.

Feeney, D. M. & Baron, J. C. (1986). Diaschisis. *Stroke*, **17**, 817–30.

Feibel, J. H. & Springer, C. J. (1982). Depression and failure to resume social activities after stroke. *Archives of Physical Medicine and Rehabilitation*, **63**, 276–8.

Folstein, M. F., Maiberger, R. & McHugh, P. R. (1977). Mood disorder as a specific complication of stroke. *Journal of Neurology, Neurosurgery and Psychiatry*, **40**, 1018–20.

Gainotti, G. (1972). Emotional behavior and hemispheric side of the lesion. *Cortex*, **8**, 41–55.

House, A. (1987*a*). Mood disorders after stroke: a review of the evidence. *International Journal of Geriatric Psychiatry*, **2**, 211–21.

House, A. (1987*b*). Depression after stroke. *British Medical Journal*, **294**, 76–8.

House, A. (1988). Mood disorder in the first six months after stroke. In *Current Approaches. Affective Disorders in the Elderly*, ed E. Murphy & S. W. Parker. Southampton: Duphar Laboratories.

House, A., Dennis, M., Mogridge, L. et al. (1990). Life events and difficulties preceding stroke. *Journal of Neurology, Neurosurgery & Psychiatry*, **53**, 1024–8.

House, A., Dennis, M., Mogridge, L. et al. (1991). Mood disorders in the first year after stroke. *British Journal of Psychiatry*, **158**, 83–92.

House, A., Dennis, M., Warlow, C. et al. (1989). Emotionalism after stroke. *British Medical Journal*, **298**, 991–4.

House, A., Dennis, M., Warlow, C. et al. (1990*a*). The relationship between intellectual impairment and mood disorder in the first year after stroke. *Psychological Medicine*, **20**, 805–14.

House, A., Dennis, M. Warlow, C. et al. (1990*b*). Mood disorders after stroke and their relation to lesion location: A CT scan study. *Brain*, **113**, 1113–29.

Jamrozik, K. (1991). Could we do more to prevent stroke? *Australian Family Physician*, **20**, 1619–26.

Johnson, G. A. (1991*a*). Research into psychiatric disorder after stroke: the need for further studies. *Australian & New Zealand Journal of Psychiatry*, **25**, 358–70.

Johnson, G. A. (1991*b*). Psychological sequelae in stroke patients. *Australian Family Physician*, **20**, 1605–11.

Johnson, G. A. & Burvill, P. W. (1990). Psychiatric sequelae of stroke. Preliminary data from the Perth Community Stroke Study. Paper presented at the Annual Meeting of the Section in Psychiatry of Old Age of the Royal Australian & New Zealand College of Psychiatrists, Melbourne.

Karliner, W.(1978). ECT for patients with CNS disease. *Psychosomatics*, **19**, 781–3.

Kolb, B. & Taylor, L. (1981). Affective behavior in patients with localized cortical excisions: role of lesion site and side. *Science*, **214**, 89–91.

Kraepelin, E. (1921). *Manic Depressive Insanity and Paranoia*. Edinburgh: E. & S. Livingstone.

Lipsey, J. R., Robinson, R. G. Pearlson, G. D. et al. (1984). Nortriptyline treatment for poststroke depression: a double blind study. *Lancet*, **i**, 297–300.

Martinot, J. L., Hardy, P., Feline, A. et al. (1990). Left frontal glucose hypometabolism in the depressed state: a confirmation. *American Journal of Psychiatry*, **147**, 1313–17.

Mayberg, H. S., Robinson, R. G., Wong, D. F. et al. (1989). PET imaging of cortical S_2 serotonin receptors following stroke: lateralized changes and relationship to depression. *American Journal of Psychiatry*, **145**, 937–43.

Mayo, N. E., Korner-Bitensky, N. A. & Becker, R. (1991). Recovery time of independent function poststroke. *American Journal of Physical Medicine & Rehabilitation*, **70**, 5–12.

Morris, P. L. & Raphael, B. (1987). Depressive disorder associated with physical illness: the impact of stroke. *General Hospital Psychiatry*, **9**, 324–30.

Morris, P. L. P., Robinson, R. G. & Raphael, B. (1990). Prevalence and course of depressive disorders in hospitalized stroke patients. *International Journal of Psychiatry in Medicine*, **20**, 349–64.

Morris, P. L. P., Robinson, R. G. & Raphael, B. (1991). The relationship between the perception of social support and poststroke depression in hospitalized patients. *Psychiatry*, **54**, 306–16.

Morris, P. L. P., Robinson, R. G. & Raphael, B. (1992). Lesion location and depression in hospitalized stroke patients. Evidence supporting a specific relationship in the left hemisphere. *Journal of Neuropsychiatry, Neuropsychology and Behavioral Neurology*, **5**, 75–82.

Murray, G. B., Shea, V. & Conn, D. K. (1987). Electroconvulsive therapy for poststroke depression. *Journal of Clinical Psychiatry*, **47**, 258–60.

Parikh, R. M., Lipsey, J. R., Robinson, R. G. et al. (1987). Two-year longitudinal study of poststroke mood disorders: dynamic changes in correlates of depression at one and two years. *Stroke*, **18**, 579–84.

Primeau, F. (1988). Poststroke depression: a critical review of the literature. *Canadian Journal of Psychiatry*, **33**, 757–65.

Reding, M. J., Orto, L. A., Winter, S. W. et al. (1986). Antidepressant therapy after stroke: a double-blind trial. Archives of Neurology, **43**, 763–5.

Robinson, R. G. (1979). Differential behavioral and biochemical effects of right and left hemisphere cerebral infarction in the rat. *Science*, **205**, 707–10.

Robinson, R. G., Bolduc, P. L. & Price, T. R. (1987). Two-year longitudinal study of poststroke mood disorders: diagnosis and outcome at one and two years. *Stroke*, **18**, 837–43.

Robinson, R. G., Bolla-Wilson, K., Kaplan, E. et al. (1986). Depression influences intellectual impairment in stroke patients. *British Journal of Psychiatry*, **148**, 541–7.

Robinson, R. G., Kubos, K. G., Starr, L. B. et al. (1984). Mood disorders in stroke patients: importance of location of lesion. *Brain*, **107**, 81–93.

Robinson, R. G., Lipsey, J. R. & Pearlson, G. D. (1984). The occurrence and treatment of poststroke mood disorder. *Comprehensive Therapy*, **10**, 19–24.

Robinson, R. G., Shoemaker, W. J., Schlumpf, M. et al. (1975). Effect of experimental cerebral infarction in rat brain: effect on catecholamines and behavior. *Nature*, **255**, 332–4.

Robinson, R. G. & Starkstein, S. E. (1990). Current research in affective disorders following stroke. *Journal of Neuropsychiatry and Clinical Neurosciences*, **2**, 1–14.

Robinson, R. G. Starr, L. B., Lipsey, J. R. et al. (1984). A two-year longitudinal study of poststroke mood disorders: dynamic changes in associated variables over the first six months of follow-up. *Stroke*, **15**, 510–17.

Robinson, R. G., Starr, L. B., Kubos, K. L. et al. (1983). A two-year longitudinal study of poststroke mood disorder: findings during the initial evaluation. *Stroke*, **14**, 736–41.

Robinson, R. G. & Szetela, B. (1981). Mood change following left hemisphere brain injury. *Annals of Neurology*, **9**, 447–53.

Ross, E. D., & Rush, A. J. (1981). Diagnosis and neuroanatomical correlates of depression in brain damaged patients. *Archives of General Psychiatry*, **38**, 1344–54.

Sharpe, M., Hawton, K., House, A. et al. (1990). Mood disorders in long-term survivors of stroke: associations with brain lesion location and volume. *Psychological Medicine*, **20**, 815–28.

Sinyor, D., Amato, P., Kaloupek, D. G. et al. (1986*a*). Poststroke depression: Relationships to functional impairment, coping strategies, and rehabilitation outcome. *Stroke*, **17**, 1102–7.

Sinyor, D., Jacques, P., Kaloupek, D. G. et al. (1986*b*). Poststroke depression and lesion location: an attempted replication. *Brain*, **109**, 537–46.

Starkstein, S. E., Boston, J. D. & Robinson, R. G. (1988) Mechanisms of mania following brain injury: twelve case reports and review of the literature. *Journal of Nervous and Mental Disease*, **176**, 87–100.

Starkstein, S. E. & Robinson, R. G. (1989). Affective disorders and cerebral vascular disease. *British Journal of Psychiatry*, **154**, 170–82.

Starkstein, S. E., Robinson, R. G., Honig, M. A. et al. (1989). Mood changes after right hemisphere lesion. *British Journal of Psychiatry*, **155**, 79–85.

Starkstein, S. E., Robinson, R. G. & Price, T. R. (1987). Comparison of cortical and subcortical lesions in the production of poststroke mood disorders. *Brain*, **110**, 1045–59.

Starkstein, S. E., Robinson, R. G. & Price, T. R. (1988). Comparison of patients with and without poststroke major depression matched for size and location of lesion. *Archives of General Psychiatry*, **45**, 247–52.

Wade, D. T., Legh-Smith, J. & Hewer, R. A. (1987). Depressed mood after stroke: A community study of its frequency. *British Journal of Psychiatry*, **151**, 200–5.

Part 9

Treatment methods

25

Geriatric psychopharmacology

BRIAN LEONARD

Introduction

The elderly person is likely to experience many socioeconomic, emotional and physiological changes which will have a major bearing on psychotropic drug treatment. Such a population is therefore more likely to be exposed to more types of drug treatments than would be found in younger age groups. This often results in drug interactions (for example, hypotension associated with diabetes mellitus and tricyclic antidepressants). Other factors which complicate therapy include age related changes in the physiological status which may be reflected in pharmacokinetic features of the psychotropic medication (Greenblatt, Abernathy & Shader, 1986). Such changes in physiological factors are summarized in Table 25.1.

It has been found that the vast majority of elderly patients being treated for a psychiatric disorder also have at least one physical disorder that requires medication (Kennedy, 1992). Thus the elderly are the most likely group to experience adverse drug reactions and interactions. Studies show that patients over the age of 70 years have approximately twice as many adverse drug reactions as those under 50.

Another problem which particularly affects the elderly population concerns compliance with prescribed medication. Factors such as impaired vision, making it difficult for the patient to recognize the various medications, impaired hearing, manual dexterity and cognition all contribute to the noncompliance. Perhaps one of the most important factors that govern noncompliance is the increased frequency and severity of the side-effects that occur with most types of medication in the elderly. This may be illustrated by the tricyclic antidepressants and phenothiazine neuroleptics, both classes of drugs having pronounced antimuscarinic activity even in the physically healthy young patient. In the elderly, there is evidence of excessive sensitivity to anticholinergic effects of drugs. This is compounded by the decline in cognitive function which accompanies aging. Thus

Table 25.1. *Effects of ageing on pharmacokinetic factors*

Factor	Effects
1. Absorption	Decrease in absorption rate and in some active transport processes in the gastrointestinal tract Decrease in gastric acidity and increased prevalence of achlorhydria Decrease in the intestinal fluid volume, gastric emptying and motility and intestinal blood flow
2. Distribution	Decrease in the total body water Decrease in the lean body mass with increased fat to muscle ratio Decreased tissue perfusion and hepatic and renal blood flow Decreased serum protein concentration (particularly albumen)
3. Metabolism	Reduced hepatic microsomal oxidase (cytochrome P450) system
4. Renal excretion	Decreased kidney weight and parenchymal cell mass Decreased renal blood flow and active tubular secretion

After Kennedy, 1991.

one must anticipate that the patient's compliance on any psychotropic drug with pronounced anticholinergic and sedative side-effects will be reduced.

Another problem which can compromize compliance concerns the hypotensive actions of many psychotropic drugs, e.g. tricyclic antidepressants, phenothiazine and neuroleptics. Due to the alpha-1 receptor antagonistic action of these drugs, they are likely to cause severe orthostatic hypotension in some elderly patients. This can cause patients to fall and injure themselves. The increased sensitivity of the elderly to the sedative effects of drugs is also well known. As hypnotics and anxiolytics are frequently administered to the elderly, the sedative effects of these drugs can be minimized by using drugs that have a short to medium half-life.

Treatment of anxiety in the elderly

Pharmacokinetic and pharmacodynamic aspects

At the present time, the benzodiazepines are still the most frequently used drugs in the treatment of anxiety symptoms in the elderly. However, the use of these drugs requires an understanding of their pharmacokinetic and pharmacodynamic characteristics that are often altered in aged patients. Thus the rate of absorption of the drug, and its volume of distribution, are the major determinants of the onset of pharmacological action and the duration of the therapeutic effect. The *volume of distribution* is the term used to relate the quantity of drug in the body relative to its concentration in the blood or plasma. The volume of distribution of any drug varies widely even within a population of patients of similar age and of the same sex. It depends on such factors as the degree of binding of the drug to plasma and tissue proteins and the solubility of the drug in adipose tissue. The volume of distribution of a drug can change as a function of the patient's age, gender, physical status and body composition. *Drug clearance* is expressed as the rate of elimination of the drugs by all routines, e.g. urine, sweat, expired air, feces, as a function of the concentration of the drug in the blood or other tissues. As psychotropic drugs are usually given for several weeks or months, the rate and extent of accumulation are determined by the half life of the drug and its clearance. The term *elimination half-life* is used as an index of the rate at which the drug is removed from the body once it has reached its steady state concentration in the blood. In general, the *half life* ($t_{1/2}$) of a drug is a function of its rate of clearance (CL) and its extent of distribution throughout the body (the volume of distribution, V). This is expressed by the formula:

$$t_{1/2} = 0.693 \times V/CL$$

In general, the older the patient the longer the $t_{1/2}$ value. This is important as such drugs as the benzodiazepines and other sedatives may accumulate and lead to adverse side-effects.

The benzodiazepines may be classified according to their elimination half-lives. Thus the *ultra short* benzodiazepines have $t_{1/2}$ values of less than 5 hours and do not accumulate. Drugs in this class include midazolam, triazolam and brotizolam which are used predominantly as hypnotics in the elderly. Such drugs are largely devoid of active metabolites which can prolong the duration of many of the older benzodiazepines, e.g. flurazepam.

The *short* and *intermediate half-life* benzodiazepines have elimination half-lives of 5–24 hours. Drugs of this type, which include lorazepam, alprazolam, temazepam and oxazepam, do not usually accumulate to any extent and accumulation of their active metabolites is not significant even in the elderly. The drug clearance of those benzodiazepines that are metabolized by the process of conjugation, e.g. oxazepam is not significantly affected by age but benzodiazepines which are metabolized by the hepatic microsomal system, e.g. diazepam, have an impaired clearance as a result of a reduction in liver function with age. The short and intermediate half-life benzodiazepines are usually used as anxiolytic agents in the elderly patient.

The *long half-life* benzodiazepines have elimination $t_{1/2}$ values greater than 24 hours and include such drugs as nitrazepam, flunitrazepam and flurazepam. Such compounds frequently have active metabolites which accumulate during chronic administration. The elimination $t_{1/2}$ values of these drugs are frequently increased, relative to healthy young controls, due to reduction in renal clearance which occurs in all elderly patients.

Table 25.2. *Pharmacokinetic characteristics of some widely used benzodiazepines*

Drug	Principal active metabolite(s)	$t_{\frac{1}{2}}$ (h) mean (range)	Comments
Midazolam		2.4 (1.5–3.5)	
Triazolam		3 (1–4.5)	Drug clearance is reduced in the elderly and by coadministration of cimetidine
Oxazepam		7.2 (6–24)	$t_{\frac{1}{2}}$ increased in patients with renal dysfunction
Temazepam		9 (4–20)	$t_{\frac{1}{2}}$ not significantly affected by age; little effect of liver damage or cimetidine coadministration
Lormetazepam		10	$t_{\frac{1}{2}}$ may increase with age
Lorazepam		14 (9–35)	$t_{\frac{1}{2}}$ increased in patients with hepatic dysfunction
Chlordiazepoxide	Desmethyl Chloridiazepoxide	10 (5–30)	$t_{\frac{1}{2}}$ increased by cimetidine and liver dysfunction
	Desmethyl diazepam	62 (51–120)	
Clobazam		24 (11–46)	$t_{\frac{1}{2}}$ increased in elderly
Nitrazepam		30 (18–57)	$t_{\frac{1}{2}}$ increase with age; little effect of liver damage
Diazepam		46 (20–70)	$t_{\frac{1}{2}}$ increases with age, liver damage and treatment with cimetidine
	Desmethyl diazepam	62 (51–120)	
	Oxazepam	7.6 (6–25)	
Clorazepate		–	Prodrug for desmethyl-diazepam
	Desmethyl diazepam	62 (51–120)	Antacids prolong $t_{\frac{1}{2}}$

After Feely & Pullar, 1990.

Table 25.2 summarizes the pharmacokinetic characteristics of different types of benzodiazepines which are used to treat anxiety and/or insomnia in the elderly.

Following short-term administration in volunteers or hospitalized patients, the elderly have higher plasma levels of any of the benzodiazepines than younger individuals and also have an increased frequency of unwanted sedative side-effects; following long-term administration, a tolerance often develops to the unwanted sedation, confusion and motor incoordination (Swift et al., 1984). Gibaldi (1987) has reviewed the effects of aging on drug dosage.

Pharmacokinetic interactions can arise following the concurrent administration of a drug which, for example, alters the gastric pH, thereby altering the absorption of the benzodiazepine. It is well established that the metabolism of benzodiazepines can be stimulated by drugs that induce liver microsomal enzyme activity, e.g. the barbiturates, while drugs such as cimetidine and disulfiram that inhibit this microsomal oxidase system have the opposite effect (Pullar et al., 1987). The benzodiazepines most affected by drugs such as cimetidine are those undergoing oxidative metabolism, while those, e.g. lorazepam and oxazepam, that are metabolized by the gluconidation pathway are largely unaffected by the concurrent administration of cimetidine. Such factors are particularly relevant in elderly patients, as the occurrence of peptic ulcers is not infrequent and cimetidine is widely used in the treatment of such conditions.

Drug treatment of anxiety and insomnia in the elderly

Most psychotropic drugs are highly lipophilic and the increased fat to lean body mass ratio in the elderly patient, and decreased metabolism and excretion mean that the half-lives of most psychotropic drugs are increased. The benzodiazepine anxiolytics and hypnotics are no exception. Following a single dose of chlordiazepoxide, diazepam or flurazepam, the time for elimination of the parent compounds and their active metabolites can be as long as 72 hours. For this reason, it is now accepted practice to administer a short acting benzodiazepine, e.g. brotizolam, oxazepam, triazolam, midazolam or temazepam only as needed and for as short a period as possible. Such drugs should usually be administered for a period not exceeding six weeks unless there is clear evidence that the patient is suffering from chronic insomnia, in which case long-term hypnotic treatment may be justified. It should be noted that even benzodiazepines which have a relatively short half-life occasionally cause excessive day-time sedation. The side-effects and dependence potential of the anxiolytics and sedative-hypnotics are well known and can usually be circumvented by slowly reducing the dose of the drug over a period of one to two weeks. Psychotherapy, either as an adjunct to drug therapy or as an alternative, has an important role to play in treating mild anxiety states in the elderly (Chapter 6).

Insomnia is a common complaint in the elderly. As people age, they require less sleep and a variety of physical ailments to which the elderly are subject can cause a change in the sleep pattern, e.g. cerebral atherosclerosis, heart disease, decreased pulmonary function, as can depression. Providing sedative-hypnotics are warranted, the judicious use of short half-life benzodiazepines may therefore be appropriate.

Because of their side-effects, there would now appear to be little merit in using chloral hydrate or related drugs in the treatment of insomnia in the elderly. The gastric irritant effect of chloral hydrate and related drugs can be particularly problematic in old age and may be a cause of peptic ulceration.

In addition to the benzodiazepines, there may be a role for nonbenzodiazepine drugs such as buspirone and zopiclone in the treatment of anxiety and insomnia in late life. Both drugs appear to be well tolerated in younger populations of patients but it is essential to await the outcome of properly conducted trials of these drugs on a substantial number of elderly patients before any conclusions may be drawn regarding their value as alternatives to the benzodiazepines.

Treatment of depression and mania in the elderly

Depression is one of the commonest psychiatric disorders in old age with prevalence rates ranging from 2–18% (see Chapter 7). Although antidepressant drugs have been the major method of treatment of depression in the elderly since the introduction of the first monoamine oxidase inhibitor and tricyclic antidepressants in the 1950s, relatively little information has been systematically collected regarding the efficacy and safety of antidepressants in the aged. There are a number of double-blind studies of both the older and some of the newer antidepressants, e.g. trazodone, nomifensine, buproprion, fluoxetine and fluvoxamine, which overall, suggest that response rates in the elderly do not differ substantially from depressed patients in young age groups (Plotkin, Gerson & Jarvik, 1987).

A disturbance in the sleep pattern is a common symptom of depression but changes in the sleep pattern also occur as a consequence of aging. Once depression has been diagnosed, there are several types of antidepressants which may be given. Because of their potent anticholinergic side-effects, there seems little merit in prescribing the older tricyclic antidepressants, e.g. amitriptyline, imipramine or dothiepin to such patients. There is now sufficient evidence to suggest that sedative antidepressants such as mianserin or trazodone given at night reduce the likelihood that the patient will require a sedative-hypnotic. For the more retarded elderly patient, a nonsedative antidepressant such as lofepramine or one of the new 5-HT reuptake inhibitor antidepressants, e.g. fluoxetine, fluvoxamine, paroxetine or sertraline may be used.

The side-effects and cardiotoxicity of the tricyclic antidepressants are well known and, while there is ample evidence of their therapeutic efficacy, it seems difficult to justify their use any longer in elderly patients who are most vulnerable to their detrimental side-effects. Of the newer antidepressants, the MAO-A reversible inhibitors such as moclobemide may also be of value in the elderly depressed patient, particularly in those patients who fail to respond to the amine uptake inhibitor type of antidepressant. It should also be remembered that ECT is a safe and effective treatment for severe depression in all patients, including the elderly (see Chapter 26).

While lithium salts have traditionally been used to treat bipolar depression, evidence for the safety and efficacy of lithium in the old has been accumulating.

However, placebo-controlled, double-blind studies of the use of lithium in the prophylaxis and management of depression in the elderly are still lacking. Nevertheless, it appears that lithium is effective in the treatment of bipolar depression, but that lower doses of the drug are required in comparison to those required by younger patients. Clearly factors such as pre-existing thyroid, renal or neurological disease must be taken into account before lithium is used in the elderly patient (Plotkin et al., 1987).

Reports are also occurring in the literature regarding the efficacy of using lithium in patients who have failed to respond to the usual course of a tricyclic antidepressant. As with younger patients, lithium carbonate can be added to the 'standard' dose of the tricyclic antidepressant in such cases in order to overcome the lack of therapeutic effect (Kushnir, 1986).

Mania can occur in any age group. Acute manic episodes in the elderly may best be managed with high potency neuroleptics. The use of lithium is not contraindicated in old age provided renal clearance is reasonably normal. The dose administered should be carefully monitored as the half-life of the drug is increased in the elderly to 36–48 hours in comparison to about 24 hours in the young adult. The serum lithium concentration in the elderly should be maintained at about 0.5 mE/l. It is essential to ensure that the older patient is not on a salt restricted diet before starting lithium therapy. The side-effects and toxicity of lithium are well established and apart from an increase in the frequency of confusional states which may be more frequent in the elderly patient, the same adverse effects can be expected as in the young patient.

Pharmacokinetic aspects

While data are generally lacking for the elderly, clinical experience indicates that such patients normally require lower doses than do younger adults. Because of changes in the physiological state of the elderly patient (see Table 25.1), there is evidence that such patients achieve higher plasma levels for a given dose of a standard tricyclic antidepressant than do younger patients (Nies et al., 1977). However, not all investigators have confirmed this relationship (e.g. Ziegler & Biggs, 1979). It must be emphasized that because of the multiple medications which may be taken by the older depressed patient, increased plasma concentrations of antidepressants can occur. For example, this could be due to co-administered neuroleptics. Conversely, changes in plasma antidepressant levels can arise because a co-administered drug increases or decreases liver microsomal oxidase activity.

In addition to the increasing frequency of the well-established anticholinergic and alpha 1 adrenoceptor antagonistic effects of the older tricylic antidepressants in the elderly patient, very occasionally more exotic side-effects may become

Table 25.3. *Potential drug interactions involving antidepressants in elderly depressed patients*

Interaction	Consequence
Tricyclic antidepressants and:	
Clonidine	Decreased antihypertensive effect
Disulfiram	Organic mental disorder
Guanethidine	Decreased antihypertensive effect
Chlorpropamide (? oral hypoglycemics)	Doxepin induced hypoglycemia
Nitroglycerin	Nortriptyline induced hypoglycemia
Nontricyclic antidepressants and:	
Tricyclic antidepressants	Fluoxetine and maprotiline may inhibit the metabolism of some tricyclics
Digoxin	Trazodone may increase the risk of digoxin toxicity
Phenothiazines	Coadministration of trazodone may cause severe hypotension
Lithium and:	
Methyldopa	Increased lithium toxicity
Phenytoin	Increased lithium toxicity
Verapamil	Bradycardia, neurotoxicity

Griffin & D'Arcy, 1984; Ciraulo et al., 1989.

apparent. Thus tricyclic antidepresssants are known to produce an acute 'jitteriness' in patients with panic disorder (Yeragani, Pohl & Balon, 1992). This syndrome is characterized by 'jitteriness', restlessness, difficulty in sitting still and increased anxiety. There is so far no evidence that the frequency of this side-effect is greater in elderly patients with panic attacks than in those from a younger age group. This is surprising in view of the apparent greater sensitivity of elderly patients to the anticholinergic effects of psychotropic drugs.

Some potential drug interactions which have been reported in elderly depressed patients when treated with antidepressants are shown in Table 25.3.

Treatment of psychosis in the elderly

Irrespective of the age of the patients, neuroleptics are usually effective in attenuating the symptoms of schizophrenia. In addition to the classical symptoms of schizophrenia, many elderly patients frequently show severe agitation, restlessness, assaultiveness and hostility. It is not unusual to observe elderly patients who are suffering from various degrees of dementia, psychosis and severe agitation simultaneously. Such conditions often can be controlled by the 'classical' phenothiazine neuroleptics such as thioridazine. Salzman (1987) has reviewed some 45 studies of the use of different types of neuroleptics in the treatment of agitation in the elderly and has concluded that while these drugs have a consistent and a reliable therapeutic effect in controlling the various features of psychotic disorder, the overall therapeutic efficacy is modest. Furthermore, despite the variety of neuroleptics used in these studies (thioridazine, trifluoperazine, chlorpromazine, haloperidol, thiothixene, prochlorperazine, mesoridazine, loxapine, molindone, melperone and fluphenazine), no single neuroleptic (or class of neuroleptics) offered any advantage as a treatment for agitation associated with psychosis or dementia.

A variety of psychotic conditions can occur in late life and it is important to remember that an old person who develops agitation, paranoid ideation or delusions may be suffering from a drug-induced delirium. The most common causes of such a condition are drugs that have potent central muscarinic blocking properties, such as the antiparkinsonian agents, antihistamines, tricyclic antidepressants and the phenothiazine neuroleptics. Witholding all psychotropic drug medication for a few days may be the most judicious management for this type of toxic psychosis!

Pharmacokinetic aspects

There are few data concerning the effect of age on the pharmacokinetic characteristics of neuroleptics. There is evidence that the elimination half-life of thioridazine is increased with age, but conflicting results occur in the literature regarding the effect of age on the steady state plasma concentrations of most of the commonly used neuroleptics (Muuze & Vanderheeren, 1977).

The pharmacodynamic aspect of neuroleptic administration is also assumed to change with increasing age. Thus due to a reduction in neurotransmitter turnover with increasing age, it has been inferred that the brain becomes increasingly sensitive to the effects of neuroleptic drugs. This could account for the increased predispositon of the elderly patient to the extrapyramidal side-effects of neuroleptics arising from a reduction in dopaminergic neurotransmission in the nigrostriatal tract (McGeer & McGeer, 1977).

While there is clear evidence of increased extrapyramidal side effects in elderly patients treated with neuroleptics (Siede & Muller, 1967), it would also appear that individual susceptibility to neuroleptics plays a major role in predisposing the patient to such effects. Thus it has been reported that the plasma concentration of a neuroleptic may vary several hundredfold between individual patients treated with the same dose either alone or together with an anticholinergic drug (Simpson & Yadalam, 1985).

Several studies have established that there is an age-associated sensitivity to the hypotensive side-effects of neuroleptics which may be associated with a reduction in central baroreceptor function (Blumenthal & Davie, 1980). The reduction in central and peripheral cholinergic function with increasing age has also been linked to a marked increase in the frequency of neuroleptic induced delirium and neurotoxicity of these drugs in the aged patient (Thompson, Moran & Nies, 1983).

One of thc more serious and persistent side-effects of prolonged neuroleptic use in the elderly is tardive dyskinesia. There is now good evidence that elderly patients are at a greater risk for the development of tardive dyskinesia than younger patients (see Baldessarini et al., 1980). It would appear that this increased incidence is unrelated to the doses of neuroleptics used or to the coadministration of anticholinergic drugs. Several factors have been described which might be important in increasing the frequency of tardive dyskinesia in the elderly.

(a) It has been shown that there is a threefold increase in the serum neuroleptic concentration in elderly patients, when compared to younger patients on the same dose of a drug (Jeste et al., 1982). It is, however, still a mattter of debate whether an increased serum level of a neuroleptic drug will predispose an elderly patient to tardive dyskinesia.

(b) Age-related brain changes, such as neuronal loss and changes in neurotransmitter receptor sensitivity, may be important predisposing factors in tardive dyskinesia (Lohr & Bracha, 1988; Waddington 1987).

(c) Tardive dyskinesia may be more common in patients with mood disorders when compared to patients with schizophrenia (Gardos & Casey, 1984), Furthermore, Waddington et al. (1990) have shown that prolonged exposure to antidepressants, particularly tricyclics, may also be an important predisposing factor to tardive dyskinesia in elderly patients.

(d) Elderly patients with physical illness are more likely to have orofacial dyskinesias than healthy subjects of the same age (Lieberman et al., 1984). This suggests that the age-related increase in physical illness may predispose elderly patients on neuroleptics to tardive dyskinesia.

In addition to neuroleptic-induced Parkinsonism and tardive dyskinesia, akathisia has also been reported to occur in 20–25% of patients on antipsychotic medication (Ayd, 1984); the high risk groups for neuroleptic-induced akathisia include the elderly, female and mentally retarded patients. The elderly appear to be at greatest risk, particularly when high potency neuroleptics are used (Steinberg, 1985).

Pre-existing brain damage and cognitive deficits appear to be risk factors for tardive dyskinesia in the elderly. Late onset, or tardive, akathisia may also occur in patients when a neuroleptic is withdrawn or the dose adminstered is abruptly decreased (Dilsaver, 1989). While the pathological cause of akathisia is unknown, there is evidence to suggest that low serum iron may induce dopamine type 2 receptor hypofunction in patients on neuroleptics which may precipitate the condition. Other factors include an imbalance between the alpha 2 and beta adrenoceptors, cholinergic supersensitivity, decreased serotonergic function and reduced GABA function (Chengappa & Flynn, 1992). It should be emphasized that neuroleptic-induced akathisia is often unrecognized as a drug induced adverse event. Indeed, as it can be misdiagnosed as a reccurance of psychosis, the dose of neuroleptic precipitating the symptoms actually may be increased thereby further exacerbating the akathisia. As there is evidence that the incidence of suicide is increased in those patients with akathisia (Ayd, 1988), it is vital that this condition be recognized in those elderly patients on high potency neuroleptics.

In contrast to the increased incidence in the elderly of side-effects involving the basal ganglia, there is no evidence that they are more prone to obstructive jaundice, agranulocytosis, weight gain, skin rashes, grand-mal seizures or the neuroleptic malignant syndrome than younger patients treated with neuroleptics (Mueller, 1985).

Conclusions

It can be seen that the types of psychotropic drug medication that may be used in the elderly are essentially similar to those used in the younger adult patient. The main difference lies in reduction in the distribution, metabolism and elimination of the drugs which necessitates their administration in lower doses initially followed by a slower escalation of the dose until optimal benefit is obtained. Side-effects, particularly sedative and anticholinergic effects, are more pronounced in the elderly and can contribute to poor compliance.

References

Ayd, F. J. (1984). High potency neuroleptics and akathisia. *Journal of Clinical Psychopharmacology*, **4**, 237–40.

Ayd, F. J. (1988). Akathisia and suicide: fact or myth? *International Drug Therapy Newsletter*, **23**, 37–9.

Baldessarini, R. J., Cole, J. O., Davis, J. M., Gardos, G., Preskorn, S. A., Simpson, G. M. & Tarsy, D. (1980). *Tardive Dyskinesia: a Task Force Report of the American Psychiatric Association*. Washington DC: American Psychiatric Association.

Blumenthal, M. D. & Davie, J. W. (1980). Dizziness and falling in elderly psychiatric outpatients. *American Journal of Psychiatry*, **137**, 203–6.

Chengappa, K. N. R. & Flynn, P. (1992). *Akathisia In Drug-Induced Dysfunction in Psychiatry*. ed. M. S. Keshavan & J. S. Kennedy, pp. 153–168. New York: Hemisphere Publishing Corporation.

Ciraulo, D. A., Shader, R. I., Greenblatt, D. J. & Greelman, W. (1989). *Drug Interactions in Psychiatry*. Baltimore: Williams and Wilkins.

Dilsaver, S. C. (1989). Antidepressant withdrawal syndromes: phenomenology and pathophysiology. *Acta Psychiatrica Scandanavica*, **79**, 113–17.

Feely, M. & Pullar, T. (1990). Pharmacokinetic differences between benzodiazepines. In *Benzodiazepines: Current Concepts*, ed. I. Hindmarch, G. Beaumont, S. Brandon & B. E. Leonard, pp. 61–72, Chichester: John Wiley & Sons.

Gardos, G. & Casey, D. E. (1984). *Tardive Dyskinesia and Affective Disorders*. Washington DC: American Psychiatric Press.

Gibaldi, M. (1987). Drug dosage in the elderly. *Perspectives in Clinical Pharmacy*, **5**, 10–15.

Greenblatt, J., Abernathy, D. R. & Shader, R. I. (1986). Pharmaco-kinetic aspects of drug therapy in the elderly. *Therapeutic Drug Monitoring*, **8**, 129–257.

Griffin, J. P. & D'Arcy, P. F. (1984). *A Manual of Adverse Drug Interactions*, 3rd Edn. Bristol: John Wright & Sons.

Jeste, D. V., Linnoila, M., Wagner, R. L. & Wyatt, R. J. (1982). Serum neuroleptic concentrations and tardive dyskinesia. *Psychopharmacology*, **76**, 377–80.

Kennedy, J. S. (1992). Adverse drug effects in the older adult. In *Drug-Induced Dysfunction in Psychiatry*. ed. M. S. Keshavan & J. S. Kennedy. pp. 93–101. New York: Hemisphere Publishing Corporation.

Kushnir, S. L. (1986). Lithium-antidepressant combinations in the treatment of depressed, physically ill geriatric patients. *American Journal of Psychiatry*, **143**, 3–4.

Lieberman, J., Kane, J. M., Woerner, M., Weinhold, P., Basavaraju, N., Kuruczi, J. & Bergmann, K. (1984). Prevalence of tardive dyskinesia in elderly patients. *Psychopharmacology Bulletin*, **20**, 382–6.

Lohr, J. B. & Bracha, H. S. (1988). Association of psychosis and movement disorders in the elderly. *Psychiatric Clinics of North America*, **11**, 61–82.

McGeer, P. L. & McGeer, E. G. (1977). Ageing and extrapyrimidal function. *Archives of Neurology*, **34**, 33–5.

Mueller, P. S. (1985). Neuroleptic malignant syndrome. *Psychosomatics*, **26**, 654–68.

Muuze, R. G. & Vanderheeren, F. A. J. (1977). Plasma levels and half-lives of thioridazine and some of its metabolites. II Low doses in older psychiatric patients. *European Journal of Clinical Pharmacology*, **11**, 141–7.

Nies, A., Robinson, D. S., Friedman, M. J., Green, R., Cooper, J. B., Ravaris, C. L. & Ives, J. D. (1977). Relationship between age and tricyclic antidepressant plasma levels. *American Journal of Psychiatry*, **134**, 790–3.

Plotkin, D. A., Gerson, S. C. & Jarvik, L. F. (1987). Antidepressant drug treatment in the elderly, In *Psychopharmacology: The Third Generation of Progress*, ed. H. Y. Meltzer, pp. 1149–1158. New York: Raven Press.

Pullar, T., Haigh, J. R. M., Peaker, S. & Feely, M. P. (1987). Pharmacokinetics of *N*-demethyl clobazam in healthy volunteers and patients with epilepsy. *British Journal of Clinical Pharmacology*, **24**, 793–7.

Salzman (1987). Treatment of agitation in the elderly. In *Psychopharmacology: The Third Generation of Progress*, eds. M. S. Keshaven & J. S. Kennedy pp. 93–101. New York: Hemisphere Publishing Corporation.

Siede, H. & Muller, H. F. (1967). Choreiform movements as side-effects of phenothiazine medication in geriatric patients. *Journal of the American Geriatrics Society*, **15**, 517–22.

Simpson, G. M. & Yadulam, K. G. (1985). Blood levels of neuroleptics: state of the art. *Journal of Clinical Psychiatry*, **46**, 22–8.

Steinberg, S. K. (1985). Drug-induced extrapyramidal symptoms in the elderly. *Modern Medicine of Canada*, **40**, 473–82.

Swift, C. G., Swift, M. R., Hamley, J., Stevenson, I. H. & Crooks, J. (1984). Side-effect tolerance in elderly long-term recipients of benzodiazepine hypnotics. *Age and Ageing*, **13**, 335–43.

Thompson, T. L. H., Moran, M. G. & Nies, A. S. (1983). Drug therapy: psychotropic drug use in the elderly. *New England Journal of Medicine*, **308**, 194–9.

Waddington, J. L. (1987). Tardive dyskinesia in schizophrenia and other disorders: associations with ageing, cognitive dysfunciton and structural brain pathology in relation to neuroleptic exposure. *Human Psychopharmacology*, **2**, 11–22.

Waddington, J. L., Brown, K., O'Neill, J. & McKeon, P. (1990). Tardive dyskinesia in bipolar affective disorder: relationship to anti-depressants, lithium, and neuroleptic exposure. In *Antidepressants: Thirty Years On*, ed. B. E. Leonard & P. S. J. Spencer, pp. 410–416. London: Clinical Neuroscience Publishers.

Yeragani, V. K., Pohl, R., Balon, R. (1992). Tricyclic antidepressant-induced jitteriness. In *Drug-induced Dysfunction in Psychiatry*, ed. M. S. Kershavan & J. S. Kennedy, pp. 169–172. New York: Hemisphere Publishing Corporation.

Ziegler, V. E. & Biggs, J. J. (1979). Tricyclic plasma levels. Effect of age, race, sex and smoking. *Journal of the American Medical Association*, **238**, 2167–9.

26

Electroconvulsive therapy in later life

SUSAN MARY BENBOW

Electroconvulsive therapy (ECT) is not contraindicated by advanced age. Indeed, over the years a number of studies have reported a more favorable treatment response in elderly people (Gold & Chiarella, 1944; Hobson, 1953; Roberts, 1959; Mendels, 1967; Coryell & Zimmerman, 1984). Reviewers have concluded, modestly, that elderly people respond to ECT at least as well as younger people (Weiner, 1982; Benbow, 1989). There are, however, particular areas of concern for clinicians who prescribe ECT for elderly people: concurrent physical illness is often present, and possible side-effects may worry doctor, relatives and patient.

This chapter will cover the following areas:

1. Indications for ECT in late life.
2. Safety of ECT.
3. Side-effects of ECT in the elderly.
4. Efficacy.
5. Treatment resistant depression, ECT and maintenance ECT.
6. Consent.
7. Practical aspects of treating older people with ECT.

Indications for ECT in late life

The American Psychiatric Association Task Force Report (1990) lists the main indications for ECT as major depression, mania and schizophrenia and other functional psychoses. In the elderly, depressive illness is the main indication for ECT (Fraser, 1981), but views vary regarding the place of this treatment in the modern therapeutic armoury. There is now a wider selection of drugs available and some authors argue that ECT should be a treatment of last resort (Malcolm & Peet, 1989). The opposing view is that elderly people may be placed 'in jeopardy' if they have to be treated with antidepressant drugs before receiving ECT (Weiss & Weiss, 1987). Only three of 205 respondents in a UK survey of old age psychiatrists agreed that ECT should be the last resort and one other person stated that the

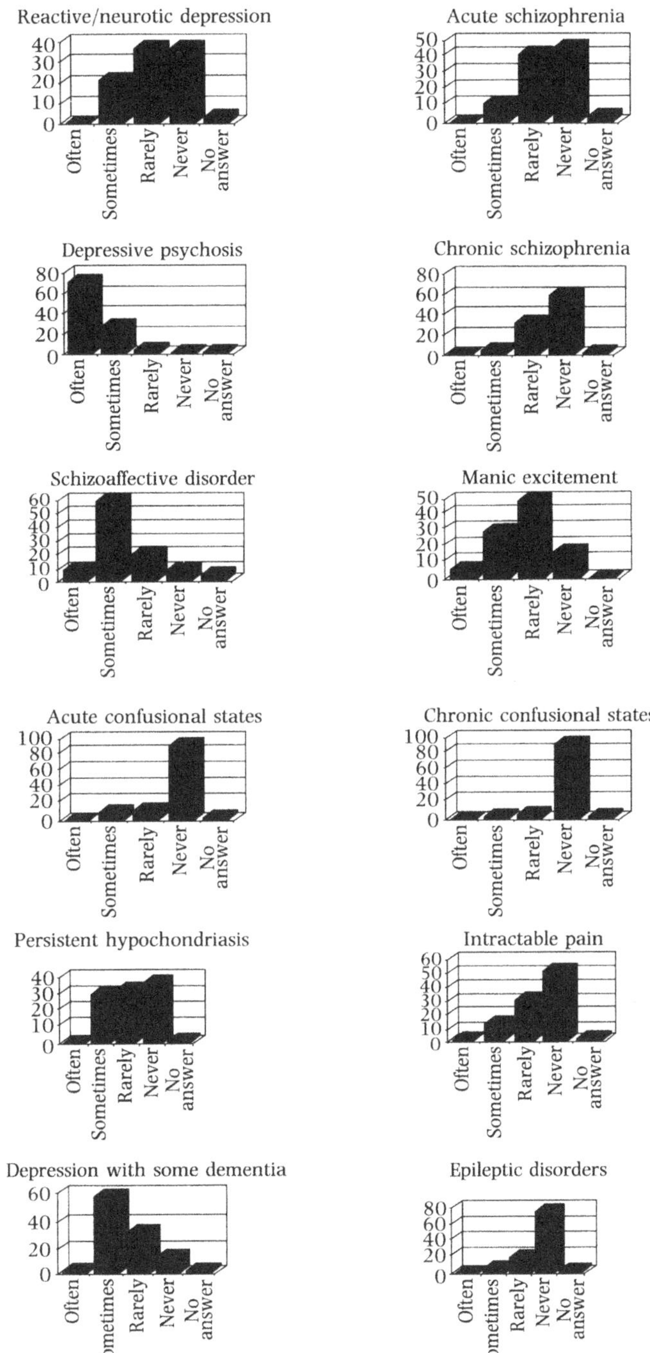

Fig. 26.1. Ratings by UK old age psychiatrists of how appropriate they regard the use of ECT in various conditions in older people.

treatment should never be used (Benbow, 1991). The majority (over 95%) of UK old age psychiatrists reported that they were in favor of ECT for appropriate patients. Figure 26.1 shows how appropriate they rated the treatment in various conditions in late life, and shows that depressive psychosis was rated most often to be the appropriate indication, although schizoaffective disorder and depression with dementia were other common indications.

In the literature there is general agreement about the features predicting a good response to ECT in later life. Many are the symptoms associated with the concept of 'endogenous depression' (Benbow, 1989). There is some suggestion of a wider potential role than earlier in life, e.g. anxiety/agitation, which has been said to be an unfavorable indicator in younger groups (Hamilton, 1982), has been linked with a more favorable response in the elderly (Fraser & Glass, 1980; Salzman, 1982). Pippard & Ellam's (1981) survey found ECT to be considered of 'especial use in the elderly', even in apparently neurotic depressive illnesses. Hobson (1953) found that an obsessional previous personality was a favorable prognostic feature and was more common in those aged over 40 years.

In some situations old age psychiatrists would regard ECT as the first choice treatment: when there has been no response to tricyclic antidepressant drugs, when previous episodes of illness have responded to ECT but not to anti-depressant drugs and when the suicidal risk is high, over 80% of old age psychiatrists would regard ECT as indicated.

Is ECT safe for physically ill old people?

In the South Manchester study of elderly people treated with ECT, fewer than 50% had no appreciable physical illness. Almost 25% had known cardiac problems and people with a wide range of other physical illnesses received treatment (Benbow, 1987). Other authors have reported similar findings (e.g. Gaspar & Samarasinghe, 1982; Gerring & Shields, 1982; Alexopoulos et al., 1984; Hay, 1989). The accumulation of physical illnesses with age is undoubtedly a concern when a frail or very elderly person is being considered for treatment, but untreated depressive illness is itself a threat to life, and experience with ECT suggests that it can be surprisingly safe for physically ill old people. Opinions amongst old age psychiatrists differ as to which conditions should be considered as absolute or relative contra-indications to treatment: Figure 26.2 displays survey findings in the UK (Benbow, 1991). The two main areas of concern are cerebral and cardiovascular conditions, in view of the haemodynamic changes induced by ECT (Huang, et al., 1989).

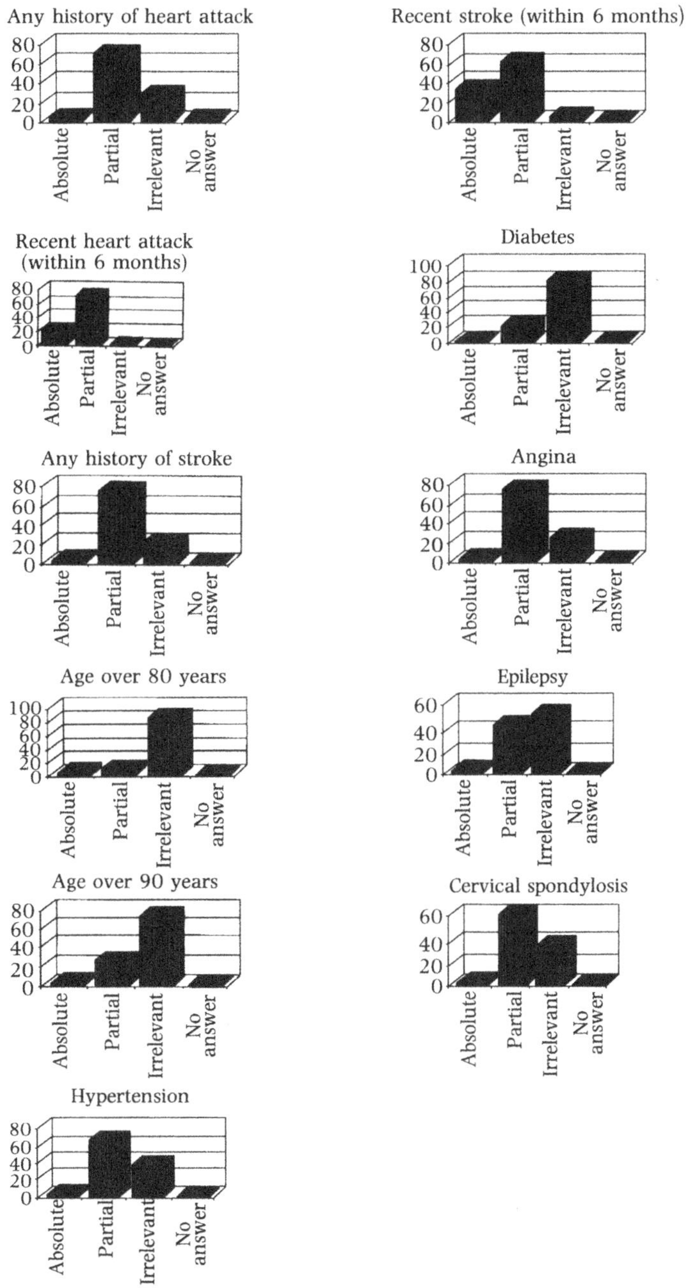

Fig. 26.2. Ratings by UK old age psychiatrists of which conditions should be considered to be absolute or relative contraindications to the use of ECT in the elderly.

Stroke

ECT has been used successfully and safely in poststroke depressive illnesses, so it is not surprising that 21% of old age psychiatrists surveyed in the UK regarded a history of stroke as irrelevant to the prescription of ECT (Benbow, 1991). 75% considered it a partial contraindication, but only 3% indicated that they would not give ECT in these circumstances. Recent stroke was more likely to be regarded as an absolute (33%) or partial (62%) contraindication. Murray, Shea & Conn (1986) have described four people (from a total of 14) treated with ECT within one month of having strokes. Alexopoulos et al. (1984) reported a patient who had received treatment four days after a cerebral infarction documented by CT scan.

Inevitably, a decision to use ECT following stroke will depend on the balance of risks and benefits. Although most clinicians would prefer to avoid its use within six months of stroke, recent stroke is not an absolute contraindication if the prognosis is grave without treatment.

Cardio-vascular disease

People with known cardiac disease have an increased rate of cardiac complications during ECT (Gerring & Shields, 1982; Alexopoulos et al., 1984). During treatment adverse effects are concentrated in older patients (Cattan et al., 1990) and those with a higher risk status using the American Society of Anesthesiologists (ASA) classification system (Burke et al., 1985). Since age and ASA rating correlate, it is likely that the increasing health problems of older people account for their increased risk. Despite this, ECT has been used safely in a range of cardiovascular diseases: people with dissecting aortic aneurysm (Devanand, Malitz & Sackeim, 1990; Rosenfeld, Glassberg & Sherrid, 1988), those on anticoagulant treatment (Loo, Cuche & Benkelfat, 1985; Tancer & Evans, 1989) and people with implanted cardiac pacemakers (Alexopoulos et al., 1984; Regestein & Lind, 1980). The cardio-vascular status of high-risk individuals must be carefully assessed prior to ECT, in collaboration with a cardiologist or other experienced physician, and ECG monitoring may be advisable during treatment. Maneksha (1991) has reviewed possible techniques for modifying the cardio-vascular response of at risk patients. Following myocardial infarction most clinicians would delay ECT for as long as possible and treatment is probably safer after 3 months (Perrin, 1961).

Dementing illnesses

Concurrent depression and dementia is a particular problem for those working with the elderly. Nevertheless 61.4% of UK old age psychiatrists rated ECT as appropriate often or sometimes in depression with dementia (see Fig. 26.1);

corresponding figures for depressive psychosis, schizoaffective disorder and reactive/neurotic depression were 96.5%, 68.3% and 22.5% respectively (Benbow, 1991). Concern about the possible effect of ECT on memory in already cognitively impaired people does not seem to dissuade specialists from using the treatment.

Over the years, case reports have described successful ECT treatment of people with various dementing illnesses (Demuth & Rand, 1980; Liang, Lam & Ancill, 1988), including Alzheimer's disease (Snow & Wells, 1981), normal pressure hydrocephalus (McAllister & Price, 1982), Huntington's disease (Perry, 1983) and Creuzfeldt-Jakob disease (McAllister & Price, 1982). Price & McAllister (1989) have reviewed and summarized relevant case material. Of a series of 122 patients treated with ECT at the University Hospital of South Manchester 4% had dementias complicating their affective illness (Benbow, 1988*a*): 31% of ECT courses given to nondemented patients were complicated by confusion or forgetfulness in comparison with 67% of courses administered to those with coexisting dementias. In Central Manchester between 1987 and 1991 the proportion of patients with dual diagnoses has been even higher at 25% (Benbow, 1992). Certainly depressive illness with concurrent dementia is not an uncommon clinical problem for old age psychiatrists.

Such people may be more likely to develop confusional states, some prolonged and lasting 6–8 weeks. Summers, Robins & Reich (1979) reported two prolonged confusional states (lasting 45 and 65 days) in the only two patients of their series (total 31) with known concurrent dementing illnesses. A three-week confusional state has also been described in a 70 year old woman with shunted normal pressure hydrocephalus (Tsuang, Tidball & Geller, 1979). The course of these confusional states is of gradual improvement and eventual recovery. Cognitive function following treatment, despite the dementia, may be better than immediately before treatment because the deficit in function related to the depressive illness responds to ECT (Greenwald et al., 1989). Thus the patient with dementia and depression may have an improved quality of life following treatment.

Nelson & Rosenberg (1991) have studied 103 patients over the age of 60 treated with ECT over a four-year period. Twenty-one had a concurrent dementia (20.4%). Response to ECT was no different in those with concurrent dementing illnesses, but confusion scores were significantly higher in the dual diagnosis group and post-ECT confusion score correlated with degree of dementia. Zwil, McAllister & Price (1992) have recently reported a review of the safety and efficacy of ECT in depressed patients with organic brain disease, with similar findings. Twenty-six of 27 courses administered produced a good affective response. Patients with diffuse or multifocal brain disease were susceptible to acute confusional states during treatment, but only one course was discontinued as a result.

The American Psychiatric Association Task Force Report (1990) notes that patients with preexisting cognitive impairments are believed to be at increased risk of cognitive side-effects during a course of ECT. It recommends that orientation and memory functions should be assessed prior to ECT and throughout the treatment course. Practical measures can be taken to minimize any cognitive side-effects during treatment, e.g. by using unilateral ECT, minimizing the use of concurrent psychoactive drugs and cutting down on the dose of anaesthetic. If a patient fails to respond to unilateral ECT, they should be allowed the opportunity of responding to bilateral treatment (Abrams, 1988*a*).

Other medical conditions

In general, whatever medical conditions are present they will need careful assessment prior to treatment, but, having said this, it is important to recognize that ECT has been used successfully in a range of serious illnesses, e.g. following craniotomy for meningioma (Hsiao & Evans, 1984), in the presence of cerebral tumour (Kellner & Rameo, 1990) and raised intracranial pressure (Dubovsky et al., 1985), treated hydrocephalus related to Paget's disease of the skull (Cardno & Simpson, 1991) and chronic subdural hematoma (Malek-Ahmadi et al., 1990). In the presence of severe unstable cervical spine disease maximal muscle relaxation and minimal neck manipulation can be employed (Kellner, Tolhurst & Burns, 1991).

What side-effects of ECT occur in the elderly?

Of possible side-effects of ECT, the effects on cognitive function are probably of most concern in older people. There has been surprisingly little research on memory in elderly people treated with ECT. Many studies have excluded older people, and naturalistic studies of older groups often exclude detailed memory tests.

Patients' experience of cognitive problems during and after ECT

Confusion is a vague complaint, which reflects an awareness of cognitive impairment and is related to memory impairment. Daniel and Crovitz (1986) query whether disorientation during ECT can be understood as a memory disorder. This is a matter of debate, but confusion and memory impairment are both noted following ECT. Table 26.1 compares patients' reports of memory problems and confusion in two studies: Freeman & Kendell's (1980) study of 166 people aged under 70 years and Benbow's (1988*b*) later study of 54 mixed age patients (41% aged over 60 years). The differences between the two studies may reflect the lack of an upper age limit in the study with more confusion (if the elderly treated with ECT are more likely to develop this side-effect than younger people) or the greater time elapsed before interview in Freeman and Kendell's study, perhaps allowing

Table 26.1. *Patients' reports of memory problems and confusion during ECT*

Symptom	Memory problems		Confusion	
Study	Freeman & Kendell 1980	Benbow 1988	Freeman & Kendell 1980	Benbow 1988
Symptom reported spontaneously	41%	20%	5%	6%
Total reporting the symptom	64%	61%	26%	43%
Symptom rated severe	25%	20%	9%	10%
Symptom rated mild/moderate	39%	41%	17%	33%
Number of patients	166	54	166	54

those who had suffered with mild symptoms to overlook reporting them, although there is no analogous tendency to report less memory impairment. The second possibility might explain why the percentage who spontaneously reported confusion is similar in both groups and also the percentage who reported the symptom to be severe. A further retrospective study of 293 patients treated with ECT found disorientation in 13% of over 65s and 10% of under 65s (Alexopoulos et al., 1984). Of the elderly group 25% had a preexisting organic brain syndrome, in comparison with none of the younger group who became disorientated.

Confusion was also the most frequently diagnosed complication in Cattan et al.'s. (1990) review of the medical records of 81 people over 65 years old who were treated with ECT. It affected 45% of 65–80 year olds and 59% of the over 80s. It was defined as 'a lack of awareness of time, place and person severe enough to interfere with patients activities of daily living or to cause delay of next ECT treatment or to persist at the time of discharge'. Memory difficulty alone and transient confusion which did not affect the patients' activities of daily living were excluded. Daniel and Crovitz (1986), in an earlier study, had not demonstrated a relationship between age and severity of postECT disorientation in an elderly population.

Fraser and Glass (1980) investigated memory in 29 elderly people treated with unilateral or bilateral ECT. Of those who completed a side-effects questionnaire, 18% reported confusion and in all cases this was mild or moderate in severity. Memory was assessed using the seven subtests of the Wechsler Memory Scale: all except the orientation scale were impaired before treatment. During treatment all scores improved, and at three weeks posttreatment scores were within one standard deviation of available age-related norms. There was no difference between unilateral and bilateral treatment groups. These findings support clinical experience that relieving the memory deficit related to depression in the elderly more than compensates for any memory deficit related to ECT. Fogel (1988) pointed this out in his clinical research agenda, and also noted that it is particularly important to know the functional consequences of any loss of memory related to ECT in older people. O'Shea and colleagues (1987) documented the improvement in cognitive function in a 91 year old woman with a psychotic depressive illness treated with ECT. Their case typifies the clinical experience of many old age psychiatrists.

Attitudes and knowledge among elderly people regarding memory and ECT

Freeman and Kendell (1980), and later Benbow (1988*b*) investigated attitudes and knowledge regarding ECT. The results of the two studies are remarkably similar, despite the differing age profiles of the two patient groups. Most people agreed that the side-effects of ECT were not severe, but felt that ECT has an effect on memory. Approximately a quarter of both series felt that ECT causes permanent memory changes and about a third reported that their memory had not returned to normal following ECT. Nevertheless 65% of Freeman and Kendell's patients and 85% of Benbow's stated that they would be prepared to have ECT again.

Malcolm (1989) found that, of 100 people assessed before starting their treatment, under 65 year olds were better informed than over 65 year olds about ECT. Younger people were, however, more fearful of treatment than older ones. Fear of permanent memory impairment was ranked as the aspect of ECT most feared partway through a course of treatment in Gomez' study (1975), and memory loss was second only to brain damage of ranked fears reported by patients before receiving treatment (46% compared with 53%) (Malcolm, 1989). Repeated explanation of the effect of ECT on memory prior to and during treatment may be helpful in reassuring people.

Relevant findings in studies of other people's attitudes to memory and ECT

Attitudes towards ECT have been studied amongst various groups. Kalayam and Steinhart (1981) questioned psychiatrists, psychiatric nurses, psychologists, psychiatric social workers and members of the general public.All groups agreed on 'the relative absence of a generalized and persistent memory loss'. Kalayam & Steinhart did not comment on the ages of their responders, nor whether they had views on age in relation to the use of ECT.

Kerr and coworkers (1982) administered a questionnaire to patients who had received ECT and to two groups of hospital visitors: group 1 were visitors to nonECT-treated patients and group 2 were visitors to ECT-treated patients. Visitors to nonECT-treated patients were more likely to agree that 'whole parts of memory are permanently wiped out' by ECT than visitors to ECT-treated patients (46% compared with 37%). The authors concluded that personal experience of ECT, either by receiving the treatment or visiting someone who has received it, improves knowledge and alleviates misconceptions. For all three groups taken together, the older the person was the more likely they were to hold correct beliefs and to be unafraid of treatment. However, almost one-third of people who had been treated with ECT agreed with what the authors described as a gross overstatement, which must be a matter of concern for doctors who prescribe ECT.

Some evidence suggests that people's attitudes to ECT become more positive as their knowledge of ECT improves. Guze and coworkers (1988) showed this in relation to attorneys, Poster, Baxter & Hammon (1985) in nursing students and Benbow (1990) in medical students. Similarly Janicak et al. (1985) showed that a more positive attitude towards ECT correlated with increased clinical experience of the treatment in four groups of mental health professionals. Since evidence suggests that people's attitudes to ECT become more positive as their knowledge improves, full explanation to patients and their relatives is important. Freeman & Cheshire's (1986) suggestion that, after receiving ECT, people should be given a further explanation of why they were treated with this form of treatment and what was involved is particularly pertinent for older people who may have memory problems related to their treatment and/or their depressive illness.

Other side-effects

In the South Manchester retrospective study of elderly people treated with ECT (Benbow, 1987), some side-effects other than confusion and forgetfulness were recorded in the case-notes: headache (1.6%), falls (0.5%) and nausea and vomiting (0.5%). Fraser & Glass (1980) used a simple ad hoc questionnaire prospectively to enquire about headache, nausea or vomiting, double vision, tremor, fatigue, drowsiness, or any other side-effect. They concluded that there was only a low incidence of side-effects and that they tended to be mild. Of their courses, 45% were free of any side-effect, 32% were complicated by headaches and 9% by nausea/ vomiting. Ataxia occurred in 41% of courses, and drowsiness (14%) and double vision (5%) were also reported. Patients were not drug free: psychotropic medication was omitted for 24 hours before treatment in their study, and was continued throughout Benbow's (1987). However, since clinical practice often involves concomitant drug usage, these results are relevant to ECT practice with older people. As with the cognitive side-effects of ECT, repeated explantaion of the nature, frequency and course of side-effects during treatment may reassure recipients.

Efficacy

Rates of response to ECT among groups of elderly people have shown a remarkable consistency and are presented in Table 26.2. Overall it is likely that 70–80% of affectively ill elderly people treated with ECT can be expected to show a marked improvement or recover fully.

There have been differences in the length of course reported in different studies. Benbow (1987) used bilateral ECT and the mean course length was 8.3 treatments, whereas Godber and colleagues (1987) used unilateral ECT with a mean of 11.2. In practice, clinicians monitor individual response as a course of treatment progresses and the total length of the course will depend on diagnosis, speed of response, knowledge of any previous response to ECT, severity of illness and quality of response to any previous treatments, as well as treatment variables (Abrams, 1988*b*). One of the main treatment issues is whether unilateral or bilateral treatment should be regarded as preferable for older people.

Some authors have suggested that unilateral nondominant ECT should be routinely administered to older people and those with coexisting physical illnesses because of research suggesting less cognitive impairment and shorter recovery time with unilateral treatment (e.g. Heshe, Roeder & Theilgaard, 1978; Fraser & Glass, 1980; Fontaine & Young, 1985). It seems that, for many depressed people, unilateral and bilateral ECT appear to be equivalent (Abrams, 1988*c*). However, there is evidence that, for some people, unilateral ECT produces less improvement than bilateral and may require more applications to produce the same outcome. Stroemgren (1973) found a comparable therapeutic effect was achieved using significantly fewer bilateral than unilateral treatments in people aged over 44 years. Heshe, Roeder & Theilgaard (1978) found similar results in people aged over 60 years. Pettinati et al. (1986) conducted a meta-analysis and demonstrated a larger bilateral over unilateral advantage for older people treated with ECT. There is also a group of people who respond to bilateral treatment, but not to unilateral (Price, 1981; Abrams et al., 1983). The case in favor of unilateral ECT in late life is not as clearcut as has been suggested in the past. The Royal College of Psychiatrists document 'The Practical Administration of Electroconvulsive Therapy' concluded that unilateral is a less effective antidepressant treatment than bilateral and that 'where the depressive illness is severe and where speed of action is important, bilateral ECT is the treatment of choice' (Freeman et al., 1989). These two conditions often apply in late life, and a case can be made for regarding bilateral ECT as preferable, given present ECT practice in the UK. The American Psychiatric Association Task Force Report (1990) states that the choice of unilateral or bilateral treatment should be made by 'ongoing analysis of applicable risks and benefits': unilateral ECT is most strongly indicated when minimization of cognitive side-effects is important, and bilateral ECT may be preferred when

Table 26.2. *Recovery rates in elderly populations treated with ECT*

Study	Year	Number of patients	Mean age	Outcome much improved/ recovered
Fraser & Glass	1980	33	73	97%
Gaspar & Samarasinghe	1982	33	73.9	78.8%
Karlinsky & Shulman	1984	33	73.2	78.8%
Godber et al.	1987	163	76	74%
Benbow	1987	122	73	80%
Rubin, Kinscherf & Wehrman	1991	46	75.9	78%

treatment is urgent or the person has failed to respond to unilateral treatment. Abrams (1988*d*) regards concurrent high-risk medical conditions, where fewer anaesthetic inductions are to be preferred, as another indication for selection of bilateral treatment.

Frequency of treatment with ECT is another practice issue. The Royal College document on ECT (Freeman et al., 1989) states that ECT should be given two or three times weekly. Fraser & Glass (1978) studied nine patients treated with a course of alternating bilateral and unilateral treatments, and demonstrated longer recovery time after bilateral compared with unilateral treatment. They also showed a cumulative effect of bilateral ECT, i.e. time for recovery after bilateral ECT became longer as the course progressed. An interval effect was also noted with bilateral treatment, i.e. recovery time was further prolonged if treatments were closer together (at an interval of one day rather than two). The authors interpreted these findings as favoring the use of unilateral ECT (although a later study did not confirm a cumulative effect (Fraser & Glass, 1980)). Alternatively, these results would support longer intervals between bilateral treatments (twice weekly rather than thrice), and the longer recovery time would suggest that bilateral ECT may not be advisable for elderly day or out-patients. Abrams (1988*b*) notes a further possible advantage of twice weekly treatment, stating that it gives time for the full effect of each treatment to develop.

ECT and treatment-resistant depression in late life

One would expect that people whose depressive illnesses are resistant to drug treatments will be more likely to receive ECT. This may explain why prolonged length of stay has been shown to be related to receipt of ECT (Herr, Abrams & Anderson, 1991). Prudic, Sackeim & Devanand (1990) found that those people who failed to respond to adequate pharmacological treatment preECT were less likely to respond to a course of treatment than those who had not failed to respond to adequate drug treatment beforehand (50% response, compared with 94% in the nonresistant group). They also showed that relapse following ECT was more likely in thc treatment-resistant group.

Despite these findings, ECT may have an important role to play in treatment resistant depression (TRD) in late life. Murphy's study (1983) of the prognosis of depressive illness in the elderly reported a poor outcome in 65% of people: only 16% of the patients followed by her received ECT. Of Baldwin & Jolley's patients (1986), 48% received ECT and only 7% had a poor outcome. Could ECT be relevant to the development of TRD in later life depressions?

A retrospective case-note study by Magni, Fisman & Helmes (1988) compared ECT resistant elderly patients with ECT responders. Before ECT, all but two patients had received a tricyclic antidepressant for a minimum of 28 days at an increasing dose until either a therapeutic dose was attained or mild side-effects developed. Of 30 ECT-treated patients 63% recovered. The remaining 27% (11) (who had all failed to respond to a minimum of seven bilateral treatments) fitted their definition of ECT-resistance: 'no significant improvement in their clinical conditions and... continued to present the clinical features of major depression'. Morris (1991) found a similar proportion of nonresponse in a prospective study of patients aged over 65 years referred for ECT.

Magni, Fisman & Helmes' nonresponders had a significantly higher frequency of onset of physical illness during the index episode, fewer life events before the onset of the index episode and a higher frequency of preceeding depressive episode of longer duration. The connection between longer duration of illness and poor treatment outcome leads Fink (1989) to argue that ECT should be considered early in the course of TRD.

These studies are intruiging, but our understanding of treatment-resistance in later life is, as yet, poorly developed. The role of ECT in TRD is an area of old age psychiatry which will benefit from further exploration in order that rational treatment programs can be developed.

Continuation/ maintenance treatment

Scott, Weeks & McDonald (1991) recently described a 67 year old woman treated with continuation ECT for recurrent unipolar depressive illness. They distinguished continuation treatment designed to minimize the re-emergence of symptoms of the index illness from prophylactic (or maintenance) treatment, designed to minimize the likelihood of further episodes of illness.

Of old age psychiatrists 20% indicated in a recent survey that they used maintenance ECT (Benbow, 1991), and others appended comments indicating that they would consider its use as an option for appropriate individuals. These figures are similar to those reported earlier by Pippard & Ellam (1981). However, maintenance ECT was not defined, and respondents probably did not distinguish between continuation and prophylactic treatment. Nevertheless, it seems that maintenance ECT is used more often than standard teaching would suggest, despite Kendell's (1981) comments that the practice is not established.

In the older literature, maintenance treatment was regarded as most effective for the depresssive illnesses of late life (Moore, 1943), and the treatment regimes used would probably be seen by modern practitioners as heroic, involving treatment programs measured in years (Stevenson & Geoghegan, 1951). There are descriptions of patients who did very well on long courses of maintenance ECT (Wolff, 1957). Despite the lack of scientific studies supporting the ongoing use of maintenance treatment, clinicians have continued to recognize a limited role for it, after the advent of lithium and newer antidepressant drugs.

The American Psychiatric Association Task Force Report (1990) has laid down criteria for maintenance/continuation ECT in the USA, but Duncan et al. (1990) pointed out that, until controlled prospective trials are carried out, clinicians can only rely on a flexible approach, tailored to each individual patient.

Consent

Murphy (1988) has claimed that psychiatrists who work with elderly people are treating patients of whom approximately two-thirds will be unable to give real consent to treatment. If this is true, consent to prescription of ECT for older people will be a particular problem.

Benbow (1987) found that 8.3% of courses administered to elderly people in South Manchester were given under the provisions of the Mental Health Act (1959). Since then the law has changed, and in Central Manchester recently 24% of a group of elderly people who received ECT did so under the Mental Mealth Act. A mixed age study found that almost one-third of patients expressed dissatisfaction with the way they had been asked to give consent, and a minority (19%) could not remember ever having consented (Benbow, 1988*b*).

Martin & Bean (1992) have addressed the issues involved in competence to consent to ECT, from a North American perspective. As they point out, there are no pass/fail criteria for competence, and the fact that capacity to consent has not been defined indicates that it is an elusive concept. Consent assumes that information has been presented to patients previously, and assessment of the person's understanding of that information and how they use it in reaching a decision about treatment forms part of the assessment of competence to consent. The Royal College of Psychiatrists document on the practical administration of ECT stresses that consent is a continuous process (or, as the American Psychiatric Association (1990) describes it, a dynamic process), and that the patient may

Table 26.3. *Modifications of ECT technique to minimize cognitive side-effects of treatments*

Technical factor	How to minimize side-effects
1. Stimulus	a. Change sine wave to brief pulse. b. Decrease dose of electricity.
2. Electrode position	Change bilateral to unilateral.
3. Frequency of treatment	Decrease frequency from thrice weekly to twice, or twice weekly to once.
4. Concomitant drugs	a. Consider whether any drugs are raising seizure threshold. If so reduce dose or stop them. b. If patient on psychotropics, decrease dose or discontinue.
5. Anaesthetic drugs	Ask anaesthetist to decrease dose if possible.

withdraw consent at any time (Freeman et al., 1989). Similarly, explanation of ECT is also continuous. UK practice emphasizes verbal explanation, whereas US practice emphasizes written information, supplemented by verbal. The best current practice should involve both. During, and after, treatment older people should be given repeated explanations of why they have been treated with ECT and what the treatment entailed, because of memory impairment related to the treatment and to the depressive illness itself (Freeman & Cheshire, 1986).

ECT in late life: practical conclusions

The main indication for treating older people with ECT is severe depressive illness, and 70–80% of people will show a good treatment response. ECT has been used despite a wide variety of physical illnesses and advanced age. There are no absolute contraindications to its use. All coexisting medical conditions should be fully assessed and, if possible, treated before administering ECT. The decision to prescribe will involve a detailed consideration of the balance between risks and benefits. Patients and their families should be involved in this process as fully as possible.

Many elderly people experience side-effects during treatment. Forgetfullness and confusion are not uncommonly observed, or complained of, during treatment. After completion of treatment, current evidence suggests that memory on testing will have improved in comparison with baseline assessments. Greater age and preexisting cognitive impairments increase the risk of these side-effects and there may be grounds for considering unilateral treatment as the preferred technique in these circumstances. Should a person treated with unilateral ECT fail to respond, however, they may respond if transferred to bilateral treatment.

ECT-related cognitive side-effects can be minimized by attention to technique (see Table 26.3). Regular assessment of memory, orientation and subjective experience is advisable throughout the course of ECT. This will allow the early detection of side-effects, and treatment technique can then be reviewed in order to minimize any possible contributory factors. These precautions are of even greater importance when a person with a known concomitant dementia is receiving treatment. Sometimes a prolonged confusional state may develop, but close monitoring should detect this early.

Maintenance ECT is still used with elderly people who respond to treatment and have an established relapsing illness. Flexible treatment regimes are preferable to the more rigid protocols of the past.

References

Abrams, R. (ed.) (1988*a*). Medical considerations: the high-risk patient. *Electroconvulsive Therapy*, Chapter 5, pp.53–78. Oxford: Oxford University Press.

Abrams, R. (ed.) (1988*b*). Technique of electroconvulsive therapy. *Electroconvulsive Therapy*, Chapter 6, pp. 79–108. Oxford: Oxford University Press.

Abrams, R. (ed.) (1988*c*). The electroconvulsive therapy stimulus: technical and theoretical considerations. *Electroconvulsive Therapy*, Chapter 7, pp. 109–116. Oxford: Oxford University Press.

Abrams, R. (ed.) (1988*d*). Unilateral electroconvulsive therapy. *Electroconvulsive Therapy*, Chapter 8, pp. 117–129. Oxford: Oxford University Press.

Abrams, R., Taylor, M. A., Faber, R. et al. (1983). Bilateral versus unilateral ECT: efficacy in melancholia. *American Journal of Psychiatry*, **140**, 463–5.

Alexopoulos, G. S., Shamoian, C. J., Lucas, J., Weiser, N. & Berger, H. (1984). Medical problems of geriatric psychiatric patients and younger controls during electroconvulsive therapy. *Journal of the American Geriatrics Society*, **32**, 651–4.

American Psychiatric Association Task Force Report (1990). *The Practice of Electroconvulsive Therapy: Recommendations for Treatment, Training and Privileging.* Washington: American Psychiatric Association.

Baldwin, R. C. & Jolley, D. J. (1986). The prognosis of depression in old age. *British Journal of Psychiatry*, **149**, 574–83.

Benbow, S. M. (1987). The use of electroconvulsive therapy in old age psychiatry. *International Journal of Geriatric Psychiatry*, **2**, 25–30.

Benbow, S. M. (1988*a*). ECT for depression in dementia. *British Journal of Psychiatry*, **152**, 859.

Benbow, S. M. (1988*b*). Patients' views on electroconvulsive therapy on completion of a course of treatment. *Convulsive Therapy*, **4**, 146–52.

Benbow, S. M. (1989). The role of electroconvulsive therapy in the treatment of depressive illness in late life. *British Journal of Psychiatry*, **155**, 147–52.

Benbow, S. M. (1990). Medical students and electroconvulsive therapy: their knowledge and attitudes. *Convulsive Therapy*, **6**, 32–7.

Benbow, S. M. (1991). Old age psychiatrists views on the use of ECT. *International Journal of Geriatric Psychiatry*, **6**, 317–22.
Benbow, S. M. (1992). Is ECT useful for depression with dementia? *Paper presented at First European Symposium on ECT*, Graz, Austria, March 26–29 1992
Burke, W. J., Rutherford, J. L., Zorumski, C. F. et al. (1985). Electroconvulsive therapy and the elderly. *Comprehensive Psychiatry*, **26**, 480–6.
Cardno, A. G. & Simpson, C. J. (1991). Electroconvulsive therapy in Paget's disease and hydrocephalus. *Convulsive Therapy*, **7**, 48–51.
Cattan, R. A., Barry, P. P., Mead, G., Reefe, W. E., Gay, A. & Silverman, M. (1990). Electroconvulsive therapy in octogenarians. *Journal of the American Geriatrics Society*, **38**, 753–8.
Coryell, M. & Zimmerman, M. (1984). Outcome following ECT for primary unipolar depression: a test of newly proposed response predictors. *American Journal of Psychiatry*, **141**, 862–7.
Daniel, W. F. & Crovitz, H. F. (1986). Disorientation during electroconvulsive therapy. *Annals of the New York Academy of Sciences*, **462**, 293–306.
Demuth, G. W. & Rand, B. S. (1980). Atypical major depression in a patient with severe primary degenerative dementia. *American Journal of Psychiatry* **137**, 1609–10.
Devanand, D. P., Malitz, S. & Sackeim, H. A. (1990). ECT in a patient with aortic aneurysm. *Journal of Clinical Psychiatry*, **51**, 255–6.
Dubovsky, S. L., Gay, M., Franks, R. D. & Hadderhorst, A. (1985). ECT in the presence of increased intracranial pressure and respiratory failure: case report. *Journal of Clinical Psychiatry*, **46**, 489–91.
Duncan, A. J., Ungvari, G. S., Russell, R. J. et al. (1990). Maintenance ECT in very old age. *Annals of Clinical Psychiatry*, **2**, 1–6.
Fink, M. (1989). The efficacy of electroconvulsive therapy in therapy-resistant psychotic patients. *Journal of Clinical Psychopharmacology*, **9**, 231–2.
Fogel, B. S. (1988). Electroconvulsive therapy in the elderly: a clinical research agenda. *International Journal of Geriatric Psychiatry*, **3**, 181–90.
Fontaine, R. & Young, T. (1985). Unilateral ECT: advantages and efficacy in the treatment of depression. *Canadian Journal of Psychiatry*, **30**, 142–7.
Fraser, R. M. (1981). ECT and the elderly. In *Electroconvulsive Therapy: an Appraisal*, ed. R. L. Palmer. Oxford: Oxford University Press.
Fraser, R. M. & Glass, I. B. (1980). Unilateral and bilateral ECT in elderly patients: a comparative study. *Acta Psychiatrica Scandinavica*, **62**, 13–31.
Freeman, C. P. L. & Cheshire, K. E. (1986). Attitude studies on electroconvulsive therapy. *Convulsive Therapy*, **2**, 31–42.
Freeman, C., Crammer, J. L., Deakin, J. F. W., McClelland, R., Mann, S. A. & Pippard, J. (1989). *The practical administration of electroconvulsive therapy (ECT)*. London: Gaskell.
Freeman, C. P. L. & Kendell, R. E. (1980). ECT: 1. Patients' experiences and attitudes. *British Journal of Psychiatry*, **137**, 8–16.
Gaspar, D. & Samarasinghe, L. A. (1982). ECT in psychogeriatric practice – a study of risk factors, indications and outcome. *Comprehensive Psychiatry*, **23**, 170–5.
Gerring, J. P. & Shields, H. M. (1982). The identification and management of patients

with a high risk for cardiac arrhythmias during modified ECT. *Journal of Clinical Psychiatry*, **43**, 140–3.

Godber, C., Rosenvinge, H., Wilkinson, D. et al. (1987). Depression in old age: prognosis after ECT. *International Journal of Geriatric Psychiatry*, **2**, 19–24.

Gold, L. & Chiarella, C. J. (1944). The prognostic value of clinical findings in cases treated with electric shock. *Journal of Nervous and Mental Diseases*, **100**, 577–83.

Gomez, J. (1975). Subjective side-effects of ECT. *British Journal of Psychiatry* **127**, 609–11.

Greenwald, B. S., Kramer-Ginsberg, E., Marin, D. B., Laitman, L. B., Hermann, C. K., Mohs, R. C. and Davis, K. L. (1989). Dementia with coexistent major depression. *American Journal of Psychiatry*, **146**, 1472–8.

Guze, B. H., Baxter, L. R., Liston, E. H. & Roy-Byrne, P. (1988). Attorneys perceptions of electroconvulsive therapy: impact of instruction with an ECT videotape demonstration. *Comprehensive Psychiatry*, **29**, 520–2.

Hamilton, M. (1982). Prediction of the response of depressions to ECT. In *Electroconvulsive Therapy: Biological Foundations and Clinical Applications* ed. R. Abrams & WB Essman. Lancaster: MTP Press.

Hay, D. P. (1989). Electroconvulsive therapy in the medically ill elderly. *Convulsive Therapy*, **5**, 8–16.

Herr, B. E., Abraham, H. D. & Anderson, W. (1991) Length of stay in a general hospital psychiatric unit. *General Hospital Psychiatry*, **13**, 68–70.

Heshe, J., Roeder, E. & Theilgaard, A. (1978). Unilateral and bilateral ECT. A psychiatric and psychological study of therapeutic effect and side-effects. *Acta Psychiatrica Scandinavica* (suppl. 275).

Hobson, R. F. (1953). Prognostic factors in electric convulsive therapy. *Journal of Neurology, Neurosurgery and Psychiatry*, **16**, 275–81.

Hsiao, J. K. & Evans, D. L. (1984). ECT in a depressed patient after craniotomy. *American Journal of Psychiatry*, **141**, 442–4.

Huang, K. C., Lucas, L. F., Tsueda, K. et al. (1989). Age-related changes in cardiovascular function associated with electroconvulsive therapy. *Convulsive Therapy* **5**, 17–25.

Janicak, P. G., Mask, J., Kestutis, M. S. W., Trimakas, K. A. & Gibbons, R. (1985) ECT: an assessment of mental health professionals knowledge and attitudes. *Journal of Clinical Psychiatry* **46**, 262–6.

Kalayam, B. & Steinhart, M. J. (1981). A survey of attitudes on the use of electroconvulsive therapy. *Hospital and Community Psychiatry* **32**, 185–8.

Karlinsky, H. & Shulman, K. T. (1984) The clinical use of electroconvulsive therapy in old age. *Journal of the American Geriatrics Society*, **32**, 183–6.

Kellner, C. H. & Rameo, L. J. (1990). Case report: dexamethasone pretreatment for ECT in an elderly patient with meningioma. *Clinical Gerontologist*, **10**, 67–70.

Kellner, C. H., Tolhurst, J. E. & Burns, C. M. (1991). ECT in the presence of severe cervical spine disease. *Convulsive Therapy*, **7**, 52–5.

Kendell, R. E. (1981). The present status of electroconvulsive therapy. *British Journal of Psychiatry*, **139**, 265–83.

Kerr, R. A., McGrath, J. J., O'Kearney, R. T. & Price, J. (1982). ECT: misconceptions and attitudes. *Australian and New Zealand Journal of Psychiatry*, **16**, 43–9.

Liang, R. A., Lam, R. W. & Ancill, R. J. (1988). ECT in the treatment of mixed depression and dementia. *British Journal of Psychiatry*, **152**, 281–4.

Loo, H., Cuche, H. & Benkelfat, C. (1985). Electroconvulsive therapy during anticoagulant therapy. *Convulsive Therapy*, **1**, 258–62.

Magni, G., Fisman, M. & Helmes, E. (1988). Clinical correlates of ECT-resistant depression in the elderly. *Journal of Clinical Psychiatry*, **49**, 405–7.

Malcolm, K. (1989). Patients' perceptions and knowledge of electroconvulsive therapy. *Psychiatric Bulletin*, **13**, 161–5.

Malcolm, K. & Peet, M. (1989). The use of electroconvulsive therapy in elderly depressive patients. In *Antidepressants for Elderly People*, ed. K. Ghose. Chapter 14, pp. 235–251. London: Chapman & Hall.

Malek-Ahmadi, P., Beceiro, J. R., McNeil, B. W. & Weddige, R. L. (1990). Electroconvulsive therapy and chronic subdural hematoma. *Convulsive Therapy*, **6**, 38–41.

Maneksha, F. R. (1991). Hypertension and tachycardia during electroconvulsive therapy: to treat or not to treat? *Convulsive Therapy*, **7**, 28–35.

Martin, B. A. & Bean, G. J. (1992). Competence to consent to electroconvulsive therapy. *Convulsive Therapy*, **8**, 92–102.

McAllister, T. W. & Price, T. R. P. (1982). Severe depressive pseudodementia with and without dementia. *American Journal of Psychiatry*, **139**, 626–9.

Mendels, J. (1967). The prediction of response to electroconvulsive therapy. *American Journal of Psychiatry*, **124**, 153–9.

Moore, N. P. (1943). The maintenance treatment of chronic psychotics by electrically induced convulsions. *Journal of Mental Science*, **89**, 257–69.

Morris, P. D. (1991). Which elderly depressives will respond to ECT? *International Journal of Geriatric Psychiatry*, **6**, 159–63.

Murphy, E. (1983). The prognosis of depression in old age. *British Journal of Psychiatry*, **142**, 111–19.

Murphy, E. (1988). Psychiatric implications. *In Consent and the Incompetent Patient: Ethics, Law and Medicine*, ed. S. R. Hirsch & J. Harris, Chapter 6, p 65–73. London: Gaskell.

Murray, G. B., Shea, V. & Conn, D. K. (1986). Electroconvulsive therapy for post-stroke depression. *Journal of Clinical Psychiatry*, **47**, 258–60.

Nelson, J. P. & Rosenberg, D. R. (1991). ECT treatment of demented elderly patients with major depression: a retrospective study of efficacy and safety. *Convulsive Therapy*, **7**, 157–65.

O'Shea, B., Lynch, T., Falvey, J. & O'Mahoney, G. (1987). Electroconvulsive therapy and cognitive improvement in a very elderly depressed patient. *British Journal of Psychiatry*, **150**, 255–7.

Perrin, G. M. (1961). Cardiovascular aspects of electric shock therapy. *Acta Psychiatrica Scandinavica*, **36**, 1–45.

Perry, G. F. (1983). ECT for dementia and catatonia. *Journal of Clinical Psychiatry*, **44**, 117.

Pettinati, H. M., Mathisen, K. S., Rosenberg, J. et al. (1986). Meta-analytical approach to reconciling discrepancies in efficacy between bilateral and unilateral electroconvulsive therapy. *Convulsive Therapy*, **2**, 7–17.

Pippard, J. & Ellam, L. (1981). *Electroconvulsive treatment in Great Britain 1980*. London: Gaskell.

Poster, E., Baxter, L. R. & Hammon, C. L. (1985). Nursing students' perception of electroconvulsive therapy: impact of instruction with an electroconvulsive therapy videotape. *Convulsive Therapy*, **1**, 277–82.

Price, T. R. P. (1981). Unlateral electroconvulsive therapy for depression. *New England Journal of Medicine*, **304**, 53.

Price, T. R. P. & McAllister, T. W. (1989). Safety and efficacy of ECT in depressed patients with dementia: a review of clinical experience. *Convulsive Therapy*, **5**, 61–74.

Prudic, J., Sackeim, H. A. & Devanand, D. P. (1990). Medication resistance and clinical response to electroconvulsive therapy. *Psychiatry Research*, **31**, 287–96.

Regestein, Q. R. & Lind, L. J. (1980). Management of electroconvulsive treatment of an elderly woman with severe hypertension and cardiac arrhythmias. *Comprehensive Psychiatry*, **21**, 288–91.

Roberts, J. M. (1959). Prognostic features in the electroshock treatment of depressive states 1. clinical features from history and examination. *Journal of Mental Science*, **105**, 693–702.

Rosenfeld, J. E., Glassberg, S. & Sherrid, M. (1988). Administration of ECT four years after aortic aneurysm dissection. *American Journal of Psychiatry*, **145**, 128–9.

Rubin, E. H., Kinscherf, D. A. & Wehrman, S. A. (1991). Response to treatment of depression in the old and the very old. *Journal of Geriatric Psychiatry and Neurology*, **4**, 65–70.

Salzman, C. (1982). Electroconvulsive therapy in the elderly patient. *Psychiatric Clinics of North America*, **5**, 191–7.

Scott, A. I. F., Weeks, D. J. & McDonald, C. F. (1991). Continuation electroconvulsive therapy: preliminary guidelines and an illustrative case report. *British Journal of Psychiatry*, **159**, 867–70.

Snow, S. S. & Wells, C. E. (1981). Case studies in neuropsychiatry: diagnosis and treatment of coexistent dementia and depression. *Journal of Clinical Psychiatry*, **42**, 439–41.

Stevenson, G. H. & Geoghegan, J. J. (1951). Prophylactic electroshock. *American Journal of Psychiatry* **107**, 743–8.

Stroemgren, L. S. (1973). Unilateral versus bilateral electroconvulsive therapy. *Acta Psychiatrica Scandinavica* (suppl. 240).

Summers, W. K., Robins, E. & Reich, T. (1979). The natural history of acute organic mental syndrome after bilateral electroconvulsive therapy. *Biological Psychiatry*, **14**, 905–12.

Tancer, M. E. & Evans, D. L. (1989). Electroconvulsive therapy in geriatric patients undergoing anticoagulation therapy. *Convulsive Therapy*, **5**, 102–9.

Tsuang, M. T., Tidball, J. S. & Geller, D. (1979). ECT in a depressed patient with shunt in place for normal pressure hydrocephalus. *American Journal of Psychiatry*, **136**, 1205–6.

Weiner, R. D. (1982). The role of electroconvulsive therapy in the treatment of depression in the elderly. *Journal of the American Geriatrics Society*, **30**, 710–12.

Wolff, G. E. (1957). Results of four years active therapy for chronic mental patients and the value of an individual maintenance dose of ECT. *American Journal of Psychiatry*, **114**, 453–6.

Zwil, A. S., McAllister, T. W. & Price, T. R. P. (1992). Safety and efficacy of ECT in depressed patients with organic brain disease: review of a clinical experience. *Convulsive Therapy*, **8**, 103–9.

27

Family therapy

BARBARA KNOTHE PETER McARDLE

Introduction

This chapter begins with the definitions of family therapy, gives an overview of the complex historical developments of the family therapy field, discusses the meager literature on the applications of family therapy to the elderly and ends with suggestions as to how the practitioner can apply family therapy concepts in their daily work. The chapter reflects the thinking of the two authors, who have been collaborating over the last three years in a project introducing family therapy into a geriatric psychiatry service.

The term family therapy can be used to describe interventions that can be added to other treatments within the framework of the biomedical model or the term can be used to describe an alternative model of helping people with problems. Family therapy as alternative model is also called the system or systemic model and it assumes that, to understand and help the older person with symptoms and signs of a functional psychiatric disorder, the clinician should have an understanding of the way symptoms and signs in an individual can be influenced by, and in turn influence interactions, behaviors and beliefs in other people, particularly in the family.

To clarify this distinction, it is useful to make the assumption that communications made by people can be understood in different ways.

Biomedical model

A clinician using the biomedical model, listening to an account given by an older person or one of their relatives would be listening for evidence and watching for behavior that helps them to decide what is wrong with the person. They are particularly interested in symptoms and signs that help to make a diagnosis of the older person's physical and mental state in order to decide from what disease, illness or syndrome they are suffering. They may also ask questions and be interested in emotional, psychological and social issues but these have less ranking in their assessment.

Family therapy model

A family therapist using a family therapy model, listening to an account given by the same older person and other family members would be listening for evidence and watching for behavior that helps them to understand how this particular family organizes itself and how the symptomatic behavior makes sense in the context of this family. To complicate this issue further, it must be said that at the present time family therapists do not yet have one coherent theoretical framework so they vary in what they pay attention to. The diversity of beliefs and orientations of family therapists probably reflects the complexity of families and the stage of development of the field. Harari & Bloch (1991) and Sluzki (1983) have attempted to integrate some of the theories.

The ways of thinking about families can be loosely grouped into five models, four of them alternatives to the biomedical model, the fifth being additive to this model. The first model describes the family as a homeostatic or cybernetic system with rules governing its functioning. Symptomatic behavior maintains the equilibrium of the system and prevents it from breaking down into its component parts (or people).

The second model considers the family as an entity which evolves over time from a less complex to a more complex state and that symptomatic behavior occurs around the transformation to a different order of complexity. Hoffman (1981) provided a detailed account of the historical development of these differing concepts.

The third model tries to combine some system understanding while incorporating evolving ideas from feminist scholarship. Luepnitz (1988) engaged in a feminist critique of the main schools of family therapy and proposed a feminist form of family therapy.

The fourth model focuses on how language itself determines how we understand our world and how we function. Our life can then be considered like a novel or a play with the narrative determining how we experience our life and the option becomes available of rewriting the plot and living a new, different story. (Lowe, 1990, Anderson & Goolishian, 1988, White & Epston, 1989).

Whichever focus the family therapist uses, the intention is to find ways of influencing family members to change, in the belief that changes in the family will be more potent than changes in the individual alone and that changes in the family will lead to changes in the individual. Family therapy as model does not include the direct cause and effect thinking that applies in the more linear biomedical model where an antecedent is believed to cause a subsequent event such as when a biological shift in an older person is believed to cause a subsequent depressive illness in that person.

Thinking about causality is replaced by thinking about circularity. Circularity implies that people, events and meanings mutually and reciprocally influence each other. How a family responds to illness in a member influences the member's illness and if the family responds differently then the illness can be influenced and modified. Both the strength and the limitations of this concept are immediately obvious and will not be discussed further.

Returning to the example of the family with a member showing symptoms and signs of depression, the family therapist wants to know how family members respond to the sad appearance and other signals of depression and what happens as family members influence each other over time, in order to intervene and change the interactions. The interventions could tackle the person's behavior or family members' responses or other aspects of family life.

It will be obvious to the reader that this use of family therapy as a model could lead to conflict between the clinician convinced of the rightness of the biomedical model of depression as illness and the family therapist convinced of the rightness of the alternative view of depression as understandable in the context of the family interactions. Their views as to the correct treatment or intervention would also be potentially in conflict. It seems to be inevitable that we believe certain views of the world to be more legitimate than others and clinicians convinced of the rightness of their world view will vary in the degree to which they are open to be persuaded of the usefulness of other world views. If both models are accepted as right in their own way, then the alternative approach of holding both models in one's mind at the same time becomes possible. Two clinicians can work together accepting that each model will have useful explanatory functions at different times with different families or with the same family at a different point in time. This has been our experience, working in close collaboration, as we tried to find out what aspects of family therapy could be applied in the geriatric psychiatry setting.

The fifth form of family therapy evolved in settings where people were using the biomedical model but addressing the influence that families can have on the progress and outcome of psychiatric illnesses. This form of family therapy has been called the psycho-educational approach and lends itself to easy application in geriatic psychiatry services.

The historical development of family therapy

It is useful to consider family therapy in an historical context as family therapy is an evolving discipline with many lessons learned that have application in working with older people.

Family therapy started in many different places more or less simultaneously.

Unlike psychoanalysis which is usually linked with Sigmund Freud as the originator, family therapists claim many people as their theoretical forebears. Family therapy theory can be thought of as an incomplete tapestry with different strands linking up for a while as some people worked together in the same work context, then diverging and moving off in different directions while remaining part of the overall whole.

One strand evolved out of work with children and adolescents. For example, John Bowlby's work on attachment theory and his (falsely) reported work in family interviews with adolescents at the Tavistock Clinic influenced John Bell to start holding conjoint family interviews in America. Meanwhile, Nathan Ackerman started to see whole families using an analytic framework. Salvador Minuchin worked with multiproblem families in the slums and later evolved the structural school of family therapy (Minuchin, 1974; Minuchin, Rosman & Baker, 1978; Minuchin & Fishman, 1981).

Another strand evolved out of the study of communications, including communications in families with a schizophrenic member. Gregory Bateson and his group including Jay Haley, Don Jackson and Virginia Satir evolved the cybernetic model of family functioning with concepts of homeostasis, patterns which connect family interactions, different levels of communication and the double bind theory of schizophrenia (Bateson & Ruesch, 1951, Bateson et al., 1956, Bateson, 1972). Satir brought into this group ideas developed in the social work field, that social context is important and went on to work with families using humanistic principles and deeply moving human experiences to create changes during sessions, these changes being maintained subsequently without further input (Satir, 1967). Jay Haley went on to focus on the importance of power in family relationships and with others who worked at the Mental Research Institute (MRI) after he left, developed strategic family therapy (Haley, 1976, 1980).

The Milan Associates, Palazzoli, Prata, Boscolo and Cecchin meanwhile developed their ideas working in private practice in Milan, Italy, seeing families with disturbed young adults (Palazolli, et al., 1978). For a long time they worked as a quartet and were influenced by Bateson and Weakland from MRI. Subsequently they separated into two pairs and have evolved along somewhat different lines (Palazzoli et al., 1989, Boscolo et al., 1987). Their model of family therapy is usually called Milan systemic therapy and incorporates circular questioning, hypothesizing and maintaining neutrality.

Murray Bowen at this time was admitting whole families with a schizophrenic member to hospital. The aim of his therapy was to help family members to differentiate from 'the undifferentiated family ego mass' which he believes is associated with schizophrenia in one family member (Bowen, 1978). The value of using the family life cycle as an organising principle was developed by his followers (Carter & McGoldrick, 1980).

Meanwhile in England two quite different strands were evolving. Laing (1960), Cooper (1971), Esterson (1970) and Szasz (1961) were describing their ideas linking schizophrenia in a causal way with the family. The idea that families 'cause' schizophrenia was a real hindrance for families who were already struggling with the difficult problem of how to deal with a psychotic member, and led to rejection of family therapy by many families and clinicians.

Much more promising and positive was the work being done at the Medical Research Council Social Psychiatry Unit in London where Leff, Vaughn and others were studying expressed emotion (EE). (Leff & Vaughn, 1981; Leff et al., 1982) They interviewed family members in the absence of the patient and measured how many critical or hostile comments were made about the patient. Relatives who made six or more critical comments, or one hostile remark, or showed evidence of marked overinvolvement with the patient were assessed as being high in EE. Relatives who showed none of these three behaviors were classified as being low in EE. Relapse of the schizophrenic illness was shown to be associated with contact with high EE families and interventions which lowered patients exposure to such behavior either by living away from the family, or by lowering the EE in the family, lowered the relapse rate. These findings of emotion being expressed by family members in the absence of the identified patient, were subsequently demonstrated to be shown to the same extent in interviews with the whole family (Szmukler et al., 1985). A completely different model of family intervention, called the psychoeducation model has evolved out of these later studies. A succinct summary of developments in the field of family therapy and its relevance to psychiatry is provided by Stagoll (1989). Some of the complex links between family theory, practice and philosophy are described by Harari and Bloch (1991).

Family therapy ideas useful for treating functional disorders in the elderly

In this section we describe the ideas which we have found to be useful and show their genesis.

The family life cycle

Like an individual, the family has an expected life cycle (Carter & McGoldrick, 1980). Biological factors in individual family members interact with social and cultural expectations as well as being altered by historical events affecting the family as a whole. For example, two major social changes which are altering the family life cycle at present include the increase in divorce leading to forms of family other than the nuclear family; and the tendency of divorced men who do not remarry not to maintain close ties with their family, leaving them at risk of isolation as they grow old. As well, the increasing number of women working outside of the family home leads to altered patterns of child-rearing and care of the aged family members. Other factors include changes in education with young adults staying at home for longer periods with consequent reduction in parental authority creating new issues to be dealt with by the family. Many western societies such as Australia are multicultural and quite diverse in their expectations of the duties of grandparents and personal care in late life (Brubaker, 1983; Browne, 1988; Bengtson & Robertson, 1985; Cherlin & Furstenberg, 1986; Denham & Smith, 1989).

The stages of the family life cycle include:

- the unattached young person
- courtship
- marriage
- a family with one child
- a family with two or more children
- a family with adolescent children
- launching of the young adults (empty nest)
- the couple in later life.

In this developmental model, the older person within the family has to negotiate a series of 'role transitions' which might include:

- the launching of young adults into the world and the re-establishment or refocusing of the marital couple's relationship,
- the empty nest or postparental stage,
- retirement of one or both members of the couple
- widowhood
- remarriage in later life
- being single because never married or divorced in later life
- grandparenthood
- relocation, a move to alternative accommodation such as a retirement village or supported accommodation such as hostels or nursing homes
- disability/personal dependency. The adaptation to physical and mental frailty of very late life (the eighth to ninth decade) with the transition to immobility from locality bound to housebound to bedbound. The last stage of the family life cycle can continue for as long as 40 years.

Elderly couples or individuals may not live with their family in the same household. The 1986 Australian Census showed 66% of 65 year olds or greater lived alone or as a couple in a private dwelling (Rowland, 1991). Close contact is often maintained with the family, with extended family often living in close proximity. This means there is often interaction between the various stages of the family life cycle operating for different generations of the extended family.

The importance of considering the family life cycle is that each stage requires a change to occur in the family relationships with different tasks having to be addressed. If the necessary changes do not occur, this may be associated with the beginning or worsening of symptomatic behavior in one family member. Such symptomatic behavior may subside if the family can be assisted with the transition. Thus a grandson may be leaving home at a time when a grandparent is retiring. Leaving home requires adjustments around loosening emotional ties whereas retirement may require re-establishing contact and new closeness. Thus two completely different developmental tasks may impinge on the extended family network at the same time.

Benbow et al. (1990) describe working with older families using the family life cycle to guide their work. Anderson & Hargrave (1990) also use this concept as does some of the work of Borzormenyi-Nagy & Spark (1973).

Problem focus and solution focus

Pottle (1984) described a geriatric psychiatry service run by using a family orientation, problem solving approaches and positive reframing. The author provides clear descriptions on how to use the family therapy concepts but does not link this description with any medical considerations of the disorders being treated.

Positive reframing means describing what is currently happening in the family and carefully considering how this could be described in positive ways or how the behavior could have positive intentions underlying it. A number of family therapy schools use this idea, (Minuchin, 1974; Minuchin & Fishman, 1981; Papp, 1983), which is also described as positive connotation (Palazolli et al., 1978; Penn, 1985). Constantine et al. (1984) and O'Brian & Bruggen (1985) give details of these techniques.

Problem-oriented methods are based on the assumption that there has been some recent change in the family or wider network which has led to referral. Another important assumption is that the relevant group will be able to solve their own problems with minimal assistance. Hence interventions are designed to encourage the family network to mobilize its own resources (Haley, 1976; Madanes, 1981; de Shazer, 1985; Watzlawick, Weakland & Fish 1974).

Family therapy concepts from adult psychiatry

There is now considerable evidence that family functioning can influence the outcome of a variety of medical and psychiatric disorders. Berkowitz (1988) reviewed studies using family therapy with patients having schizophrenia and depression; Kahlweg & Goldstein (1987) report studies employing the vulnerability-stress model of mental disorders, including several longitudinal prospective studies of high risk goups in which family relationships were studied before the onset of the disorder. Measures used were based on direct observation of the families. Leff & Vaughn (1981) and Leff et al. (1982) described a number of studies which monitored the effects of social and family interventions on high EE in families and on relapse rates in the patients. They consistently obtained results confirming a causal role for relatives' EE on patients' relapse and provided confirmation for the therapeutic effectiveness of social interventions in combination with drug treament. Miklowitz et al. (1988) showed a link between family affective style and EE and the course of mania. Negative affective style and high expressed emotion increased relapse rate by five to six times. Hooley, Orley & Teasdale (1986) studied the predictive validity of EE in a clinically depressed sample and examined the interactional correlates of high and low levels of EE in patient–spouse dyads. They found patients with unipolar depression living with a spouse high in EE to be significantly more likely to relapse within nine months after discharge from hospital than patients living with a spouse low in EE. Keitner & Miller (1990) reviewed the relevance of families in major depression. They found that family pathology present during an acute episode of depression persists after the patient's recovery. They found that the course of a depressive illness, relapse rates and suicidal behavior are affected by the functioning of the family. There is also evidence that the children of depressed patients are at high risk for psychopathology. Family and marital interventions were found to be effective particularly in the treatment of depressed women. Gonzalez, Steinglass & Reiss (1989) noted the usefulness of information and problem solving opportunities provided for families with a variety of medical disorders.

Although these and many other studies have not specifically addressed an elderly population, many of the principles can be applied to older people and in fact, some of the cohort of patients included in the above studies were elderly. Gonzalez et al. (1989) used a highly structured discussion group to provide information and problem solving opportunities to families with members with chronic medical conditions. Of the 24 patients involved, five were aged 60 or over. Hooley et al. (1986) studied patients between the ages of 27 and 70 years to show clear links between high EE and greater relapse of depression after discharge from hospital.

From studies such as these some assumptions have become accepted and form the basis for family interventions easily applicable to old people suffering from functional disorders:

(1) The vulnerability–stress model of schizophrenia which states that schizophrenia occurs when there is a combination of genetic vulnerability for the condition and disturbed family relationship patterns which are present prior to the development of the condition. (Goldstein, 1985)

(2) Family interactions affect the course of schizophrenia after its onset and modification of family interactions can affect the subsequent course of the illness (Leff & Vaughn, 1981). There is now substantial literature indicating that family interventions aimed at reducing high expressed emotion reduces relapse rates in schizophrenics treated with medication, living with their families. A good review of the psychoeducational model of family therapy is given by Anderson, Reiss & Hogarty (1985).

(3) Family interactions affect the course of affective disorders and modification of family interactions can decrease relapse rates (Miklowitz et al., 1988). Keitner & Miller (1990) in their recent overview of family functioning and major depression, noted in their conclusion (paraphrased). 'Family dysfunction accompanies acute depression and often persists after remission. Ongoing family problems, particularly if associated with criticism of the patient are associated with a prolonged course and a higher risk of relapse.' It is clear that family interventions can improve the outcome although it is not clear exactly how this happens.

(4) Marital discord is associated with poorer recovery from depression and marital therapy can improve the subsequent course of the patient. This is so for women but not so for men (Keitner & Miller 1990).

Application of family therapy methods to functional disorders in a geriatric psychiatry setting

Although it is not uncommon for some functional disorders to present for the first time in late life, many have been present for some time and run a chronic, relapsing pattern, often with associated physical or organic pathology. Families naturally organize themselves around these problems and develop certain responses, some of which are not helpful. Family therapy interventions seek to help families organize themselves better and find alternative, 'better' solutions to their problems. Brodaty & Gresham (1989) use a similar approach in their educational programs for the carers of dementia sufferers. Another good description of the psycho-educational model is provided by McFarlane (1991).

In outline this program involves:

1. Engaging the family early in the crisis of the acute episode.
2. Providing education and information about the disorder and its treatment using the stress/diathesis model.
3. Providing advice about handling illness-related behavior and handling deficits.
4. Specifically reducing negative or hostile affects.
5. Seeing families either individually or as a group of four to five families and continuing contact with the families on a regular basis for periods up to two years after discharge.

Practical suggestions

Logistics

In our experience, the psychoeducational approach was not adequate in every case so that we have added eclectically various other techniques from the range of available family therapy interventions. At this time experience is inadequate to be able to be clearly prescriptive, neither does the material from the literature allow this. What follows is based on our current thinking and level of experience.

Family therapy interventions can be introduced into the geriatric psychiatry setting in the spirit of scientific progress, using a more or less well defined trial and error method. For this to be most effective, a family interviewing area should be available with a two-way mirror and video camera to enable close study of interventions made and results obtained.

A team of interested clinicians needs to be formed, with the most senior consultant psychiatrist being involved and a visiting clinician with family therapy expertise being available at least some of the time. The use of two-way mirrors and video allows team observers to watch family interviews, form different perspectives, generate new hypotheses and ask different types of questions. This kind of open team work has its uncomfortable moments but has useful functions for improving techniques, increasing self monitoring skills and leading to better understanding of the work of other team members. Such an arrangement also greatly facilitates peer review and quality assurance.

Genograms

Drawing a genogram on which all family members are clearly identified is a fundamental first step in thinking about the family as a whole (Stagoll & Lang, 1980). While working on the genogram, family issues can be easily explored and defined. Such information as the later life experience of family members in this and other generations, family life cycle issues, beliefs about caring, transgenerational obligations, resentments and guilt, cultural norms and expectations and beliefs about illness behavior become available for discussion.

Giving of diagnosis and prognosis

Thorough clinical evaluation of the individual patient needs to be made prior to the family interview so that clear demonstrations can be made of what behavior is part of the illness and what is not. Family questions about diagnosis, results of investigations such as CT scans, neurophysiological data, reports of assessment of daily living skills and physical capacities need to be clearly given to family members so that everyone knows exactly what is wrong and what can be expected of the patient. This is different from more traditional family therapy where such biomedical data is not usually provided. With elderly patients making available clear accessible information about the total state of the patient is a crucial part of the family interview.

Such detailed feedback means that there has to be careful planning before the family interview to make sure all relevant information and reports are available and that all relevant staff members attend. There needs to be a clear agenda set about the purpose of the family meeting and it must be decided who is in charge of the family interview as well as what issues will be taken up with the family. This involves close liaison between different staff members with clear lines of responsibility being developed.

Structuring of interviews

The meeting is arranged by telephone with an explanation about the purpose of the meeting and preparation about the context in which the interview will occur. The presence of the two-way screen and the video camera is described and their purpose clarified.

The identified patient would generally attend the family meeting. Family members have to feel sure that the clinician knows how the patient acts in the family context. In the initial part of the meeting all family members are identified, rapport is established with everyone, the genogram is commenced and information is given and sought. Family members are asked about their perceptions of the problems, who was involved in the referral process, their attempted solutions and their expectations and beliefs. Common themes that emerge and can be addressed include myths about old age. For example that the aged are always set in their ways or that institutionalization is needed when it clearly is not. Family members often jump to the conclusion that psychiatric symptoms in the elderly are due to senility. A frequent occurrence is the marginalization of the patient during discussions as they are talked about as if not present. It is important to include the patient in the discussion as much as is feasible. Decisions made in the presence of all family members are implemented with much greater success.

A detailed discussion of the diagnosis, treatment planning and use of medication or electroconvulsive therapy (ECT) and advice about how to respond to altered behavior resulting from psychosis or depression can be elaborated. Specific help is provided to the family to reduce their stress and fear. Family members are supported in minimising critical or hostile responses to the identified patient or to each other.

This approach seeks to provide information for the family and gain their collaboration in assisting the identified patient's recovery or to ensure prevention of relapse. Even a single meeting can have surprisingly useful effects although preventing relapse may require frequent meeetings over lengthy periods and the literature suggests multiple family groups are also likely to be helpful (Gonzalez et al., 1989).

Clinical examples

1. This case vignette has been chosen to illustrate how the family life cycle, problem orientation and positive reframing can be used in practice.

A woman in her 70s tried to commit suicide because she was really fed up with the quality of her life. She had always said to everyone that when her time came she would kill herself.

She lived on her own and had limited contact with her only son and his wife. They were in their early 40s, and were unable to have children. Her husband had died over 10 years earlier, slowly and painfully, of cancer and she had nursed him at home. She tried seriously to kill herself, and to cause as few problems as possible to anyone. She had all her affairs in order, wrote a letter to her son telling him she would be dead and to get the doctor to come and deal with her body. She lay on the made-up bed after she took tablets and thought she had taken care of all the details.

The reason for her plan's failure was totally unpredicted. Her letter to her son arrived within the day instead of the day after.

From a medical framework, the obvious diagnosis to consider is whether this woman is suffering from a depressive illness. Once this is treated, her depression would lift and she would find a reason for living again. This diagnosis was carefully considered and excluded.

This left the treating team unsure how to proceed. Using ideas from family therapy provided new factors to consider and other possibilities for treatment.

Using the family life cycle analysis it was clear that this family was arrested at a transition point. The younger generation had not had children and the patient had been deprived of her opportunity to have grandchildren and to define herself as useful in this way. There had not been the usual opportunities for nurturing that arise out of the birth of young children. Helping family members to discuss these issues led to new solutions becoming available as the patient and her son became more involved with each other.

Using problem orientation in this case brought out the facts that the son and daughter-in-law were furious with the patient for her action, not so much out of concern for her but because of the guilt feelings generated in each of them as they tried to blame each other for what happened. One problem was their inability to come to terms with the fact that there had not been sufficient love and care exchanged for the patient to want to live any longer. This problem focus enabled family members to clarify what they could reasonably expect from each other, and how they could keep this up in the future.

Using reframing enabled staff gently to point out that whilst the attempted suicide had been upsetting and frightening for the son, it had served the positive function of bringing the family closer together and had certainly given the son a chance to show that he was truly concerned for his mother.

2. This vignette has been chosen to exemplify the use of a psychoeducational approach. Mr F, aged 66, was admitted to the assessment ward with a diagnosis of 'late paraphrenia' or late onset schizophrenia.

Mr F lived with his wife and bachelor son, aged 35. Over the previous two years he had developed persecutory delusions regarding terrorists. He worked as a filing clerk in a high security area of the Public Service. His imminent retirement had become a focus of anxiety for him and appeared to be related to the onset of his psychiatric symptoms.

Following his retirement some 12 months previously, his psychiatric symptoms had gradually escalated. He believed cars were patrolling his street, bodies were being buried under the house, that he heard the voices of various men threatening him with elaborate schemes of a persecutory and at times, quite terrifying nature. Outpatient antipsychotic therapy and general clinical support had only partially ameliorated the problem.

An admission was precipitated when his son became increasingly angry and upset with his father's behavior and deluded beliefs. Over a period of weeks, he had tried to talk his father out of his beliefs, cajole him and threaten him. This was associated with an escalation in his father's psychotic symptoms and disturbed behavior, and distress in Mrs F until a crisis occurred and admission was organized by the local doctor.

Within two days of admission, Mr F was free of hallucinations and his delusions had become quiescent and were generally focused on his home and not the ward. He was relaxed, appropriate and independent in the ward setting.

It was postulated that his son's, and to a lesser degree his wife's lack of understanding of the nature of his psychiatric illness and their subsequent fearful response to this, generated increasing arousal and expressed emotion which may have acted to exacerbate his psychosis. Based upon this hypothesis, a number of family meetings were arranged including Mr and Mrs F and in particular, the son who lived with them.

Detailed explanations of the nature of the psychosis, descriptions of delusions and hallucinations and theories of their biochemical nature were provided. The behavior disturbances were explained in terms of a psychotic illness and information about schizophrenia was provided. Follow-up interviews were established, again particularly focusing on the question of Mr F's disturbed behavior and their response to this. The effect of arousal and fear were noted and recommended responses to this behavior disturbance were provided. It was clear that Mr F's son had no idea what was wrong with his father, while Mrs F also had a very limited idea of what was going on with her husband up until this time. These discussions led to the patient and family developing a more positive view of the benefits of medication and treatment and a feeling of optimism and control about the future treatment and outcome.

3. This clinical vignette has been chosen to describe some of the features relevant to patients with depression.

Mrs H, a 69 year old woman with no children was referred from another psychiatric service with a history of recurring depressive stupor, requiring urgent ECT. Mr and Mrs H had a marriage characterized by a pattern of Mrs H growing more passive and dependent in the latter years of her marriage and Mr H taking over more and more responsibilities for household duties. Especially with the onset of retirement, such areas as cooking, cleaning, shopping and financial management were taken over to be managed by the husband.

Mrs H's episodes of illness were characterized by her gradually ceasing to talk, taking herself to bed and over one or two weeks reducing her food and fluid intake until her husband contacted local medical services and admission was arranged.

Admission usually resulted in a course of urgent ECT being given for a diagnosis of catatonia. Recovery often occurred within one to three treatments, with Mrs H complaining of depressed mood but appearing to respond well in groups and social programs.

She was referred to the day hospital where she appeared sociable, in a quiet way and interacted with other attenders. This contrasted with her husband's reports of a very withdrawn state in her home life.

Again, the initial thrust of treatment was psychobiological, with lithium and antidepressants being prescribed for Mrs H and support being provided for husband and wife. Despite this, the relapse pattern persisted and Mr and Mrs H were referred to the family assessment program. At the assessment it was hypothesized that the behavior pattern reflected the disturbance in the marital relationship and the social worker on the inpatient team, who had undertaken some family therapy training, contracted to work with the couple.

This required negotiation on the part of the inpatient team to support the work of the social worker, particularly to monitor readmissions and discharges. Mr and Mrs H were engaged in a program to promote some change in roles at home with Mr H placing less emphasis on his caring and domestic role and Mrs H being encouraged to take more responsibility for herself and her personal life. This was achieved through family meetings and also home visits.

This treatment led to a greatly reduced number of admissions, a complete cessation of ECT treatment and also brought out more explicit marital disharmony and clear ambivalence about the future of the marriage, leading to discussion between the couple.

It is important to note that this approach to the management of Mrs H led to some tensions with the general practitioner and the consultant psychiatrist had to reassure him and explain the treatment rationale to him.

Conclusion

This chapter has dealt with the definitions of family therapy, its historical development and has sought to clarify for clinicians how family therapy can be useful to help them treat functional psychiatric disorders in elderly people. We point to a rich body of literature on theory and technique, making attempts to be as inclusive as possible while remaining selective. We have emphasized the usefulness of consulting experts in family therapy and establishing family therapy teams within geriatric psychiatry services. We hope clinicians will apply some of the material presented and in turn add to the development of more specific interventions with the elderly and their families.

References

Anderson, C. M., Reiss D. & Hogarty, G. (1985). *Schizophrenia and the Family*. New York: The Guilford Press.

Anderson, H. & Goolishian, H. (1988). Human systems as linguistic systems: preliminary and evolving ideas about the implications for clinical theory. *Family Process*, **27**, 371–93.

Anderson, W. T. & Hargrave, T. D. (1990). Contextual family therapy and older people: building trust in the intergenerational family. *Journal of Family Therapy*, **12**, 311–20.

Bateson, G. & Ruesch, J. (1951). *Communication: The Social Matrix of Psychiatry*. New York: Norton.

Bateson, G., Jackson, D., Haley, J. & Weakland, J. (1956). Towards a theory of schizophrenia. *Behavioral Science*, **1**, 251–64.

Bateson, G. (1972). *Steps to an Ecology of Mind*. New York: Ballantine.

Benbow, S., Egan, D., Marriot, A., Tregay, K., Walsh, S., Wells, J. & Wood, J. (1990). Using the family life cycle with later life families. *Journal of Family Therapy*, **12**, 321–40.

Bengtson, V. L. & Robertson, J. F. (1985). *Grandparenthood*. Beverley Hills: Sage Publications.

Berkowitz, R. (1988). Family therapy and adult mental illness: Schizophrenia and Depression. *Journal of Family Therapy*, **4**, 339–56.

Boscolo, L., Cecchin, G., Hoffman, L. & Penn, P. (1987). *Milan Systemic Family Therapy: Conversations in Theory and Practice*. New York: Basic Books.

Boszormenyi-Nagy, I. & Spark, G. M. (1973). *Invisible Loyalties*. New York: Harper & Row.

Bowen, M. (1978). *Family Therapy in Clinical Practice*. New York: Jason Aronson.

Brodaty, H. & Gresham, M. (1989). Effects of a training program to reduce stress in carers of patients with dementia. *British Medical Journal*, **299**, 1375–9.

Browne, E. (1988). The Australian family: 1788–1888–1988. *Australian and New Zealand Journal of Family Therapy*, **9**, 1–8.

Brubaker, T. (Ed.) (1983). *Family Relationships in Later Life*. Beverley Hills: Sage Publications.

Carter, E. A. & McGoldrick, M. (1980). *The Family Life Cycle: A Framework for Family Therapy*. New York: Gardner Press.

Cherlin, A. J. & Furstenberg, F. F. (1986). *The New American Grandparent: A Place in the Family, a Life Apart*. New York: Basic Books.

Constantine, J. A., Stone Fish, L. & Piercy, F. P. (1984). A systematic procedure for teaching positive connotation. *Journal of Marital and Family Therapy*, **10**, 313–15.

Cooper, D. (1971). *The Death of the Family*. London: Penguin.

Denham, T. E. & Smith, C. W. (1989). The Influence of grandparents on grandchildren: a review of the literature and resources. *Family Relations*, **38**, 345–50.

de Shazer, S. (1985). *Keys to Solution in Brief Therapy*. New York: Norton.

Esterson, A. (1970). *The Leaves of Spring. Schizophrenia, Family and Sacrifice*. London: Tavistock Publications.

Goldstein, M. J. (1985). Family factors that antedate the onset of schizophrenia and related disorders: the results of a fifteen year prospective longitudinal study. *Acta Psychiatrica Scandinavica*, **71** (Suppl. 319), 7–18.

Gonzalez, S., Steinglass, P. & Reiss, D. (1989). Putting the illness in its place: discussion groups for families with chronic medical conditions. *Family Process*, **28**, 69–87.

Haley, J. (1976). *Problem-Solving Therapy: New Strategies for Effective Family Therapy*. San Francisco: Jossey-Bass.

Haley, J. (1980). *Leaving Home: The Therapy of Disturbed Young People*. New York: McGraw-Hill.

Harari, E. & Bloch, S. (1991). Family therapy: conceptual, empirical and clinical aspects. *Current Opinion in Psychiatry*, **3**, 359–67.

Hoffman, L. (1981). *Foundations of Family Therapy. A Conceptual Framework for Systems Change*. New York: Basic Books.

Hooley, J. M., Orley, J. & Teasdale, J. D. (1986). Levels of expressed emotion and relapse in depressed patients. *British Journal of Psychiatry*, **148**, 642–7.

Kahlweg, K. & Goldstein, M. J. (1987). *Understanding Major Mental Disorder: The Contribution of Family Interaction Research*. New York: Family Process Press.

Keitner, G. I. & Miller, I. W. (1990). Family functioning and major depression: an overview. *American Journal of Psychiatry*, **147**, 1128–37.

Laing, R. D. (1960). *The Divided Self*. Chicago: Quadrangle Books.

Leff, J. P. & Vaughn, C. E. (1981). The role of maintenance therapy and relatives expressed emotion in relapse of schizophrenia: a two year follow-up. *British Journal of Psychiatry*, **139**, 102–4.

Leff, J. P., Kuipers, L., Berkowitz, R., Eberlein-Vries, R. & Sturgeon, D. (1982). A controlled trial of interventions in the families of schizophrenic patients. *British Journal of Psychiatry*, **141**, 121–34.

Lowe, R. (1990). Re-imagining family therapy: choosing the metaphors we live by. *Australian and New Zealand Journal of Family Therapy*, **11**, 1–9.

Luepnitz, D. A. (1988). *The Family Interpreted. Feminist Theory in Clinical Practice*. New York: Basic Books.

Madanes, C. (1981). *Strategic Family Therapy*. San Francisco: Jossey-Bass.

McFarlane, W. R. (1991). Family psychoeducational treatment. In *Handbook of Family Therapy*, Eds. A. Gurman & D. Kniskern, Volume II. New York: Brunner/Mazel.

Miklowitz, D. J., Goldstein, M. J., Neuchterlein, K. H., Snyder, K. S. & Mintz, J. (1988). Family factors and the course of bipolar affective disorder. *Archives of General Psychiatry*, **45**, 225–31.

Minuchin, S. (1974). *Families and Family Therapy*. Cambridge, Mass: Harvard University Press.

Minuchin, S., Rosman, B. L. & Baker, L. (1978). *Psychosomatic Families: Anorexia Nervosa in Context*. Cambridge, Mass: Harvard University Press.

Minuchin, S. & Fishman, H. C. (1981). *Family Therapy Techniques*. Cambridge, Mass: Harvard University Press.

O'Brian, C. & Bruggen, P. (1985). Our personal and professional lives: learning positive connotation and circular questioning. *Family Process*, **24**, 311–22.

Palazzoli, M. S., Cecchin, G., Boscolo, L. & Prata, G. (1978). *Paradox and Counterparadox*. New York: Jason Aronson.

Palazzoli, M. S., Cirillo, S., Selvini, M. & Sorrentino, A. M. (1989). *Family Games: General Models of Psychotic Processes in the Family*. London: Karnac Books.

Papp, P. (1983). *The Process of Change*. New York: Guilford Press.

Penn, P. (1985). Feed-forward: future questions, future maps. *Family Process*, **24**, 299–310.

Pottle, S. (1984). Developing a network-oriented service for elderly people and their carers. In A. Treacher & J. Carpenter (Eds). *Using Family Therapy* Oxford: J. Blackwell.

Rowland, D. T. (1991). *Ageing in Australia*. Melbourne: Longman Cheshire.

Satir, V. (1967). *Conjoint Family Therapy*. Palo Alto: Science and Behavior Books.

Sluzki, C. E. (1983). Process, structure and world views: towards an integrated view of systemic models in family therapy. *Family Process*, **22**, 469–76.

Stagoll, B. & Lang, M. (1980). Climbing the family tree: working with genograms. *The Australian Journal of Family Therapy*, **1**, 161–71.

Stagoll, B. (1989). Aspects of family therapy. *Current Opinion in Psychiatry*, **2**, 377–83.

Szasz, T. S. (1961). *The Myth of Mental Illness: Foundations of a Theory of Personal Conduct*. New York: Hoeber-Harper.

Szmukler, G. I., Berkowitz, R., Eisler, I., Leff, J. & Dare, C. (1985). 'Expressed emotion' in individual and family settings: a comparative study. *British Journal of Psychiatry* **151**, 174–8.

Watzlawick, P., Weakland, J. H. & Fish, R. (1974). *Change: Principles of Problem Formation and Problem Resolution*. New York: Norton.

White, M. & Epston, D. (1989). *Literate Means to Therapeutic Ends*. Adelaide: Dulwich Centre Publications.

28

Group therapy in the elderly

SANFORD I. FINKEL PAUL METLER WENDY WASSON KAREN BERTE NANCY BAILEY DIANE BRAUER JAMES GANDY

Introduction

In recent years a great deal has been written about the value of group psychotherapy for older people (Tross & Blum, 1988; Finkel, 1991; Leszcz, 1987, 1991; Lothstein & Zimet, 1988). Few clinics or programs, however, devote extensive resources providing group therapy services to a wide range of older adults. At the Older Adult Program of Northwestern Memorial Hospital, nine diverse group therapy experiences are provided both on-site and in the community at large. Over 80% of this population have diagnoses of functional psychiatric disorders, with depression being the most prevalent. The group therapy modalities include insight-oriented family support, cognitive behavioral, supportive, institutional, activities-oriented, creative, and bereavement groups.

Because there is a shortage of mental health professionals devoted to treating the increasing number of older people with functional disorders, group therapy is a logical and important treatment modality. Besides the obvious economic benefit compared to individual therapy, therapy groups provide nurturance, a sense of sustenance and support that allows older people to enhance their coping mechanisms, to resolve conflicts, and to diminish the disabling symptoms of functional disorders.

Group therapy offers the following special opportunities for older people:

1. To re-establish well-functioning defenses and coping mechanisms via interactions with other group members and to enhance a sense of usefulness in one another.
2. To establish a sense of identity as part of a social entity.
3. To become part of a family unit with a nurturing supportive system that would translate to other environmental situations.
4. To resolve old conflicts via reflection, reminiscence, re-enactment, resolution, and growth.
5. To enhance self-esteem by ameliorating a harsh superego that lends itself toward shame.

6. To adapt to, and accept, losses that cannot be reversed without expending excessive energy.

There are obvious differences in conducting group therapy for older patients versus younger ones. The elderly prefer late morning and mid-afternoon times and generally do not wish to participate in night sessions or therapy immediately after lunch. This is in contrast to the preferences of the younger population who generally favor attending therapy after work. In addition, it is much easier to obtain an equal male/female balance in younger age groups. In late life it is not atypical to have groups predominantly of women. Transportation problems, inclement weather, illness, or winter vacations also complicate outpatient group therapy with older people.

In contrast, alliances between the therapist and elderly group members tend to form more quickly. Older group therapy patients tend to be more patient and tolerant of monopolistic or silent group members. At times, their patience may exceed that of the therapist. Goldfarb has pointed out that 'younger persons in group psychotherapy break, remake, test, and consolidate relationships with others ... older people do not seem to go through this process in their groups, no matter what the interests or the skills of the therapist' (Goldfarb, 1972). After-group socialization and touching between patients and therapists are considered appropriate for older group members, in contrast to younger group therapy participants.

Although the ideal number of patients for a group is between five and eight, a range up to 12 is considered acceptable. This is especially true in an older group in which absence may significantly reduce the number of attendees. Special attention to lighting, comfort of the furniture, room temperature, and handicapped accessibility is essential. The allocated time can range from 30 to 90 minutes, depending on the setting and the functioning level of the patients.

Themes include social losses, physical illness and sensory decrement, autonomy versus dependence, loneliness, intergenerational conflicts, seeking of information about one's illness, and attempts to sustain a level of hopefulness. Common goals include providing information, finding ways to help individuals re-engage with others, concrete problem solving, enhancing self-esteem, provision of narcissistic supplies, and halting regression.

The Older Adult Program of Northwestern Memorial Hospital has a long-established tradition of providing psychotherapy experiences to older adults in the Chicago community. Among the approximately 5400 patients per year who visit the clinic, one-third receive only psychotherapy, one-third receive medication management, and one-third receive a combination of these services. Established in 1977, the underlying philosophy of the clinic has been psychodynamic, with a traditional emphasis on individual psychotherapy. In 1988 a commitment was made to add group psychotherapy to the available services and to develop an expertise in group psychotherapy experiences utilizing a variety of conceptual frameworks. The following groups represent the current group psychotherapy services for those with functional disorders.

Expressive, insight-oriented group psychotherapy

Insight-oriented group psychotherapy is of special value to older adults with anxiety and depressive disorders that are combined with character pathology. Accompanying aging are narcissistic injuries, which can lead to losses of self-object relationships and coping abilities, resulting in diminished self-esteem and a variety of psychological symptoms (Kohut, 1984; Lazarus, 1980; Schwartzman, 1984; Yalom, 1985). Group therapy can provide relationships that serve necessary self-object functions, as well as a feeling of group cohesion, which, in turn, can restore a sense of vitality and self-stability by providing idealized self-objects, mirroring self-objects, and twinning self-objects (Leszcz, 1991). By establishing these self-objects, individuals feel valued, protected, and of worth. Individual vulnerability is better understood within the group context, which allows for understanding of interpersonal problems and their resolutions.

The primary goal in creating an insight-oriented psychotherapy group is to: 1) assist older adults establish meaningful connections within the group, with the intent that this process, together with an increase in self-knowledge, would help in negotiating relationships outside the group more successfully; 2) concomitantly reduce signs and symptoms of psychiatric illness. Individual and pharmacological therapy are also used, as needed to resolve the functional psychiatric disorder(s).

Members were either referred by other professionals to this out-patient group, or they were self-referred. Led by two middle-adult female psychologists, the group met for one and one-half hours weekly for 12 months. Each prospective member was screened individually by the co-therapist team. Interestingly, all of the group members had previously been in some type of group experience which they had found helpful. It was also striking that the members had many more factors in common than being older and depression-prone. All were women in their late sixties and early seventies who had experienced considerable conflicts with at least one child. Five had been divorced, and the one married woman experienced considerable conflict with her husband. All tended to see themselves as 'the strong mother' who had denied her own needs while receiving little emotional support from those surrounding her.

Despite these similarities, there were important differences among members. There were differences in cultural and racial backgrounds, socioeconomic status, styles of relating, and patterns of dealing with problems. One woman in the group was extremely quiet and passive, while others were verbal and dominant; some tended to become immobilized and withdrawn, seeing 'the cup as half empty', while others used activity to avoid feelings as they tried (often unsuccessfully) to cling to the positive.

The themes that emerged concerned losses (of health, independence, or significant relationships), intergenerational conflicts, conflictual feelings about dependency, difficulty asserting needs or interests, and feeling that older adults are not understood or held in esteem by 'younger people' (e.g. their children, health care workers).

A strong focus for the group emerged over time. While some 'complaining' and ventilating of angry and depressed feelings was tolerated, a strong norm of active problem solving developed. In other words, in the face of change or loss, what could the group member do to reduce her sense of powerlessness and impotence? Members of the group would share their ideas of 'different things you can do', as well as underline the importance of caring, while setting limits on those who made unreasonable demands. The tension between expressing feelings versus doing something to improve the situation was an ongoing group issue and led to considerable feeling and, at times, outright antagonism among members.

The presence of two members with significant health problems was a powerful force within the group. Members responded to the physical and psychological neediness of these two peers with an initial outpouring of support and suggestions. The two 'identified patients' responded to the group in different ways: one eagerly took in the attention, support and suggestions of the group, while the other often rejected her peers' suggestions. However, both of these women ultimately became targets of conflict to a degree not observed with any other members. In addition, the 'healthier' group members described, in various ways, a sense of being overwhelmed by the behaviors of these two women, perhaps due to a projection of their own dependency conflicts and fears.

Conflicts over dependence–independence were apparent in certain transference responses. Periodically the wish to be rescued by the expert authority figure would emerge, often during a period of conflict or frustration, as an expressed desire for more 'direction' from the therapists. However, at other times the members assumed the parental role, noting that the group served a teaching function in helping the 'young' therapists to better understand older adults.

Relationships with children were often reflected in the evolving transferences. In particular, one woman who talked of her childrens' lack of empathy for her age-related problems would sometimes admonish the therapists if she felt their comments did not reflect an understanding of her status as an older adult. At the same time she also noted ' ... when I was young I didn't understand either. I had no sympathy for my parents ... '

The therapists' countertransference responses were not dissimilar to those experienced with younger patients. However, both therapists recalled struggling in interpreting when a member's problems or complaints were a reflection of a reality of older adulthood or were an indication of individual psychological process. For example, when was the absence of a member truly due to transportation difficulty or illness, and when did it reflect resistance? How should the co-therapists respond to the absence? Member absences with this outpatient group were significant at various times throughout the year and questions remain for the co-therapists regarding reasonable expectations and norms concerning an attendance criterion for continued membership in an insight-oriented therapy group for older adults.

In summary, this experience with expressive, insight-oriented psychotherapy with older adults has found few age-related factors that bear consideration. Content themes may reflect some of the more immediate concerns of the older adult, such as increased health changes, or societal or personal conditions that threaten continued independence. Group management must include responsible reflection on how to balance the age-related realities that can affect attendance with the therapeutic impact of absence in this type of group. Nonetheless, group member responses at the conclusion of this group supported the professionals' observations that insight, self-reflection, and change are desired, valued, and obtainable goals for older adults.

A group for cognitively intact residents in the nursing home

Though most nursing home residents have dementia, many others have functional psychiatric disorders. In particular, depressive disorders are unrecognized and thus undertreated in the nursing home setting, where the prevalence ranges from 18–20% for major depression to 27–44% for other dysphoric states (Katz et al., 1989). Even when depression is recognized by nursing home staff, many patients refuse nonpharmacological treatment, not wishing to be confronted with their illness and situation. Yet, with much persistence outreach liaison staff were able to form a group of five residents, four women and one man. All five had severe physical disabilities. One member had amyotrophic lateral sclerosis (ALS), one had Parkinson's disease and one had multiple physical disabilities secondary to a major stroke. Almost all of the residents in the group had a diagnosis of major depression or dysthymia with mixed personality disorders.

All of the group members had been resident in the nursing home for more than one year. Most were socially isolated, inasmuch as most residents seldom converse or socialize with each other. Many residents have very little contact with family or friends, leaving them feeling withdrawn, lonely, and depressed. The residents needed a place in which they could feel a sense of connectedness to their environment and to each other and could express their thoughts and feelings. Further, many needed an opportunity to work through some issues, such as resentment at family and friends, fear of decline, and regrets from past experiences.

The group thus became a place for the residents to reflect on their personal histories and to come to terms with some of these experiences. Residents – even those in nursing homes – have potentials not yet realized. During this stage of life new learning and growth can take place. It was this firm belief that supported the rationale and commitment to having group therapy in the home. More than simply support groups or reminiscent groups, this group was psychotherapeutic in nature.

Several themes surfaced throughout the course of the group. One that emerged repeatedly was the residents' feelings of being powerless and having little control in their life. This took many forms, including control over privacy; control over sleeping and waking schedules; control over food they ate; control over safety and security; and control over body and bodily functions.

Mr S., age 76, has Lou Gehrig's disease (ALS). Three years prior to the group's beginning, this man was able to walk without a cane, feed, bathe and clothe himself. He had control over all of his bodily functions. When he entered the group, he was bound to a wheelchair, had very little control over the muscles in his neck (needed a neck brace), and little control over the muscles in his arms, hands, and legs. He could not scratch his face when it itched or wipe the sweat off his brow. During the first session, when asked about himself, he began to cry. He stated that he wished he was dead for he felt that he was 'a slave to his own body, trapped in hell'. Once the group began, he reported to the group that he did not feel that he could talk to the staff about these feelings for fear that they would take this as complaining and this would lead to being sent to a floor for those more regressed. Consequently, he was left harbouring these thoughts and feelings without any forum to express them. The group became a place where he could express these feelings without fear of any potential retribution.

Another theme that emerged during the course of the group dealt with the residents' early histories, childhoods, and relationships with parents, as well as their relationships with their children. Two of the members had never married. The other three had married and were divorced. The three married residents had children. One woman had a son who was diagnosed as schizophrenic. Another woman had had no contact with her eldest daughter for the past 15 years after having a 'disagreement and a fight'. For those members who had never married, the group became a place where they could talk about what that was like and gain some insight about why they had remained single. For those who had married and had a family, the group became a place to attempt to work out or better understand these conflicts. For both married and single residents, gaining some insight into their relationships with their parents was extremely helpful for understanding their own intimate relationships or lack thereof.

Mrs J., age 60, had never married and had very few intimate relationships with men. Through the course of the group she began to talk about her early childhood and her relationship with her father. He did not want a girl and always expressed his disappointment in her. He was verbally abusive and would humiliate and degrade her in front of others. When she began to date, she had very little confidence that any man would like her. She realized in the group that she never allowed any man to get close to her out of fear that they would expose her vulnerabilities and ultimately reject her. Not only did she lack confidence, she felt much conflict about her own sense of being a woman. Her fear of intimacy was rooted in this early relationship with her father.

Issues related to parenthood became a highly sensitive issue in the group, leading to conflicts among group members.

Mrs A, age 78, had a schizophrenic son. Often, she would get very angry and argumentative whenever someone in the group was critical of someone else's parent. Through group intervention she developed insight into how guilty she felt because of her son. She believed that she was to blame for his emotional problems and felt responsible. She once reported to the group that when her son was originally diagnosed, the doctors insinuated that she was to blame for her son's schizophrenia. She gradually accepted that there were many potential causes of her son's illness, and she could not assume responsibility.

Lastly, the issues of change and its painful association with one's physical and mental deterioration were a primary focus in the group. For most members there was a constant fear that if their condition 'changed', it meant being sent to a floor where residents are in much worse condition. Not only was this like being sent to Dante's Purgatory, it also was a sign that the end was near. Change meant less control over their lives, less independence and autonomy, and less of their 'old' identity. Obviously, the group could not prevent 'change'. However, talking about their fears, hearing how other people cope with them, and, most importantly, getting realistic feedback about their conditions was very helpful.

The group members felt a connectedness to one another that did not exist among most residents outside the group. Even for group members who did not always get along, there was a closeness due to shared experiences in the group that was unique for a nursing home setting. Further, the group was a place where these residents felt in control. They decided what to discuss and the process by which the discussion took place. It was ultimately their group. It became a forum for many members to discuss hidden fears and worries and to discover pieces of themselves that they had never known. Finally, the group was a place in which the members felt wanted and needed – a feeling most nursing home residents lack. Before entering the nursing home, these people were productive, capable, competent individuals. Through the group, they felt needed and realized their contributions to other group members. During this stage of life, especially for those in a nursing home, most individuals do not feel very needed, competent or important. However, in this group, when one member was gone for a session, it was noted, and his or her absence was felt. The group depended on each member, and each member was important to the group as a whole.

A senior achiever's group: a cognitive–behavioral approach

The Senior Achiever's group at the Older Adult Clinic at Northwestern Memorial Hospital chose their name years ago. The name reflects an underlying value held by the members – that as older adults they are contributing in some way to their families, their communities, and to society. Coming together each week in a group serves to create an environment to rekindle those values, even in the midst of weighty realities of functional psychiatric illness, physical deterioration, flagging spirits, and financial worries.

The emphasis of this group is on conscious cognition in using behavioral strategies and cognitive therapy application to promote mastery and maintenance of positive affects, to confront cognitive distortions and the meaning of life events, and to clarify and identify reactions in particular situations. Role-playing, didactic discussions, modeling, and active group feedback also are commonly utilized (Gallagher, 1981; Rush, 1983).

The formal goals of the Senior Achiever's group are to:

1. promote a sense of control at a time when events and losses strike randomly;
2. offer emotional support;
3. encourage active mastery and problem solving;
4. develop more adaptive ways of coping; and
5. enhance self-esteem.

Self-expression is encouraged. Reminiscing is often a vehicle for reviewing past achievements and for tapping into skills, strengths, and energies that built earlier lives. Maintaining positive self-images and correcting negative self-perceptions are our objectives so that group members view themselves as vital individuals, capable of leading vigorous, meaningful lives.

A planned program is used, balancing group members' interests and suggestions with the objectives. The following topics have served as past weekly programs:

1. Dried flower arrangements (both men and women enjoyed this and took arrangements home)
2. Current events (always a favorite)
3. Senior Benefit Day – sharing various information about special services for seniors
4. Discussion of volunteer opportunities
5. Writing to a pen pal in a nursing home
6. Favourite photo (encouraging reminiscing and sharing)
7. Performing a short play on the inpatient unit
8. Poetry reading, writing experience
9. Treasured object (time to reflect and promote group cohesion)
10. Senior nutrition (hospital nutritionist educates and informs group)
11. Fire safety provided by Chicago Fire Department firefighter

The Senior Achiever's group is ongoing and is composed of individuals with various psychiatric problems, adjustment disorders, obsessive disorders, depressive disorders, schizophrenia, and anxiety disorders. Currently, one man and seven women are members. Most have had at least one psychiatric hospitalization in the past and are fairly stable at present, due to a combination of factors that may include medication and individual treatment.

This group is open to new members, with tolerance for individuals 'trying out' the group for one session prior to making a commitment. Screening is done by the group leaders prior to acceptance into the group. It is felt that 12–14 members is the top limit, with 8–10 actually attending on any given day. Weather and illness are the main reasons for absences. Members are asked to call to cancel in order to strengthen their commitment and to highlight the importance of the group in their lives.

This group is led cooperatively, by a staff member and an experienced volunteer who is a senior citizen in her seventies.

Tailored to the goals of Senior Achievers, the programs from week to week reflect themes of mastery and accomplishment concerning struggles with psychiatric illness, failing health, financial worries, and losses that often characterize older adulthood. Depression is common to all members and is discussed and acknowledged as an ongoing problem.

Mutual support produces a sense of well-being and control over circumstances and spurs members to carry out the tasks of daily living.

Ms B, age 82, is plagued by a debilitating medical condition compromising seriously her energy level, strength, and endurance. Her list of medications seems endless. Her money worries are ever present, as she attempts to follow special dietary restrictions and make ends meet on a very limited income.

Ms. B sees herself as a woman committed to helping others and pushes herself to remain active in the community and at church. She takes a leadership role in the group and receives affirmation and support which helps her continue. Her spirit is unflagging and serves to inspire other members. Her defined role lends a sense of purpose and meaningfulness which has therapeutic benefit.

This example of perseverance and courage stimulated feelings of inadequacy and worthlessness in one of the members, who claimed favoritism when she thought Ms B was coming to the group without registering. She thought Ms B got in 'free'. She was cold to Ms B in the waiting room when Ms B attempted to chat prior to the group session. Group leaders cleared up this misconception and were aware of the angry feelings of this patient toward Ms B. This incident also reminded them of their own reactions to Ms B's struggle, and they resolved to be more mindful of this in the group process.

Supportive group therapy

Continuity of care is of special importance for patients with severe functional disorders who have been psychiatrically hospitalized. Unfortunately, many such patients are discharged without sufficient support to allow for continued community adjustment. For this reason, recidivisim is high for such patients, particularly for those with medical comorbidity and a paucity of community social and health support. Accordingly, the older adult program (OAP) has established a supportive group therapy program to provide encouragement, information, direction, and emotional support during the transition from the hospital to the community and beyond. The recidivism rate is substantially lower than for the rest of the discharged geropsychiatric inpatients.

The goal of the support group is to monitor day-to-day functioning for patients who have a variety of severe functional psychiatric illnesses – especially depression, schizophrenia, and anxiety disorders. The group members share similar fears and adjustment problems. Although all of the current members have been in the hospital for psychiatric reasons, this is not a criterion for membership of the outpatient group. In an atmosphere of respect and understanding, expression of feelings is encouraged as members face often overwhelming changes and challenges. The group is a supportive adjunct to individual therapy. The members learn from each other different new ways of coping and share feelings and common values of perseverance, affirming each other through encouragement and listening.

This group is particularly useful in these times of shortened hospital stays. It can help to maintain the delicate balance between an individual's optimum functioning and decompensation. The group offers support, structure, and socialization. The shared experience of either psychiatric hospitalization or struggle with profound mental disorders encourages group cohesion. As a supportive adjunct to individual therapy and pharmacotherapy, the group provides additional attention at a time of high vulnerability for the older adult members. The past hospitalization or current acute distress of new members serves to remind others of strides made in recovery from their illnesses. The longer-term members, in turn, offer concrete suggestions, encouragement, and often take the initiative in problem solving with newer members. Thus, this group is particularly valuable for strengthening coping mechanisms, thereby helping people to remain in the community.

Originated four years ago, the group currently has six members (one male and five females) who range in age from 62 to 90. One original member still attends.

Psychiatrically hospitalized individuals typically attend one group session prior to discharge. This allows for continuity of care, and an opportunity to process feelings about joining a group. Members of the treatment team also review the course of hospitalization and the discharge plan. When referrals come from non-hospital sources, screening proceeds, with case assignment made to a group leader who assesses appropriateness. The group meets twice a week, with a nurse from the inpatient unit and a social worker from the outpatient program serving as co-leaders.

Recurring topics are various fears, somatic complaints, depressed feelings, and day-to-day events of interest or concern. The most common fear is of relapse resulting in rehospitalization. Often, there is a lack of understanding about the etiology of the illness and concern that, without warning, one might be struck down again. The loss of control and fear of dependency generally coexist. The group tries, therefore, to educate its members about their illnesses.

Another common theme relates to losses such as hearing problems, gait difficulties, joint pains, and cataract surgery. Coping with the effects of loss of friends or family, family conflict, and environmental stresses generates suggestions, advice, and sharing among members.

Miss H, age 82, entered the group with a degenerative medical condition as well as an improving major depression. Articulate about her struggle with these illnesses, she credits the group with helping her maintain a more positive outlook and strength in the face of adjusting to physical disabilities. She took courses at the City College and hoped to secure a job, when her physical illness flared up again. She was hospitalized and found herself increasingly depressed, as a result of this disruption in her uphill climb. She enjoyed hearing from group members who wrote to her during the group meeting time to encourage her. She received an outpouring of support when she returned to the group a few weeks later. Her temporary relapse provoked a discussion about depression and the contributing factors and touched on others' fears of relapse.

Family caregiver's group

Family members often have difficulty following a decision to place a loved one in a home. Caregivers are prone to guilt, anger, remorse, and anxiety, as well as depressive disorders. Some struggle to find a balance between an overdriven need constantly to be at the nursing home overseeing the care of their relative versus staying away and focusing on their own physical and emotional well-being. Attempts to cope with the tremendous pain and suffering from seeing the deterioration of a lifelong mate or parent were often unsuccessful. All of the family members complained that they felt 'stuck' in their role as caregiver, unable to move forward.

This group, conducted at the Lieberman Geriatric Health Centre by an older adult program psychiatrist and Lieberman Geriatric Health Centre social worker, was comprized of two adult children and three spouses (three women and two men). Two of the men, both spouses, had a diagnosis of major depression. The two adult children, both daughters, had Axis II diagnoses as well as anxiety disorder.

The other spouse, a woman, had a diagnosis of adjustment disorder with depressed mood. The two adult children had their own families, including children. The three spouses also had children, although one of the men had lost a son in a fatal car accident a few years earlier. The greatest difficulty and challenge for the group was establishing cohesiveness with these two very distinct sets of caregivers each with unique issues, problems, and concerns. Given the limited number of family members seeking group therapy, only one group was formed.

In general, the adult children were dealing with unresolved childhood conflicts. They tended to feel more anxious and more ambivalent in regard to being a caregiver. The spouses were dealing with losing a lifelong mate. They tended to feel much more depressed, more isolated, more fearful about the future. For the most part, they had little ambivalence about being a caregiver. On the contrary, being a caregiver was central to their daily existence. They needed that role. The adult children expressed more resentment; the spouses expressed more sadness. The adult children focused on the negative aspects of their relationships with their parents; the spouses focused more on the positive aspects of their marriages and the pain of loss, while minimizing the suffering they endured while giving care to a spouse at home.

The gap between the adult children and spouses was bridged by focusing on underlying themes. When one of the adult children would talk about anger at a parent for not being there when the the adult was younger, the group leaders would comment on the pain one feels when one's needs are not met by those one depends on. Both the adult children and the spouses could identify with this issue.

The group provided not only support, but served as a forum for learning and coping. Questions included the following: 'How do I leave after each visit without feeling tremendous guilt and without creating a major scene on the floor?' 'How do I work with the staff at the home without alienating myself from them?' 'How do I begin throwing away my loved one's clothes?'

In serving as a forum, group members could gain insight into their own particular struggles.

One of the major themes that emerged during the course of the group, especially for the adult children, dealt with this struggle between feeling guilt and rage. Both daughters (ages 57 and 61) were visiting their mothers on a frequent basis. After each visit, however, the daughters would leave feeling unhappy, frustrated, anxious, and angry. The etiology of these feelings came from more than simply the result of caring for a sick parent. Both daughters felt tremendous turmoil. Neither particularly wanted to visit her mother and neither felt any relief after her visit. However, neither could bring herself to visit any less. One daughter, in particular, could not understand why she did not want to visit and why she was so reluctant to stay once she came. After several group sessions it became clear that both women felt intense rage toward their mothers, which had been repressed as children. Placing their mothers in the nursing home triggered unresolved childhood conflicts with their parents. As described by the group members, both daughters were very narcissistic. They were demanding, demeaning, and self-absorbed. Neither daughter ever felt 'good enough' or ever felt she had pleased her mother 'enough'. It appeared that these women spent much of their adult life trying to gain their mother's love, nurturance, and approval to no avail. Both parents were very angry with their daughters for placing them in the nursing home. Consequently, the need for approval gained momentum after the placement, and the repressed childhood rage pushed forth. By placing them in a nursing home, their unconscious rage and sadism found relief, leaving them with tremendous guilt. The more these two group members were able to allow these angry and rageful feelings to surface, the less guilt they experienced. Each daughter gained insight by observing and understanding the other daughter's situation. Once they began to let the anger come forth, they were then able to make sense of it and come to some understanding. It was as if they were able to begin soothing themselves for their painful experiences.

Rather than unconsciously punish themselves for these feelings, they consciously put the anger and rage in perspective and worked through it.

The men had different experiences. Both had been principally invested in their work and had few friends of either gender and few social supports. Their wives had planned social events, maintained social relations, and established social networks. For one of the men, this included maintaining the relationships with his children. Consequently, these men were isolated once their wives became ill, accentuating their loneliness and anger and contributing to their depression.

Women had very strong social networks and social support systems. They all had close women friends and had many activities to fill their days. In comparison to the men, the women seemed better able to cope without a spouse. Consequently, the group worked with the men to help them establish social networks and support systems. In sum, the men seemed more dependent than the women on the group as a main source of support and connectedness. Interestingly, the women seemed to feel very maternal toward the men, tending to be very supportive, concerned, and even nurturing.

The poetry group

Group therapy can allow members to begin to alleviate psychological symptoms through sharing creative efforts in a safe and structured environment. Further, members experience a learning process, allowing for conflict resolution via a creative process. This process allows for a feeling experience that is an antidote to apathy and withdrawal. It elicits a response at some level of inner cognition, and, finally, in interaction with the older person's external world (Saul, 1988).

Using poetry writing and discussion, this group develops the capacity for self-observation and an awareness of internal life. It encourages self-expression and, in the context of mutual respect, a support for each other to find the words to express a unique and common wisdom. Concomitantly, there is a reduction and prevention of recurrence of functional psychiatric illness.

While much has been explored regarding the use of reminiscence in individual and group therapy with older adults, the poetry therapy group adds another dimension to the process of life review. Besides the unearthing and sharing of memories, the older adult's poem is a product. This generativity, then, builds something new and lasting out of the past. The poem is also an expression and a representation of Erikson's challenge of integrity versus despair, a conduit for integrity as well as its living symbol.

The Northwestern Older Adult Poetry Therapy Group is an ongoing group that has met for three years. The five original members each has a history of severe personality disorder, as well as a variety of other diagnoses (depression, schizophrenia, obsessive disorder, anxiety disorder). Each of the original members was in individual treatment at the Older Adult Program as well as the poetry group. Three of the original members are still in the group, and new members have been added, bringing total current membership to seven.

No effort to limit members of this group to a particular diagnosis was made, but the high percentage of concomitant borderline personality disorder appeared to be a result of the new members' own interest (most were needy, verbal, and very bright) and their individual therapist's need to have more support in working with very difficult patients. The group was composed of one male and four females ranging in age from 63 to 75.

Throughout its existence the group has had one staff member – an individual with experience at writing poetry as well as with poetry therapy. In addition, the group has had several student co-therapists, each staying with the group for about six months. The format involves reading a 'famous' poem chosen by the leader, discussing it in terms of the issues and feelings it provoked, and then, perhaps, writing a group poem dealing with these same issues. Finally, each member (and leader) reads a poem that he or she has written during the week on a topic assigned at the previous meeting. The group then comments on each poem read.

The most common themes are of loss, death, love, sibling rivalry, impermanence, regrets, and 'roads not taken'.

Themes of rage and sibling rivalry were expressed after a rather explosive incident between two group members, both with great unfulfilled academic strivings, who were in constant competition for the leadership role and quite openly hostile to each other. The topic of childhood memories produced poems about younger more successful siblings from both of these members, and poems about rage and fears of being unprotected from other members and the leaders (!) When the poems were examined as an unconscious statement by the group about their feelings regarding the previous week's outbursts and rivalries, members were able to discuss these issues in a far more modulated and effective manner. Poems written in the group, then, can reflect themes and issues of transference and countertransference that are occurring presently in the group process.

Bereavement group

The death of a spouse evokes the strengths and vulnerabilities of the surviving partner. Suicide rates in widowhood are $2\frac{1}{2}$ times greater than for the population at large. When relatives, friends, and others who do not understand the grief process treat the widowed person as sick or incompetent, they may be undermining attempts of the survivor to reestablish the usual coping mechanisms (Hainer, 1988). Further, grieving individuals rapidly develop a sense that they are saturating their support system with their mourning. Identifying themselves as a burden to others, they begin to isolate from social networks. Concomitantly, friends and family frequently avoid extensive discussions of death in order to prevent unpleasant responses.

Ironically, the supporting individuals avoid the very process that offers the greatest assistance in working through grief. Further complicating matters, friends and family often select a healing rate that is mismatched for the needs of the mourner. A major thrust of this group was therefore directed at providing an environment that minimized the sense of burden and respected the individual's pace of recovery.

The group was initiated with the expectation that a group environment might temper the usual suffering of bereavement as well as shorten the recovery period associated with it. A time limited format was adopted (weekly sessions × 5 months) to send a direct message to members. The expectation was that they would achieve some resolution of their grief. Later group sessions were most productive. Members reached greater intimacy and shared more painful material in anticipation of the group's impending termination.

A blend of a cognitive–behavioral approach and an insight-oriented process, relying on a bereavement manual (Spangler, 1988) accepted by local hospice agencies was utilized. The group members were educated about mourning phases and symptoms and were given home assignments to facilitate the process of sharing with others. These assignments involved writing letters both to fictitious or real people as well as to the deceased themselves, describing their loss. A personal journal was encouraged and referred to in group discussion.

Initially each session was scheduled for one hour; however, the group rapidly moved to expand this to ninety minutes in order to more fully develop topics of each session. While another initial attempt involved bringing refreshments to each session, this also yielded to the group's disfavor. Perhaps group members were declaring that group sessions were not merely social gatherings.

Each of our group members was white and widowed aged between 68 and 80 years. Grieving the losses of children and siblings was also a focus. Members were a highly educated group recruited directly from the community via a public medical newsletter. Recent history of major depression existed in four of the six group members in the earlier stages of their bereavement. Two members had concomitant anxiety features manifesting with panic episodes. Three group members were receiving individual psychotherapy and/or pharmacotherapy while enrolled in the group. Cognitive impairment was minimal among members.

Each group member was individually screened by the two group leaders (a psychology intern and a geriatric psychiatry fellow) prior to entry. A firm commitment was sought in order to minimize the disruption of member turnover. Only one individual had previous group experience. In response, early sessions were instructive with regard to group process as well as the grieving process itself.

Members of the group spent considerable time discussing the loneliness and emptiness they experienced, often referring to themselves as out of place in their previous social spheres: 'Like a man who arrives to a formal affair dressed in a black tuxedo with brown shoes', as one member described it. All agreed they were struggling for new social identity.

While sadness was an important area of discussion, the primary affect was anger. It was apparent that they were reluctant to share their anger within their support systems, and thus the group served as an outlet. Often anger was displaced on to fellow group members for infractions of group rules such as tardiness. Anger reached its greatest level, however, in response to a group member failing to respond to another member in an empathic manner. This anger was readily understood in the context of the anger felt toward the loss of the dead family member (Freud, 1964), as well as toward the medical system. The members were angry at a system that failed to defy death and had been insensitive to their emotional suffering at the time of their loved one's death. The circumstance of death was also a relevant factor in understanding anger. Those members whose loved one died after a chronic course seemed to harbor greater anger. This usually involved issues of nursing home placement, and the perceived injustices of that system, as well. In response to this, the group members seemed quick to validate their struggles, and often praised each other for courage in dealing with a prolonged death. This seemed to attenuate the guilt associated with utilizing the nursing home.

In order to temper the emotional pain incurred in the discussion of death, group members made frequent use of favorable reminiscing. At times, this was intentionally prompted by inviting members to bring photographs and memorabilia so the group could better share each other's emotional attachment. Members of the group thus made use of memories of how their loved ones lived as well as how they died.

There was general agreement among the group that this five month process did a great deal to allay their sense of isolation. Clearly, their loss and their subsequent involvement in a group helped them to identify a sense of trust in others that they had not previously recognized. Those members who made the greatest use of sharing techniques, namely the letter writing and journal recording, developed the most in establishing a 'new sense of identity'. These techniques were acknowledged as tools that would be used long after group termination.

A few confounding factors that seemed to interfere with people benefiting from group work became apparent. First, if group members had anxiety or depressive disorders predating their loss, the tendency was to try to get these 'solved' in the group setting. This distracted from grief work. However, it did prompt individual and pharmacotherapy which, in turn, facilitated the group work. Second, timing of the death and when the individual entered the group was relevant. Only one member dropped out of the group. This was believed to be, in part, due to the fact that she entered within a few weeks of the death of her husband. The intensity of group sharing seemed too much in the early stages of her grief. It does not appear that the group process is best suited for the marked reaction often encountered in the earliest stages of bereavement.

Those members who utilized the structured exercises of the group found greater resolution of their grief, as well as reduction in anxiety and suffering. This resolution perhaps is best represented by Ms A, a semi-retired social worker, who stated 'I'm almost ashamed to admit that I'm enjoying my newfound freedom'. The love of a new life is not synonymous with the abandonment of a previously loved one.

Caregivers of demented elderly

The suffering of those caring for a demented relative is enormous. The pain of witnessing decline is accentuated by the caregiver's isolation. Thus, group therapy is highly advised. This group consisted of seven members (five women and two men) ranging in age from 62 to 82. Each of the members had a spouse with dementia in the middle or later stages of the illness. The length of caretaking time varied from two to eight years.

All but one of the group members had either a major depression or dysthymia with anxiety features. One group member had an adjustment disorder with depressed mood. At least four of the group members had fairly serious physical illnesses including heart disease, high blood pressure, diabetes, and history of strokes. One group member was hospitalized with bone cancer during the group experience.

The focus of the group was the caregiver, not the identified patient at the Day Care Center. The group's orientation was insight-oriented/supportive psychotherapy, not psycho-educational. The caregivers needed to learn how to sort out and better understand their complex feelings and to improve their care for themselves.

Thus, these patients had capacity for insight and introspection, and could focus on their own needs. Many caregivers initially have difficulty focusing on themselves, however. During the process, each caregiver was asked to 'describe one incident in which you responded to your spouse or parent in a manner that afterward you regretted'. Those that were capable of examining their experiences were included in the group.

The ultimate two goals were:

1. to help caregivers better cope with their life situation by reducing psychosocial symptoms;
2. to help caregivers sort out and understand their feelings and conflicts regarding the potential placement of a loved one in a nursing home or the acquisition of full-time in-home care. All caregivers were extremely dedicated, and such decisions were very painful to make.

Initially, members felt angry and guilt-ridden and had difficulty discussing their own needs. It was much easier to talk about their demented relative; how their spouse wanders in the middle of the night or how their parent forgets where the bathroom is. To express anger or sorrow was much more difficult. However, after several months of meeting together, there was a distinct shift in the group process. Once the members were able to concentrate on their experiences, there was a drastic change in the momentum of the group. As if a dam had broken, a flood of thoughts, feelings, concerns, fears, and anxieties pushed forth. For many years these caregivers put all of their energy into caring for someone else; they had lost touch with their own needs.

Once this shift occurred, there was a sense of relief in the group. Now there was discussion about their needs, frustration, and feelings of neglect. They expressed resentment and anger and talked about feeling abandoned. As one woman said, 'I still have a life to live and I'm not ready to give it up'. Many members began to discuss the possibility of having their relative in a nursing home. For a long time they had had the enormous pressure of the '36-hour day', and they were feeling depleted and incompetent to continue the responsibility of full-time management. During the next several months, several members began the process of visiting nursing homes. By the time the group ended, two members had placed their spouses in nursing homes, one member had full-time in-home care, two members had part-time in-home care, and one member had her spouse in respite care for two weeks.

Several themes emerged in the group. The most significant of these dealt with the pain associated with watching a lifelong mate or parent deteriorate while feeling helpless to 'make things better'. For the most part, these caregivers were competent in their work, and private lives. These were people used to having control over their lives, who had always been able to solve most problems. Given their personal histories, it was extremely difficult to watch loved ones deteriorate and to feel powerless in being able to 'make them better'. Many longed for a past life that was far better. Men mourned the wives who were nurturing and concerned, who used to cook the meals, clean the house and make plans with family and friends. Women mourned the husbands who were adoring, successful, competent, and took care of their needs. All caregivers were resentful. One woman reported how angry she was at her husband for never saying 'I love you' anymore.

One woman in particular had special difficulty with her anger. She had been caring for her husband for over seven years. Her diagnosis was major depression with a mixed personality disorder. When she first came to the group, she tended to project her anger at those around her. She was mistrustful and hypervigilant and talked about how everyone was mistreating her. She was intermittently delusional, accusing people around her who were talking negatively about her.

Generally, the group was very supportive of her. They acknowledged her feelings and were empathic with her fears. In many respects, the group gave her what was missing in her relationship with her husband. Like a surrogate husband/father, the group members gave her attention, warmth and concern. The group felt a need to take care of her and to watch over her. This helped to relieve some of her depressive, anxious, and paranoid symptoms, and helped her to confront her painful feelings.

As she received the support and concern of the group, she began to experience more rage at her husband. She felt safe in the group to express these feelings, and as she was more able to express her anger, she became more independent and autonomous. She felt more empowered. By the end of the group she was able, with a minimum of guilt and turbulence, to make the decision to place her husband in a nursing home.

Conclusions

Approximately 80% of the patients participating in the above groups had diagnoses of functional psychiatric disorders, the most common being a depressive disorder. The percentage of previously psychiatrically hospitalized patients exceeded 25%, whereas the considerable majority had previous psychiatric treatment. The vast majority had character pathology, which either contributed to or derived from the functional psychiatric disorder. For many, individual psychotherapy and/or pharmacotherapy would be provided simultaneously to the group psychotherapy. Research on group psychotherapy is in an embryonic phase. However, the clinical impressions of both the staff and the patients, combined with overt improvement in functioning and diminished psychiatric symptoms, strongly suggest that group psychotherapy is a modality that benefits many older adults with functional psychiatric disorders and character pathology.

References

Finkel, S. I. (1991). Group psychotherapy in later life. *New Techniques in the Psychotherapy of Older Patients*, ed. W. A. Myers, pp. 223–44, Washington, DC: American Psychiatric Press, Inc.

Finkel, S. I. (1990). Group psychotherapy with older people. *Hospital and Community Psychiatry*, **41**, 189–91.

Freud, S. (1964). Mourning and Melancholia. In *Standard Edition of the Complete Psychological Works of Sigmund Freud*, volume 14. ed. J. Strachey. London: Hogarth Press.

Gallagher, D. (1981). Behavioral group therapy with elderly depressives: an experimental study in behavioral group therapy. *Behavioral Group Therapy*, eds. D. Upper and S. Ross. Champaign, Illinois: Research Press.

Goldfarb, A. I. (1972). Group therapy with the old and the aged. *Group Treatment of Mental Illness*, eds. H. I. Kaplan & B. J. Sadock, pp. 623–42. New York: Dutton.

Hainer, J. (1988). Groups for widowed and lonely older persons. In *Group Psychotherapies for the Elderly*, eds. B. W. Maclellan, S. Saul & M. B. Weiner, pp. 131–8. Madison: International Universities Press.

Katz, I. R., Lesher, E., Clevin, M., Jethanandani, V., & Paramelee, P. (1989). Clinical features of depression in the nursing home. *International Psychogeriatrics*, **1**, 5–15.

Kohut, H. (1984). *How does Analysis Cure?* Chicago: University of Chicago Press.

Lazarus, L. W. (1980). Self-psychology and psychotherapy with the elderly: theory and practice. *Journal of Geriatric Psychiatry*, **13**, 69–88.

Leszcz, M. (1987). Group psychotherapy with the elderly. In *Treating the Elderly with Psychotherapy*, eds. J. Sadavoy & M. Leszsz, pp. 527–46. Madison: International Universities Press.

Leszcz, M. (1991). Group therapy. In *Comprehensive Review of Geriatric Psychiatry*, eds. J. Sadavoy, L. W. Lazarus & L. F. Jarvik, pp. 527–546. London: American Psychiatry Press, Inc.

Lothstein, L. M., & Zimet, G. (1988). Twinship and alter ego self-object transferences in group therapy with the elderly. A reanalysis of the pairing phenomenon. *International Journal of Group Psychotherapy*, **38**, 303–17.

Rush, A. J. (1983). Cognitive therapy of depression. *Psychiatric Clinics of North America*, **6**, 105–27.

Saul, S. (1988). The arts as psychotherapeutic modalities with groups of older people. In *Group Psychotherapies for the Elderly*, eds. B. W. Maclellan, S. Saul & M. B. Weiner, pp. 139–48. Madison: International Universities Press.

Schwartzman, G. (1984). The use of the group as self object. *International Journal of Group Psychotherapy*, **34**, 229–42.

Spangler, J. D. (1988). *Bereavement Support Groups: Leadership Manual*. Denver: Grief Education Institute.

Tross, S. & Blum, J. E. (1988). Review of group therapy with the older adult: practice and research. In *Group Psychotherapies for the Elderly*, eds. B. W. Maclellan, S. Saul & M. B. Weiner, pp. 3–32. Madison: International Universities Press.

Yalom, I. B. (1985). *The Theory and Practice of Group Psychotherapy*. New York: Basic Books.

29

Integrated psychotherapy of the elderly

JOEL SADAVOY

Introduction

Psychotherapy for the elderly is a rich but all too infrequently utilized modality of treatment. The data on efficacy and descriptions of technique reveal the depth and flexibility of approaches including cognitive therapies especially for depression and anxiety disorders (Thompson et al., 1991), psychotherapy in the institution (Sadavoy, 1992; Goldfarb & Turner, 1953), psychoanalytic psychotherapy (Rechtschaffen, 1959) psychoanalysis (Meerloo, 1953), and interpersonal psychotherapy (Scholomskas et al., 1983).

Elderly patients arrive at treatment on a variety of pathways either through self-referral or, perhaps more commonly, because the individual is brought by his or her family. Frequently, the first contact is with a caregiver in the community such as a general practitioner or social worker. This initial contact offers a special opportunity for psychotherapeutic intervention, because the older person may accept more easily the medical context of the general practitioner's office or the service context of the social worker's office as opposed to the psychiatric context. Geriatric patients often feel that they will be branded as 'crazy' if they see a psychiatrist (Lazarus & Sadavoy, 1991) and frequently they are frightened of the meaning of the referral. The practitioner's awareness of the potential efficacy of these treatments is important since the elderly tend substantially to underutilize psychiatric outpatient services, not only because of their own shame and embarrassment, but equally because of practical problems in arranging transportation, the presence of comorbid medical conditions which may interfere with therapy, and scepticism about such treatment by too-narrowly focused practitioners.

The functional perspective

The decision about which is the most appropriate psychotherapeutic intervention for a given patient is best made based on a functional rather than chronological perspective. This is so because the aged are a heterogeneous population who traverse the period of old age on a long path that begins with normative aging at one extreme and ends with physical and mental frailty at the other (Kahana, 1979). At the normative end of the aging process generally are the young–old and the middle–old (Neugarten, 1979), 65 to 75 years of age, who are relatively healthy and often able to mobilize a variety of strengths and capacities to deal with the problems of aging as they arise. At the far end of the continuum are the frail elderly, often the old old, over age 80, frequently institutionalized and coping with a multiplicity of diseases, as well as cognitive decline. When deciding how to intervene psychotherapeutically with a given patient, it is helpful to try to place the patient at a point along this continuum since the more normative elderly should be encouraged to develop autonomous control over their environment to the limits of their capacity, while the more frail elderly are in need of a greater degree of environmental support. Similarly, during psychotherapy, the normative elderly are more likely to be able to reflect on their problems and work through psychological stressors (e.g. grief) with the expectation that they will be able to reconstitute and carry on with their lives (Kahana, 1987). The frail elderly, however, are less able to use insight and self-reflection. They are much more in need of supportive interventions, wherein the therapist and other caregivers must be prepared to take on an advocacy role, for example, contacting community support agencies to make sure that the patient has adequate home care, meals on wheels, and so on.

The psychological tasks of aging

With this perspective in mind it is an obvious first step to look beyond the initial physical or other crisis presentation of the patient to determine the interacting psychological issues. This is especially important for geriatric patients who often struggle with concurrent relational, social and physical problems.

The most difficult and basic psychological and adaptational tasks of old age include coping with grief, anxiety, depression and demands upon adaptational skills in order to deal with losses associated with physical, relational and social decline. In addition to coping with loss, the elderly generally must cope with a variety of fears and anxieties often associated with facing the unknown, as well as an awareness of their own mortality.

In some respects clinical experience of elderly patients is surprising in that fear of death and death anxiety is not a prominent finding. This is particularly so in the old–old cohort who often have come to terms with their mortality and, indeed, may welcome it or at least accept it with equanimity. The author's experience parallels the theoretical position of Elliott Jacques (1965) who proposed that death anxiety is most evident in middle age when the first glimpses of the finite horizon of life emerge. In contrast, the elderly struggle more significantly with fears of pain, being left alone, placed in an institution or becoming dependent.

Because loss is one central issue in the psychological presentation of the elderly, an important developmental task for the aging individual is to work through and accept the multiple biopsychosocial losses associated with this stage of life. This is a grieving process which Pollock (1987) has labelled mourning-liberation. It goes on throughout life but becomes most important in old age. Unless losses are dealt with effectively, the aging individual may find all of his or her psychological energy taken up with coping with alterations in self-image, bitterness over abandonment and so on. This is a daunting process for some, since the troubles of old age often come in 'battalions'. What seems to be so overwhelming for some elderly patients is the speed and cumulative effect of multiple losses occurring close together before enough time has elapsed to allow them to deal with the preceding crisis. The author recently saw a survivor of the Nazi Holocaust who was depressed following a disabling stroke, trying to cope with this devastating change at the same time as her husband lay dying in a hospital bed down the hall. When coping with loss the elderly often must adapt to a new level of dependency. Family relationships change as children become more dominant in the caretaking relationships. The elderly must sometimes give up some control and self-reliance in keeping with declining capacities, an especially difficult task when care must be taken over by professionals or other strangers, as occurs, for example, after institutionalization.

Patients react to physical and other disabilities in old age with a variety of psychological responses which often interact. Some patients have a strong need to deny their problems. A particularly problematic example of denial occurs when a dependent elderly person is reliant upon a husband or wife who will not acknowledge the nature or severity of their spouse's illness. It is common to find that, despite being told over and over again what the problems are, a spouse will continue to expect their dementing husband or wife to behave normally, becoming frustrated, enraged and even physically abusive when this does not happen. A gentle, caring and educative stance on the part of the therapist is needed and the therapist should beware of becoming angrily confrontational and feeling frustrated because good advice is not heeded. However, if after a trial of intervention and education there is no change in the pattern of denial and if the welfare of the patient is threatened, it may be necessary for the therapist to intervene to separate a vulnerable elderly person from an unyielding caregiver.

Many elderly patients become acutely anxious, and fear that they are going to be abandoned in the face of their difficulties, often assuming that others will not want to tolerate their illnesses. They may express the fear that they will become a burden on their families. However, this fear is often a thinly disguised anxiety that their children or spouse will reject them. In the face of often overwhelming illness or incurable disease, such as dementia or a stroke, patients and/or caregivers may become enraged both with themselves and their illness and displace this feeling onto the physician or the caretaking system. The therapist must be sensitive to the fact that such angry feelings may cover over more basic feelings of depression and hopelessness.

The therapist should keep in mind that some elderly patients do not understand the nature of their problems, although they are capable of forming an understanding if educated. Ignorance about disease will breed fears and fantasies which may become overwhelming and lead to undue pessimism.

Especially with chronic illnesses, withdrawal and depression are a common accompaniment. Sometimes major affective disorder develops, and more often these are dysthymic reactions which resemble depression, and more accurately, should be seen as struggles to adapt to loss and grief.

Similarly, patients frequently develop anxiety states or even panic which may be characterized by sleeplessness, frequent calls for help and assistance or the development of a helpless, importuning, sometimes demanding stance which has been termed 'the exaggerated helplessness syndrome' (Breslau, 1987).

Making contact

Psychotherapy, like any other treatment, relies on careful evaluation and diagnosis. Initial contact, therefore, is characterized by a complete physical and psychiatric history with attention to the patient's social and economic cohort, educational level, retained physical and cognitive capacities and family relationships.

In the initial evaluation of the elderly patient it is important to define who is the patient, who is in need of psychotherapeutic intervention. Sometimes it is the individual patient presenting with an acute problem who is the one who is in need of psychotherapy, but it is also true that other members of the patient's system, especially a spouse or a child who is a primary caregiver, will be equally or more in need of psychotherapy (Goldstein, 1991).

When the presenting problem is an acute crisis, the issues are often relatively clearcut. However, when the problem is more chronic, one may ask why the patient is presenting in distress at this time. For example, a 72-year-old man sought therapy at the urging of his daughter, three years after triple bypass surgery. He was concerned about his temper outbursts, although his temper had been a lifelong problem and apparently he had adapted reasonably well following his operation. Hence, the reason he was now seeking help was not immediately evident. It was only on close questioning that two factors came to light. The first was that the patient had been increasingly resentful of his wife's sexual and emotional unavailability and he had started to feel more angry with her. In this context, he came across an article in *Readers' Digest* which warned that patients with anger and temper outbursts were more prone to heart attacks. He became acutely anxious that his rage would kill him and he sought help.

During the initial assessment it is helpful and instructive to explore and form a picture of the patient's current self-perception. The physically ill patient may be asked what does your illness mean to you? How does it make you feel to have the illness? Does it change your image of yourself and the way that you relate to others? Do you feel capable of coping with this or does it feel as though it is going to be overwhelming? Similarly, important information about the possible course of therapy and the types of interventions which will be helpful may be obtained by asking the patient about their perception of the therapist. In particular, one wants to know what the patient expects from the therapist, and what kind of information the patient wants to have (some patients want complete explanations, while others want to leave the care and decision-making entirely in the hands of the doctor). During the process of this inquiry, the therapist will get a sense of how reliant the patient wants to be, and, in turn, how fearful the patient is of having to deal with the illness alone.

Early on, the therapist explores the realities of the patient's current and future needs and how those realities stack up against the patient's expectations. The patient is often helped if the therapist summarizes what he or she has heard the patient say during the assessment with regard to their self-perception, perceptions of the therapist and statement of needs and expectations. This feedback summary to patients gives them the knowledge that they have been heard and understood and that the therapist is truly aware of their difficulties. It is a first step in cementing the alliance between patient and therapist. Patients derive immense support if the physician also outlines a realistic treatment program based on their new understanding of the patient that takes into account the patient's physical, interpersonal and psychological stressors.

The psychotherapeutic perspective also demands an evaluation of the patient's developmental history (often omitted during a work-up on elderly patients) with particular reference to the nature of the psychological defense mechanisms (which they have always employed) and the impact of life stressors on their personality structure. This part of the inquiry is more than a sterile gathering of lists of peers, school attainments and milestones. It is a lively investigation of the emotional tone of the patient's relationships – what was gratifying and what angering. How did the patient obtain pleasure and gratification from activities; was it the creativity, the recognition of others, or the obsessional concern with perfection?

General principles of psychotherapy

Once the therapist has assessed the patient's presenting problems and determined some of the components of the psychological reaction with which the particular patient is struggling, the next question is how to intervene. Any effective intervention for the elderly must be informed by complete physical diagnosis with the use of pharmacology as necessary. However, for many of the anxiety syndromes, depressive withdrawal and reactions that stem from ignorance, avoidance or denial, psychotherapeutic intervention may be very helpful.

Psychotherapy, at this point in the life cycle, may be the only avenue open to satisfying the basic human need to be known and understood as an individual. Illness and other alterations of life in the final stage of human development all interact to create feelings of being lost, unacknowledged and unknown.

If regular psychotherapy is to be instituted, the therapist should set aside a specific time which is kept free of interruptions. However, because geriatric patients often have difficulties with transportation and coping with unforeseen problems, the therapy time should also be somewhat flexible and meet the needs of the patient.

In certain instances, patients who cannot come to the office may have to be seen at home depending upon the availability of the therapist.

The therapist should expect to meet the patient. Geriatric patients, particularly, are vulnerable to feeling that the therapist does not want to see them or that they are a burden. The therapist should beware of retreating into unresponsiveness or a 'classical' stance that the therapy is solely the responsibility of the patient. Patients who fail to come may be called to find out why and to re-book the next appointment. This concept of regularity and reliability in sessions is one of the most important elements of the psychotherapeutic endeavour, but one which often is paid insufficient attention (Sadavoy, 1992).

The heterogeneity of the elderly patient group requires flexibility of technique and careful attention to individualizing the approach to each patient. The common wisdom that old people like to be touched, sat close to and spoken loudly at is often true, but, equally many patients find it demeaning. In the words of a fictional patient: 'nothing is more humiliating than to be given a bed pan by a stranger who calls you by your first name'.

In choosing a psychotherapeutic intervention, the therapist must keep in mind the importance of blending psychotherapy with other modalities. This is best illustrated in the management of depression. The depressions of old age often appear to be 'reactive' because of the concurrent problems of the patient and may be labelled 'neurotic' or 'reactive' depression. Some therapists erroneously believe that such 'reactive' depressions are less responsive to antidepressants and that psychotherapy is primarily indicated. This may be true particularly if the patient is seen to have a concurrent longstanding personality problem. However, if a geriatric patient presents with signs of severe depression sufficient to fulfil criteria for a major affective disorder, and is substantially disabled by these symptoms, the biological therapy must be the treatment of first choice with psychotherapy a necessary initial adjunct, regardless of the presence of precipitant. A notable exception is bereavement which is difficult to distinguish from a depressive syndrome. When the symptoms of bereavement are still in the acute phase (less than three months old), even if there is a relatively severe picture, psychotherapy may be utilized as a trial without medication. However, the therapist should watch for prolongation of these symptoms, and if they continue for beyond four to six months, either worsening or not improving, then active pharmacologic or other intervention often is necessary. The picture can be quite confusing as illustrated in this case.

Clinical example

Mrs. A, a 66-year-old woman who was widowed approximately two months prior to assessment was referred for treatment of depression. Her symptoms included withdrawal from all activities, marked sleep disturbance, $5\frac{1}{2}$ pound weight loss with appetite disturbance, loss of energy and interest, frequent fits of crying, hopelessness about the future and feelings of being a burden to others and 'hating myself'. She had occasional wishes for death but was not actively suicidal. Her mood was pervasive and according to her never lifted. She had a concurrent comorbid condition of mitral insufficiency leading to occasional episodes of tachycardia. In the past history was an episode of severe depression when she was in her 30s, which was self-limiting, remitting spontaneously after several weeks. She also described a number of psychodynamic issues relevant to the development of this severe depressive picture. Clearly, the diagnosis of major depression was virtually indistinguishable from that of bereavement. In this case the therapist elected to delay the institution of antidepressant medication, although noting that this would be added to the treatment if she did not begin to respond. Fortunately, psychotherapy alone was effective over a period of several weeks.

Bereavement, therefore, is a special instance in evaluating the indications for psychotherapy. While symptoms may be severe in the early stages following the loss, it is the author's experience that psychotherapy is often an effective mode of intervention which does not necessarily require concurrent use of medication.

In taking a psychotherapeutic approach to the geriatric patient the therapist should be aware that integration of treatments rather than choosing the purity of one therapeutic modality is likely to be most effective. Broadly, four individual interventions are commonly used in this age group, supportive psychotherapy, reminiscence therapy, cognitive and behavioral therapy and psychodynamic psychotherapy. Additionally, therapists must be prepared to offer therapy in the family or group setting.

Supportive psychotherapy

Supportive therapies are useful for all patients, but are particularly so for the frail elderly. Using this mode of intervention the therapist is active and interventive. He engages frequently with the patient, encouraging them to go on, and asking questions which elicit the expression of feeling states, rather than just practical information. For example, instead of asking simply 'how is your energy' the therapist asks: 'how does it feel when you cannot do the things you used to, what goes through your mind when you are alone, how do you react and feel about the response of your family?'

Promoting ventilation of feelings is one element of supportive therapy. The process is encouraged when the therapist creates a safe and nonjudgmental atmosphere coupled with very specific inquiries about areas of emotional importance – physical illnesses, family relationships or living arrangements. In this process, especially if the patient has some cognitive impairment, the therapist must be able to tolerate repetition and recurrence of themes. Such repetition is common, but far from being useless, it may be an important mechanism for an otherwise emotionally restricted patient to make contact with their emotional self, thereby enhancing reintegration and healing.

Supportive techniques include a patient-centered stance which may be developed by listening attentively and then rephrasing the patient's thoughts for them to demonstrate that they have been heard and understood.

When distorted ideas emerge or there is a need for practical solutions the therapist should not hesitate to suggest other ways of thinking or explore problem solving mechanisms. However, paternalism, if too strong, impairs the patient's sense of control. For the elderly, who often feel that their opinions about their own life are not valued, this is especially important, and the therapist should take pains to respect the patient's control to the limits of their capacity.

Reassurance may be confused with support. Perhaps most importantly, therapeutic reassurance must convey realistic hope. This requires of the therapist a genuine concern with uncovering and understanding the depth and complexity of the issues. To say 'don't worry' when clearly there is much to be concerned about creates distance. While momentarily relieved, patients rapidly realize the hollowness of this approach and lose faith in the therapist's willingness to be fully involved with their problems. Indeed, reassurance may fulfil the function for the therapist of staying at an emotional distance from the pain or demandingness of the patient.

Reminiscence therapy

The purpose of reminiscence therapy is to help enhance the patient's sense of self, by encouraging life review, which has been said to be a normal process in aging. Since reminiscence or life review therapy was proposed by Butler (1963) it has received considerable research attention. Tobin and Lieberman (1976) found that, while reminiscence is a common, perhaps normative process in old age, it is not universal nor, in itself, does it seem to lead to a resolution of longstanding conflicts. However, in controlled circumstances in therapy it can be effective.

This technique seems to exercise its effect by promoting cohesion of the sense of self, enhanced self-esteem and improved interaction with others. The mechanism of change lies in the retrieval of remembered past experiences which derive from a time of greater vigour, strength and involvement. The contact with a part of themselves that, in the past, was healthier and perhaps more capable of coping, when guided in therapy, helps patients to work through losses and to put their current situation into a lifelong perspective.

While this approach may be used effectively for most elderly patients including depressed elderly, caution should be exercised with patients whose current perspectives are focused entirely on bad images of the past or recreations of intense traumatic experiences. One such patient, with a recurrent unipolar depression seen recently by the author, was a survivor of the holocaust. Reminiscence for her was a painful process and her depression in itself was already re-evoking traumatic memories from the war. Since such massive trauma is virtually impossible to work through or to put into a more enhancing context, a more appropriate approach is to help the patient encapsulate or focus her thoughts on nontraumatic events and memories. Similarly, patients who harbour depressive psychotic delusions will not be helped by reminiscence because of the distortions which are firmly fixed. One elderly depressed patient was convinced that she had misrepresented herself on her tax return by failing to sign her name correctly. She ruminated repeatedly about this delusional misdeed and all thoughts of the past served only to actuate further self-accusation. Clearly, reminiscence is contraindicated during the early stages of therapy of such patients.

In other situations, however, reminiscence may be very helpful. An example of using this technique in a group setting occurred in a psychotherapy session for depressed patients in a psychiatric day hospital. The patients, who averaged about 75 years of age, began to speak about their past swimming experiences. Three of these women, it turned out, had been high divers and they spoke with obvious intense pleasure about the memories of their exhilaration and pride in the physical accomplishments of their youth. Concurrently, their mood and sense of self-esteem visibly changed as they became filled with the remembered self-assurance.

The basic technique of this therapy is to guide the patient's memories to various important images of the past, especially satisfying relationships, productive and creative work, physical ability and spiritual faith.

In addition to verbal interventions, techniques of reminiscence include asking patients to make audiotapes, written records or even video records of their lives.

In keeping with this technique, patients may also be encouraged to take up previously enjoyed activities or to develop new ones.

Despite how common reminiscence is in the early stages of therapy, as elderly patients become more comfortable with the therapist, memories may give way to working on more immediate, age-related conflicts. This evolution appears to occur when the patient develops confidence in the therapist's acceptance of their current role and abilities. In other words, while reminiscence serves a healing function in therapy, it is also a manifestation of the elderly patient's fear of rejection and sense of alienation caused by age-related changes. Reminiscence is an initial method of presenting the aging self in a better light as though to say, 'I may not seem to be much now, but just listen to what I used to be'.

Cognitive therapy

Cognitive therapy has been shown to be especially useful for treatment of dysthymic disorders, depression and anxiety although, despite the impression conveyed in some research it is not a substitute for medication, especially in severe depressions. This approach is based on the theory that ideas produce feelings and that various situations may provoke distorted ideas about oneself which, for example, lead to depressive or anxiety producing conclusions, thereby inducing symptomatic behavior. The theory and therapeutic approach was first described by Beck et al. (1979). Training manuals have been developed and more recently the approaches have been adapted to the elderly (Thompson et al., 1991).

The first step in treatment is to help the patient identify the major source of depressive conflict (distorted belief systems). For example, patients may feel 'I am bad because I do not do enough for my husband' or 'I can't perform my work the way I used to and I am useless'. Such distortions may arise in response to loss of relationships, work roles, health, economic stability, or home. Using this technique, the therapist keeps the patient focused on the here and now, gently interrupting the tendency to reminiscence. In step two, the therapist examines with the patient the pros and cons of the idea and of the reality versus the fantasy. Part of this process is to help the patient correct distortions in thought and to introduce reality, for example 'this aspect of what you feel may be true, but perhaps this other element is not'. In order to consolidate the learning process that goes on in therapy, some therapists strongly advocate that the patient be given homework, often comprised of trying a simple specific action (Gallagher & Thompson, 1983). However, the therapist should beware that in more severe depressions, even simple actions may be beyond the capacity of the patient and care must be taken not to advise what the patient cannot do.

Thompson et al. (1991) suggest some modifications of technique specific to treating the elderly. These include enhancing the relationship by encouraging the patient to teach the therapist (as well as vice versa) attending to sensory deficits such as hearing loss, and presenting feedback in several different sensory modalities, e.g. auditory and written. In one Day Hospital Program (Steingart, 1991) all discussions are accompanied by written summaries prepared throughout the group sessions on flip charts.

A detailed discussion of cognitive behavioral techniques is beyond the scope of this chapter and may be found elsewhere (McMullin, 1986; Burns, 1989). Specific useful approaches include (Thompson et al., 1991): (a) constructing a dysfunctional thought record, i.e. a list of thoughts that produce symptoms; (b) the patient is then encouraged to develop new alternate or adaptive thoughts in response to each dysfunctional thought; (c) in the process of developing new perspectives (alternate thoughts) the patient's belief system is carefully examined (evaluating the evidence) and distortions dissected along the patient's chain of reasoning until the core erroneous premise is revealed (vertical arrow technique).

Concurrent approaches include encouraging engagement in pleasant activities, journal writing, assertiveness training, and relaxation training.

Dynamic and interpersonal therapy

Intensive psychodynamic psychotherapy or even psychoanalysis has been attempted with geriatric patients with success. In general, appropriate geriatric patients resemble those who are appropriate at any age. Techniques are also similar although some age specific modifications and geriatric specific themes are evident.

As noted above, the centrality of loss places heavy strain on the ability of the aging individual to maintain self-esteem, value and purpose. Inevitably everyone must face diminishing ego capacities and increased vulnerability to narcissistic blows. In psychotherapy these losses emerge as various themes: early on during aging, marriages evolve and may come under strain as children become increasingly involved in their own lives; role change is an important component in facing retirement, often accompanied by fears of loss of status and reduced economic resources; individuals confront the reality of their life achievements and the potential disappointment in failing to realize long held ambitions and idealized aspirations; physical changes leading to loss of sexual attractiveness coupled with changing demography cause difficulties in finding appropriate relationships, especially for women. As aging continues, bereavement inevitably ensues, individuals having to face the loss of spouse, other family members, and friends. Perhaps most traumatic is the experience of those who outlive their adult children.

A variety of theories of the psychological tasks of aging have been developed. Erikson (1968) understood the eighth and last phase of his developmental theory as characterized by the need to attain ego integrity. Failure to do so leads to despair and self-loathing.

Development theorists (Nemiroff & Colarusso, 1985) have stressed the perspective that intrapsychic change can continue throughout adult life. In this theoretical model adult experience acts to modify intrapsychic structures of the individual (in contrast to classical theorists who hold that the structure of the psyche is fixed in early life).

Pearl King (1980) has described her view of old age as a time when adolescent conflicts are reworked, the difference being that the direction of the energy is reversed. For example, issues of autonomy and dependence are central to old age as to adolescence but, in contrast to adolescence, the direction is not toward expansion and individuation, but rather toward the acceptance of restriction and increased reliance on others.

Age-specific issues that are central to traditional psychoanalytic theory of aging include anxieties generated by physical incapacity and dependency; anxiety over loss of sexual potency and reactivation of infantile castration fears; and various resistances to accepting age specific changes with the emergence of regressive or otherwise inappropriate behaviors.

Transference and countertransference issues

Central to psychodynamic psychotherapy is an understanding of the basis for the patient's reactions in the therapeutic encounter (transference) as well as an examination of the reactions of the therapists which derive from their own psychological conflicts (countertransference).

Because the unconscious is timeless (Berezin, 1972), it is not affected by the patient's age. Hence, regardless of the difference in the chronological age of patient and therapist, elderly patients often experience themselves as small, childlike and helpless. The therapist, therefore, may become a substitute parent whose idealized and unrealistically viewed power becomes a magical shield against the forces of old age. For some patients, negative transferences may emerge and therapists may be rejected, patients viewing them as intrusive, voyeuristic or otherwise dangerous to their self-esteem. As in treatment of younger patients, transference may become eroticized, the older patient developing sexual feelings and fantasies about the younger therapist. This can be an acutely uncomfortable experience for the therapist who must confront his own feelings about the taboos of sexuality in old age and, at a deeper level, the sexuality of parents.

Frequently, the patient will begin to deal with the therapist as though he or she is a child, (so-called filial transference). In this constellation of feeling, the therapist may begin to feel the indirectly expressed demands of the patient for the therapist to care for and treat them as a loving child would treat a parent.

The classical transference paradigm is one in which the infantile feelings of the patient are acted out with the therapist who then takes on the parental role. With geriatric patients, the opposite paradigm temporarily develops (so-called reverse transference) in which the patient acts out the parental role and imposes a child-like relationship on the therapist.

Countertransference is an important element in therapy in that it may be responsible either for the therapist avoiding treatment of the aging patient or, conversely, initiating an unrealistic and overzealous treatment approach. In the former case, the therapist may feel, sometimes unreasonably, that the aging patient is unsuitable for therapy, rationalizing that treatment may be ineffective or non-productive. These feelings are often reinforced by therapists' feelings that the patient is at the end of life and therefore does not warrant intense therapeutic effort. Additionally, therapeutic avoidance may be fostered by the therapist's sense that he or she is incompetent to deal with the overwhelming problems of the patient, particularly if they are severely physically ill or dying.

A variety of reactions may emerge during psychotherapy of the elderly including anxiety about the therapist's own mortality, shock at experiencing sexualized feelings toward the patient, emergence of conflicts with their own parents, fears of being overwhelmed by unmanageable destructive forces of aging, and over-idealization of the patient with unconscious desires to become the favored child.

All of these conflicts may make it difficult for therapists to deal with the issue of termination of psychotherapy with older patients. Therapists may begin to feel that they must continue therapy to protect the patient from the decline of ageing. This may not be a conscious idea but, rather a manifestation of anxiety about the fate of the wellbeing of the patient should therapy end. Indeed, termination is a difficult matter in psychotherapy of the elderly. However, those patients who retain sufficient ego strength and flexibility in their lives are able to end therapy. Others, whose physical, intellectual and social circumstances produce a greater degree of dependency, often require long term or indefinite intermittent therapy.

Integration of therapies

While psychodynamic, cognitive, reminiscence and supportive therapies comprise four separate approaches, in practice it is useful to use ideas from all four models at the same time.

Case example

The case of Mrs A described above who presented with a picture of acute grief continued with an exploration of her background which served as a framework to understand her current symptomatology. She had grown up in a home in which she assumed the role of the 'good child' performing rigidly to high standards of behaviour in order to maintain the love and approval of her parents, in particular her mother. She harbored a lifelong sense of inferiority and jealousy particularly in relationship to her sister and gradually developed coping methods which led her to become highly compliant, keeping all feelings of anger and rejection to herself. Consequently, she was a model child and adolescent carrying on this pattern into her married life, all the while secretly feeling angry and taken advantage of. Her husband's attention was diverted to his own mother during their marriage, sacrificing his own family including his wife. The patient felt abandoned to look after her two children but never overtly complained. In the final 18 years of her marriage her husband developed a chronic cardiac condition which left him disabled, thereby increasing the patient's self-imposed demands. Her life became highly restricted in that she had to devote herself to her husband and to her work, unable to spend time with her friends. Consequently these relationships gradually diminished and by the time she entered therapy, she asserted that her friends were 'long gone'.

At the death of her husband she was left with very ambivalent feelings toward him which made it difficult for her adequately to grieve. Because of her longstanding self-sacrifice it was hard for her to conceptualize herself as an independent person capable of looking after herself. The concept of giving to herself was foreign and when she thought of doing so she reexperienced childhood feelings that she would be rejected and abandoned. Moreover, since her life had always been defined by the things that she did for others, when her sick husband finally died she no longer had a focus for these efforts and she felt useless and valueless.

After assessment, a treatment plan was suggested based on intensive psychotherapy twice a week. The patient readily agreed saying she 'had a lot to work out'.

In subsequent early sessions she began to speak of a secret and longstanding wish to be more independent but at first was unable to talk about herself without adopting the self-attacking stance which she had utilized throughout her life. Initially, the therapist took a supportive and relatively reflective stance with her, encouraging her to talk about the feelings of injustice which she felt both related to the recent past, i.e. her husband, as well as similar feelings about her family and her distant past. She welcomed the opportunity to begin to talk about these feelings because she had never revealed them to anyone before. Parenthetically, it is important to note that many geriatric patients will confide in a therapist that they have harbored longstanding secret feelings which only come out in this last stage of life.

In the early phases of therapy the patient recounted events but did not connect them with feeling states. As the combination of anger and depression surrounding her self-imposed and externally imposed emotional imprisonment throughout her life became evident, therapy began to focus on material that highlighted to her that it must have been very hard for her to have to give up her own dreams and ambitions because of the needs of her husband and others. This type of nonjudgmental and gently interpretive stance helped establish a safe alliance in therapy. As she became more convinced that I was not going to reject her or judge her for her feelings she slowly started to reveal herself more deeply. Person by person she spoke of virtually everyone in her life who had always 'taken advantage of me'. During this process she became more firmly attached in the therapy and on several occasions repeated her sense of how much work had to be done and how much she needed to understand about herself. As therapy progressed she showed an eagerness and excitement to know more about herself, and began to make important changes in the way that she dealt with herself and her life. While her depression fluctuated in intensity, it gradually moderated through therapy and in the process the patient began to become more self-assertive. The change was promoted utilizing two techniques. The first was psychodynamic interpretation of her need to protect herself from parental rejection by always complying with the wishes of others. This approach was coupled with a more cognitively based intervention which explored the distorted belief that she held about her need to please others because of her fear that they would not continue to respond to her in her time of bereavement and need. Additionally, the therapist encouraged her to take active control of certain situations. For example she was trying to cope with a highly demanding sister-in-law who frequently called and asked her to chauffeur her to various places. The patient, in the past, always complied immediately with these requests. With encouragement and armed with increased knowledge about herself the patient began to refuse. She returned to her following sessions quite exhilarated by the fact that she had been able to confront her sister-in-law without the expected consequences and gradually began extending her degree of control to all the relationships in her life.

In summary, the therapeutic approach in this case was a combination of supportive, cognitive/interpersonal, practical intervention and more laterally psychodynamically based interventions. This is a potent armamentarium in psychotherapy which, in this case, led to the remission of depressive symptoms and active reinvolvement of the patient both in her life and in the continuing treatment.

Behavioral interventions

Behavior therapies generally are used to target specific behaviors which are troublesome to the patient or to those in the environment. Indications for such intervention may include depressive or even psychotic disorders, disorders with a physiological component such as incontinence or wandering and socially inappropriate behavior (Carstensen & Edelstein, 1987; Hussian & Davis, 1985; Lewinsohn and Teri, 1983).

Treatment technique includes a clear definition of a target behavior and an analysis of the environmental precipitants which produce the behavior. This analysis is then followed by the introduction of specific alterations in environmental response, such as staff reactions, or the introduction of reinforcers to encourage and shape behavioral change in the desired direction.

Problems with behavior therapy include the fact that treatment programs often must be maintained in order for their efficacy to continue. Sometimes behavior programs are successfully introduced on a time-limited basis but once the program has ceased the principles often do not generalize. Equally important is the fact that 'troublesome' behavior is often an external evaluation of a caregiver or staff member. Despite the best of intentions, there is a danger that such an externally imposed value will not take into consideration the actual need and benefit of the patient, rather imposing a mechanistic instrumental change. The ethical and moral issues involved in such circumstances must be carefully weighed.

Family intervention

With the elderly, it is common wisdom that the family generally should be involved. This is particularly true for patients at the frail end of the developmental continuum but may be less so at the normative end. How then should this be done?

First the patient must be informed by the therapist that he or she wants to see the family and secondly, the patient should consent to this process. Some patients cannot give consent because of cognitive incapacity. However, the therapist should resist the temptation to bypass the patient and turn directly to the family, either in the interview situation, or by telephone, without recognizing that some patients do not wish to have their families involved.

Once consent to involve the family has been obtained, the therapist should attempt to determine who is the primary caregiver. Generally, there is one individual who was more responsible for the patient than others. This step is important because it identifies not only that person who will often be the most helpful ally in the treatment process but also that relationship which is potentially the most conflictual in the patient's system. Where possible and appropriate, discussions about the patient and the treatment should be conducted jointly, especially when discussing initial plans.

The therapist should avoid making unilateral or secret decisions with the family. Often families will conspiratorially tell the therapist something which they want held in confidence from the patient. This should happen very rarely and only in special circumstances. Otherwise, the therapist should inform the family (if the patient is competent), that it is his obligation to discuss everything openly. The fact of old age does not take away the personhood and rights to confidentiality that exist in the therapist/patient relationship.

Group psychotherapy

Supportive groups have been used in a variety of settings, in particular in the institutional setting with both cognitively impaired and intact members. Such groups enhance peer relationships and provide a forum for patients to discuss their issues with those who have had similar experiences. Group techniques include reality orientation, resocialization, orientation, as well as a variety of activity-oriented groups including movement and dance, crafts and music. The goals include enhancing self-esteem, improving social contact with peers, increasing activity level and instilling hope. For a review of this area see Leszcz (1991).

Conclusion

Overall, the myth of aging is that the elderly cannot change and that psychotherapy is not effective. This is an erroneous concept for many geriatric problems. Psychotherapy with the elderly can be both fruitful and rewarding for patient and therapist.

References

Beck, A. T., Rush, A. J., Shaw, B. F. et al. (1979). *Cognitive Therapy of Depression*, New York: Guilford.

Berezin, M. (1972). Psychodynamic considerations of aging and the aged: an overview. *American Journal of Psychiatry*, **128**, 33–41.

Breslau, L. (1987). Exaggerated helplessness syndrome. In *Treating the Elderly with Psychotherapy: The Scope for Change in Later Life*, ed. J. Sadavoy & M. Leszcz. Madison: International Universities Press.

Butler, R. N. (1963). The life review: an interpretation of reminiscence in the aged. *Psychiatry*, **26**, 65–70.

Burns, D. D. (1989). *The Feeling Good Handbook: Using the New Mood Therapy in Everyday Life*. New York: William Morrow.

Carstensen, L. L. & Edelstein, B. A. (eds) (1987). *Handbook of Clinical Gerontology*, New York: Pergamon Press.

Erikson, E. H. (1968). The human life cycle. In *International Encyclopedia of the Social Sciences*, ed. D. L. Sills, pp. 186–292. New York: Macmillan.

Gallagher, D. E. & Thompson, L. W. (1983). Effectiveness of psychotherapy for both endogenous and non-endogenous depression in older adult outpatients. *Journal of Gerontology*, **38**, 707–12.

Goldfarb, A. I. & Turner, H. (1953). Psychotherapy of aged persons, II: utilization and effectiveness of 'brief' therapy. *American Journal of Psychiatry*, **109**, 916–21.

Goldstein, M. (1991). Family therapy. In *Comprehensive Review of Geriatric Psychiatry*, ed. J. Sadavoy, L. Lazarus & L. Jarvik, pp. 513–526. Washington: American Psychiatric Press, Inc.

Hussian, R. A. & Davis, R. L. (1985). *Response Care: Behavioural Interventions with Elderly Persons*. Illinois: Champaign Research Press.

Jacques, E. (1965). Death and the mid-life crisis. *International Journal of Psychoanalysis*, **46**, 502–14.

Kahana, R. (1979). Strategies of dynamic psychotherapy with the wide range of older individuals. *Journal of Geriatric Psychiatry*, **12**, 71–100.

Kahana, R. (1987). Geriatric psychotherapy: beyond crisis management. In *Treating the Elderly With Psychotherapy: The Scope for Change in Later Life*, ed. J. Sadavoy & M. Leszcz, pp. 233–263. Madison: International Universities Press.

King, P. M. H. (1980). The life cycle as indicated by the nature of the transference in the psychoanalysis of the middle-aged and elderly. *International Journal of Psychoanalysis*, **61**, 153–9.

Lazarus, L & Sadavoy, J (1991). Individual psychotherapy. In *Comprehensive Review of Geriatric Psychiatry*, ed. J. Sadavoy, L. Lazarus & L. Jarvik, pp. 487–512. Washington: American Psychiatric Press.

Leszcz, M. (1991). Group therapy. In *Comprehensive Review of Geriatric Psychiatry*, ed. J. Sadavoy, L. Lazarus & L. Jarvik, pp. 527–546. Washington: American Psychiatric Press.

Lewinsohn, P. M. & Teri, L. (eds) (1983). *Clinical Geropsychology: New Directions in Assessment and Treatment*, New York: Pergamon Press.

McMullin, R. E. (1986). *Handbook of Cognitive Therapy Techniques*. New York: Norton.

Meerloo, J. A. M. (1953). Contribution of psychoanalysis to the problem of the aged. In *Psychoanalysis and Social Work*, ed. M. Hermann, pp. 321–337. New York: International Universities Press.

Nemiroff, R. A. & Colarusso, C. A. (eds) (1985). *The Race Against Time*. New York: Plenum Press.

Neugarten, B. (1979). Time, age and the life-cycle. *American Journal of Psychiatry*, **136**, 887–94.

Pollock, G. H. (1987). The mourning-liberation process: ideas on the inner life of the older adult. In *Treating the Elderly With Psychotherapy: The Scope for Change in Later Life*, ed. J. Sadavoy & M. Leszcz, pp. 3–29. Madison: International Universities Press.

Rechtschaffen, A. (1959). Psychotherapy with geriatric patients: a review of the literature. *Journal of Gerontology*, **14**, 73–84.

Sadavoy, J. (1992). Psychotherapy in the institutionalized elderly. In *Practical Psychiatry in the Nursing Home*, ed. D. Conn, N. Herrmann, A. Kaye, D. Rewilak, A. Robinson & B. Schogt, pp. 217–235. Toronto: Hogrefe and Huber.

Scholomskas, A. J., Chevron, E. S., Prusoff, B. A. & Berry, C. (1983). Short term interpersonal therapy (IPT) with the depressed elderly: Case reports and discussion. *American Journal of Psychotherapy*, **37**, 552–66.

Steingart, A. (1991). Day programs. In *Comprehensive Review of Geriatric Psychiatry*, ed. J. Sadavoy & L. Lazarus, pp. 603–612. Washington: American Psychiatric Press.

Thompson, L. W., Gantz, F., Florsheim, M., Del Maestro, S., Rodman, J., Gallagher-Thompson, D. & Bryan, H. (1991). Cognitive–behavioral therapy for affective disorders in the elderly. In *New Techniques in the Psychotherapy of Older Patients*, ed. W. A. Meyers, pp. 3–19. Washington: American Psychiatric Press Inc.

Tobin, S. & Lieberman, M. A. (1976). *Last Home for the Aged: Critical Implications of Institutionization*. San Francisco: Jossey-Bass.

30

Management of the treatment team in a multidisciplinary framwork

EDMOND CHIU

Introduction

With the introduction of modern drug treatment methods in psychiatry, the custodial mental hospitals opened their doors in the late 1950s. The ability to control disturbed behavior and discharge patients back into the community led to the realization of rehabilitation possibilities; the emergence of programs aimed at restoring the psychiatrically disabled person to full functioning and reintegration into home and community. This period coincided with the development of health care professions additional to medical and nursing. Social work, occupational therapy, physiotherapy and psychology evolved and emerged into distinct and autonomous health care disciplines. Music therapy, psychodrama and recreational therapy followed them to achieve health care profession status.

Recognising that the effective operation of a psychiatric treatment program requires the active participation and cooperation of members of these health care disciplines, psychiatrists gradually included them in treatment teams. The rise of the community psychiatry movement in the 1960s and 1970s gave further impetus to the concept and practice of multidisciplinary teams. Now, the concept of team work in psychiatry has evolved to such a degree, that multidisciplinary team work has become axiomatic in psychiatric care.

Definition

The word 'multidisciplinary' is not easily found in textbooks of psychiatry published in the 1970s and 1980s. There are few references to multidisciplinary team work in standard psychiatric texts. The term is not found in the major medical dictionaries. In the 1990 Third Edition of *Mosby's Medical, Nursing and Allied Health Dictionary*, 'Multidisciplinary health care team' is defined as 'a group of health care workers who are members of different disciplines, each one providing specific services to the patient'.

Perhaps the most useful discussion of the multidisciplinary team in psychiatry can be found in *Current Themes in Psychiatry*, Volume 2 (Gaind & Hudson, 1979) where the role of these teams in community psychiatry, the ethical issues confronting their working and clarification of the clinical responsibilities of team members are well considered. Freeman addressed the role of teams in community psychiatry and the integration of the hospital and community based staff into the same organizational structure. 'It should therefore come within the responsibilities of a multidisciplinary professional team, which is also concerned with acute care, home visiting, rehabilitation and all the other facilities which make up an integrated service' (ibid, p.7). Anthony Clare, in his chapter on Ethics in Psychiatry discussed the issue of clinical responsibility (ibid p. 79–81) in operating in a multidisciplinary setting as expressed in the Royal College of Psychiatrists (1977) report, which debated the medical/legal responsibilities of clinicians and where the final responsibility in the context of 'multiprofessional expansion' create the imperative for various professional groups to examine these issues using as the guiding mainstay the fundamental interest of the patient.

In the area of geriatric psychiatry the seminal publication of Enoch & Howells' *Contemporary Issues in Psychiatry* (1974), a collection of writing on issues pertinent to the British psychiatric scene in 1970–1973, provided a very clear picture of team work in geriatric psychiatry. The chapter on 'The Organization of Psychogeriatrics' served as a blueprint for the development of service delivery systems to the elderly. In this chapter, Enoch and Howells commented: 'There is a contemporary tendency to emphasize cooperation and coordination as sufficient in themselves. Without denying their importance they are futile in the absence of trained personnel, each with a defined role, trained for that role and personally responsible for the part each plays. Personal responsibility and coordination are equally important'.

Although the term 'multidisciplinary team' was not used by the study group which prepared the basis of the chapter, this comment highlighted the essentials of multidisciplinary team work – cooperation, coordination and personal responsibility.

In the United States, the Group for Advancement of Psychiatry published its report on 'The Dimension of Community Psychiatry' in 1968 (Report No. 69) which addressed a parallel concern. The rise of the community psychiatry movement, which operates on a foundation of multidisciplinary team work, confronts the psychiatrist with certain dilemmas as he or she collaborates with other health care professionals and lay persons in developing community mental health services and programs. Such multidisciplinary team work varies from the simple availability but separate functioning of each autonomous discipline group, to more complex arrangements contributed to by all disciplines, sharing clinical functions in the care of patients.

The balance between cooperation, collaboration, coordination and responsibility can be at best delicate and at worst chaotic and destructive. Political battles in struggles of leadership with resultant 'demedicalization' of community mental health teams was a common scenario in the community mental health movement of the 1970s and 1980s in the United States. As each discipline vied for leadership, frequently the patients become the victims of team discord.

The multidisciplinary team in geriatric psychiatry practice

Observers of medical practice with the elderly will quickly note the phenomenon of the multidisciplinary team in operation. The core and basis of geriatric medicine and geriatric psychiatry is comprehensive assessment at the elderly patient's place of residence. Comprehensive assessment of the elderly has been established as an effective strategy for improving patient outcome in the hospital setting. The 'manifesto' of Enoch & Howells (1974) clearly advocated comprehensive assessment both in the community and inpatient, outpatient and day hospital settings. Outreach and day hospitalization are the other essential components. Cohen (1980) wrote that 'outreach teams should be multidisciplinary in the mental health and medical sense. Certain types of day hospitalization, depending on the nature of the clinical problem, ... require the medical/mental health mix. Institutional settings such as hospitals and nursing homes clearly require this mix'.

The best organization of resources usually follows the establishment of a 'psychogeriatric team' (Arie, 1971; Pitt, 1974) which can provide a comprehensive assessment of medical, psychiatric, social, community, lifestyle and other aspects of an elderly person's needs and thereby planning and providing services appropriate to serve these needs. The 'psychogeriatric team' also serve to liaise extensively with all sectors of the community through the wide network of professional and nonprofessional contacts.

It is generally accepted that such a multidisciplinary team is an essential given of any geriatric psychiatry program which wishes to claim effectively to meet the multiple and often interacting needs of the elderly psychiatrically ill. This section of the book therefore includes contributions from those health care professions which contribute to the function of the multidisciplinary team.

The effective working of such a team requires more than cooperation, collaboration and coordination. A very high level of mutual respect, understanding and appreciation of each discipline's strengths and limitations, as well as the overlapping expertise which may cause interprofessional tensions, is necessary.

A professional's status is integrally linked to his or her personal identity. Modification of such status thus threatens that identity and self-worth. Security and fulfilment of personal aspirations and ambitions are intimately enmeshed with the ability to satisfy and gratify these desires which motivate the professional to achieve full potential and fulfilment. Some necessary ingredients leading to such fulfilment include participation, control, effective contribution and recognition of one's expertise. Thus the appreciative acceptance of each member's contribution, integration of all members expertise to form a coherent management plan, sharing and taking responsibility to achieve a common goal mutually agreed upon, are all elements in making the multidisciplinary team work effectively. The leader of the team must be able to clarify the sphere of activity in which each member has a personal as well as professional competence and responsibility, looking beyond disciplinary prerogatives and allocating professional tasks which best fit each team member. Thus a careful reading of the following chapters will provide an insight into the extent of the professional competence of other health care disciplines and provide a basis for effective functioning of multidisciplinary teams in geriatric psychiatry.

References

Arie, T. (1971). Morale and the planning of psychogeriatric services. *British Medical Journal*, 3, 166–70.

Cohen, G. (1980). *Handbook of Mental Health and Ageing*. eds. J. E. Birren & R. B. Sloane. Englewood Cliffs: Prentice Hall.

Enoch, M. D. & Howells, J. G. (1974). The Organization of Psychogeriatrics. In *Contemporary Issues in Psychiatry*. ed. J. G. Howells. London: Butterworth.

Gaind, R. N. & Hudson, B. C. (1979). *Current Themes in Psychiatry, 2*. London: Macmillan.

Group for Advancement of Psychiatry (1968). *The Dimension of Community Psychiatry* (*Vol. VI*). Report No. 69, April. New York: Mental Health Materials Center Inc.

Mosby's Medical, Nursing and Allied Health Dictionary (1990). 3rd Edition. St. Louis: Mosby.

Pitt, B. (1974). *Psychogeriatrics*. Edinburgh & London: Churchill Livingstone.

Royal College of Psychiatrists. (1977). The responsibilities of consultative psychiatry within the National Health Service. *British Journal of Psychiatry*, News and Notes Supplement. September, pp. 4–7.

31

Occupational therapy

KRISTINE J. ALEXANDER

This chapter describes the contributions made by occupational therapy to the treatment of elderly patients with functional psychiatric illnesses. The domain of concern of occupational therapy is defined, which provides the parameters of evaluation and intervention. The tools of practice used by occupational therapists for assessment and treatment are explained in detail. The phases of intervention, namely prevention, rehabilitation and maintenance are presented with examples of different treatment procedures.

Definition of occupational therapy

Occupational therapy has been defined as the art and science of directing an individual's participation in selected activities and tasks in order to evaluate that person's functional ability, and subsequently, to develop skills, restore function, maintain ability and prevent dysfunction (Health & Welfare Canada and CAOT, 1986; Mosey, 1986). The primary emphasis of occupational therapy with elderly patients who have a functional psychiatric disorder is restoration, maintenance and prevention (Wagman and Kennedy, 1988).

The occupational therapist is concerned with a particular domain of an individual's functional ability. The domain of concern of occupational therapy has been described by Mosey (1986) as consisting of areas of occupational performance and the performance components of these occupations, within the context of the individual's age and cultural, social and physical environment. This is illustrated in Fig. 31.1.

The occupations, or roles, which an occupational therapist may investigate during evaluation and subsequently provide therapeutic intervention are:

- activities of daily living (self-care, homemaking)
- work (paid and volunteer or schooling)
- leisure and recreational pursuits or interests

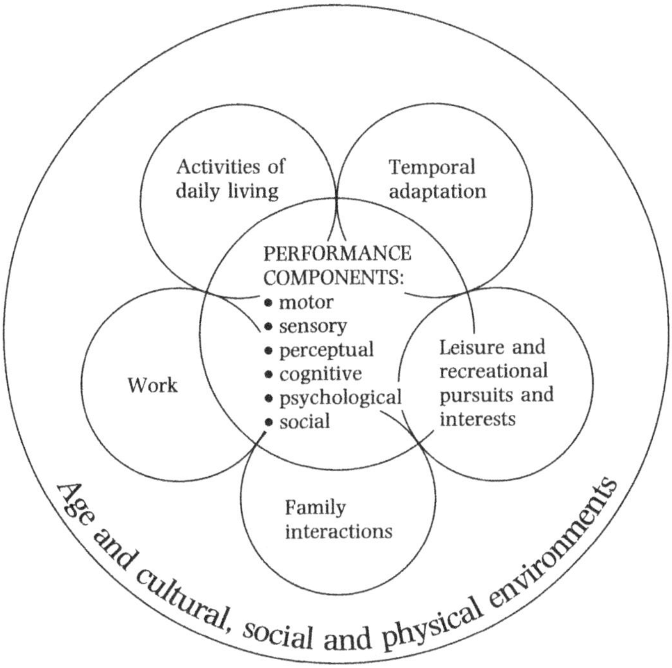

Fig. 31.1. Domain of concern of occupational therapy.

- family interactions, and
- temporal adaptation (the ability to organize one's time)

It is, however, the performance components that are often considered to be the core of occupational therapy, as this is where the evaluation and intervention process usually begins (Mosey, 1986). The performance components consist of:

- motor function (includes balance, mobility, coordination, manipulation, endurance)
- sensory function (particularly visual, auditory, tactile, vestibular, and proprioceptive sensation)
- perception (for example, figure-ground discrimination, visual gnosis, stereognosis, praxis)
- cognitive function (includes memory, concentration, problem solving and organizational skills)
- psychological function (for example, motivation, mood, insight, anxiety, self esteem, stream of thought)
- social interaction (for example, cooperativeness, communication, confidence, nonverbal behavior, social skills, assertiveness)

These aspects of occupational performance and components may be expressed differently if the occupational therapist follows a particular school of thought, for example Kielhofner's Model of Human Occupation (1989). In this case the five areas of occupation performance will be evaluated as the patient's roles and habits.

Performance components will be evaluated as personal causation (belief in oneself and feelings of control), values (personal standards and goals), interests, and skills (includes interpersonal, sensorimotor, perceptual, and cognitive skills).

The body of knowledge of occupational therapy consists of selected theories from the biological sciences, psychology, sociology, the arts, and medicine as well as theories generated through the practice of occupational therapy. Most occupational therapists are eclectic in their clinical work, and draw from specific theories and models of occupational therapy according to the needs of their clientele.

Occupational therapy evaluation

Introduction

Evaluation is the essential, first step in the process of occupational therapy intervention. Before planning the objectives and program of occupational therapy treatment, the therapist must first evaluate the patient's functional status. The goal of evaluation is to identify the individual's strengths and weaknesses in order to identify those aspects of dysfunction which can be remedied by occupational therapy (Mosey, 1986). Evaluation is not only carried out at the beginning of the intervention process. Periodic review of the patient's functional status is required to monitor the effects of treatment and adjust intervention to match the patient's changing needs (Solomon, 1990).

Reasons for evaluation

Evaluation is undertaken for a variety of reasons. As stated earlier, evaluation enables the occupational therapist to identify areas of strength and areas of dysfunction, in order to establish a baseline of information about the patient (Tiffany, 1978). This, in turn, will enable the occupational therapist to establish treatment priorities and will guide the therapist in planning an individualized treatment program. Evaluation gives some indication of the patient's potential for change (Smith & Tiffany, 1983). The most appropriate method of occupational therapy intervention is determined through evaluation. The therapist is able to determine if the patient is suitable for individual or group-based intervention. The occupational therapist should evaluate the individual for group compatibility (Hoff, 1988). Re-evaluation following a period of occupational therapy intervention, provides an indication of changes in the patient's functional status, and the effectiveness of treatment.

Occupational therapy evaluation, along with evaluation results from other team members, aids the setting of overall goals (Smith & Tiffany, 1983). The results of occupational therapy evaluation may contribute to diagnosis, for example in

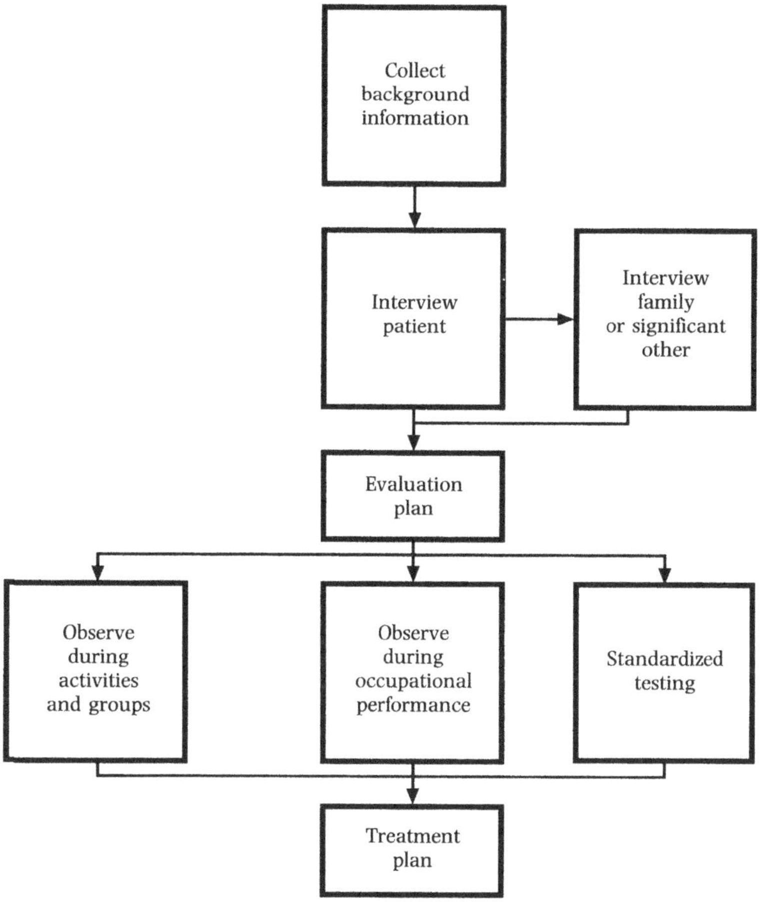

Fig. 31.2. Occupational therapy evaluation procedure.

differentiating depression presenting as psuedo-dementia, from an organic dementia (Miller, 1987). It is a method of monitoring the effects of medication, and other treatments, on the patient's functional status. The presence and effects of medication side effects can also be assessed by occupational therapy procedures (Denton, 1988), for example, identifying the presence and effects of parkinsonism in a patient taking antipsychotic medication.

Evaluation of a patient's functional status helps answer questions related to discharge planning. For example, for a patient with an affective disorder examination of their performance during domestic activities of daily living, provides answers to such questions as:

- Does the patient neglect their personal care or nutrition?
- Is the patient able to make decisions and solve routine household problems? Is the patient safe in their own home?
- Is the patient motivated to perform daily living tasks?

- Is the patient able to look after themselves, independently, in their own home?
- What community supports are needed to enable the patient to return home and remain there?
- What is the most appropriate future accommodation for the patient?

Areas assessed

The areas commonly evaluated by the occupational therapist are the five areas of occupational performance, which reflect the domain of concern of the profession described by Mosey (1986) (refer to Fig. 31.1). Within each area of occupational performance, the occupational therapist may be required to assess the performance components which contribute to the patient's ability to engage in these occupations. Of special relevance when evaluating performance of the elderly patient with a functional psychiatric illness, is the necessity to take into consideration the individual's age and cultural group membership in order to 'determine whether the client's functioning... is within the range of what is considered to be acceptable' (Mosey, 1986, p. 9).

Evaluation of the human and nonhuman factors in the environment is essential in order to determine how they facilitate or inhibit the patient's function (Fidler & Fidler, 1978, cited in Mocellin, 1982). This refers to social aspects such as the patient's cultural group or the support offered by family and friends. Alternatively, it may focus on the physical aspects of the environment such as the patient's housing situation or the availability of transportation.

Evaluation procedure

Any valid evaluation of a patient's functional status must be based on several sources, yielding a multidimensional picture of the patient (Smith & Tiffany, 1983). Typically, the steps that an occupational therapist undertakes in the evaluation procedure involve the collection of background information, often from the patient's medical record. Rogers (1987) described that the next steps include the therapist obtaining the individual's perceptions of their situation and needs. At some point the occupational therapist seeks to liaise with the patient's family, or caregiver, for further information and corroboration of the data obtained from the patient. Lastly, the occupational therapy evaluation process hinges on assessment of the patient's practical performance of activities. The latter in particular provides information about the patient's performance components. Fig. 31.2 illustrates the process of occupational therapy evaluation.

There are some special considerations of which the occupational therapist should be cognisant when evaluating the elderly patient with a functional psychiatric disorder. These include possible hearing and vision deficits which may adversely affect evaluation results if not taken into account. Burton (1989*b*) advised that the therapist should take into account the elderly patient's vulnerability to fatigue, their slowed response time, slowness in changing mental set, and difficulty in dealing with more than one item at a time. It was recommended that performance be assessed by practical demonstration rather than by self report, due to elderly persons' tendency to incorrectly estimate their abilities (Krugman, 1959, cited in Burton, 1989*a*).

Evaluation tools

The methods employed by the occupational therapist are varied according to the area of function which is to be assessed, and the purpose of the evaluation. The tools that the occupational therapist uses in the evaluation process include use of medical records, interviewing, observation of the patient's functional performance during informal assessment situations, and use of standardized tests.

Documents

The medical record is a resource of valuable background information about the patient. It is often after consulting the medical record that the occupational therapist formulates a initial evaluation plan. The medical record may also provide indications of precautions that must be considered when planning and carrying out other methods of evaluation (Smith & Tiffany, 1983). For example, it may provide information of an individual's physical illnesses and disabilities, such as rheumatoid arthritis or hemiplegia. The occupational therapist may then need to broaden the evaluation plan to determine the effects these disabilities have on the patient's functioning, for example, in activities of daily living or leisure pursuits.

Interviewing

Interviewing the patient is often the first step in developing rapport between the patient and the therapist. It provides an opportunity for the patient to develop an understanding of occupational therapy and the role it will play in their treatment (Smith & Tiffany, 1983).

As stated by Rogers (1987), an interview with the patient enables the occupational therapist to ascertain the individual's self-perceptions of their functional status. The therapist is interested in the patient's perceptions of those tasks they can perform easily, those which they perform with difficulty, and those which they are unable to perform. The patient's perception of the reasons for their difficulties is important information to obtain. For example, a patient with a chronic psychotic illness who has never learnt a task would be viewed differently from a patient with an affective disorder who has, but no longer uses the skill. The patient's level of motivation, degree of self esteem, and anxiety are important factors to discern during the interview. Questioning is also orientated to how the patient spends their time. This provides information about the patient's temporal adaptation (for example, has the patient with an affective disorder recently abandoned previous activities and routines?)

Interviewing the patient's family members is a valuable part of the evaluation process. A number of authors cited by Intagliata, Willer & Egri (1986) acknowledged that the family was an extremely important source of information about the patient's history of illness and their current functioning. Mosey (1986) agreed when she described that the family provide valuable information when the patient is unable to give a clear account of their present and past situation, for example in the case of a patient in the acute phase of a psychotic episode. The family may also serve as a check on the reliability of the patient's reports. Family members may shed light on the motivation and interest of a depressed patient towards social contacts and leisure pursuits. Denton (1988) echoed this belief, but warned that caregiver reports may be biased by a myriad of feelings. Therefore the occupational therapist must carefully appraise the validity of information received. The family may also help to identify needs of the patient that are not otherwise apparent to the occupational therapist (Intagliata et al., 1986).

Observation

Observation of the patient's functional performance of activities and tasks is the core of the occupational therapy evaluation process. Observation of an individual's function during activities may provide the occupational therapist with information regarding the patient's performance components, in other words, their motor skills, sensory perception, cognitive functioning, social skills, and/or psychological functioning. Informal observation may provide information regarding the impact of deficits (for example, physical deficits which may have been identified via formal tests) on the patient's functioning level.

Activities may be especially altered or adapted by the occupational therapist in order to focus on one particular skill (for example, decision making) or one particular performance component (for example, social interaction). The success of the use of activities as evaluation tools relies upon the accuracy and detail of activity analysis, and observation can become more objective by planning ahead and by obtaining consensual validation from co-therapists or the patient (Tiffany, 1978). In contrast, spontaneous interaction with a patient may provide information that would otherwise be difficult to glean (Smith & Tiffany, 1983), for example, information regarding the delusional system of a psychotic patient, or regarding hallucinations they may experience.

Evaluation using projective techniques, such as painting, clay work and collage, enables the patient with a functional psychiatric disorder to express otherwise inexpressible parts of their personality. This can be a useful technique to employ with patients who are withdrawn, unable, or unwilling to verbally present feelings or experiences. The occupational therapist must be sensitive to the symbolic as well as the concrete representations in all aspects of doing activities, as this is the hallmark of good observation (Tiffany, 1978).

Performance testing in the actual or simulated environment provides the occupational therapist with information about the patient's performance components (Rogers, 1987). Trace & Howell (1991) illustrated how the reasons for unsafe behavior can often be identified through observation. For example, unsafe use of cooking facilities may be due to failing eyesight, memory problems, poor judgement, poorly designed or unsafe equipment. Rogers advised that evaluation in the actual situation (such as, the patient's home) is generally preferable, as the elderly are more dependent on the environment than are young people. When evaluation is done in a simulated environment (for example, the occupational therapy department), the therapist must take into account the patient's unfamiliarity with the test environment.

'The continuing observation of a client's performance is the key to the essential process of ongoing evaluation' (Tiffany, 1978, p. 307). Thus evaluation may continue, in an informal fashion, during the treatment phase of intervention as the occupational therapist is sensitive to changes in the quality of the patient's performance during tasks and activities.

Standardized tests

Formal tests are used by the occupational therapist when a standardized measure is required (for example, to quantify differences pre- and post-treatment) or to investigate an area of occupational performance or component in more detail. Examples of standardized tests used include:

- *Driving assessment* (Gregory, 1987), patients with a psychotic illness may be assessed to determine the effects of medication side-effects on their driving reactions and safety; patients with an affective disorder may be assessed with particular emphasis on their anticipation and problem solving abilities.
- *Self-care assessments* such as the Barthel Index (Mahoney & Barthel, 1965) are useful in the elderly population to screen for the effects of physical deficits, but also to determine the level of motivation to attend to their personal care in individuals with functional psychiatric disorders.
- *Instrumental activities of daily living assessments* such as the Domestic and Community Skills Assessment (Collister, Alexander & Wood, 1986), the Milwaukee Evaluation of Daily Living Skills (Leonardelli, 1988), or the Scorable Self-Care Evaluation (Clark & Peters, 1984) are used to assess patients' knowledge of, familiarity with, and motivation toward, domestic or community activities of daily living.
- *Leisure assessments* such as the Interest Checklist (Matsutsuyu, 1969) are important for patients with a psychotic illness and those with an affective disorder, to enable the occupational therapist to tailor treatment to their interests, and ensure referral to appropriate community activities when this becomes relevant.

- *Cognitive assessments* such as the Mini-Mental State examination (Folstein, Folstein & McHugh, 1975), or Allen's Cognitive Level test (Allen, 1985) are used to determine the type and extent of cognitive deficits which may be experienced by an individual with a chronic psychotic illness, or a patient presenting with pseudo-dementia.
- *Physical assessments* such as measuring range of movement with a goniometer, measuring grip strength with a dynamometer are used to objectively measure physical deficits of the elderly patient.
- *Functional assessments* such as the Bay Area Functional Performance evaluation (Williams & Bloomer, 1987) evaluate a variety of functional skills such as problem solving, organizational and social skills.
- *Projective assessments* such as the Azima Battery and the Magazine Picture Collage (Hemphill, 1982) are available for the occupational therapist to assess psychological functioning and personality traits in patients who have functional psychiatric disorders.

The primary purpose of evaluation is to guide treatment planning and implementation. Without this next step evaluation can be a pointless exercise. Similarly, without evaluation, treatment plans will be ill formed and inefficient. Thus evaluation is a vital part of the occupational therapy process.

Occupational therapy intervention

Introduction

The occupational therapist holds a unique position amongst the members of the treatment team due to the deliberate and planned use of goal-directed activity towards a specific aim. It is the role of the occupational therapist to structure intervention to match the needs, skills and deficits of the patient. Just as the occupational therapist evaluated the patient's level of functioning, so must the activity to be employed be analysed. The outcome of this analysis is skilfully structured and treatment graded within the most facilitative environment.

Butin & Heaney (1991) recognized the important role that occupational therapy has to play in the rehabilitation of the elderly patient. They described a population of geriatric psychiatry patients who were largely treated by biological interventions with the addition of family and individual therapy. While these individuals were discharged generally free of psychiatric symptomatology, maladaptive behavior patterns and skills dysfunction remained present and contributed to non-compliance and relapses. With the contribution of occupational therapy, significant effects can occur in developing adaptive behavior patterns and skill retraining.

Based on the results from evaluation with the patient, and consultation with other members of the therapeutic team, the occupational therapist devises a plan of intervention. The plan consists of the objectives of therapy, the methods by which the therapist intends to achieve these objectives, and a sense of the priorities of the objectives. Intervention with the elderly patient with a functional psychiatric disorder aims to assist the individual to recover past skills and to encourage the use of present skills (Solomon, 1990). The main goal of therapy should be to help the elderly person regain some control and independence (Molinari, 1991; Smith, 1987; Trace & Howell, 1991). In some cases it may not be possible to restore the elderly patient to full independence, therefore the goal of optimizing function may be a more realistic objective (Smith, 1987).

Tools of practice

During the intervention planning phase, the occupational therapist identifies the patient's need for individual and/or group-based intervention. The therapeutic activities best suited to the individual are also formulated. The therapist is able to choose from the five tools of occupational therapy practice. The tools of occupational therapy practice may be defined as:

- the conscious use of self
- the teaching–learning process (or training)
- the use of purposeful activities (including activity analysis)
- the use of therapeutic groups, and
- the use of the nonhuman environment (Mosey, 1986).

Conscious use of self

The manner in which the occupational therapist behaves and the attitude which is held permeate all aspects of intervention. The general milieu created by the therapist is considered to be one of the most important factors in treatment (Mosey, 1986). Curative factors in the therapeutic relationship between patient and therapist are acceptance, nonpossessive warmth, genuineness, hope and accurate empathy (Miller, 1987). 'A further expectation in any treatment program is that the patient ... is able to function at a level higher than the level at which he/she currently functions.' (Solomon, 1990, p. 45). If the occupational therapist genuinely believes and transmits a positive attitude to the patient, it will consequently promote positive expectation in the patient. This is an important approach to use with the depressed patient who has negative self-esteem.

Conscious use of self also refers to use of nonverbal behavior and use of the therapist's body to alleviate anxiety, provide reassurance, provide physical support, for physical manipulation and maintenance of appropriate positioning (Mosey, 1986). The latter points are especially relevant for dealing with the physically disabled older patient.

During treatment, the occupational therapist should be a facilitator, resource person, observer and listener (Love, 1988). The therapist should be a role model of appropriate behaviors for patients with a psychotic illness, in particular those patients who have been institutionalized. In group-based treatment, the therapist should consciously adapt an appropriate style of group leadership (that is, autocratic, democratic or *laissez-faire*), according to the purpose of the group and the needs of the group members (Bruce, 1988). However, group involvement may be a threatening concept to the elderly patient 'who has never previously been involved in discussing and sharing personal problems [or experiences] with a group. Therefore sensitivity, patience and the development of a trusting relationship with the therapist are required before they will even consider joining a group session.' (Docherty & Harley, 1987, p. 121–122; cited in Norman & Crosby, 1990).

The teaching–learning process

Learning by doing is central to occupational therapy with mentally ill patients (Harwood & Wenzl, 1990). The teaching–learning process, or training, is designed to teach the patient new skills, knowledge and attitudes (Mosey, 1986). Training may occur in a one-to-one or in a group situation. It typically involves the use of educational activities such as lectures, audiovisual materials, handouts, simulated exercises and home work (Bruce, 1988).

Training may focus on developing compensatory strategies in the elderly patient (for example, learning the principles of work simplification and energy conservation); teaching new skills (for example, assertiveness training); or in revitalising old skills (for example, social skills training). When planning this type of intervention with the elderly, especially those with a psychotic illness, the following requirements should be included. Classes require more active trainers, more social reinforcements for less skill increments, shorter and more repetitive sessions, fewer patients per group and more relative attention to the simpler levels of a given skill (Goldstein, Gershaw & Sprafkin, 1979; cited in Agacinski & Stern, 1984, p. 18).

Purposeful activities

Fidler (1963; cited in Bruce, 1988) stated that task accomplishment is not the purpose of activity, but the means by which the therapeutic purpose is realized. In other words, the task that the patient performs is less important than the process of how the individual performs it (Denton, 1988). The purpose of involvement in an activity will be decided by the occupational therapist in the objectives of intervention. Through activity analysis the occupational therapist considers the sensory, motor, social, cognitive and psychological aspects of the activity. Based on this analysis the therapist selects the appropriate activity, and adapts it to suit the treatment goals. In this way activity analysis serves as a precursor to the design of activity adaptations. These adaptations are required to optimize the patient's capabilities and to work on, or compensate for, their disabilities (Levy, 1990).

The activities that are used during therapy must be age appropriate for the elderly patient and matched to their specific, individual interests. Consideration of the physical demands of an activity is of particular relevance to the older patient, who may be experiencing physical decline associated with aging (for example, reduced vision, hearing difficulties) or disability associated with a specific illness (for example, emphysema resulting in reduced stamina and endurance). Different activities will elicit different affective responses and levels of interest from individuals (Boyer et al., 1989). The occupational therapist must ascertain the activities which will be most meaningful and motivating for an individual. For example, woodwork has often been found to be an acceptable and motivating activity with elderly men.

Therapeutic groups

Group-based therapy is a common form of intervention in psychiatry. Although the structure and purpose of a group may vary, the therapeutic factors that are common to each group and influence the outcome of the group experience are universal and have been described by Yalom (1983). The occupational therapist uses group-based intervention to achieve specified treatment goals. The therapist's knowledge of group dynamics and skill in planning the group program will directly impinge on the successful outcome of the group process. For example, in activity groups where the patients tend to direct most of their communication to the occupational therapist, rather than to one another, the group loses much of its potential for learning (Mosey, 1973; cited in Love, 1988).

Groups must be structured in such a way that they are appropriate for the patients in the group, in order that the patients achieve their particular objectives (Mosey, 1973; cited in Love, 1988). There is considerable theoretical agreement (Yalom, 1983; Kernber, 1976 cited in Cole & Greene, 1988) that the degree of structuring of therapeutic groups should follow levels of psychological impairment of the group members. Thus greater structure and explicitness of norms, rules and roles must be provided for the more severely disturbed patients. Many occupational therapy authors (Agacinski & Stern, 1984; Harwood & Wenzl, 1990; Bowers, 1967, cited in Parham, Priddy, McGovern & Richman, 1982; Lushbourgh et al., 1988; Hoff, 1988; Butin & Heaney, 1991) have described activity group programs where the patients have been allocated to separate group programs, or streams, according to their level of functional ability. In particular, cognitive functioning level has often been the critical determinant (Agacinski & Stern, 1984; Harwood & Wenzl, 1990; Lushbourgh et al., 1988; Hoff, 1988). For example, patients with a chronic psychotic illness such as schizophrenia, and patients who have an anxiety disorder may be programed into seperate groups.

Research into the type of groups offered to patients with functional psychiatric illnesses supports the occupational therapist's use of activity over a verbally orientated approach (Schwartzber, Howe & McDermott, 1982 and Kanas, 1986, cited in Cole & Greene, 1988). Comparison of group means showed that patients receiving activity-based group therapy achieved a four times greater symptom reduction than those receiving a verbally orientated approach (Klyczek & Mann, 1986, cited in Lushbourgh et al., 1988). Similarly Decarlo and Mann (1985, cited in Lushbourgh et al., 1988) found that activity therapy was significantly more effective than verbal therapy in improving self-perception of interpersonal communication skills with psychiatric patients.

Environment

The occupational therapist should be concerned about the physical environment in which therapy is to take place. The environment should be structured or modified to ensure that it is safe and that it facilitates function (Mosey, 1986). Levy (1990) reported a number of examples of environmental adaptations for use with the elderly patient. These included the use of extra illumination of the activity environment, magnifying or large print lettering for patients with visual decline; the use of supplementary visual and tactile cues for patients with hearing impairment. Removal of dangerous items that could be misused by the suicidal patients may decrease the risk of harm (Trace & Howell, 1991). Minimizing environmental distractions (both visual and auditory) is an important consideration for patients with a psychotic illness.

The environment is an important consideration if the patient is to return home. The occupational therapist must carry out a home visit to the patient's home in order to assess safety of the environment and to prescribe any adaptive equipment or home modifications. Examples of home modifications are the provision of rails in the toilet or bathroom to assist with safe transfers; provision of a flexi-shower hose and shower stool for independent showering; marking stove dials for increased visibility; automatic kettle shut off to compensate for forgetfulness; the removal of rugs and provision of handrails at external accesses to prevent tripping and falls; provision of a personal alarm system may make sufficient difference to permit an individual to return to independent living.

Stages of intervention

Intervention can be divided into three main subtypes or stages. These are prevention, rehabilitation and maintenance (which includes follow-up and quality of life programs).

Prevention

Mosey (1986) described the ultimate goal of prevention in psychiatry as a more satisfying and effective life for people, with a reduction in the strains and stresses that appear to contribute to psychosocial dysfunction. Prevention may be conceptualized as reducing the incidence of disease and disability in a given population, reducing the severity and duration of disorders, and preventing any secondary difficulties that may arise from existing disease or disability (Mosey, 1986).

Occupational therapists may contribute to reducing the incidence of psychiatric illness by developing health promotion and health education programs such as retirement planning groups to prevent a depressive reaction upon retirement from paid employment, or stress management programs to enable anxious patients to remain in the community. The role of occupational therapy in prevention of mental illness in the elderly is becoming more developed with the advent of community-based geriatric psychiatry assessment teams. 'To prevent chronic psychological problems and psychiatric recidivism from occurring in the elderly, it is important for the occupational therapist to provide outreach programs to identify and evaluate those who have emotional problems before they become incapacitated' (Molinari, 1991, p. 28).

The severity of a disorder may be reduced by providing activity programs where otherwise withdrawn patients can participate, thus maintaining practical and social skills. Also occupational therapists have a significant role to play in preventing any secondary difficulties that may arise from psychiatric illness. For example, support groups for caregivers of patients who have a chronic psychotic illness, are important to prevent carer 'burn-out' which may result in the patient being admitted to institutional care. The prevention of hospitalization occurs by enabling psychiatric patients to remain in their own homes where therapy and support may be provided to the patient and their family (Bumphrey, 1989). This is an important part of the role of the occupational therapist on the geriatric psychiatry assessment team.

Rehabilitation

Rehabilitation is a process of change. Mosey (1986) described this process as being orientated to the acquisition of knowledge, skills and attitudes that will be required for future functioning. Intervention is directed at using current abilities to overcome or compensate for deficits due to illness.

Intervention in occupational therapy with the elderly patient focuses on the five areas of occupational performance (see Fig. 31.1). However, the areas of activities of daily living (primarily homemaking activities, but also including self-care) and leisure interests and pursuits are the most commonly addressed during rehabilitation. Similarly, while all types of performance components may require intervention, addressing social and psychological dysfunction predominates in occupational therapy treatment plans with the elderly psychiatric patient.

Activities of daily living. Difficulties in the area of activities of daily living (ADL) may be addressed during individual or during group sessions. Individual sessions typically focus on retraining the patient in domestic or community tasks, or personal care. The elderly patient may suffer from a physical illness and disability which impinges on their ability to care for themselves. In such cases the occupational therapist may prescribe aids and adaptive equipment to assist the elderly person to shower and dress (for example, long-handled back scrubber, stocking gutter or long handled shoe horn), and the individual will require a certain amount of training in the use of this equipment. Similarly, if the occupational therapist prescribes equipment for use in the home, during meal preparation for example, training is also necessary. Individual sessions would also be the appropriate way in which to train a patient to use public transport in their local area, if this need has been indicated during the evaluation process.

The need for home modifications must be considered by the occupational therapist if the patient has difficulties with personal or domestic ADL. A home visit is indicated, not only to assess the physical environment, but to enable accurate recommendations for structural changes or additions to the home. Alternatively, Solomon (1990) described how a home visit may be used as a means of building self-confidence and self-esteem in the patient with a functional psychiatric disorder. Home visits may also be undertaken to consider the social environment at the patient's residence, to discuss with family members, or caregivers, the changes that are being encouraged in the patient, and to enlist their support in cooperating and facilitating the rehabilitation process.

ADL problems may be addressed in a group setting if there are a number of patients with similar needs. An example of this type of group is a cooking group. Through their involvement in the cooking group the patient may learn new skills if they have never cooked before, for example in the case of a recently widowed man. Where the patient possesses the skills but does not use this ability, confidence and motivation can be facilitated. The other group members may support the individual's attempts to return to cooking outside the group situation. A budgeting group is another example where patients may be trained in a skill in a setting which is time efficient for the therapist, and supportive for the patient. The availability of new responses, ideas and handy hints is increased if such a skill is dealt with in a group setting.

Leisure interests and pursuits. Art, craft, and hobby activities have been traditional media in occupational therapy programs. These types of activities are usually performed in a group setting to promote personal expression and increase self esteem (Lushbourgh et al., 1988), to introduce individuals to new leisure pursuits, or rekindle old interests. Other media used for these purposes include music, gardening, creative writing or sports and games.

Solomon (1990, p. 47) advised that 'groups that train or retrain patients in the use of leisure time should focus on a wide variety of options in the community, ranging from senior centres to art museums, concerts or sports events.' Discharge planning groups emphasize the focus on involvement in the community which, for the elderly, primarily involves recreational and leisure pursuits. Lushbourgh et al. (1988) described a goals group where the group members set personal goals for community living. Impediments to reaching these goals were discussed and strategies were formulated for reaching the goals.

Social interaction and skills. Folts (1988) described how social skills are hampered in the psychiatric patient due to a number of reasons. It could be due to the presence of psychotic symptoms resulting in thought disorder; disuse of social skills due to noninteraction and social isolation, often seen with depressed patients; and institutionalization of patients with a chronic mental illness erodes their social skills with apathy and passivity characterizing their interpersonal style (Lushbourgh et al., 1988).

A formalized social skills training program may not always be the most appropriate method of developing social skills in the elderly psychiatric patient. Less formal and more natural settings can be effective. The use of activity groups has been firmly established in the literature (cited in Love, 1988) as a means of enhancing patients' social skills. These groups are structured in such a way that will facilitate social interaction between group members and therefore, provide opportunities for individuals to practice and learn more effective social behaviors (Love, 1988). Other types of groups such as discussion groups, current affairs/newpaper groups, cooking groups, social games (for example, the 'Ungame', the 'Social Skills' game) or even chatting over morning tea maybe structured by the occupational therapist to meet the aims of encouraging and developing patients' social skills. Videotaping discussions has been a useful way of providing feedback to patients regarding their social skills. Elderly patients have found this technique acceptable and insightful.

It is important for the occupational therapist also to consider the psychiatric patient's social environment when providing intervention in this area. Inservice training sessions can be held to educate staff members on how they can help patients to practice outside the group setting. Family meetings can aid in enlisting the help of those who will come in frequent contact with the patient after discharge (Folts, 1988).

Psychological functioning. Occupational therapy intervention in this area may focus on one or a number of psychological functions, including cognitive functioning, mood, emotional state, and level of tension or anxiety. Intervention may be individual or group based.

Some patients with depression become so disabled that they present with cognitive dysfunction, in other words, psuedo-dementia. Patients with psychotic illnesses, particularly schizophrenia, often exhibit cognitive dysfunction. These patients have been found to benefit from sensory or cognitive stimulation groups. For the depressed patient such stimulation may be only required until their depression lifts, and the cognitive dysfunction resolves. Then, they may move on to a more demanding program suited to their changing needs. But for the chronically mentally ill, sensory stimulation may remain as an appropriate and effective intervention.

Occupational therapy with the depressed patient usually aims to break the inactivity cycle, increase motivation, increase self-confidence, increase functional ability and increase self-esteem (Miller, 1987). Many elderly people become depressed in reaction to the death of a loved one or another type of loss (for example, retirement, loss of function through illness). Individual grief counselling may be the first step for the occupational therapist. Ancillary interventions include involving the patient in a discussion group such as a loss support group (Norman & Crosby, 1990) or a life review group (Miller, 1987).

Life review therapy, of which reminiscence is a part, can allow older people to express guilt, fear, grief and uneasiness along with a range of positive emotions. Life review is characterized by the return to consciousness of past experiences, especially unresolved conflicts and preoccupations with the death of others. Providing an opportunity for the patient to unburden himself by talking freely, and gaining insight into their problems and rebuilding self-esteem are also key components of this approach (Miller, 1987). Life review activities may involve writing down thoughts; writing poetry; compiling a scrapbook of memorabilia; compiling a family photo album; searching and preparing a family genealogy; making a history of one's life experiences; expressive art; group discussions and activities where memories and experiences are shared; use of audiovisual material that act as memory aids and triggers for reminiscing (Mosey, 1986).

Projective techniques can be used, often in a group situation, to encourage self expression, to ventilate feelings, to constructively redirect feelings, and develop insight through imagery and association (Miller, 1987). Group therapy which uses projective activities may incorporate expressive painting, collage, other forms of art, working with clay, music, and drama.

Another specific technique used by occupational therapists is the use of sports, physical games and exercises for therapeutic psychological effects. A review of the literature (cited in Chamove, 1986) highlights the consistent effects of moderate levels of physical exercise in reducing depression. Benefits specified included improving self-concept, promoting relaxation, and improving sleep. Positive effects were quite consistent in the few studies on geriatric populations (for example, Clark et al., 1975, cited in Chamove, 1986). For schizophrenic patients, the reported primary benefits have included increased adjustment, higher activity level, increased initiation of social interaction, and reduced levels of agitation (literature review in Chamove, 1986). In the study by Chamove (1986, p. 131) the 'results have shown that when long-term schizophrenic patients were rated on days when they were relatively more active and compared with ratings on days when they were less active ... almost all categories [of the rating scale] showed a significant improvement on more active days. Patients showed significantly less psychotic features, less movement disorder, were less irritable, less depressed, less retarded, less tense and showed more social interest and more social competence ... This is not to suggest that inactivity is the cause of their illness, simply that altering their behavior towards more activity improves it.'

Individual sessions of relaxation training may be indicated for the highly anxious patient who is distractable with poor concentration. When the patient has improved to the point that they can tolerate a group situation, the training can continue in that setting. The occupational therapist will also have to consider the most appropriate type of relaxation method to teach to an individual patient. Some patients present with largely physical symptoms possibly requiring a muscle relaxation based approach. Others present with difficulties which are largely cognitive, requiring a treatment approach based on cognitive restructuring methods. Those with discrete phobias may not require the general approach of stress management programs as a more specific desensitization program may be required (Keable, 1988). A stress management program is more comprehensive than relaxation training as it includes a number of additional aspects. Keable (1988) described the components that might be included in an occupational therapy stress management program as:

1. General education about the causes and effects of anxiety upon the mind, body and behavior
2. Various relaxation methods (for example, contrast muscle relaxation, biofeedback, physiological relaxation, or a combined approach)
3. Cognitive restructuring or rational emotive therapy approaches
4. Realistic goal setting
5. Problem-solving techniques
6. Social skills and assertiveness training.

Maintenance

Maintenance is the process of preserving and supporting an individual's current level of functioning (Mosey, 1986). Maintenance of functioning may occur after rehabilitation, where new skills have been learned or old ones rekindled. Maintenance may occur simultaneously with rehabilitative intervention, in order to maintain those skills which the patient still retains despite illness.

The quality of life programs often offered by occupational therapists may be seen as maintenance of patient's functional skills. This type of therapy is often dismissed as diversional when in fact, it has a vital role to play in treatment. Mosey (1986) stated that it appears that an individual is less likely to change in an environment that does not gratify human health needs. Quality of life programs aim to fulfil inherent health needs so that the individual may experience well being. This is of particular relevance for chronically mentally ill patients, or those who live in institutions. These health needs are akin to Maslow's hierarchy of needs (1962, cited in Mosey, 1986) and include the following:

- the need for adequate food, clothing, shelter and optimum balance of work, rest and play.
- the need for love, acceptance and group association
- the need for mastery, the ability to have control over one's environment
- the need for self-esteem and recognition from others
- the need for pleasure and fun
- the need for self-actualization

As the patient moves toward discharge the occupational therapist should ensure that the individual's health needs are satisfied within the community (Mosey, 1986), for example, by referral to community activities, groups and clubs, or volunteer services. Follow up and monitoring requires that the occupational therapist assess whether the services to which the patient has been linked seem to be appropriate and effective. This may entail the occupational therapist visiting the individual at home, at the facility where the patient attends and/or liaising with family members or caregivers (Intagliata et al., 1986).

Conclusions

Occupational therapists provide their services to elderly patients with a psychiatric illness in a variety of settings. Occupational therapists may be members of a community-based assessment team, where evaluation and intervention are provided in the patient's residence. The occupational therapist is traditionally employed in psychiatric hospitals where they may work in acute or long-term care wards. Occupational therapists often make up a significant part of the staffing of day hospitals due to their focus on rehabilitation. While day centres are often confused with day hospitals, occupational therapists also work in these settings or in other community clubs or groups (for example, local government operated activity or social groups, as consultants to self-help groups or senior citizen centres). Privately run residential facilities, such as supported residential homes and nursing homes, also employ occupational therapists for psychosocial programs.

This description of the role of occupational therapy in the treatment of functional psychiatric disorders in the elderly has focused on evaluation and intervention. Occupational therapists play a role in diagnosis of the illness, highlighting patients' strengths and deficits for treatment, and contribute to discharge planning.

Intervention concentrates on prevention of disability and dysfunction, rehabilitation to the patient's optimum level of functioning, and maintenance of skills and abilities. The occupational therapy profession is unique in its use of purposeful, directed activity for evaluation and treatment.

Acknowledgements

The author wishes to sincerely thank the following occupational therapists – Michael Loh, Julie Meehan, Anne-Marie Wright, Sarah Kosmin, Jane Verity and Marion Glanville – for their support and assistance during preparation for this chapter.

References

Agacinski, K. & Stern, D. (1984). A two track program enhances therapeutic gains for chronically ill in a day hospital population. *Occupational Therapy in Mental Health*, **4** (2), 15–22.

Allen, C. (1985). *Occupational Therapy for Psychiatric Diseases: Measurement and Management of Cognitive Disabilities*, Boston: Little, Brown & Co.

Boyer, J., Colman, W., Levy, L. & Manoly, B. (1989). Affective responses to activities: a comparative study. *American Journal of Occupational Therapy*, **43** (2), 81–8.

Bruce, M. A. (1988). Occupational therapy in group treatment. In *Occupational Therapy in Mental Health: Principles in Practice*, eds. D. W. Scott and N. Katz, pp. 116–132. London: Taylor & Francis.

Bumphrey, E. E. (1989). Occupational therapy within the primary health care team. *British Journal of Occupational Therapy*, **52** (7), 252–5.

Burton, J. E. (1989*a*). The model of human occupation and occupational therapy practice with elderly patients. Part 1: Characteristics of ageing. *British Journal of Occupational Therapy*, **52** (6), 215–18.

Burton, J. E. (1989*b*). The model of human occupation and occupational therapy practice with elderly patients. Part 2: Application. *British Journal of Occupational Therapy*, **52** (6), 219–21.

Butin, D. N. & Heaney, C. (1991). Program planning in geriatric psychiatry: a model for psychosocial rehabilitation. *Physical & Occupational Therapy in Geriatrics*, **9** (3/4), 153–71.

Chamove, A. S. (1986). Positive short-term effects of activity on behavior in chronic schizophrenic patients. *British Journal of Clinical Psychiatry*, **25**, 125–33.

Clark, E. N. & Peters, E. (1984). *The Scorable Self-Care Evaluation*. Thorofare, New Jersey: SLACK Inc.

Cole, M. B. & Greene, L. R. (1988). A preference for activity: a comparative study of psychotherapy groups vs. occupational therapy groups for psychotic and borderline patients. *Occupational Therapy in Mental Health*, **8** (3), 53–67.

Collister, L., Alexander, K. & Wood, S. (1987). *The Domestic and Community Skills Assessment*. Melbourne: Mont Park Hospital.

Denton, P. (1988). Occupational therapy update: assessing the patient's functional performance. *Hospital and Community Psychiatry*, **39** (9), 935–6.

Folstein, M. F., Folstein, S.E. & McHugh, P. R. (1975). 'Mini mental state': a practical guide for grading the cognitive state of patients for the clinician. *Journal of Psychiatric Research*, **12**, 189–98

Folts, D. J. (1988). Social skills training. In *Occupational Therapy in Mental Health: Principles in Practice*, eds. D. W. Scott & N. Katz, pp. 144–156. London: Taylor & Francis.

Gregory, S. (Ed.). (1987). *Occupational Therapy Driver Assessment Course: Reference Manual.* Shepparton: Driver Education Centre of Australia.

Harwood, K. J. & Wenzl, D. (1990). Admissions to discharge: a psychogeriatric transitional program. *Occupational Therapy in Mental Health*, **10** (3), 79–100.

Health and Welfare Canada and the Canadian Association of Occupational Therapists (1983). *Guidelines for the Client-Centred Practice of Occupational Therapy.* Ottawa, Ont.: Department of National Health and Welfare, H39–33/1983E.

Hemphill, B. J. (Ed.). (1982). *The Evaluative Process in Psychiatric Occupational Therapy.* Thorofare, New Jersey: SLACK Inc.

Hoff, S. (1988). The occupational therapist as case manager in an adult day health care setting. *Physical and Occupational Therapy in Geriatrics*, **6** (1), 21–32.

Intagliata, J., Willer, B. & Egri, G. (1986). Role of the family in case management of the mentally ill. *Schizophrenia Bulletin*. **12** (4), 699–708.

Keable, D. (1988). Relaxation training in occupational therapy. In *Occupational Therapy in Mental Health: Principles in Practice*. eds. D. W. Scott & N. Katz, pp. 1–18. London: Taylor & Francis.

Kielhofner, G. & Nichol, M. (1989). The model of human occupation: a developing conceptual tool for clinicians. *British Journal of Occupational Therapy*, **52** (6), 210–14.

Leonardelli, C. A. (1988). *The Milwaukee Evaluation of Daily Living Skills: Evaluation in Long-term Psychiatric Care.* Thorofare, New Jersey: SLACK Inc.

Levy, L. L. (1990). Activity, social role retention and the multiply disabled aged: strategies for intervention. *Occupational Therapy in Mental Health*, **10** (3), 1–30.

Love, H. H. (1988). Concept and use of the social skills game to facilitate group interaction: a case study. *Occupational Therapy in Mental Health*, **8** (3), 119–33.

Lushbourgh, R. S., Priddy, J. M., Sewell, H. H., Lovett, S. B. & Jones, T. C. (1988). The effectiveness of an occupational therapy program in an inpatient geropsychiatric setting. *Physical and Occupational Therapy In Geriatrics*, **6** (2), 63–73.

Mahoney, F. I. & Barthel, D. W. (1965). Functional evaluation: the Barthel index. *Maryland State Medical Journal*, **14**, 61–5.

Matsutsuyu, J. S. (1969). The interest check list. *American Journal of Occupational Therapy*, **23**, 323–8.

Miller, P. (1987). Models for treament of depression. *Physical and Occupational Therapy in Geriatrics*, **5** (1), 3–11.

Mocellin, G. (1982). The use of activities in the treatment and rehabilitation of psychiatric patients: an overview. *Australian Occupational Therapy Journal*, **29** (3), 109–17.

Molinari, V. A. (1991). The mentally impaired elderly. *Physical and Occupational Therapy in Geriatrics*, **9** (3/4), 23–30.
Mosey, A. C. (1981). *Occupational Therapy: Configuration of a Profession*. New York: Raven Press.
Mosey, A. C. (1986). *Psychosocial Components of Occupational Therapy*. New York: Raven Press.
Norman, A. N. & Crosby, P. M. (1990). Meeting the challenge: role of occupational therapy in a geriatric day hospital. *Occupational Therapy in Mental Health*, **10** (3), 65–78.
Parham, I. A., Priddy, J. M., McGovern, T. V. & Richman, C. M. (1982). Group psychotherapy with the elderly: problems and prospects. *Psychotherapy: Theory, Research and Practice*, **19** (4), 437–43.
Rogers, J. C. (1987). Occupational therapy assessment for older adults with depression: asking the right questions. *Physical and Occupational Therapy in Geriatrics*, **5** (1), 13–33.
Smith, H. (1987). Mastery and achievement: guidelines using clinical problem solving with depressed elderly clients. *Physical and Occupational Therapy in Geriatrics*, **5** (1), 35–46.
Smith, H. D. & Tiffany, E. G. (1983). Assessment and evaluation – an overview. In *Willard and Spackman's Occupational Therapy*, 6th edition. (eds) H. L. Hopkins and H. D. Smith. pp. 143–147. Philadelphia: J. B. Lippincott Co.
Solomon, K. (1990). Learned helplessness in the elderly: theoretic and clinical considerations. *Occupational Therapy in Mental Health*, **10** (3), 31–51.
Tiffany, E. G. (1978). The occupational therapy process: treatment, maintenance, rehabilitation and prevention. In *Willard and Spackman's Occupational Therapy*, 5th edition. (eds.) H. L. Hopkins & H. D. Smith. pp. 304–318. Philadelphia: J. B. Lippincott Co.
Trace, S. & Howell, H. (1991). Occupational therapy in geriatric mental health. *American Journal of Occupational Therapy*, **45** (9), 833–8.
Wagman, J. & Kennedy, M. (1988). Position paper on occupational therapy with the elderly population. *Canadian Journal of Occupational Therapy*, **55** (2), Centrefold 1–4.
Williams, S. L. & Bloomer, J. (1987). *The Bay Area Functional Performance Evaluation*. 2nd edn. Palo Alto, CA: Consulting Psychologists Press.
Yalom, I. (1983). *Inpatient Group Psychotherapy*, New York: Basic Books.

32

Nursing management

JAN TINNEY

'The first requirement in a hospital is that it should do the sick no harm.'
Florence Nightingale (Quoted by Barritt, 1935)

This chapter outlines nursing principles and detailed procedures adopted in the care of elderly patients with a functional psychiatric illness and deals in turn with depression, anxiety neurosis and paranoid states.

Introduction

It is strongly felt that 'unless nurses have knowledge of the elderly's unique and specialized needs', acutely ill elderly people will not receive the care they need and deserve, with the result being a potential difference between continued life and death.

Many studies have raised broad issues about the nursing care of the elderly who are acutely or chronically ill, the preparation of nurses to care for the hospitalized elderly, their attitudes and understanding towards the care delivered and the specific needs required. Nurses must be prepared to examine alternative methods and models of caring and practice, and recognize that the elderly comprise a vulnerable and high risk population, very often open to abuse. It is essential to have an understanding of life experiences, loss, dependency, grief, and how many features of a psychiatric illness in the elderly can be masked by an underlying physical illness and that physical illness can be a contributing factor of a psychiatric disorder in the elderly.

Historically, nurses who have chosen to work in old age psychiatry have been viewed as the 'poor relations' of the nursing profession. It is only now that nurses specialising in this area are being recognized for their skills and contribution. Although nurses recognize the need for continuing improvement in service delivery, *they are also determined* to raise the standard and quality of care provided and to investigate alternative approaches to management. This chapter reflects the changes in attitude that have led psychiatric nurses to respond to the elderly with a psychiatric illness and their families in a sensitive and caring way.

The approach to caring must be holistic with greatest regard for status and culture. It is essential in the overall caring program and planning for management of the elderly ill person that it be recognised that the nurse has a key role in the treatment and care delivered. Many professionals have the opportunity to be actively involved at varying stages of the person's illness but the nurse has the privilege to be involved throughout the total process. It is vital that nurses no longer view the complexities and presenting illness of the elderly as merely 'a part of growing old'. A positive attitude and understanding towards the treatment of the elderly person must be adopted and concentration made on what abilities have been retained. The approach to management must be innovative, realistic and empathetic with the optimum quality and standard of care being delivered, recognizing the need for constant evaluation.

The generalized formulated nursing care plan proposed does not give consideration to the individual's cultural or religious beliefs, although this is an area that is now increasingly being given greater consideration when providing and planning for services. For far too long nurses and others neglected the needs of the elderly migrant population. Nurses giving direct care and formulating management plans must orient themselves to the specific needs of the person from an ethnic background, equipping themselves to provide a comprehensive service. As the general population ages so does the migrant population. Poor communication skills, integration into society, coming to terms with the loss of the extended family unit and consequent isolation are just a few of the problems that the elderly migrant person may experience. No longer is the elderly migrant person necessarily cared for in the extended family unit. In psychiatry, some transcultural psychiatry units are emerging but often nurses have little or no knowledge of the existence of these services. Traditionally the members of the multidisciplinary team have consisted of nurses, medical staff, and allied health professionals but interpreting services also have an important role to play within the management team.

Depression

The literature informs us that depression in the elderly is one of the most misdiagnosed illnesses and often masked by other conditions. Depression in later life can be severe, debilitating and deadly. Depression is a state of mind that most people will experience at some stage or other in their lives. Its severity may range from a feeling of sadness to total withdrawal. To feel totally isolated, alone with what is perceived as no quality to one's life must be devastating. The elderly person may present having suffered a number of losses as a contributing factor to their depressive state. The impact of this accumulation of losses may be greater in the elderly adult because unlike the young, the elderly often do not have their losses offset by gains although it must be recognized that treatment of the elderly person with depression is as successful as in any other age group.

Listed below are a number of identified losses:

- loss of job
- loss of status
- loss of independence
- loss of health
- loss of home
- loss of spouse, family etc.
- altered self-image

Assessment

Before attempting to formulate any management plan the nurse has to have gained a comprehensive assessment of the physical, mental and social status of the patient due to the wide variety of factors impacting upon the presentation of the patient with depression. The assessment must be uniquely thorough as no other profession has 24-hour contact with the patient. The observations documented over this period will assist other members of the multidisciplinary team to have input into the overall management plan. The nurse should view every interaction with the patient as an opportunity for observation and assessment. The approach needs to be sensitive to the individual's needs, demonstrating warmth, understanding and empathy, which will lay the foundation for a trusting relationship between the nurse and the patient. Throughout this 24-hour assessment there will be an opportunity to observe the patient during a variety of activities. This will allow assessment of the patient's changing moods, reactions, interactions, responses and physical state. Over recent years the emphasis has shifted from a purely psychiatric approach to one that encompasses all aspects of the patient's presentation. Attention to assessment, management, diagnosis and care is equally as important for both the physical and psychological components of the person's presentation. Nurses need to be aware of the impact of physical symptoms when approaching the formulation of a management plan. This is important not only in the acute phase of illness but may require strategies to be put into place for continuing care management. The formulation of a care plan is an accepted means of documenting the nursing process in a variety of forms.

The care plan should reflect the patients individual need, with an accurate statement of identified problems, management strategies, goals to be achieved and evaluation criteria. There should be incorporated into this plan a method of ownership by the patient, caregiver and family members. This will assist all involved to understand the goals to be pursued and achieved. Goals set must be realistic and achievable and therefore must be defined as both short and long term. Contracts are sometimes entered into based on the assumption that patients have the right to make decisions regarding their health care and that nurses are responsible in negotiating with patients the care they will provide. Historically, nurses have been quite successful in this process but there has been little or no documentation of this.

The nurse must obtain the following information:

- medical history
- physical examination
- psychiatric history
- clinical observation status
- legal status
- medication history, past and present
- electrocardiograph
- urinalysis
- order for investigations
- family assessment
- mental status examination
- nutritional history
- psychosocial assessment

Listed below are a number of presenting problems that may be identified during psychiatric assessment:

- feelings of worthlessness
- feelings of isolation
- feelings of anger
- low self-esteem
- disturbed sleep pattern
- loss of weight
- loss of appetite
- no motivation
- poor concentration
- irritability
- suicidal ideation
- tearfulness
- anxiety
- restlessness
- somatic complaints
- delusions
- hallucinations

Depressive illness

Depressive illness is well discussed in Section 4. The nursing management of specific problems in depressed elderly patients is illustrated in Table 32.1.

Table 32.1. *Nursing management of problems identified in depressed patients*

MAINTAINING ADEQUATE NUTRITION/HYDRATION

Goal

- To provide optimum level of nutrition/hydration
- To improve interest in dietary needs and involve patient in on-going educational program

Management

- Commence on fluid balance chart
- Closely observe patient at meal times
- Ascertain likes/dislikes
- Refer to dietician
- Partake in meal with patient
- Encourage good food intake
- Ensure food is presented well, e.g. portions not too large
- Involve patient in planning of meals, later involve patient in preparing meal
- Refer patient to occupational therapist for assessment of level of independence
- If weight lost, supplement accordingly
- Provide positive feedback for even the smallest achievement. Do not be condescending

FEELINGS OF LOW SELF-ESTEEM

Goal

- To develop and increase feelings of self-worth and self-esteem by participation in a variety of management program, both on individual and group basis
- To establish patients access to other members of the treating team

Management

- Be sincere, conveying care and concern. Spend time with patient, identify feelings
- Provide low stimulus environment at times throughout the day, protecting patient from being too overwhelmed
- Encourage patient into appropriate activity programme with achievable goals
- Refer patient to occupational therapist for inclusion in appropriate sessions
- Consider environment, e.g. colours, lighting, flowers, noise level, personalised items will influence patient's mood
- Have agreed time to spend with patient on one to one basis, developing trust and rapport
- Follow through on agreed activities, tasks to be achieved
- Refer to psychologist, discuss involvement on individual or group basis
- Following consultation involve patient in specific discussion groups
- Monitor understanding, engage in on-going education if necessary
- Give written information on rights issues and services available

PATIENTS' RIGHTS

Goal

- Ensure patient/family has a clear and concise understanding of rights issue and how to access appropriate services

Table 32.1. (*cont.*)

Management
- Involve interpreter if necessary
- Act as advocate on patient's behalf
- Inform patient of how to access options/services, e.g. public advocate, legal representation, appeals process

RISK FACTORS

Goal
- To provide a safe and secure environment by ensuring attention to all aspects of patient's presentation

Management
- Assess severity of patient's symptoms, e.g. withdrawn, isolated behaviour, content of conversation
- Assess potential for self-harm through conversation and observation, if concerned, Conduct appropriate search of area for reason for self-harm with patient's permission and review category observations
- Explain interventions to patient
- Continually reassess patient's presentation
- Obtain previous history, premorbid personality

APATHETIC/WITHDRAWN BEHAVIOR

Goal
- Reintegrate into groups and eventually community setting

Management
- Spend a designated period of time with patient each day, e.g. walking in the garden
- Spend time in nonverbal setting
- Offer reassurance, support by physical contact (placing hand on shoulder) if tolerated
- Be alert for nonverbal 'cues'
- Provide sensory low stimulus environment, e.g. soft music, flowers, noise level, lighting and outlook for rooms
- Obtain premorbid personality history
- Allow personal space – consider with whom patient may be sharing facility
- Do not allow patient to spend long periods of time in isolation, encourage interaction, even nonverbally, with selected copatients

INABILITY TO COMMUNICATE

Goal
- Encourage patient to feel comfortable in communicating with others and to ascertain any other causes and alleviate barriers, e.g. symptoms of illness
- To alleviate problems
- Establish routine

Management
- Encourage patient to express feelings in other nonverbal ways, e.g. drawing, painting or writing
- Encourage patient to verbalize on one to one basis initially but do not overwhelm patient

Table 32.1. (*cont.*)

- Assess level of communication skills
- Refer patient to psychologist
- Monitor patient's behavior and responses to environment, copatients, family
- Involve patient in progressive physical activity programme, e.g. short walks, gentle exercises
- Commence on-going education programme

SLEEP DISTURBANCE

Goal

- To establish a restful sleep pattern and to assist the patient in identifying contributing factors

Management

- Monitor/chart sleep pattern, alert night staff to problems
- Consult with patient regarding problems related to sleep disturbance, e.g. difficulty getting off to sleep, early morning awakening. Ask night staff to monitor problem
- Monitor effects of sedation, decrease as soon as is acceptable
- Encourage degree of physical activity to promote physical tiredness
- Discourage sleeping for long periods during the day, be gentle but firm in establishing routine for resting and rising
- Provide a quiet milieu, ensure noise levels are lessened
- Limit coffee/tea consumption late evening/night. Offer alternative
- Encourage patient to alert staff if awake
- Provide night light, if patient wakes, light can be reassuring
- Establish good sleep hygiene

DECREASED ATTENTION TO PERSONAL HYGIENE/APPEARANCE

Goal

- To promote self-worth, increase self-esteem and pride in self-image
- To assess patient's capabilities to carry out procedures themselves
- If patient not capable, involve support services prior to patient's discharge

Management

- As necessary, assist patient with personal hygiene needs as symptoms of amotivation/ambivalence may be present
- Assist in organizing items necessary to complete procedure
- Be supportive, reassuring, give patient time
- Ensure attention to personal clothing
- Refer to podiatrist, hairdresser as appropriate
- Attend to details of self-care, e.g. shaving, nails, make-up etc.
- Attend to accessories, e.g. hearing aid, watch, jewellery, toiletries
- Refer to occupational therapist for ADL assessment if necessary

MEDICATION

Goal

- Effective stabilization of patient. Monitoring of side-effects and seek effective management of same

Table 32.1. (*cont.*)

Management
- Monitor response/side-effects of medication regime
- Observe signs of defaulting or hoarding (especially as mood uplifts)
- Commence educational programme with patient on medication benefits/side-effects
- Place patient on clinical observation chart, observe side-effects of medication, e.g. hypotension

SOCIAL ISOLATION

Goal
- To establish appropriate resocialization programme to meet individual needs
- To integrate into community support services following hospitalization, e.g. community centre, day hospital

Management
- Consult with family/friends regarding history, interests and hobbies
- Discuss with patient past social interactions/interests
- Refer to occupational therapist
- Initially involve patient in one-to-one interaction, promoting relationship, then group socialization program

ANXIETY/FEAR RELATED TO HOSPITALIZATION

Goal
- To assist the patients transfer into the hospital setting with the minimal distress occurring
- Involve other family members so they may also be supportive of the patient and assist in relieving associated anxiety/fear

Management
- Offer reassurance/support
- Conduct a thorough orientation to the environment, this may need to be repeated
- Encourage patient to ask questions to seek clarification
- Limit the number of personnel in admission procedure, patient may feel overwhelmed
- Introduce the primary nurse and other key staff only
- Do not overload patient with information, be clear and concise, clarify other issues later

INCREASED ANXIETY

Goal
- To educate patient to observe for 'cues' that could heighten anxiety
- To cope with feelings of anxiety in a constructive way
- To develop strategies to cope with anxiety

Management
- Assess degree of anxiety being experienced
- Monitor contributing factors, e.g. pressure in group, overwhelmed by tasks, requests, interviews
- Be an active listener, sit with patient
- Recognise anxiety, be supportive but firm
- Discuss with patient possible identified cause/causes
- Attempt to divert patient, e.g. walking with patient, one/one activity

Table 32.1. (*cont.*)

- Refer to psychologist
- Educate patient/or even participate in relaxation techniques/sessions with patient
- Reduce stimulus provide quiet area
- Communication should be clear and concise
- Be supportive
- Involve in small group sessions as patient's anxiety decreases
- Assist patient to ventilate feelings, talk patient through situations step by step

PHYSICAL PROBLEMS

(e.g. chest infection, UTI, cardiac problems, renal problems, vitamin deficiencies, visual impairment, auditory impairment)

Goal

- To ensure holistic approach to management is given. All aspects of patient's needs are met
- Commence preventative health program
- Refer to other agencies for continuing monitoring of physical state

Management

- Ensure investigations are completed
- Monitor clinical observations, report abnormalities
- Involve other agencies, e.g. blind/deaf society
- Instigate management strategies according to results, e.g. UTI push fluids
- Refer to other disciplines, e.g. dietitian, physiotherapist

GRIEF/LOSS/FEAR/ANGER

Goal

- Identify loss through phases, adapt lifestyle, develop new strategies
- Promote return to community
- Positive attitude to the future

Management

- Establish rapport/trust by assisting patient to feel comfortable. Nurse patient initially on one to one basis
- Discourage continual rumination on one aspect of grief/feelings
- Discourage avoidance by patient continually involving themselves in alternative activities
- Have a designated agreed time to spend with patient
- Encourage patient to ventilate feelings verbally or nonverbally, e.g. writing feelings down
- Facilitate patient's expressions of anger, guilt, resentment through conversation, activity, both individually and as a group, recognize feelings as 'normal'
- Encourage independence, allow patient to make decisions, develop ownership
- Involve patient in activities that allow ventilation/expression of concerns, fear, etc
- Commence discussion (as appropriate as to his/her expectations from hospitalization)
- Encourage patient to identify his/her goals

Table 32.1. *(cont.)*

DISCHARGE PLANNING

Goal

- To prepare patient for discharge, then refer back to the appropriate environment with support/services
- To support family/patient in transition from hospital to community setting

Management

- Involve family members in predischarge discussions
- Involve social worker, involve other agencies who will be involved in supportive/continuing care
- Introduce patient to the people involved in his/her on-going care
- Promote self-confidence and independence, by encouraging patient to have leave prior to discharge
- Involve patient in discharge planning groups
- Involve occupational therapist in discussing with patient involvement in community support/leisure services
- Ensure patient has on-going assessment of any outstanding physical problems and use of medication
- Involve community nursing service in the initial post discharge visit

Anxiety disorders

Anxiety disorders in the elderly have not been as extensively studied as have other disorders (see Chapter 6). It is sometimes felt that anxiety and fearfulness are inevitable in old age. Anxiety disorders tend to be chronic once established (Schepira et al., 1972, Agars et al., 1972) and in the majority of cases in the elderly are probably of longstanding duration. Anxiety disorders can however, occur for the first time in old age. Other disorders associated with anxiety may be depression, panic disorder, phobias, dementia, delirium and paranoid states. Anxiety disorders may often be associated with a physical disorder in the elderly. A thorough assessment including a physical examination needs to be undertaken. Generalized anxiety disorder is characterized by symptoms such as tension, inability to relax, trembling, hyperactivity, frequency of micturation, stomach upsets, diarrhea, anticipation of misfortune, difficulty in concentrating, insomnia, impatience, impending doom and feelings of worthlessness (American Psychiatric Association, 1987). Some causes of anxiety in the older person can be readily identifiable but others may not be as obvious. The nurse requires to be particularly familiar with events prior to the patient's hospitalization and to any factors that could contribute to an increase in the patient's anxiety level. The management of specific problems in the anxious elderly patient is illustrated in Table 32.2.

Table 32.2. *Nursing management of patients with anxiety disorders*

PATIENTS' SAFETY

Goal

- To create an atmosphere within the environment that will demonstrate to the patient a feeling of safety and security

Management

- Be reassuring and supportive
- Spend time with patient on one-to-one basis
- Reduce stimulus to create milieu endeavouring to create a feeling of security
- Monitor patient's level of anxiety, be aware of escalation
- Provide a safe, secure, well-lit environment
- Ensure environment is stable and familiar
- Encourage patient to follow a routine

SLEEP DISTURBANCE

Goal

- To establish an appropriate sleep hygiene and eliminate any contributing factors

Management

- Use night light to assist patient in alleviating increasing anxiety by being in a darkened room
- Involve night staff in monitoring sleep pattern, commence on sleep chart
- Encourage use of relaxation techniques prior to retiring
- Encourage use of stress management techniques prior to retiring
- Encourage patient to inform nurse if awake
- Educate patient on dietary consumption, e.g. caffeine intake late at night
- Review contributing factors in the environment
- Monitor effects of sedation, reduce as sleep pattern more established
- Involve patient in activities during the day to increase fatigue

ASSESSMENT OF PHYSICAL STATE

Goal

- Eliminate any other causes for presentation
- Educate and assist patient/family to cope with results if any

Management

- Commence on clinical observation chart
- Monitor dietary intake
- Be honest but not overinclusive with explanation, therefore not heightening patient's anxiety level
- Complete physical work-up
- Follow through on results
- Investigate increase in bowel movements/urinary output

Table 32.2. (*cont.*)

MEDICATIONS

Goal

- To assess effectiveness of medication regime
- To educate patient regarding desirable alternatives
- Assist patient in transit period from medication to other therapies

Management

- Monitor closely effect and side-effects of medication
- Monitor for withdrawals
- Medication to be effectively utilized, e.g. if anxiety increases out of control, feelings related
- Medications to be used in conjunction with other therapies
- Check history for abuse of medications
- Cohesive team approach is essential

RISK ASSESSMENT

Goal

- Ensure patient safety and security

Management

- Observe patient for fears, e.g. impending doom, increase in somatic complaints
- Reassess category observations
- Observe for signs of depressive themes

SOCIAL ISOLATION

Goal

- To assist patient to develop resocialization skills
- To investigate community support services available following discharge, introduce patient into community programmes during hospitalization

Management

- Refer to occupational therapist
- Gradual introduction to small group activity
- Monitor outcomes, reassess effectiveness of activities on an ongoing basis
- Encourage participation in daily activities
- Participate with patient initially in group activities
- Assess patient's lifestyle, activities and interactions
- Ascertain any interests or hobbies, investigate the possibility of pursuing same while in hospital
- Involve patient in activity that may initially require only short term concentration preferably with positive outcome
- Promote self-confidence and independence through group activities, recognise achievements, e.g. self-awareness groups

DISCHARGE PLANNING

Goal

- To commence discharge planning at the beginning of hospitalization
- To integrate patient into community setting with support services and networks having been established

Table 32.2. (*cont.*)

Management

- Commence discussion, as appropriate, as to patient's expectation to hospitalization
- Encourage patient to identify goals
- On-going education regarding management of illness
- Assist patient to deal with anxiety related to discharge
- Involve patient's family in pre-discharge discussion
- Involve social worker/occupational therapist
- Discussion with patient about leisure activities
- Involve support services prior to patient's discharge
- Link in to community support services if relevant

Paranoid disorders

The elderly person suffering from a paranoid disorder may present with persecutory or grandiose delusions that influence their behavior, mood and thinking. Often they are hostile, angry, suspicious, guarded, fearful, grandiose, even suicidal. The disorder may be of a short or long time duration (American Psychiatric Association, 1987). Paranoid states may affect individuals from all social classes and educational backgrounds. Social isolation, and the aging process may tend to increase suspiciousness and paranoid thoughts (Burnside, 1988). The physical complications of aging such as hearing and visual deficits can be contributing factors. Many feelings of suspiciousness and paranoia are responses to relationships and situations in which the older person feels powerless and unimportant. (Ebersole & Hess, 1989). Paranoid features can present in a number of illnesses affecting the elderly, including paraphrenia, psychotic depression, dementia, substance abuse, sensory deprivation and delirium.

When caring for a person with a paranoid illness, the nurse needs to be extremely skilled during the assessment period. It may be necessary to obtain a history from significant others. As the patient becomes less anxious, angry, additional details can be obtained from the patient directly. In eliciting information from the patient, clear, concise communication and an empathetic, honest approach are vital. An authoritarian approach will only evoke a hostile angry response. The underlying anxiety needs to be recognized and reduced, and not appear to impose a threat to the person. Personal space should be recognized and respected. As a trusting relationship develops and barriers are reduced an increase in the length of contact will emerge.

The paranoid person may be generally angry, and the nurse should accept the angry attitude as a reaction to the person's perceived threatening environment. It is best to acknowledge the question without reacting with anger in turn and to accept criticism without becoming defensive (Ebersole & Hess, 1989).

The management of specific problems affecting paranoid patients is illustrated in Table 32.3.

Table 32.3. *Nursing management of paranoid disorders in the elderly*

POOR DIETARY INTAKE

Goal
- Prevent dehydration
- Adequate dietary intake
- Gain optimum level of weight
- Optimum level of health

Management
- Monitor all dietary intake
- Commence on fluid balance chart
- Monitor weight
- Refer to dietitian
- Supplement lack of food intake if patient accepts
- Ascertain likes/dislikes
- Offer reassurance
- Sit with patient if necessary, even partake of same meal
- Food may be brought in from home, discuss with relatives
- Serve foods in sealed containers, e.g. milk, the patient can open the carton themselves
- Let patients see other patients eating first
- If patient restless offer frequent drinks, finger foods, these can be ingested while walking
- If appropriate involve family in food planning and service
- Consider cultural background and culturally appropriate foods

SUSPICIOUSNESS

Goal
- To alleviate anxiety and fears related to suspiciousness
- To develop a trusting relationship
- Set and maintain a therapeutic relationship

Management
- Be nonthreatening in all approaches
- Offer support and reassurance
- Do not be judgmental
- Do not intrude upon personal space
- Be honest
- Develop rapport by spending time with patient
- Be firm but caring and responsive
- Obtain good premorbid history
- Consider cultural background

PATIENTS' RIGHTS

Goal
- To ensure patients rights are adhered to, and patient has a clear, concise understanding of how to access information and services

Table 32.3. (*cont.*)

Management
- Ascertain level of understanding of rights issue
- Give written information to patient in own language
- Undertake on-going education if patient unsure
- Be honest
- Inform patient of services and appeal processes available, e.g. Public Advocate, Legal Services
- Assist patient in accessing services
- Work as an advocate on behalf of patient

DELUSIONS **(e.g. persecutory/grandiose)**

Goal
- To return patient to a reality-based functioning level
- To discharge patient back into a community setting with support mechanisms in place

Management
- Cohesive team approach to management
- Do not argue with patient
- Attempt to return patient to reality base when appropriate
- Do not joke with patient
- Reinforce to patient that the origin of their fears is internal not externally based
- Spend time with patient, recognise fears
- Reinforce safety and security
- Use night light if persecutory ideas present at night
- Nurse patient close to nurse's station
- Be aware of contributing factors in the environment
- Consider cultural background
- Ensure appropriate monitoring of effectiveness of medications
- Observe for escalation and ideas

SOCIAL ISOLATION

Goal
- To reduce isolation by integrating into hospital/community based activities endeavouring to reduce rehospitalization

Management
- Attempt individual contact only initially
- Progress from small to larger groups for increased interaction
- Introduce patient to social and occupational therapy groups
- Consider interests and hobbies, if any
- Involve patients in tasks where there is achievement and which are achievable
- Discuss ongoing activity/group interests when discharged

MEDICATION

Goal
- To ensure patient compliance with prescribed medications and understanding of the necessity for compliance after discharge from hospital
- To reduce anxieties and fears associated with long-term medication regime and possible associated side-effects
- To educate patient regarding coping with possible long illness

Table 32.3. (*cont.*)

Management
- Ensure patient ingests all prescribed medication. Initially liquid form may be preferred
- Ensure patient does not default on medication. Check mouth, under tongue
- Be honest, direct, and firm. Do not enter into bargaining situation
- Involve patient in ongoing educational program regarding medications, e.g. dosage, name, side-effects
- Monitor and report any side-effects of medications

AGGRESSION

Goal
- To ensure the safety of patient and others
- To ensure the optimum level of management
- To assist patient to cope with feelings of aggression appropriately

Management
- Encourage patient to ventilate fears and feelings in socially acceptable forms
- Reinforce the safety and security of the environment
- Observe for 'cues' that could indicate escalation in patient's aggressive presentation
- Introduce appropriate management strategies
- Provide low stimulus environment if contributing factor in patient's behavior
- Continually re-assess patient's presentation

ATTENTION TO PERSONAL HYGIENE NEEDS

Goals
- To ensure optimum standard of hygiene maintained in accordance with individual's personal preferences, capabilities and cultural needs
- To involve support services prior to discharge to ensure maintenance of standard of health care

Management
- Ensure all aspects of patient's hygiene needs are attended to
- Involve patient in discussion regarding when they would wish their needs to be attended to, e.g. AM/PM, alternate days etc.
- Ensure oral hygiene attended to
- If necessary refer patient to appropriate services, e.g. dentist, podiatrist, hairdresser
- Consider patient's cultural background. Can influence hygiene habits
- Ascertain whether shower/bath preferred
- Refer to occupational therapist for ADL assessment
- Ensure patient has adequate personal clothing, refer to social worker, investigate cultural aspects

PHYSICAL NEEDS

Goals
- To evaluate patient's physical state through assessment and investigation
- To ensure optimum level of health, to treat any underlying causes and maintain patient at optimum functioning level

Management
- Do not overwhelm patient with urgency of investigation unless necessary
- Ensure investigations are complete to eliminate any other causes for presentation, with explanation to patient

Table 32.3. (*cont.*)

- Involve other team members
- Observe patient for symptoms that could be a contributing factor, e.g. infection
- Commence patient on clinical observations
- Monitor ongoing physical state
- Assess patient for any underlying bruising or abrasions

RISK ASSESSMENT

Goals

- To ensure patient safety through implementing appropriate management

Management

- Commence patient on risk category observations
- Review frequently in accordance with presentation
- Institute management of risk behavior in consultation and with collaboration of other team members

Conclusion

A problem orientated nursing approach is described in this chapter which provides a detailed analysis of necessary goals of nursing care and management strategies to assist the patients to achieve them.

Nursing management is the central pillar in a total management plan, the application of such must be accompanied by sensitivity, empathy and understanding of the elderly person's life journey. A holistic and flexible approach is essential in developing a therapeutic relationship with the older person. Participating in a multidisciplinary team, the nurse can contribute very detailed, relevant and significant observation of behavior, emotional and mental status, response to treatment and relationship to family and formal carers. The 24-hour contact with the patient places the nurse in a valuable and valued position in effecting successful management of problems arising out of functional psychiatric disorders. Therefore a sensitive, warm and well-trained nurse who efficiently atttends to details is a crucial member of the multidisciplinary treatment team in geriatric psychiatry.

References

Agars et al. (1972). *Behavior Modification: Principles and Clinical Applications*. Boston, Mass: Little Brown & Co.

American Psychiatry Association (1987). *Diagnostic and Statistical Manual of Mental Disorder*. Edition Revised, Washington, DC: American Psychiatric Association.

Burnside, I. (1988). Paranoid State. *Nursing and the Aged*. Chapter 24, pp. 795–807. McGraw-Hill.

Ebersole & Hess (1990). *Towards Healthy Aging. Human Needs and Nursing Responses*. 3rd edn. St Louis: Mosby.

Greist, J. H. & Jefferson, J. W. (1983). *Depression and Its Treatment. Help for the Nation's Mental Problems*. American Psychiatric Press Inc.

33

Social work and the psychiatry of late life

ELIZABETH OZANNE

New directions in mental health services in the 1990s and implications for geriatric psychiatry

Worldwide changes in the provision and focus of mental health services in recent decades have been via initial efforts to deinstitutionalize large psychiatric institutions and later attempts to build up a comprehensive regional infrastructure of community based mental health support services including the mainstreaming into general health of psychiatric services (Health Department of Victoria, 1992*b*).

The direction of the changes being implemented has been to shift the focus of service from separate centralized institutions to integrated regionalized community facilities that will assist in maintaining those with psychiatric disabilities in the community via more effective outreach, advocacy and support, rehabilitation and case management (Rosen, 1992). This shift from largely institutionally based to community provided services is requiring new skills and capacities of mental health personnel and a cultural change in the focus of service intervention to facilitate community coping capacity and competence in clients/consumers.

The direction of contemporary changes has been towards:

1. shorter stays in institutional settings
2. more episodic care for the acutely mentally ill
3. the creation of more innovative and humane long-term care settings
4. increased relative allocation of resources to community-based facilities
5. a greater focus on assertive community outreach and rehabilitation
6. greater liaison with general practice, local government and other community agencies to facilitate better primary prevention and ongoing community support.
7. provision of a comprehensive range of community care programs including assessment, case management, rehabilitation, vocational guidance and housing support.

These changes in mental health service delivery reflect wider changes in health systems towards a greater emphasis on primary intervention and prevention, and the development of tertiary rehabilitative technologies for new long-term care populations to balance the substantial investment in the acute care system (National Health Strategy, 1991).

The international rights movement and several UN Covenants (UN, 1992) have also put emphasis on the need for greater focus on innovation in service planning and delivery as well as a greater partnership orientation in treatment modes with consumers (Burdekin 1991; National Health Strategy, 1993*a*).

Increasing recognition is also being given to issues of resource allocation in mental health and the need for public mental health services to focus primarily on the seriously mentally ill and interventions that support this population in terms of rehabilitation services that foster social recovery and community reintegration in work and housing (Health Department of Victoria, 1990). The role of the community and private and not-for-profit sectors in service provision is also under review and new public–private mixes of service delivery are being explored (McKenzie, 1992; National Health Strategy, 1991). Research into the etiology and progress of mental illness and the outcome of existing interventions is highlighting the lack of efficacy of many present treatment approaches and the need to shift focus to viewing mental illness as a 'problem of living' which requires a more social rehabilitative interventive technology (Wilson, 1992).

Geriatric psychiatry as a relatively new field of practice has emerged in this changing context (Health Department of Victoria, 1988), partly responsive to the aging of the population but also responsive to new government policy thrusts in relation to mental health, aging, disability and dementia (Australian Health Ministers, 1992; Commonwealth Department of Health, Housing and Community Services, 1991, 1992; Commonwealth of Australia, 1986). The development of geriatric psychiatry has, however, occurred at a time of considerable cost constraint and restructuring which has meant that the early specific focus on the psychiatric needs of the elderly is now having to be viewed within the overall restructuring and integration of mental health services in mainstream general medical services. Though this presents some new opportunities (Lebowitz, 1993), it also carries with it particular risks in relation to specific resource allocation and continued positive discrimination for what has been a relatively neglected area in the past (Healy, 1992).

The social work orientation and new directions in geriatric psychiatry

The value orientation of social work is essentially humanistic. The primary unit of attention is not the individual alone, or a particular symptom picture, but the total transactional unit or gestalt of the 'person in their environment'. This orientation is generally referred to as 'ecological' (Germain & Gitterman, 1981). From this perspective, individuals are seen to be in continual interaction with their immediate networks and wider environment, adapting to and coping with internal and external changes towards the goal of greater effectance and/or competence (Maluccio, 1981) and they are more or less successful in this pursuit.

The ecological orientation of social work fits well with more recent directions in mental health policy in terms of the greater recognition being given to a social rehabilitation orientation (Anthony & Liberman, 1986) in the provision of services. This orientation puts emphasis on mental illness as a 'problem of living' (more than just a nosological symptom picture) and the need for interventions to improve the community coping capacity and quality of life, particularly for the chronically mentally ill, via a supportive infrastructure of community services and assertive community outreach.

A social work perspective emphasises strategies to enhance an individual's adaptation and coping capacity via supportive casework, group work, family work and case management in clinical settings of institution and community, while also actively working at tasks of organizational change, community linkage and resource mobilization on behalf of elderly mentally ill persons.

It would, in fact, seem that all professions are moving towards a more 'ecological' or 'systems' perspective as presenting problems become more complex, health care more multidisciplinary and health systems are more preoccupied with long-term care populations.

The specific aims of social work intervention

Reflecting this ecological perspective, the aim of social work intervention is to facilitate the individual's capacity for effectance and environmental mastery, often in situations and with populations where there are particular constraints, both internal and external, that undermine coping capacity and mastery (Lawton & Nahemow, 1973; Kahana, 1975). The social worker thus works with both individuals and service systems in endeavouring to achieve better person/ environment fit (Coulton, 1981).

The goals of social work intervention with individuals and in service systems are stated by Monk (1981) as:

1. to help people enlarge their competence and increase their problem-solving and coping abilities
2. to help people obtain resources
3. to facilitate interaction between individuals and others in their environment
4. to make organizations responsive to people and to influence interactions between organizations and institutions
5. to influence social and environmental policy

These principles of practice in relation to social work intervention with the aged and the elderly mentally infirm are elaborated in Table 33.1, which is an excerpt from Monk (1981).

Table 33.1. *Objectives of social work practice with the elderly*

Help people enlarge their competence and increase their problem-solving and coping abilities

(a) Social work practice with the aged should be based on a positive attitude toward the intrinsic value of old age and its validity as a distinct state of the life cycle that is endowed with its own meaning and developmental tasks. Practitioners working with older people perceive and encourage the expression of their client's potential to enrich and contribute to the cycle of generations. Social workers in general seek to understand the meaning of aging, free from the distortions of stereotypical beliefs, through an examination of their own feelings about the process of growing old and a sense of life's value within its inevitable limits.

(b) No two older people are exactly alike. The principle of individualization and the concomitant avoidance of age-related biases are the cognitive and ethical foundations of practice. Social work intervention requires an understanding of each person's lifelong ways of coping. Some individuals may be engaged in nostalgic reminiscences. Others obstinately retain an orientation toward the future. Like individuals of any other age, older people are capable of varying levels of adaptation and self-expression.

(c) Social workers identify and assess the extent and quality of an older person's remaining strengths. They strive to help the individual maximize the use of these strengths, even in the face of loss and progressive deterioration.

(d) Treatment objectives aimed at enhancing the older person's coping skills must be realistically scaled down to the level of his or her remaining strengths. This should be done on the understanding that even micro-behavioral changes are positive indications of the outcome of the treatment.

(e) Although an older individual may never regain his or her waning strength, it is the social worker's task to bolster the person's sense of personal integrity. The dependence that accompanies the receipt of protective services should injure the person's self-esteem as little as possible and should not carry a price tag of moral degradation or infantilization.

Help people obtain resources

(a) Older people are especially intimidated by complex eligibility requirements and the discouraging bureaucratic maze of existing services. In addition, because of value-related conflicts, a sense of pride, or fear of surrendering their personal autonomy, they often refuse services to which they are entitled. Social workers strive to understand the source of such culturally based considerations and personal anxieties that older clients experience regarding the receipt of services. They then attempt to build up the client's trust, facilitate access to services, and make sure that the client knows about and obtains the services to which he or she is entitled.

Table 33.1. (*cont.*)

(b) Because most older people have several chronic conditions, they may require services on a continuous basis. In such cases, social workers must focus on case management and co-ordination with the aim of linking older clients to services, monitoring the delivery of services, reassessing the individual client's condition and needs at regular intervals, and making sure that available services are continued to meet the particular needs of the client.

Facilitate interaction between individuals and others in their environment

(a) As people grow older, members of their lifelong support systems – spouse offspring, relatives and friends – die or move away. Both the onset of widowhood, spelling the probability that loneliness will be a permanent part of life, and the individual's bombardment by repeated losses point to the need for intervention that is geared to circumstances of bereavement and the client's potential for resocialization. In dealing with bereavement, social workers are called on to provide support to the client and help him or her through the process of grieving resulting from the loss of a spouse, close relatives or friends.
(b) When helping to resocialize the bereaved client, social workers assist in the development of new support systems and facilitate the individual's adjustment and integration to new social contexts, such as self-help groups, multiservice centres, and lifelong learning programs.
(c) To the same purpose, social workers facilitate instrumental and expressive interaction between individuals of different generations. They promote mutual helping efforts that are responsive to the needs of everyone involved.
(d) Resocialization is also a challenge for the aging nuclear couple when the last of their offspring leaves home. Social workers facilitate clients' adjustments and their search for meaning in a new family situation that they may never have experienced before.
(e) Social workers are increasingly called on to provide relief to those who are middle-aged, most especially when these individuals find they can no longer attend to the needs of aging, ailing parents or grandparents. In such instances, workers facilitate the integration of a family's strengths and resources through formalized personal care services.
(f) Ultimately, the activities of social workers enable older people to remain in their familiar environment for as long as possible and thus to retain a sense of competence and continuity in their relationship with the environment. Workers efforts in this regard may call for enriching the environment with architectural and other supports and ensuring access to services. When it is no longer possible for the older person to remain in his or her home and neighborhood, it is incumbent on the social worker to help the person prepare for the impending transition to institutional care as carefully and smoothly as possible, thus avoiding the trauma of a sudden uprooting.

Table 33.1. (*cont.*)

Make organisations responsive to people

(a) As the number of aged people grows in this society, social service agencies are experiencing a relentless increase in their gerontological caseloads. A major task for social workers is to promote an awareness of who these clients are and what their specific service requirements may be. Workers within agencies must develop treatment modalities that take into account the cumulative losses undergone by older clients, the social, mental and physical limitations that affect an older person's request for help and the difficulty that many older people experience in making use of services.

(b) Social workers must interpret for agencies the need to define service priorities in ways that are congruent with major geriatric needs. For example, services for the aged must be geared to the reduction of stress and the alleviation of the client's sense of helplessness rather than to personality reconstruction. In addition, service systems should include an 'early warning' component attuned to the major crises of old age.

(c) Workers must also make sure that older people, like competent clients of all ages, remain the masters of their own destiny and are involved in making determinations concerning their own future. Service systems should provide older clients with alternative courses of action from which they can choose. Furthermore, these systems should be coordinated to form comprehensive networks with multiple points of entry and, when possible, 'one-stop' stations or centres that provide multiple services.

(d) Given the contradictory evidence about whether services are best provided in an age-integrated or age-segregated system, social workers should retain a flexible, open-minded attitude. It is likely that some services obtain better outcomes when they are offered in multigenerational situations but that others may be more effective when delivered to clients of one age group only. In either case, the preferences of clients should be consulted, but when a given course becomes inevitable, such as institutionalization in a long-term care facility, proper counselling and adequate preparation of the client should especially prevail.

Influence social and environmental policy

(a) Though many government programs that benefit the aged directly or indirectly have been generated in recent years, their apparent abundance is not a valid indication of their adequacy. Social workers must critically examine whether existing programs are relevant and appropriate in the light of the changing social, economic and demographic conditions related to the ageing.

(b) As formulated in the program implementation stage, provision of eligibility, program restrictions, and determinations of service priorities are at times inconsistent with the intent of legislation. Social workers critically examine whether there is continuity between programs and policies and assist in the improvement of needs assessment and the setting of priorities.

Table 33.1. (*cont.*)

(c)	Most public funds for the aged are used to provide cash supports, and this overshadows the provision of services. Workers must correct this imbalance by defining the extent and nature of clients' needs related to such areas as housing, nutrition, physical and mental impairment, isolation, transportation and employment. They may then assist in the formulation of cogent, innovative policies.
(d)	Because of the increase in the number of aging people relative to the rest of the population, neither families nor the public at large can be called on to assume total and exclusive responsibility for those who are aged. Social workers must therefore devise incentives to be given to families and communities for assuming a wider responsibility for other people. In a similar vein, they can design and promote co-operative and communal living arrangements as well as opportunities for work that promote the self-sufficiency of aging.

Mental health and mental illness in late life and service utilization patterns of the elderly

Old age is usually accompanied by some deterioration in sensory and cognitive functions, but personality tends to remain relatively stable in normal aging and stable mental health is the norm in late life (Hooyman & Kiyak, 1992). This is not to diminish the public health importance of the sizeable elderly minority who have significant mental health problems and psychopathology. Mental health problems in later life are significant in frequency, in their impact on mental state, emotional state and behavior of the elderly and they have the potential to influence the course of physical illness (Cohen, 1990). Personality disorders and psychiatric symptoms may also emerge among some older persons who showed no signs of psychopathology earlier in their lives. Although such conditions are not a normal process of aging, in some individuals, the stresses of old age may compound an existing predisposition to psychopathology. These stresses may be internal, resulting from physiological and psychological processes, perhaps the onset of chronic illness, or external, relating to role losses, for example, the death of a spouse and friends. These conditions significantly impact on older people's competence, so that they become more vulnerable to environmental stress. The study of personality and adjustment, stress and coping in old age shows that the role of social support is of paramount importance in late life adaptation. Haug et al. (1989) in a 9-year study of people over 65 found that the level of social support and physical health were major determinants of the prevalence of mental illness and the work of House et al. (1988) and Antonucci & Akiyama (1991) at the Institute of Social Research in Michigan is increasingly highlighting the direct impact of social support on health and mental health status throughout the life course.

Typical client pathways and trajectories of the elderly in psychiatric services and service responses

A number of different populations among the over 65 age group tend to present to psychiatric services. These can be roughly grouped into

1. the old deinstitutionalized population currently being supported in community residential units or independent community living via case management strategies and supportive services.
2. crisis or emergency presentation cases requiring immediate assessment or action and possible hospital admission. These may be related to psychotic conditions, suicide attempts or other indicators of severe depression and the breakdown of care arrangements in relation to dementia.
3. community consultation in relation to cases of self-neglect/abuse/risk.
4. supportive casework, groupwork and program development with the long-term institutional population.

Pritchard and Brearley (1982) classify the major types of presenting situations and types of service system responses needed in relation to work with the elderly mentally ill as follows:

1. Situations where there is imminent and serious danger and urgent action is needed or requested
2. Situations where a major loss has been sustained and there is need for personal help with feelings, attitudes and emotions as in the situation of bereavement
3. Situations where the major need is for maintenance and protection and acquiring and making operative appropriate community supports.

Primary, secondary and tertiary intervention with the elderly mentally infirm

Social workers encounter the elderly mentally ill in a range of settings in both institutions and the community and are involved in intervention at primary, secondary and tertiary level. Table 33.2 sets out some of the major contexts, roles and tasks of intervention in a variety of these settings.

Social work intervention in depression and confusional states

Depressive conditions of all grades of severity are common among older people, though are often poorly recognized and diagnosed. Suicide rates increase in the fifth decade and remain high in later life, the rate for men exceeding that for women.

The intervention issues in depression relate firstly to accurate recognition and diagnosis of the causative factors in the person and in the immediate social situation and choosing the most appropriate intervention strategy of either a supportive and/or pharmacological nature. The major risks to be considered with severe depression relate to suicide and self-neglect. This may necessitate hospital admission, close social support, development of a confiding professional relationship and ongoing active treatment of the underlying depressive illness. Those living alone are more vulnerable to self-neglect in the areas of personal hygiene, nutrition, personal and financial affairs and self-care and may require close monitoring and regular supportive contact by the social worker.

Careful clinical assessment, documenting onset and differentiating out other conditions is again critical in the case of confusion as is the role played by key informants in filling out the history of onset.

Acute confusional illness is usually of short duration with a fairly abrupt onset and recovery and is usually associated with underlying physical illness. It can lead to rapid deterioration in physical health and death, disturbed paranoid behavior or major self-neglect and will usually require urgent medical intervention, hospital admission, sedation, reassurance and close supervision either at home or in a semisupported environment.

Chronic confusional illness usually has a slow insidious onset and may manifest itself in early difficulties with employment and relationships. As the confusion progresses however, the responsibility on families and carers becomes more profound and interventions need to be primarily directed at supporting the family caregiver as principal 'case manager' in the task of psychosocial management in the absence of medical cure (Berman & Rappaport, 1984).

The issues raised by chronic confusion are again self-neglect, safety and accidents in the home, the dangers of wandering and road accidents, physical illness, safety of carers and ultimately admission to long-term care. Intially the social worker focuses primarily on the confused person themselves to the degree that they have insight into the progressive cognitive losses they are sustaining. Ultimately, however, work is primarily with the carers – assisting them in their daily care tasks, eventually enabling them to detach from direct care work and make an institutional placement when deterioration is profound.

Various degrees of paranoid symptomatology are common among older people whether provoked by lifelong circumstances or current stressors. Severe delusions may be ameliorated by pharmacological intervention and a more structured 'contractual' case work relationship.

Table 33.2. *Primary, secondary and tertiary interventions with the elderly*

Target populations in an aging society	Primary service need	Level of inter-vention	Aims of intervention	Types of intervention	Roles adopted by social worker	Contexts of intervention
Well elderly in community	1. Good primary care 2. Specific protection 3. Health promotion	Primary	Prevention: to ward off and prevent problems before they occur	Information and referral Education Consultation Community Development Self-help/mutual aid Specific preventative programmes, e.g. diet, exercise, medical management, crime, accident and abuse prevention	Educator/Consultant Advocate/Broker Community Developer Group Worker Policy Planner Administrator	Local government Community health Centre General practice Community service Agencies Community advice Bureaus Adult education Centres Self Help/advocacy organizations Senior citizens' Centres Resource centres

At risk elderly presenting with acute problems/ trauma	1. Early diagnosis and prompt treatment 2. Support of functionally dependent via assistance with coping methods	Secondary	Treatment: 1. avoiding further breakdown 2. aid with development of coping methods	Functional Assessment and Diagnosis Range of therapeutic interventions with individual and resource mobilization in their environment	Diagnostician Clinician/Caseworker Enabler/Broker/Advocate Policy Planning Research Evaluation	Hospital outpatients Emergency departments Geriatric assessment teams Community police Local government Domiciliary service Guardianship Board Office of Public Advocate
Long-term care populations in institutions and community	1. Disability limitation 2. Rehabilitation 3. Maintenance and prosthetic approaches 4. self-health management of chronic conditions	Tertiary	Rehabilitation maintenance	Full range of clinical and prosthetic supports in institutional settings and community Group Work/protective practice for disabled individuals and families	Care/case manager Broker/advocate Long-term care Administration Policy/planner Program Developer/evaluator	Hospitals/nursing homes Hostels/hospices Rehabilitation Centres Psychiatric hospitals Special dementia units Home nursing service Respite programs Home care services

Service utilization and presentation patterns of the older mentally ill person

The research literature on service utilization by older persons is limited. It suggests older subjects are less likely to report the symptoms of mental illness and are generally more inhibited in expressing negative feelings. They are more likely to utilize general medical than psychiatric service and express a preference for a general practitioner in dealing with depression and dementia than a psychiatric professional (Waxman Carner & Klein, 1984; Brody & Kleban, 1981; Hooyman & Kiyak, 1991). This may be related to the older person's reluctance to interpret their problems as psychological due to the perceived social stigma of such admission (German, 1985), limited knowledge of the psychiatric conditions of late life and lack of confidence in and easy access to mental health workers. Studies show that older persons are less likely to use community health services and more likely to end up in hospital and chronic long-term care facilities (Redick & Taube, 1980; Butler & Lewis, 1982; Kahn, 1975). For instance elderly persons are less than 6% of the load of psychiatric outpatient units but take up 25% of the beds in long-term care facilities. Some studies of the ethnic aged show that they are twice as likely to enter mental hospitals, but less likely to use nursing homes. The emergency and crisis presentation of many older people to psychiatric services, particularly hospitals, suggests that early identification and primary care systems are inadequately screening presenting symptoms. The literature suggests that there is in fact an overreliance on pharmacological treatments with the elderly and an underutilization of other forms of more socially oriented treatment technologies by both the aged themselves and the professionals with whom they are in contact.

Most studies conclude that there is considerable underutilization of mental health services by the elderly compared to the general population (Gurin, Veroff & Feld, 1960). In a period when there is a major push towards community-based care, it therefore seems important to locate the barriers to effective service utilization that relate to the elderly person themselves, professional practitioners and the general service system. These factors might be grouped as follows:

Factors related to the elderly themselves

The elderly would appear to:

(a) both underreport and discount their own symptoms.
(b) prefer physical to psychiatric explanations of their condition.
(c) have more trust in general practitioners than psychiatric professionals.
(d) have limited knowledge/education about the major psychiatric conditions of late life.
(e) have limited understanding and connection with or access to the service system of geriatric psychiatry.
(f) lack any specific advocacy on their behalf to inform them of their options.

Factors related to professional practitioners

(a) There would appear to be considerable 'professional ageism' evidenced in the underservicing and discounting of presenting symptoms.
(b) This is often coupled with 'therapeutic pessimism' in relation to the efficacy and effectiveness of intervention with the aged.
(c) Most practitioners lack specific education in the psychiatry of late life.
(d) There are considerable difficulties in accurately diagnosing complex multiple conditions.
(e) There is an overreliance on pharmacological interventions over other forms of more socially oriented treatments because practitioners are unfamiliar with these other options or how to refer to them.

Factors related to the service system

(a) Lack of sufficient active outreach in the area of primary care
(b) Though the general practitioner is the most accessible primary carer, they may often be the least well informed about other community services
(c) Psychiatric services in the past have been forbidding/institutional services by and large – not community integrated and not regionally located
(d) The special needs of the aged have generally been underrepresented in psychiatric services
(e) Lack of coordination and integration between different types of services for the aged
(f) Problems of access in terms of location/architecture/transport
(g) Lack of utilization of appropriate technologies/programs that relate specifically to the needs of the elderly.
(h) Lack of outreach to special needs groups, non-English speaking and aboriginal populations, for instance.

Issues that need to be addressed in service design and delivery for older people with mental illness

From the above it is apparent that there is a need to address specifically the service needs of the elderly mentally ill via:

1. Improving early identification, diagnosis and assessment of mental illness in the elderly living in the community. This could no doubt be achieved by better education of, and liaison with, primary care providers, particularly general practitioners, local government home care departments, home nursing services, community health centres, day care providers and senior citizens' centres. This may require formal input to basic training as well as post-basic and inservice options.
2. Developing the community outreach and liaison psychiatry functions of mental health services so they are able to actively consult and advise.

3. Increasing the ability of regional services to respond appropriately and quickly to crises and emergencies via either mobile response teams or direct 24-hour consultancy.
4. Better service integration and coordination of psychiatric services with health, welfare, employment and housing agencies as well as other services specifically set up to cater for the needs of the elderly e.g. senior citizens'centres, day care services.
5. More effective case management of chronic mental illness in the community.
6. Design and implementation of new community support programs and their evaluation.
7. More active work and collaboration with families and carers of the elderly mentally ill individually and as an interest group advocating for the needs of the older mentally ill.
8. Improving the quality of care in long-term care settings by greater attention to quality assurance and standards in long-term care settings.
9. Improving the access of underserved populations amongst the mentally ill elderly (e.g. the ethnic aged/aboriginals).
10. Specific advocacy for the large group of elderly still predominantly in institutional settings.

Though some of these issues have been addressed in recent reviews and reforms of geriatric psychiatry services with the establishment of geriatric psychiatry assessment teams, specialist geriatric psychiatry units with day respite, acute, hostel and nursing home facilities, mobile emergency response teams and the availability of more decentralized and community integrated psychiatric consultation and the setting up of transcultural consulting units, the aged, compared to the general population, continue to underutilize community mental health services and overutilize hospital and long-term care facilities.

Traditional and new social work roles in psychogeriatric services

Traditional roles social workers have taken in geriatric psychiatry services have included psychosocial assessment and casework with older individuals and their families, group work both with the older person and their carers, and discharge planning and referral from acute to home care and semisupported accommodation. Social workers in community agencies have similarly acted as primary care agents in identifying and supporting older people with a psychiatric disability in the community or referring them to public psychiatric services when emergency or inpatient care was indicated. The major locations for practice have predominantly been public psychiatric institutions and general community agencies.

Emergent roles in contemporary reforms of geriatric psychiatry services have seen a shift of many social work positions from segregated hospitals to community and regionally based services where they have become members of multidisciplinary geriatric psychiatry assessment teams, ageing specialists on community mental health teams, service coordinators of new purpose-built regional geriatric psychiatry day, hostel and nursing home services and policy planners with significant input into program innovation and policy development at regional and state level.

The growing interest in case management and assertive community outreach in geriatric psychiatry is also providing challenging opportunities for social workers to utilize their casework, community development and program planning skills in new settings.

Ongoing reform of the long-term care setting in remaining psychiatric institutions and the development of new geriatric psychiatry units in general hospitals and new community facilities continues to require attention to program innovation and service development in these settings. To some degree this is facilitated by better regulation of standards and quality assurance but it also requires ongoing commitment to research, program development and evaluation by each of the professional groups involved.

Future developments in the education of social workers for practice in geriatric psychiatry services

Much greater attention is now paid to issues of aging and mental health and mental illness in the curriculum of social work education. At the University of Melbourne, students may opt to do specialist electives in their second year on either or both gerontology and/or mental health (specializing in geriatric psychiatry) and also have considerable input on mental health throughout the lifecourse in their first year. The aged and the mentally ill are considered as major target populations in casework, group work and family work seminars, and students are also introduced to several models of case management appropriate to different long-term care populations. The legal context of social work practice, particularly in relation to the Mental Health legislation, the Disability Services Act, the operation of the Guardianship and Administration processes, the Office of the Public Advocate, the Health Services complaint bodies, the Ombudsman and the Mental Health Review Board are specifically addressed. Course content on program design, development, and advocacy also address specifically the needs of the aged and those with psychiatric disability. The development of policy appropriate to an aging society is examined across a range of practice areas, including mental health. A significant number of field placements undertaken during social work training are in gerontological and/or mental health agencies.

At the postgraduate level, aging and mental health units are offered at the masters level and the School of Social Work is presently working on the establishment of a major mental health postgraduate research and practice unit which will work closely with the new major teaching mental health and general hospitals and associated services, providing training in practice research and evaluation. Such a unit will be staffed by several faculty members working jointly in the academic and clinical setting and will involve a number of both masters and PhD students undertaking postgraduate research. The development of such units is considered critical to the ongoing generation and evaluation of practice-relevant programs and research that will impact positively on better outcomes for older psychiatrically disabled clients.

References

Anthony, W. A. & Liberman, R. P. (1986). The practice of psychiatric rehabilitation: historical, conceptual and research base. *Schizophrenia Bulletin*, **12**, (4) pp. 542–59.

Antonucci T. C. & Akiyama, H. (1992). *Social Relations and Mental Health Over the Life Course*. Michigan: Institute of Social Research.

Australian Health Ministers' Conference (1992). *National Mental Health Policy*. Canberra: Australian Government Publishing Service (April).

Babigian, H. M. & Lehman, A. F. (1987). Functional psychoses in later life: epidemiological patterns from the Monroe County psychiatric register. In *Schizophrenia and Ageing*, ed. N. E. Miller & G. D. Cohen, pp. 9–21. New York: Guilford.

Berman, S. & Rappaport, M. M. (1984). Social work and Alzheimer's disease: psychosocial management in the absence of medical cure. *Social Work in Health Care*, **10**, (2) 53–70.

Blazer, D. (1980). The epidemiology of mental illness in late life. In *Handbook of Geriatric Psychiatry*, ed. E. Busse & D. Blazer. New York: Van Nostrand Reinhold.

Blazer, D. (1986). Depression. *Generations*, **10** 21–3.

Blazer, D. Hughes, D. C. & George L. K. (1987). The epidemiology of depression in an elderly community population. *The Gerontologist* **27** (3) 281–7.

Brody E. N. & Kleban M. H. (1981). Physical and mental health symptoms of older people: who do they tell? *Journal of the American Geriatrics Society* **29**, 442–9.

Brody E. M. & Kleban M. H. (1983). Day-to-day mental and physical health symptoms of older people. A report on health logs. *The Gerontologist*, **23**, 75–85.

Burdekin B. (1991). Human rights and mental illness. *Mental Health in Australia* 3 December pp. 4–10.

Burdekin B. (1990). Human rights and the mentally ill. *Mental Health in Australia* December pp. 41–5.

Butler, R. N. & Lewis, M. (1982). *Ageing and Mental Health: Positive Psychosocial Approaches*. (3rd edn). St. Louis: C. V. Mosby.

Cohen, G. D. (1990). Psychopathology and mental health in the mature and elderly adult. Chapter 22. In *Handbook of the Psychology of Ageing* Third Edition. New York: Academic Press.

Commonwealth of Australia (1986). *Disability Services Act*. Austrialian Government Publishing Service, Canberra.

Commonwealth Department of Health, Housing and Community Services (1991). *Aged Care Reform Strategy Mid-Term Review 1990–91.* September, Australian Government Publishing Service.

Commonwealth Department of Health, Housing and Community Services (1992). *Putting the Pieces Together: A National Action Plan for Dementia Care* Australian Government Publishing Service.

Commonwealth Rehabilitation Service (1991). *Vocational Rehabilitation for People with Psychiatric Disabilities* February.

Coulton, C. J. (1981). Person–environment fit as the focus in health care *Social Work*, **1**, 26–35.

Eisen, P. & Wolfenden K. (1988). *A National Mental Health Services Policy.* Report to Commonwealth, State and Territory Health Ministers, Canberra.

Evashwick C., Rowe, G., Diehr, P. & Branch, L. (1984). Factors explaining the use of health care services by the elderly. *Health Services Research*, **19**, 357–82.

Feister, A. & Neigher, W. (1979). *Client Outcome: Overview Evaluation in Practice* Bethesda MD: National Institute of Mental Health.

Germain, C. B. & Gitterman, A. (1981). Ecological perspective. *Encyclopaedia of Social Work.* National Association of Social Workers, Silver Springs Maryland, pp. 488–499.

German, P. S., Shapiro, S. & Skinner, E. A. (1985). Mental health of the elderly. *Journal of the American Geriatrics Society*, **33**, 246–52.

Goldney, R. D. & Hugo M. (1984). Factors associated with 'masked' psychological illness in the elderly. *Psychopathology* **17**, 228–32.

Gurin, G., Veroff, J. & Feld, S. (1960). *Americans View their Mental Health.* New York: Basic Books.

Gurland, B. J. & Meyers B. S. (1986). Geriatric psychiatry in *Textbook of Psychiatry* ed. J. A. Talbott, R. E. Hales & S. C. Yudofsky pp. 1117–1139 Washington DC: American Psychiatric Press.

Haug M. R., Breslau, N. & Folman, S. J. (1989). Coping resources and selective survival in mental health of the elderly. *Research on Ageing*, **11**, 468–491.

Health Department of Victoria, Office of Psychiatric Services (1988). *Psychiatric Services for Older People in Victoria.* Policy and Program Statement, May.

Health Department of Victoria, Office of Psychiatric Services (1990). *Rehabilitation Services for People with Psychosocial Disability in Victoria*, Policy and Program Statement, April.

Health Department of Victoria, Office of Psychiatric Services (1992*a*) *Clinical Practice and Service Standards for Psychiatric Inpatient Services.*

Health Department of Victoria, Office of Psychiatric Services (1992*b*) *Policy and Strategic Directions for Public Psychiatric Services in Victoria*, January.

Healy, (1992). *The Impact of Mainstreaming and Integration on Psychiatric Services.* Report of a Consultative Project, Department of Social Work, La Trobe University.

Hooyman, N. R. & Kiyak, H. (1991). Mental disorders and the use of mental health services, in *Social Gerontology: A Multidisciplinary Perspective*, 2nd edn. Chapter 10 Boston: Allyn and Bacon.

House, J. S., Landis, Karl R. & Umberson, D. (1988). Social relationships and health. *Science* **241**, 540–5.

Kahana, E. (1975). A congruence model of person–environment interaction. In *Theory Development in Environments and Ageing*, ed. M. P. Lawton. New York: Wiley.

Kahn, R. L. (1975). The mental health system and the future aged. *The Gerontologist*, **15**, 24–31.

LaRue, A. Dessonville, C. & Jarvik, L. (1985). Ageing and mental disorders. In *Handbook of the psychology of Ageing* 2nd Edition, eds J. E. Birren and K. W. Schaie, pp. 664–702. New York: Van Nostrand Reinhold.

Lawton, M. P. & Nahemow, L. (1973). Ecology and the ageing process. In *Psychology of Adult Development and Ageing*, ed. C. Eisdorfer & M. P. Lawton. American Psychological Association.

Lebowitz, B. D. (1993). Mental health and ageing: federal perspectives. *Generations Journal of the American Society on Ageing*, Winter/Spring V.XVII (1) 65–8.

McKenzie, L. (1992). The nongovernment psychiatric disabilities sector: strategies for the future. *New Paradigm* September.

Maluccio, Anthony N. ed. (1981). *Promoting Competence in Clients: A New/Old Approach to Social Work Practice.* New York: Free Press.

Mechanic D. (1991). Strategies for integrating public mental health services. *Hospital and Community Psychiatry*, **42** 797–801.

Miller, N. E. & Cohen, G. D. (1987). *Schizophrenia and Ageing*. New York: Guilford.

Monk, A. (1981). Social work with the aged: principles of practice. *Social Work* January 26, 1, 61–8.

Mortimer, J. A. (1983). Alzheimer's disease and senile dementia: Prevalence and incidence. In *Alzheimer's disease*. ed. B. Reisberg, pp. 141–148 New York: Free Press.

National Community Advisory Group on Mental Health (1992). A first ever national mental health policy. *Newsletter* No. 1 December.

National Better Health Program (1991). *The Role of Primary Health Care – Improving Australia's Health*. National Centre for Epidemiology and Population Health September.

National Health Strategy (1991). *The Australian Health Jigsaw: Integration of Health Care Delivery*. Issues Paper No. 1, July.

National Health Strategy (1993*a*). Healthy participation: achieving greater public participation and accountability in the Australian health care system, *Background Paper No. 12*, March.

National Health Strategy (1993*b*). Help where help is needed – continuity of care for people with chronic mental illness, *Issues Paper No. 5*, February.

Pritchard, S. & Brearley P. (1982). Risk and social work, Chapter 4 in *Risk and Ageing*. ed. C. P. Brearley, Routledge and Kegan Paul: London.

Redick, R. & Taube, C. (1980). Demography and mental health care of the aged. In *Handbook of Mental Health and Ageing*, eds J. E. Birren & R. B. Sloane. Englewood Cliffs NJ: Prentice Hall.

Rimmer, J. R., Buckingham, W. J. & Farhall, J. F. (1988). Achieving continuity of care in comprehensive psychiatric service systems – Victoria's approach. Paper delivered to invited symposium: The Community Emphasis in Mental Health Policy and Practice, 24th International Congress of Psychology, Sydney, August.

Robins L. N. (1984). Introduction to the ECA Project as a source of epidemiologic data on alcohol problems. In *Nature and Extent of Alcohol Problems Among the Elderly*, eds. G. Maddox, L. N. Robins & N. Rosenberg. DHHS Publication No. ADM 84–1321, pp. 201–216. Washington DC: US Government Printing Office.

Rose S. M. & Black B. L. (1985). *Advocacy and Empowerment: Mental Health Care in the Community*. London, Boston: Routledge and Kegan Paul.

Rosen, A. (1992). Community psychiatry services: will they endure? *Current Opinion in Psychiatry*, **5**, 257–65.

Roth, M. (1976). The psychiatric disorders of late life. *Psychiatric Annals*, **6**, 57–101.

Rovner, B. W., Kafonek S., Filipp L., Lucas M. J. & Folstein M. F. (1986). Prevalence of mental illness in a community nursing home. *American Journal of Psychiatry*, **143**, 1446–9.

Sadavoy, J. & Leszcz M. (eds) (1987). *Treating the Elderly with Psychotherapy: The Scope for change in Later Life*. Madison CT: International Universities Press.

Schuckit, M. A., Miller, P. L. & Berman J. (1980). The three year course of psychiatric problems in a geriatric population, *Journal of Clinical Psychiatry*, **41** 27–32.

Talbott, J. A. (1983). A special population: the elderly deinstitutionalized chronically mentally ill patient. *Psychiatric Quarterly*, **55**, 90–105.

Teeter, R. B., Garetz, F. K. Miller W. B. & Heiland, W. F. (1976). Psychiatric disturbances of aged patients in skilled nursing homes. *American Journal of Psychiatry*, **133** (12), 1430–4.

United Nations Charters (1992). *International Covenant on Civil and Political Rights. Declaration on the Rights of Disabled People. The Declaration for the Care of the Rights of the Mentally Ill.*

Victorian Mental Illness Awareness Council (1990). *Unlocking the System: Consumer Participation Strategies in Mental Health*, Melbourne.

Victorian Mental Illness Awareness Council (1992). *Declaration of Rights by and on Behalf of all People with Psychiatric Disabilities*. Melbourne.

Waxman, H. M., Carner, E. A. and Klein, M. (1984). Underutilization of mental health professionals by community elderly. *The Gerontologist*, **24**, 23–30.

Wilson, S. F. (1992). Community support and community integration: new directions for client outcome research, Chapter 18. In *Case Management and Social Work*, ed. S. Rose, pp. 245–257.

34

Music therapy

RUTH BRIGHT

Introduction

There are several definitions for music therapy; the shortest runs thus: '... the planned use of music to reach nonmusical goals'. A longer definition describes music therapy as '... the planned use of music to improve the functioning in their environment of those with social, cognitive, emotional and/or physical disadvantage.'

Both of these indicate the nature of music therapy:

* It has potential uses in a very broad range of difficulties experienced by groups or individuals.
* It is based upon planning, which entails assessment of the patient(s)' needs.
* Assessment leads to the identification of individual or group goals.
* The music therapy intervention is planned in order to reach the goals identified in the assessment.
* On-going evaluation may lead to reappraisal of the goals and the treatment approach.

Tertiary educational programmes in music therapy are planned in accordance with the various principles outlined above, and involve both theoretical knowledge and practical skills.

Although some work in private practice in the community, music therapists commonly work as members of a team in a hospital, a clinic or in special education.

Music therapy differs from recreational music in the establishing of specific non-musical goals. Thus in music therapy the music is not an end in itself but a means to an end. In recreational music there may be chance therapeutic benefits, as when a lonely individual finds friendship with members of a choir because of mutual interests, but these benefits are not the designated goal of the music activity. Music therapy, in contrast, has stated therapeutic goals for which the music is the facilitator.

In the care of the aged, the goals of music therapy include:

* catharsis of unresolved grief, e.g. over disability or bereavement; this may be a recent loss or one which has remained unresolved over many years;
* acceptance of impending death and separation;
* the management of depression or other psychiatric illness;
* establishing or reestablishing social skills;
* cognitive therapy in reorientation, reminiscence, etc;
* eye–hand coordination;
* the relearning of communication skills in aphasia;
* improvement of gait, e.g. in Parkinson's disease;
* relearning of motor skills following hemiplegia;
* reestablishing awareness of body schema;
* pain management (postoperatively, in conditions such as arthritis, or in terminal illness);
* emotional benefits such as enjoyment, decision-making and freedom of choice, the dignity of individuality.
* reestablishing of impaired human relationships with family members.

Why does music therapy 'work'?

It is known that the auditory function remains active even when other aspects of communication have been lost, so that there is substantial anecdotal evidence of people, unconscious or even apparently moribund, who have later recovered consciousness and have been able to repeat comments which were made in their hearing.

The fact that, in simplistic terms, music is represented in the non-dominant hemisphere whereas speech is mediated from the dominant hemisphere (Gates & Bradshaw, 1977), may explain the observations that dysphasic persons may be able to sing songs, which is observed in stroke patients as well as in the dysphasia of dementia.

It has been suggested that the hippocampus, which is the rehearsal centre of the brain, retains music function even in advanced dementing conditions so that people whose usual channels of communication have been lost are able nevertheless to sing melodies of musical items which were frequently rehearsed earlier in life (Tomaino, 1991). But in view of recent investigations of dysfunction in the hippocampus, including the possibility that atrophy may be a marker for Alzheimer-type dementia (Leon et al., 1989) one must assume that there is 'multi-wiring' for music, and that no one explanation can account for its undoubted sparing in dementing conditions.

Thus, because music is essentially nonverbal and because it has emotive qualities, it may 'get through' to people who are otherwise unresponsive or who are blocking emotional responses. Even if the response appears to be temporary (as in advanced Alzheimer-type dementia) we should not for this reason dismiss as valueless its contribution to the quality of life for the sufferer and family (Bright, 1992).

In what situations is music therapy useful?

In old age, it is perhaps in the management of depression that music has its strongest application. We may see depression in old age as a response to loss in those who are cognitively intact and have not previously been depressed, as a new episode in a lifetime of recurring depression, or as a complicating factor in the management of dementing processes. All of these cause distress to sufferer and family, and all need empathic management (Bright, 1986).

In pseudo-dementia depressive illness appears to masquerade as an organic brain syndrome, and appropriate therapy may help to reverse the condition (McAlister, 1983; Bulbena & Berrios, 1986).

There is evidence to support a belief that some depression following cerebrovascular accidents has a biochemical origin, and a self-limiting life history (Robinson et al., 1984), but here too music therapy is useful. We may observe psychiatric illness such as depression or a manic episode following a major bereavement, and psychosis of late onset is not uncommon. All of these difficulties will complicate an existing or incipient dementing process, with possible confusion in diagnosis and assessment.

In the practice of geriatrics, it is often impossible entirely to separate conditions into organic and functional processes, but music therapy always has something to offer irrespective of the classificatory problems.

Assessment

Assessment must be based upon preliminary information as to:

* general health
* cognitive level
* psychiatric diagnosis
* interventions already used, for how long and with what success.

Music Therapy Assessment is based upon the foregoing but also includes observations as to:

* patient's interest in music
* perception of own health, especially losses experienced
* special problems, not necessarily pathological, which may affect musical participation.

It is necessary to decide which patients may benefit from music therapy and what form the intervention should take. For those whose illness permits insight, music in therapy can provide a means of facilitating that insight, but for others its first role is to provide emotional support and empathy until such time as medication or other forms of treatment lead to greater accessibility.

The information contained in the referral is included in the assessment, although this information is not always complete. It is not uncommon to have a patient referred because she is depressed following the death of her husband only to find that the picture is far more complex than this simple statement, with, e.g. highly ambivalent feelings about the death, strong feelings of guilt, extreme feelings of anger, any or all of which complicate the situation.

The standard items for assessment include any evidence of hallucinations and delusional thinking, thought disorder etc. Even if these are already noted in the patient's clinical records, it is important to observe whether they are also apparent in the music therapy session.

One also listens, when talking to the patient about their life, for indications of nihilistic or suicidal ideation revealed by responses such as these, in reply to the therapist's comment that it was nearly lunchtime: 'Maybe but there is no point in my going – my insides have all rotted away.' 'I don't deserve to eat, I'm too wicked.' 'I'll be dead tomorrow so why bother.'

Assessment of other aspects of the person's well-being includes body language and verbal style when speaking of relationships and of the self, observations of emotional tension and rigidity, tremor other than Parkinsonian, eye-contact and general posture. These are common to all interviews with those judged to be psychiatrically ill, but must not be neglected by the music therapist. This is also true of indications of transference as the relationship progresses and a personal awareness of countertransference.

One must be aware, too, of concomitant illness which may affect the music therapy process, as well as sensory losses such as defects of sight and hearing.

Observations of patients' conversation, health and general behavior are common to all who work in psychiatry, but the music therapist needs to be equally aware of them because inner attitudes may be more clearly revealed in the music therapy session, when the guards are down, than in the formal psychiatric interview.

Assessment of music skills

The degree of musicality is of importance in the assessment, not because musical skills are necessary for music therapy to be appropriate but in order to find out musical preferences and taste. Even for a given age range there will be those whose preference is for church hymns, for operatic excerpts, for 'easy listening' items, for the classical repertoire, for brass bands, or for no music at all, and such preferences must be recognized.

One can then work from this basis when using music in communication, although one may ultimately move into improvised rather than precomposed music, to know the initial preference is of value.

Even for those who say they hate music, music therapy is not necessarily contra-indicated, because there may well be past unhappy events which have led to this statement, and to deal with these experiences may well benefit the patient. For example, an elderly man who said he hated music later revealed that he had been unable to sing in tune at school and had been made to feel stupid because of this problem, so that he grew up associating music with rejection and personal feelings of stupidity. The same man, given adequate reassurance and explanation about the physiological mechanisms of singing in tune, joined happily in the group by playing a drum to lead the rhythm, and thereby gained new self-esteem.

Strategies which may be included in a planned program of individual music therapy

1. Choice of items for listening or participation.
2. Discussion of reasons for choice.
3. Links between music and relationships, with especial reference to relationships which have been lost and which loss may have contributed to the current illness.
4. Improvised music, shared between therapist and patient. This may be: keyboard only, vocal, keyboard and vocal, or may include percussion instruments if these are acceptable to the patient.
5. Improvised music as a simple projection test – is the music played perceived as angry and threatening? Sad and lonely? Frightening and obscure?
6. Song-writing, either word-substitution in known songs or totally creative (using tape-recorder so that music can be written onto paper later).

The choice of strategies, the preference for one rather than another or for the order in which they are employed, is determined by the degree of empathy achieved as well as the possibilities for insight and therapeutic discussion.

Case histories which illustrate some specific uses of music therapy in dealing with functional psychiatric illness in the elderly

Case history 1

Mr A. seemed to demonstrate two levels of depressive response to his stroke, which had caused right-sided hemiplegia and aphasia. He had been a lifelong perfectionist, and at first rejected all attempts at rehabilitation. He was willing sometimes to try to play the electric keyboard with his left hand, following the movement of his fingers to the far right-hand end of the keyboard with head-scanning movements which helped to deal with the problems created by a homonymous hemianopia. Unfortunately, however, progress in rehabilitation was not fruitful owing to his depression, which caused him to withdraw to his room rather than stay in the rehabilitation area, to wish to be in bed and to be angry when attempts were made to persuade him to stay up and 'have a go'. Mr A. went to a nursing home because his wife was not able to care for him.

Following reassessment, Mr A. returned nine months later, for a second period of rehabilitation in the day hospital of the hospital in which he had been an in-patient. At this time it was noted that his level of depression was greatly diminished; he was still easily discouraged and displayed some depressed behaviour with loss of eye contact, slumped posture with sighs and crying when things went wrong, but he was usually willing to make some efforts.

He joined the five-member group for music and speech therapy, and enjoyed the group activities, making moderately successful attempts at communication in several modalities: verbally, by gesture, by drawing and by writing. He smiled at and made eye contact with fellow group members, laughed quite often, and was on occasion able to laugh at himself.

The work in the weekly session of one hour included using musical instruments to enhance the rhythm of speech and for auditory discrimination; mime of actions to represent words of songs; gestures and appropriate social behavior to express emotion; sketches combined with well-known songs to use the visual and auditory pathways for word recognition (bypassing, initially, attempts at verbal communication). Sessions also included singing, movement, laughter, and encouragement of physical contact between group members.

This program thus combined therapy designed to reach speech therapy goals with work to reach music therapy goals, i.e. improving general communication and self-esteem, thereby diminishing the social isolation and lowered self-image which is such a common feature of the aphasic person's existence. Videos taken over six weeks, rated for target behaviors by independent observers, revealed significant improvement in all members, including Mr A.

Case history 2

Mrs B. was a 65 year old widow admitted for rehabilitation to an alcohol-related brain damage unit in a psychiatric hospital. Her case illustrates the fact that some depressive illness which comes to attention in the latter part of life has its origins in middle age or in early adult life and also shows that there is hope for change even when the person has reached the later stages of living.

The referral for music therapy described how Mrs B's hazardous intake of alcohol had started after the death of her husband in a motor vehicle accident which she had witnessed some 19 years earlier. Information from the family confirmed her own statements that before the death of her husband she had drunk alcohol only on rare occasions. It was assumed that the use of alcohol had been an attempt at self-medication for depression because she had been unable to resolve her sadness over her husband's death.

The initial assessment in music therapy revealed a very anxious lady, who had preserved a relatively youthful appearance despite her alcohol intake. Neuropsychological testing in the Regional Brain Damage Unit showed some memory loss but frontal lobe skills of insight and planning were relatively intact, so that a music therapy approach was planned emphasising insight and the possibility of change.

The story revealed to the therapist differed significantly from the assumptions by her family and by the referring staff in that her predominant feeling about her husband's death was not (as had been assumed) simple sadness but extreme and burning anger with him for not having had the car repaired when she asked him to do so, which failure had led to his death.

Music was played which she associated with him, and the picture of the relationship which emerged was that of an unloving marriage between two people whose childhoods had lacked role models for warmth or affection; one partner had been brought up in an institution, the other by strict 'cold' grandparents in conditions of extreme poverty.

Mrs B. was reassured that it is all right to be angry with someone who is dead, and that her anger over the needlessness of her husband's death was a normal reaction. Discordant music was improvised by therapist and patient to suggest feelings of rage, and changes were then made in the affect of the music to suggest regaining of control, so that Mrs B. did not retain a concept of anger as something to fear.

Sketches were drawn for her to take from the session; these showed

(a) Her being weighed down by a burden on her back, which she identified as containing anger and guilt. The anger was with her husband for dying in that way and with herself for having damaged herself by drinking. The guilt was over the coldness of the marriage and her drinking. It was strongly suggested that a way would be found to cut her loose from those burdens and a pair of scissors was drawn next to the sketch.
(b) A second sketch was drawn showing her no longer burdened but standing straight, with the load on the ground behind her.

Simple sketches are useful in providing continuity from one session to the next, giving a visual reminder of what has been achieved. The concrete imagery is especially useful for persons with alcohol-related brain damage who may have lost part of their capacity for abstract thought (Walsh, 1978).

As she left the session, Mrs B was told that even this preliminary conversation might help her to feel better about herself, and this was confirmed in the second session, when she described great feelings of relief from having spoken openly for the first time of the real reasons why she had begun to drink after her husband's death, and the comfort of being reassured that she had not been wicked to feel angry.

The Gestalt technique of the empty chair was used, preceded by improvised music to express feelings of anger and stress, which gave the patient permission to shout and rage at her dead husband for having been (as she saw it) too mean to spend money on getting the car repaired and anger for his therefore having left her to bring up the teenage children alone.

Mrs B. was too apprehensive to take on her husband's role in this empty chair approach, but instead began to speak of her own responsibility in the coldness of the marriage, gradually coming to see in the course of the hour-long interaction that she had been in part responsible for the lack of closeness in the relationship. She also volunteered the idea that perhaps it was the extreme poverty of his upbringing which had made it a frightening prospect for her husband even to consider paying for car repairs.

It was concluded from these discussions that Mrs B. was ready to forgive her husband as well as forgive herself for her anger and her drinking, and arrangements were made to take her the next week to the cemetery for a symbolic session of forgiveness and separation. (She had only once visited the crematorium, for an extremely formal family visit, devoid for herself of any personal emotion.)

The visit proved cathartic; Mrs B. spent over an hour crying at the wall where the ashes were interred, speaking directly to her husband, asking his forgiveness, giving him her forgiveness, and praying that he might know of this.

Mrs B's self-assessment revealed a marked improvement in her mood, her choice of music changed to reflect greater optimism even though in the first week immediately following the grave visit she cried frequently. It was necessary for staff to reassure family members that Mrs B. was doing the grief work which had been blocked for 19 years, that she was in fact 'better' and not 'worse'!

Follow-up has shown that Mrs B. is living competently in sheltered accommodation, with occasional times of self-doubt and anxiety, but with no return of her feelings of anger and no return to using alcohol.

Case history 3

Mrs C., a widow in her early 70s, was a day-hospital patient attending physiotherapy for a painful left arm and shoulder. When, at Case Conference, it was found that her daughter had only recently died, and the physiotherapist suggested that her pain might have a psychosomatic component, she was referred for music therapy in the hope that she might deal with her apparently blocked grief.

Assessment revealed an anxious lady, who spoke first in somewhat unemotional tones of her daughter's death. Such quasi-objectivity is often linked with the hiding of what are perceived as discreditable feelings and thoughts about a death, and permission is needed for such responses to be ventilated. This is achieved by a two-fold approach:

(a) The first step is to play music which is associated with the person and/or the relationship; this counteracts intellectualization when emotional responses have been denied, and restores the 'gut feeling' about the true nature of the relationship. (In the rare instance of a person who has no such associations, a song such as the theme from the film 'The Way We Were' has proved helpful, since it speaks of remembering the things we want to remember, forgetting the things we want to forget and asks whether we can ever go back and relive the past.) For Mrs C. there was a useful piece of associative music, connected with her daughter's first name, and this song elicited tears.

(b) The next stage is to offer open-ended comments (rather than direct questions) which leave the patient free to agree, disagree or ignore the opening which is offered. e.g. 'When we look back on a relationship, we remember many different feelings, don't we, and sometimes these are quite difficult to talk about ...'

Mrs C. accepted the offered opportunity and spoke very angrily of her daughter's death. She described a shopping expedition a week before her daughter's death which Mrs C. had found tiring and irritating because she had been left holding heavy parcels whilst her daughter tried on one dress after another. So, when her daughter invited her to come out the next week, she had flatly refused; her daughter had gone alone and had died of a heart attack.

Mrs C. was angry and hurt because she found that the daughter already knew of the cardiac problem but had not told her mother; she also felt guilty, believing that if she had gone on the shopping expedition to carry parcels her daughter would not have died. Mrs C. said angrily 'If only she had told me, of course I would have gone with her!'

After some reflective conversation, in which Mrs C's feelings were acknowledged and accepted as valid, music associated with the daughter's babyhood was played and discussion followed about how much easier it seems to be for a mother when children are infants and parents can protect them from harm, but that we want children to become independent, even though it can be hurtful at times. The session was then brought to a close, and an informal contract was established for a total of six sessions.

In this and subsequent interactions, several significant facts were revealed:

1. As the result of her guilty feelings, Mrs C. had moved into her daughter's house, sat in her daughter's seat at the top of the dinner table and cooked from her recipe book.
2. She had found conflict in trying to change her teenage grand-daughter's style of dress and behavior, expressing disapproval of the girl's friends. This suggested that there had been substantial conflict with the girl's mother about parenting methods, and this belief was supported by Mrs C's account of her son-in-law's antagonism to her presence in the home. This reinforced the view that the conflict and anger with her daughter was not confined to the circumstances surrounding the death.

3. Mrs C. had given up her ordinary friendships and no longer attended outings with her women friends to play lawn bowls, go to the cinema and go out to lunch. It seemed that Mrs C. was somewhat resentful about this separation from her normal social activities, blaming her daughter for it, but continued trying to take the place of her daughter in order to expiate her guilt over her death.

Mrs C. was again reassured that it was acceptable to feel angry with her daughter, understandable that she had felt hurt in not being told of the cardiac problems. She came to realize that she need not feel compelled to take over the role of her daughter in the family, and that her daughter's upbringing of the grand-daughter was probably little different from that of the girl's peers at school.

This brought up feelings of fear about changes perceived in the world today, a sense of helplessness in society's altered attitudes on social and family behavior, and it became clear that her daughter's death (although the most important) was only one of many sources of disquiet.

Gradually, over the weekly sessions, involving familar and improvised music with counselling, Mrs C. was helped to regain her self-esteem, work through her feelings of guilt, hurt and anger about her daughter, and on the fifth session she arrived to describe how she had moved out of her daughter's house, was once more playing lawn bowls and had made arrangements to return to her previous patterns of social outings with her women friends. She still had times of sadness over her daughter's death, but no longer experienced disabling guilt and anger.

Because of this change and because of Mrs C.'s own need for decision-making, it was decided that she could be regarded as having 'graduated' a week earlier than had been planned, and the sixth and final session of the original contract did not take place. This was highly pleasing to her and separation was achieved satisfactorily.

The pain in her shoulder was no longer a problem and discussion with the physiotherapist revealed that it had diminished progressively as Mrs C. achieved catharsis of her painful emotions associated with her daughter's sudden death. The fact that the pain had been in her left shoulder, i.e. the arm which had carried the parcels one week and had not carried them the week her daughter went shopping alone (and also probably the arm on which she had carried her daughter when the daughter was a baby) was considered to be significant by the staff of the Day Hospital, and discharge from both physiotherapy and music therapy was completed.

Case history 4

Mr D. was in his late 70s when he was admitted to a psychogeriatric unit suffering from a manic illness, apparently as a consequence of the death of his wife whilst he was out of the house. He showed flight of ideas with some grandiosity (delusions as to the books he was going to have published and their effects upon the world), pressure of words, and irritability with suspected suicidal ideation.

Although (because of Mr D.'s transfer to another unit) the music therapy intervention was limited to two sessions, he showed good response to the effects of familiar music and was able to understand to some extent that his feelings of tension were probably the result of his guilty feelings that his wife had died whilst he had been out shopping. He was able to talk about this calmly, in marked contrast to the agitation observed in most other situations.

Some two years later Mr D. was admitted with a similar manic episode following the death of his grand-daughter when a drunken driver's car mounted the footpath and she was killed. He found this an even more difficult loss to resolve and his anger was the more readily expressed. The music he had sung to the child was eventually used, after trust had been re-established, in order to facilitate some measure of grief-work, since he expressed some bewilderment that all he had felt about the death was anger. Medication, group work and continued individual music therapy over approximately one month combined to give him some measure of relief.

Psychosis in the elderly

From time to time music therapy techniques have been used for persons suffering from late-onset psychosis as well as for those with long-established psychotic illness. Observations support a view that although music therapy cannot effect major changes in delusional beliefs or hallucinations, we are able to provide patients with at least temporary relief from their distress. The details of past experiences which are ventilated as a consequence of the music therapy session are frequently useful for other clinicians in providing background information and personal history.

Music which is familiar and which has happy associations from the past produces a calming effect, probably by distraction and by providing a stronger stimulus than at least some of the intrusive thoughts, ruminations and beliefs.

In music therapy for psychosis in elderly people we are working with the person's wellbeing rather than their illness, and although this may be classified as palliative rather than curative, the sense of peace and individuality which many patients have obtained has been significant.

Musical content in music therapy: the skills of the therapist

The choice of music for the type of work discussed here will depend on circumstances; hearing significant music and discussing relationships will be best for one patient; others, suffering mainly from social isolation, may benefit from group activities such as singing. Some enjoy creativity through playing instruments but others see this as childish; possible apraxia in those with brain damage will render impossible the planned movements needed to play instruments (Geschwind, 1985). Whatever musical material or method is used, the primary focus is upon the patient's need and the therapist is constantly developing new skills in order to meet those needs.

Familiar and significant music

The music therapist needs to have an extensive repertoire of music which can be played on request immediately, rather than having to say 'I'll try to get it for you for next week.' This is not always possible but remains the ideal.

A patient suffering from agitated depression with hyperventilation (who was referred for music therapy because it was believed by her psychiatrist that she was broken-hearted over the recent death of her husband) was asked what music they had danced to during their courtship. She said they had danced to the waltz of the 1930s, 'Fascination', but when this was played on a portable keyboard her facial expression suggested that she had very mixed emotional responses to hearing this.

The therapist therefore said 'Things must be very different for you now that your husband is dead.' Such open-ended comment allows the patient freedom to acknowledge a painful relationship if indeed it was a difficult bond, but does not prevent the person speaking of happy times if the relationship was in fact one of uniform happiness.

What emerged initially was anger, that the dead man had sung this song during their courtship and had promised a happy relationship. He had, however, been a secret drinker who physically abused her, but she had never allowed the neighbors to know that this was happening. Thus when he died, would-be sympathizers had said 'You must miss him!', thereby locking the widow into a false position of grief when relief was actually her predominating emotion.

Hearing again the music, which reminded her of the anger and disappointment she had felt, allowed her to bring to the surface the long-hidden feelings, and this in turn allowed the music therapist to provide what was necessary in reassurance and permission.

When someone asks for an item which is totally unkown to the therapist, it is important to acknowledge that one cannot play it, and if the therapist has a feeling of incompetence about this, it can be extraordinarily encouraging to the patient to know that someone else can experience a sense of failure! The next step may be to ask whether the person can sing the tune (this is not uncommon and to tape this singing then permits one to learn the music before the next session as well as giving the patient a sense of satisfaction) or, if this is impossible, to talk about why the piece is important to the patient, the circumstance of life in which that importance was acquired, what the words of a song mean to him or her.

It is often possible to play a related item which has the same theme, or to improvise a melody which conjures up the same mood, so that the discussion has the benefit of the nonverbal means of communication.

It must be noted that perception of mood in music is culturally determined, so that, although people who share the same cultural background may perceive the same emotional content in any given piece of music, ethnic origin (with all that this implies in terms of musical structure, tonal system, etc) has strong influences upon one's perception of the mood of any item of music (Bright, 1993*b*).

Improvisation by the therapist, sometimes joined by the patient, will be helpful for some patients to express emotions, although the use of percussion instruments is deemed by many adult Australians to be childish and humiliating!

In this there appears to be a difference between Australia and Europe, where (according to anecdotal reports by European music therapists) percussion work is well received by elderly patients, especially by those with mild cognitive impairment. Nevertheless, once a trusting relationshp has been established, some people do enjoy playing adult-type instruments such as large Bongo drums, sets of chime bars, and have participated with benefit in group improvisation on a theme such as 'change and adaptation'. This has been used to good effect with persons suffering from mild depressive reactions to acquired disability.

Ideas of sadness, loss, anger, frustration and peace all lend themselves to improvised music, and this, usually for individual patients, leads comfortably into relaxation work, although with no changed state of consciousness. For example one might start with a visualization thus:

> While you listen to this, imagine that you are a bird floating high on a thermal, looking down at a quiet stretch of beach; people are down there and you watch them.

This is evocative of insight as well as calm, and people often describe seeing themselves on the beach and discuss quite objectively their feelings about their situation, in a way which ordinary question and answer interchanges do not promote.

Ideas of a constructive nature can then be inserted into the words which accompany the music, helping people to cope with particular feelings of anger, loss, despair and confusion over what is happening to them or about a specific life event.

Such relaxation techniques which involve listening to music with visual imagery will be more effective for some people than for others, and assessment does not always reveal the advisability or otherwise of such work. It is therefore important to try out such a technique in a preliminary way before deciding whether or not it is appropriate. It seems likely that it would be contra-indicated for patients with hallucinations or systemized delusional beliefs, since the visualizations are too easily incorporated into those hallucinations or delusional thinking.

As mentioned above under 'strategies', song writing can be helpful for ventilating feelings, and many achieve this by word substitution in known songs. Whatever musical material or method is used, the primary focus is upon the patient's needs (Bright, 1991).

Summary

The case histories which have been given support the view that music therapy has much to offer in the management of functional psychiatric illness in the elderly.

Assessment in music therapy usually supports assessment made by others, but may sometimes reveal a different, lower level of impairment by demonstrating that a patient is capable of more change than had otherwise been deemed possible.

The music therapist is able to offer most for the elderly patient when working in a clinical milieu in which observations can be shared, leading to better assessment of the patient's disabilities and assets, with all that this implies for present treatment and future management.

References

Bright, R. (1986). *Grieving: A Handbook for Those Who Care*. St Louis: MMB Inc.

Bright, R. (1991). *Music in Geriatric Care: a Second Look*. Wahroonga: Music Therapy Enterprises.

Bright, R. (1992). Music therapy. In *Caregiving in Dementia*, B. Miesen & G. Jones (eds.). London: Routledge.

Bright, R. (1993). Cultural aspects of music in therapy. In *Music Therapy in Health and Education*. M. Heal & T. Wigram (eds). London: Jessica Kingsley.

Bulbena, A. & Berrios, G. E. (1986). Pseudodementia: facts and figures. *British Journal of Psychiatry*, **148**, 87–94.

Gates, A. & Bradshaw, J. L. (1977). The role of the cerebral hemispheres in music. *Brain and Language*, **4**, 403–31.

Geschwind, N. (1985). Apraxia. In *Handbook of Clinical Neurology*, P. J. Vincken & G. W. Bruyn (eds.), pp. 423–32. Amsterdam: Elsevier.

Leong, M. J. de, George, A. E., Stylopoulos, L. A., Smith, G. & Miller, D. C. (1989). Early marker for Alzheimer's disease; the atrophic hippocampus. *Lancet*, **ii**, 672–3.

McAlister, T. W. (1983). Pseudodementia: an overview. *American Journal of Psychiatry*, **140**, 528–33.

Robinson, R. G., Starr, L. B., Lipsey, J. R. et al. (1984). A two-year longitudinal study of poststroke mood disorders. *Journal of Nervous and Mental Disorders*, **173**, 221–6.

Tomaino, C. (1991). The use of music therapy in the treatment of patients with neurological disorders. *Proceedings of Canadian Association of Music Therapy*. (In press)

Walsh, K. W. (1978). *Neuropsychology – a Clinical Approach*, pp. 110–152. London: Churchill-Livingstone.

35

The role of the physiotherapist in management of functional psychiatric disorders

KAREN WEBSTER   JOAN McMEEKEN

Introduction

The physiotherapist has a range of responsibilities in functional psychiatric disorders. In addition to treating the physical conditions encountered in an aging population and those more specific to this group of patients, the physiotherapist is responsible for the education of patients, their family, carers and fellow staff members. As a member of the multidisciplinary team, the physiotherapist contributes a sophisticated understanding of normal and abnormal movement and the means of therapeutic intervention for movement problems to the treatment program.

Role of the physiotherapist

In the management of all psychiatric disorders a mature approach is required to assist patients with lack of motivation, cognitive problems and a variety of functional deficits. Physiotherapists undertaking the management of patients with functional psychiatric disorders should possess comprehensive knowledge and skills in cardiothoracic, neurological and musculoskeletal physiotherapy and in techniques of behavioral management. They must understand the normal psychophysiology of aging and the effects of superimposed pathology.

Patients are seen in the context of all the factors impinging on their lives and all health professionals should be aware of the integration between mind and body. Moon (1988) argues that the increasing knowledge in mental health should be absorbed into physiotherapy so that 'all treatment approaches acknowledge the intrinsic unity between the mind and the body'. This is supported by Katona (1991) who reports that depression is found more often in the elderly with poor physical health than in the physically healthy. Therefore, it is essential that nonphysiotherapists acknowledge the importance of the body in contributing to the management of disorders of the mind. Improvements in both physical capacity and social behavior have been demonstrated in a controlled study of physiotherapy management of long-term psychiatric patients (McEwan, 1983).

The role of physiotherapy in psychiatry is addressed by a number of authors (Crews, 1990; Fookes, 1980; Sen & Hustwayte, 1989; Hare, 1985, 1986; Evans, 1980; Ward, 1980). Although physiotherapy is addressed in the context of different aspects of psychiatry, the authors emphasize the importance of gaining and maintaining maximum functional independence, contributing to the total health of the individuals by active participation in the health care team and providing education and support to families, care givers and the community. There is limited information on physiotherapy in functional psychiatric conditions in the elderly, such as depression, bipolar disorder, paranoid states, and personality disorders. This situation reflects Moon's (1988) 'body/mind split' model of health care in which physiotherapists have worked mainly in general hospitals. Although physiotherapists have been involved with psychiatric services for many decades (May, 1954), it is only in recent times that physiotherapy has been recognized as an important component of the multidisciplinary team approach in geriatric psychiatry, and the psychological benefits of physical activity on the institutionalized geriatric psychiatry patient established by controlled clinical trials (Powell, 1974).

The physiotherapist working with functional psychiatric illness in the elderly will fulfil several roles: as a specialist physiotherapist, as a member of the multidisciplinary team and as an adviser and educator.

Specialist role

The specialist role of the physiotherapist comprises the following elements:

* Neuromusculoskeletal assessment of patients' suitability for specific physical activity programs.
* Assessment, diagnosis and management of individual patients with a variety of physical conditions.
* Development of programs to improve, maintain or slow the deterioration of the patient's present functional level; their general and specific mobility and strength; and prevent or minimize postural deformities.
* Provision of specialized equipment necessary for patient's function and care.
* Education of family, carers and other members of the community in the physiotherapy management of elderly people with functional psychiatric disorders.
* Promotion of the treatment elements of physiotherapy to the multidisciplinary team for the management of specific functional psychiatric disorders.
* Education of health professionals in the recognition of these disorders in the elderly living within the community.

With aging there is the advent of increased physical problems and this is evident in the population who suffer from psychiatric conditions. The physiotherapist will be responsible for the assessment and treatment of patients with both the wide variety of physical conditions found within the general community and the added complications of the functional psychiatric disorders. Those conditions frequently coexisting with the psychiatric condition include:

* Neurological conditions such as stroke, Parkinson's disease.
* Musculoskeletal conditions such as rheumatoid or osteoarthritic joints, soft tissue injuries or disorders, painful neck or back, and fractures especially of the neck or femur.
* Cardiothoracic conditions, myocardial infarction, ischaemic heart disease, acute bronchitis or pneumonia, chronic obstructive airways disease.
* Circulatory conditions such as venous insufficiency, oedema, ulcers, pressure sores and amputation.
* Other conditions such as stress incontinence.

Although these problems have not caused the psychiatric condition they make life more complicated for both the patient and carers and if these physical conditions can be alleviated or improved the patient may improve mentally. There may be a depression secondary to a severe physical disability such as the late stages of a progressive neurological disorder or a dense hemiplegia after a cerebral vascular accident. In managing patients with these multiple problems the physiotherapist must be aware that their grieving process may need to be considered.

A further group of clinical problems may be directly or indirectly caused by the psychiatric condition. These include:

* The results of self-inflicted injuries in depressed patients such as nerve and tendon injury and nerve palsies from pressure on peripheral nerves due to a prolonged period of immobility in one position after a drug overdose.
* Physical weakness, loss of function, mobility and postural problems resulting from depression or delusional ideation of psychotic patients. Many depressed patients have poor posture illustrating their sad, disillusioned state. Those suffering from chronic schizophrenia may also have adopted bizarre postures. Postures may become habitual and lead to contractures, joint stiffness and muscle weakness with biomechanical inefficiency and pain. Postural assessment may reveal both short- and long term defects and with suitable treatment pain and dysfunction may be prevented or alleviated.
* Side-effects of neuroleptic drugs may cause balance and gait problems in extrapyramidal symptoms or dystonias (see Chapter 25).

The physiotherapist will also manage those conditions that arise as a secondary complication of the psychiatric condition, such as lack of physical fitness and loss of confidence in the ability to undertake normal daily activities.

Generalist role

The physiotherapist is responsible for the design and supervision of group programs of relaxation and appropriate exercise to improve general well-being, cardiovascular fitness, strength and mobility, activities of daily living and to promote socialization and independent functioning.

Members of the multidisciplinary team should participate in fulfilling the aims of programs such that there is some blending or overlap of professional roles. If this is successful then the members of the team will complement each other; for as reported by Fookes (1980), 'Each member must be aware of when he is working at the centre of his professional role, and when at the periphery. At the periphery of his own role he is close to the periphery of someone else's.'

The physiotherapist provides either group or individual programs using physical treatments to achieve psychiatric benefits (Evans, 1980). Such physical treatments include relaxation for individual patients suffering from anxiety neurosis or agitated states, or as a group activity for the inpatient unit. The goal of relaxation is to teach control of muscular tension. For many patients this is a new skill which must be learnt. Physiotherapists choose a method of relaxation most suitable for the individual patient or group which may incorporate ideas from progressive muscular relaxation, autogenic training, physiological relaxation or electromyographic feedback. The techniques evolved are adapted to the needs of each patient and may change with each group.

It is well established that exercise is beneficial for maintaining the function of body systems of the aging population (Walker, 1986; Shephard, 1985) as well as providing psychological rewards (Eide, 1982). The physiotherapist has a unique compendium of detailed knowledge of applied anatomy and kinesiology, biomechanics, normal and abnormal physiology and the pathology of trauma, illness and disease. Behavioral management strategies are employed to encourage cooperative participation in appropriate activities to maximize performance without leading to further pathology. It is essential that participation in exercise programs is encouraged in geriatric psychiatry units and this can be achieved by the physiotherapist in group or individual programs. The physiotherapist involved in these activities will frequently detect physical conditions, such as loss of range of shoulder joints, postural problems, or decreased exercise tolerance, which have been missed in earlier assessment.

An apathetic and unresponsive group may be motivated by the provision of pleasurable activities such as croquet, bowls or putting. The aims of these activities are similar to the aims of exercise programs for they improve flexibility of joints, soft tissue mobility and muscle strength as well as increasing motivation, improving self-esteem and encouraging socialization. Pleasurable activities removed from the context of 'treatment' are nonthreatening and have the potential for increased participation. If a patient has participated in these activities before admission, it may rekindle the individual's interest. The physiotherapist should endeavour to contact community facilities for resumption of the activity when the patient is discharged.

Dance and movement with music will often give patients who are unable to express their emotions verbally an opportunity to do so through another medium, namely movement. Music can be used to elicit different types of movement responses while giving the group an opportunity for more creative self-expression. Music may also be used for the relief of pain (Melzack & Wall, 1988).

Advisory and educational role

The advisory and educational role encompasses:

* promotion of health and provision of education on matters relating to health for patients, families and carers.
* teaching techniques of physical management, such as lifting and manual handling to family members, carers and staff.
* advising on specialized equipment necessary for patient care.
* community education to groups such as to elderly citizens' clubs.

This role involves advice and education of patients, carers and other members of the multidisciplinary team. For patients this will take the form of promotion of health education covering such topics as maintaining a healthy lifestyle, the benefits of exercise, maintaining good posture, osteoporosis, coping with chronic physical conditions, prevention of falls, and incontinence prevention and management. Patients who will be discharged back to their home in the community or to supported accommodation can participate in health education programs during their admission period.

With the discharge of a patient with a physical disability, advice must be provided to the carer on the physical needs of the patient and the relationship this has to ongoing mental health. Specific continuing treatment needs must be addressed either by referral to relevant health professionals or by specific education of the carer. Items of equipment, such as walking aids, orthotics, seating, and footwear which are required to maintain the patient's independence must be obtained and provision made for ongoing review and maintenance. To ensure safety in the home, matters such as the wearing of appropriate footwear rather than soft slippers often needs to be reinforced. The importance of self-care, appropriate dressing and planned activities for the day, in order to maintain self-esteem and health is addressed. It is important to ensure that carers are able to handle and transfer the patient safely and with minimal energy costs to themselves.

Education and training in suitable techniques to prevent injury to the carer, who may also be elderly, is essential.

Education of other health care staff in lifting and manual handling techniques has long been an accepted role of the physiotherapist in a hospital setting. The disciplines of medicine and nursing rarely incorporate these skills into undergraduate training programs and it is a requirement that all staff are proficient in manual handling in a safe manner. In the psychiatric hospital staff require instruction in procedures for the continuing management of the patient, such as postural drainage in chest infections, splinting and positioning for prevention of contractures and passive movements for immobilized patients.

Physiotherapists contributing to the multidisciplinary team in geriatric psychiatry must have had a thorough postgraduate generalized training in physical conditions as well as a comprehensive knowledge of the psychiatric conditions encountered in functional psychiatric disorders. Knowledge of the psychiatric management of these conditions, the medication used in treatment, its side-effects and how these may impinge on the physiotherapy treatment program is required. The physiotherapist must be able to set realistic goals with patients, carers and team members. Because the physiotherapist is working with a patient with dual disability, physical as well as psychiatric, the expectations of the outcome of treatment may have to change. Consequently more physiotherapeutic sessions will usually be necessary as treatment programs can seldom be carried out without supervision. The physiotherapist must be particularly competent in assessment skills as it is frequently difficult to gain accurate information from the patient about the symptoms or condition. Aggressive behavior may be displayed by the patient suffering from a paranoid state, or the patient may misinterpret what a physiotherapist is doing when carrying out a technique such as chest percussion. Therefore the physiotherapist must be tolerant to all types of behaviors and have time to sit, talk and listen sympathetically in order to gain the patient's confidence and cooperation.

The physiotherapist must have a knowledge of group dynamics and sound interpersonal communication skills. In the group situation it is important to be able to cope with a patient in the hypomanic stages of a bipolar disorder or encourage some responses from a severely withdrawn patient. As a group leader the physiotherapist must be aware when delusional material is being introduced into a group discussion and take appropriate measures to ensure the focus of the group is being maintained. An understanding of the skills and boundaries of the other members of the multidisciplinary team will enable the physiotherapeutic programs to be undertaken within the context of the total care program provided by the team.

In order to provide a high-quality physiotherapy service to geriatric psychiatry patients appropriate physiotherapy education at undergraduate and postgraduate levels and within health and community services is required. Education must develop an understanding of the etiology and management of psychiatric disorders and incorporate psychiatric topics in all relevant subjects and areas of clinical practice. Physiotherapy academics and clinicians working in areas of psychiatric practice should be involved in teaching to ensure that physiotherapists on graduation will have appropriate theoretical knowledge, practical skills and professional attitudes to manage the patients suffering from psychiatric problems. The increasing proportion of older people in the community and the integration of psychiatric and general hospitals will increase the likelihood of all physiotherapists managing geriatric psychiatry patients. After graduation, specific continuing education programs for physiotherapists and course work multidisciplinary studies, combined with discipline specific research, is required to provide an ongoing research base to identify appropriate therapeutic intervention and to disseminate information to physiotherapists and their clinical colleagues (Mead, 1985).

A more effective physiotherapy service is desirable in most psychiatric hospitals and for those people whose psychiatric health-care needs are integrated into community and health care facilities. To ensure this service, a clear career structure should enable new graduates to perceive adequate promotional pathways in which experienced physiotherapy staff provide opportunities for the further development of knowledge and skills. Physiotherapy involvement in community services for the mentally ill and especially in geriatric psychiatry is rare, despite the ability of physiotherapists to encompass the psychosocial and physiotherapeutic needs of people with psychiatric disorders and to encompass the accepted frames of reference for patient management (Filer, 1988; French, 1992). Furthermore, guidelines for good practice are available to enable the development of quality assurance tools to evaluate physiotherapy practice in geriatric psychiatry and to determine the outcome of management (Dunn, Johnstone & Kelly, 1991).

Physiotherapists have not always been supportive of their own colleagues working professionally in psychiatry. Any perceived stigma associated with physiotherapy professionals working in these areas must be addressed and the profession must accept and support geriatric psychiatry as an appropriate occupational environment (Fookes, 1980; Moon, 1988). The lack of sufficient physiotherapists over many years to fill available positions in all areas of psychiatry has also strongly mitigated against provision of an optimal or even adequate service (Parker, 1964; McMeeken, 1992). Integration of psychiatric patients into mainstream health care is unlikely to redress this situation without adequate resourcing. The acknowledged growth requirement for physiotherapists within all parts of the community (Melvin, 1988; DEET, 1990; DEET, 1991) will also reduce the likelihood of enhanced physiotherapy management of the geriatric psychiatric patient unless this is specifically addressed.

Conclusion

The physiotherapist undertakes a specialist role in the assessment, diagnosis and management of physical problems in the geriatric psychiatry patient and in the education of others involved in the patient's care. The particular physiotherapy expertise is invaluable when neurological, musculoskeletal, cardiothoracic or circulatory conditions coexist with the psychiatric disorder or there are secondary physical complications as a result of the disorder. As a member of the multidisciplinary team managing the patient, the physiotherapist takes a leadership role in designing the physical components of group activities and participates in a complementary manner with other group or discipline programs. Education of undergraduate and postgraduate students, other health professionals, patients' families, carers and members of the community is a significant professional activity required to provide an optimal service to geriatric psychiatry patients.

References

Crews, B. (1990). A physiotherapist's contribution to the formation of an acute mental health team. *Physiotherapy*, **76**, 296–8.

Department of Employment, Education and Training (1990). *Physiotherapy in New South Wales. A labour market report, prepared by Occupational Research and Information Section of the Department of Employment, Education and Training*. Canberra: Australian Government Publishing Service.

Department of Employment, Education and Training. (1991). *Australia's Workforce in the Year 2001, prepared by the Economic and Policy Analysis Division of the Department of Employment, Education and Training*. Canberra: Australian Government Publishing Service.

Dunn, C., Johnstone, J. & Kelly, M. (1991). *Guidelines for Good Practice for Physiotherapists in Mental Health Services*. London: Association of Chartered Physiotherapists in Psychiatry.

Eide, R. (1982). The relationship between body image, self-image and physical activity. *Scandinavian Journal Sociological Medicine Supplement*, **29**, 109–12.

Evans, D. I. (1980). The role of the physiotherapist in a psychiatric hospital. *Physiotherapy*, **66**, 398–400.

Filer, A. J. (1988). The role of the physiotherapist in the psychiatric team. *Fisioterapei*, **44**, 42–4.

Fookes, B. H. (1980). The physiotherapist in geriatric psychiatry. *Physiotherapy*, **66**, 405–7.

French, S. (1992). *Physiotherapy: A Psychosocial Approach*. Oxford: Butterworth Heinemann.

Hare, M. (1986). *Physiotherapy in Psychiatry*. London: Heinemann.

Hare, M. (1985). The physical problems of depressive illness. *Physiotherapy*, **71**, 258–61.

Katona, C. L. E. (1991). Depression in old age. *Reviews in Clinical Gerontology*, **1**, 371–84.

May, F. (1954). The changing face of physical medicine. *Australian Journal of Physiotherapy*, **1**, 6–10.

McEwan, B. (1983). An evaluation of the need to the long-stay psychiatric patient for organized exercise. *Australian Journal of Physiotherapy*, **29**, 202–8.

McMeeken, J. M. (1992). Physiotherapy – movement for life. Dean's Lecturer Series, Faculty of Medicine, Dentistry and Health Sciences, The University of Melbourne.

Mead, P. (1985). The advisory role of the physiotherapist in mental illness. *Physiotherapy*, **71**, 261–2.

Melvin, J. L. (1988). Rehabilitation in the year 2000. *American Journals Physical Medicine and Rehabilitation*, **67**, 197–201.

Melzack, R. & Wall, P. (1988). *The Challenge of Pain*. Harmondsworth: Penguin Books.

Moon, M. I. (1988). Body, mind and soul; a route to integration. *New Zealand Journal of Physiotherapy*, April, 16–17.

Parker, D. W. L. (1964). The past and future of physiotherapy. *Australian Journal of Physiotherapy*, **10**, 41–6.

Powell, R. R. (1974). Psychological effects of exercise therapy upon institutionalized geriatric mental patients. *Journal of Gerontology*, **29**, 157–61.

Sen, K. & Hustwayte, J. (1989). Physiotherapy in the Brent mental health project for elderly people. *Physiotherapy*, **75**, 185–6.

Shephard, R. J. (1985). Physical fitness: exercise and ageing. In *Principles and Practice of Geriatric Medicine*, ed. M. S. J. Pathy. John Wiley & Sons Limited.

Walker, J. M. (1986). Exercise and ageing. *New Zealand Journal of Physiotherapy*, April, 8–12.

Ward, D. (1980). Setting up a physiotherapy service in a psychiatric hospital. *Physiotherapy*, **66**, 401–2.

Part 10

Conclusion

A concluding overview

BRIAN DAVIES

In everyday clinical work, whether in family or specialist practice, management of functional psychiatric disorders in the elderly is of prime importance. This importance lies in the number of patients presenting with these complaints and the effective treatments that are now available. The early 1990s are an appropriate time to review our present knowledge of these disorders. The editors have asked a group of workers from different parts of the world to write about their particular areas of expertise. Contributors have been asked not only to focus on current knowledge but on areas where research is needed and would be possible with available methods of study. These research ideas are amongst the most interesting aspects of this book.

Until the 1950s mental illnesses in the elderly were synonymous with organic brain disease. Even depressive and paranoid syndromes were attributed to underlying brain disease. Martin Roth's study of the natural history of mental disorders in old age, published in the *Journal of Mental Science* in 1955 showed two important findings. Firstly, a two-year outlook for a senile/arteriosclerotic group of patients in hospital was quite different to that of a depressed/paranoid group of hospital in-patients. There was a very high mortality in the first group and a very low mortality in the second.

The study also showed that these depressed/paranoid syndromes – the functional illnesses – accounted for more than half of hospital admissions. In Britain these findings were the impetus for the development of further studies of psychiatric disorders in the elderly and the subsequent development of services to deal with them.

Epidemiological studies have now shown that most functional illnesses in the elderly occur in the community and are not in fact treated, even at a family doctor level. The development of antianxiety, antidepressant and antipsychotic drugs from the 1950s has progressed. In particular in the 1980s new compounds with fewer side-effects – a very important consideration in the elderly – have been introduced and are now available for prescription by family doctors. In general psychiatric practice, the indications for psychotherapy and behavior therapy have become more closely defined but their values in the elderly are less clear, as discussed in chapters 25 and 26.

In this book, the number of chapters has been related to the extent of the particular clinical problem. Mood disorders get eight chapters, while late onset paranoid disorders get only two. British psychiatry has had a preoccupation with these paranoid disorders, yet their clinical importance is small, compared with the mood disorders.

However, the attention of trainees in psychiatry should be drawn to these two chapters on paranoid disorders because they clearly show the current approach to psychiatric problems. In Chapter 18, Part I on the late paraphrenias, Almeida et al. review the history, epidemiology, clinical features, diagnosis, role of personality, sensory impairment, genetics, neuropsychological and imaging findings, as well as management and treatment. In addition 'what needs to be done' is clearly stated. Rabins and Pearlson, in Chapter 18, Part II have compared and contrasted organic and functional syndromes using available data and this approach emphasizes the fact that clinical syndromes in psychiatry are not the same as specific diseases in general medicine. Specific biological markers have not been discovered, though the dexamethasone suppression test was a major advance in the study of depressive syndromes.

The problem of chronic depression in the elderly is one important focus of this book. How much of the chronicity is due to inadequate treatment? Side effects of anti-depressants and reluctance to strongly recommend ECT and to continue with ECT beyond the normal six or eight treatments are important factors in the treatment of elderly depressed patients. How much of this chronicity is, in fact, related to brain changes that modern imaging techniques seem to suggest – though normative data of brain imaging in the elderly is not large. The practical approaches to these problems and the needs for further studies are all to be found in this book.

In the 1980s, Alzheimer's disease became a particular focus of medical and public attention. The application of the molecular biologists' methods to the study of amyloid plaques and tangles has produced new and interesting results. In 1992 radio and television programs frequently drew attention to these findings. Yet in clinical work, basic treatment for these profound pathological changes must be years away. It is the functional illnesses in the elderly that we should be able to help now. This text clearly outlines our 'core knowledge' about the clinical problems, discusses appropriate treatments and also describes gaps in the knowledge where future research is needed.

Reference

Roth, M. (1955). The natural history of mental disorder in old age. *Journal of Mental Science*, **129**, 281–301.

Index

Page numbers of tables, illustrations and figures are in italics